Key Topics in Otolaryngology and Head & Neck Surgery

3rd Edition

Nick Roland, MBChB, MD, FRCS (ORL)
Consultant ENT/Head and Neck Surgeon
University Hospital Aintree
Liverpool, UK;
Southport and Ormskirk NHS Trust
Lancashire, UK

Duncan McRae, MD, FRCS (ORL)
Consultant ENT Surgeon
Colchester General Hospital
Colchester, UK

Andrew W. McCombe, MD, FRCS (ORL)
Consultant ENT Surgeon
City Hospital
Dubai Healthcare City;
Adjunct Clinical Professor of Surgery
Mohammed Bin Rashid University Medical School
Dubai, UAE

58 illustrations

Thieme
Stuttgart • New York • Delhi • Rio de Janeiro

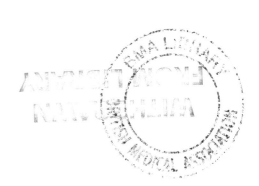

Library of Congress Cataloging-in-Publication Data

Names: Roland, N. J., author. | McRae, R. D. R. (Robert Duncan Roderick), author. | McCombe, A. W. (Andrew Wightman), author.

Title: Key topics in otolaryngology / Nick Roland, Duncan McRae, Andrew W. McCombe.

Other titles: Key topics in otolaryngology and head and neck surgery

Description: Third edition. | Stuttgart; New York: Thieme, [2019] | Preceded by Key topics in otolaryngology and head and neck surgery / N. J. Roland, R. D. R. McRae, A. W. McCombe. Second edition. 2001. | Includes bibliographical references and index.

Identifiers: LCCN 2018052322 (print) | LCCN 2018053752 (ebook) | ISBN 9783132406872 (ebook) | ISBN 9783132404779 (softcover: alk. paper) | ISBN

Subjects: | MESH: Otorhinolaryngologic Diseases | Handbooks

Classification: LCC RF56 (ebook) | LCC RF56 (print) | NLM WV 39 | DDC 617.5/1—dc23

LC record available at https://lccn.loc.gov/2018052322

© 2019 by Georg Thieme Verlag KG

Thieme Publishers Stuttgart
Rüdigerstrasse 14, 70469 Stuttgart, Germany
+49 [0]711 8931 421, customerservice@thieme.de

Thieme Publishers New York
333 Seventh Avenue, New York, NY 10001, USA
+1-800-782-3488, customerservice@thieme.com

Thieme Publishers Delhi
A-12, Second Floor, Sector-2, Noida-201301
Uttar Pradesh, India
+91 120 45 566 00, customerservice@thieme.in

Thieme Publishers Rio de Janeiro,
Thieme Publicações Ltda.
Edifício Rodolpho de Paoli, 25º andar
Av. Nilo Peçanha, 50 – Sala 2508
Rio de Janeiro 20020-906 Brasil
+55 21 3172 2297 / +55 21 3172 1896

Cover design: Thieme Publishing Group
Typesetting by DiTech Process Solutions Pvt. Ltd., India

Printed in Germany by CPI Books   5 4 3 2 1

ISBN 978-3-13-240477-9

Also available as an e-book:
eISBN 978-3-13-240687-2

Important Note: Medicine is an ever-changing science undergoing continual development. Research and clinical experience are continually expanding our knowledge, in particular our knowledge of proper treatment and drug therapy. Insofar as this book mentions any dosage or application, readers may rest assured that the authors, editors, and publishers have made every effort to ensure that such references are in accordance with **the state of knowledge at the time of production of the book.**

Nevertheless, this does not involve, imply, or express any guarantee or responsibility on the part of the publishers with respect to any dosage instructions and forms of application stated in the book. **Every user is requested to examine carefully** the manufacturer's leaflets accompanying each drug and to check, if necessary in consultation with a physician or specialist, whether the dosage schedules mentioned therein or the contraindications stated by the manufacturer differ from the statements made in the present book. Such examination is particularly important with drugs that are either rarely used or have been newly released on the market. Every dosage schedule or every form of application used is entirely at the user's risk and responsibility. The authors and publishers request every user to report to the publishers any discrepancies or inaccuracies noticed.

Some of the product names, patents, and registered designs referred to in this book are in fact registered trademarks or proprietary names, even though specific reference to this fact is not always made in the text. Therefore, the appearance of a name without a designation as proprietary is not to be construed as a representation by the publisher that it is in the public domain.

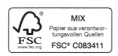

Contents

Contents

Contents

Preface

Otolaryngology is a rapidly changing discipline that encompasses a broad range of sub-specialties. Many weighty texts exist, which give exhaustive coverage of the subject, but they risk hiding the wood from the trees. Common problems occur commonly, and this is as true for post-graduate examinations as it is for clinical practice. Certain 'key' topics tend to present themselves far more frequently than others. The aim of this book has always been to give a succinct overview of the key topics in otolaryngology and head and neck surgery in a comprehensible, easy-to-read style. This is the third edition of this very successful format and aims to refresh and update on previous editions.

Basic information is contained in some topics (e.g. examination of the ear, nose and throat), and a symptom-orientated approach is used in others (e.g. epistaxis, foreign bodies, otalgia, otorrhoea). The breadth and simple style should make the book an ideal introduction to the specialty for medical students, and an accessible source of reference for general practitioners and junior doctors cross-covering ENT Surgery.

The text is up-to-date and provides sufficient detail to be used as a valuable revision aid for those studying for post-graduate examinations in otolaryngology and head and neck surgery. Scrutiny of past papers and discussion with candidates reveal that there are certain key areas which tend to be repeated. We have endeavoured to cover these areas using a common framework for each topic. It is hoped that this will engender an approach which will be of use to the candidate considering questions that are not discussed in this book.

A text of this size cannot pretend to be all-inclusive and this one does not set out to be so. Anatomy is only described in the context of a particular clinical topic and the principles of surgical techniques are covered only when deemed appropriate. Clarity and brevity have been our aim. We suggest the book be used early in the revision process before turning to more major texts. The reader is encouraged to refer to the articles and texts which are recommended for further reading at the end of each topic. We are confident, following feedback from past readers and candidates, that *Key Topics in Otolaryngology* will be of particular value in those overwhelming days just before examination, for which we wish you every success!

Nick Roland, MBChB, MD, FRCS (ORL)
Duncan McRae, MD, FRCS (ORL)
Andrew W. McCombe, MD, FRCS (ORL)

Contributors

Martin J. Burton, MA, DM, FRCS
Professor of Otolaryngology
Nuffield Department of Surgery
University of Oxford
Oxford, UK

Peter Charters, FRCA
Consultant Anaesthetist
Department of Anaesthesia
University Hospital Aintree
Liverpool, UK

Seema Charters, FRCA
Consultant Anaesthetist
Warrington and Halton Hospitals NHS Trust
Warrington, UK

Linnea Cheung, MBChB, MRCS-DOHNS
ENT Specialty Registrar
Department of ENT
Gloucestershire Royal Hospitals NHS Trust
Gloucester, UK

Raymond W. Clarke, DCH, FRCS (ORL)
Consultant Paediatric Otolaryngologist
Royal Liverpool Children's Hospital
Liverpool, UK

Declan Costello, MA, MBBS, FRCS (ORL-HNS)
Consultant Ear, Nose and Throat Surgeon
(Voice Disorders)
ENT Department
Wexham Park Hospital
Slough, UK

Soumit Dasgupta, MS, FRCS
Consultant Audiovestibular Physician/
Neurotologist and Clinical Lead
Department of Paediatric Audiology
Alder Hey Children's NHS Foundation Trust
Liverpool, UK;
Honorary Lecturer
Manchester Centre for Audiology and Deafness
University of Manchester
Manchester, UK

Camilla Dawson, DClinP
Clinical Lead Speech and Language Therapist
Therapy Services
University Hospitals Birmingham NHS
Foundation Trust
Birmingham, UK

Lesley Dempsey
Clinical Nurse Specialist in Head and
Neck Cancer
University Hospital Aintree
Liverpool, UK

Mike Dilkes, MS, FRCS (ORL-HNS)
Consultant ENT Surgeon
HealthHub
London, UK

Muriel Donaldson, MSc, RD
Head and Neck Clinical Specialist Dietitian
Department of Dietetics and Nutrition
QMC Campus Nottingham
University Hospitals NHS Trust
Nottingham, UK

Rachel Donnelly, MSc
Head of Nutrition and Dietetics
Department of Nutrition and Dietetics
Guy's and St Thomas' NHS Foundation Trust
London, UK

Alwyn D'Souza, FRCS
Consultant ENT/Facial Plastic Surgeon
Department of ENT
University Hospital Lewisham
London, UK

**Angeles Espeso, FRCS (ORL-HNS), DONHS, MRCS
GLAS, AFRCSI**
Otology and Paediatric ENT
Consultant Surgeon
Department of ENT
East Suffolk and North Essex NHS Foundation
Trust (ESNEFT)
Essex, UK

Johannes Fagan, MBChB, MMed, FCS (ORL)
Chairman
Division of Otolaryngology
University of Cape Town
Cape Town, South Africa

Simon Freeman, MBChB, MPhil, FRCS (ORL-HNS)
Consultant Otolaryngologist and
Skull Base Surgeon
Department of Otolaryngology
Salford Royal NHS Foundation Trust
Salford, UK

Andrew C. Hall, MD
Specialist Registrar
Department of Otology and Auditory Implantation
Royal National Throat, Nose and Ear Hospital
London, UK

Rebecca Hanlon, FRCR
Consultant Radiologist
Department of Radiology
University Hospital Aintree
Liverpool, UK

Jarrod J. Homer, MD, FRCS
Professor of Otolaryngology-Head and Neck
Surgery and Consultant Surgeon
Department of Otolaryngology-Head and
Neck Surgery
Manchester Head and Neck Centre
Manchester University NHS Foundation Trust
Manchester, UK

Tony Kay, registered with RCCP, MSHAA
Audiologist
Head of Audiology Services
Audiology Department
Aintree University Hospital NHS Foundation Trust
Liverpool, UK

Andrew J. Kinschuk, MBChB, DOHNS, FRCS (ORL-HNS)
Consultant of Otorhinolaryngology
Department of Otolaryngology and Head and
Neck Surgery
University Hospital Aintree
Liverpool, UK

Kevin Kulendra, DOHNS, FRCS (ORL-HNS)
Consultant ENT Surgeon
ENT Department
Chelsea and Westminster Hospital NHS
Foundation Trust
West Middlesex University Hospital
London, UK

Samuel C. Leong, MPhil, FRCSEd (ORL-HNS)
Rhinologist and Anterior Skull Base Surgeon
Department of Otorhinolaryngology-Head and
Neck Surgery
Aintree University Hospital NHS Foundation Trust
Liverpool, UK

Tristram Lesser, FRCSEd, FHKCORL, MS (Lon)
Consultant ENT Surgeon
ORL-HNS Ltd.
Renacres Hospital NHS Treatment Centre
Lancashire, UK

Simon Lloyd, MPhil (Cantab), FRCS (ORL-HNS)
Professor of Otolaryngology
Manchester Royal Infirmary and
Salford Royal Hospital
Manchester, UK

Christopher Loh, FRCS (ORL-HNS)
Consultant ENT Surgeon
Department of Otolaryngology
Aintree University Hospital NHS Foundation Trust
Liverpool, UK

Kate McCombe, MRCP, FRCA, MA
Consultant Anaesthetist
Mediclinic City Hospital;
Adjunct Assistant Professor
Mohammed Bin Rashid University of Medicine
and Healthcare Sciences
Dubai, UAE

Andrew W. McCombe, MD, FRCS (ORL)
Consultant ENT Surgeon
City Hospital
Dubai Healthcare City;
Adjunct Clinical Professor of Surgery
Mohammed Bin Rashid University Medical School
Dubai, UAE

Don McFerran, MA, FRCS
Consultant ENT Surgeon
ENT Department
East Suffolk and North Essex NHS
Foundation Trust
Colchester, UK

Duncan McRae, MD, FRCS (ORL)
Consultant ENT Surgeon
Colchester General Hospital
Colchester, UK

James Mitchell, FRCS (ORL-HNS)
Consultant ENT Surgeon
ENT Department
Frimley Park Hospital
Surrey, UK

Christopher Nutting, MD, PhD, FRCP, FRCR
Professor of Clinical Oncology
Head and Neck Unit
Royal Marsden Hospital
London, UK

Vinidh Paleri, MS, FRCS (ORL-HNS)
Consultant Head and Neck and Thyroid Surgeon
The Royal Marsden Hospital
London, UK

Paul Pracy, MBBS, FRCS (ORL-HNS)
Consultant
Department of Otolaryngology, Head and Neck
Surgery
University Hospital Birmingham
Birmingham, UK

M. Shahed Quraishi, OBE, FRCS
Consultant ENT Surgeon
Department of Head and Neck Surgery
Doncaster Royal Infirmary
Doncaster, UK

Simon Rogers, MD
Consultant Maxillofacial Surgeon
University Hospital Aintree
Liverpool, UK;
Professor
Edge Hilll University
Ormskirk, UK

Nick Roland, MBChB, MD, FRCS (ORL)
Consultant ENT/Head and Neck Surgeon
University Hospital Aintree
Liverpool, UK;
Southport and Ormskirk NHS Trust
Lancashire, UK

Shakeel R. Saeed, MD, FRCS (ORL)
Professor of Otology/Neuro-otology
University College London Ear Institute
London, UK

Julia Selby, PhD
Consultant Speech and Language Therapist
Voice, ENT and Respiratory Services
The Royal Brompton Hospital
London, UK

Richard Shaw, MD, FDS, FRCS (OMFS)
Professor
Department of Molecular and Clinical
Cancer Medicine
University of Liverpool Cancer Research Centre
Liverpool, UK

Ricard Simo, FRCS (ORL-HNS), PhD
Consultant Otorhinolaryngologist Head,
Neck and Thyroid Surgeon
Honorary Senior Lecturer KCL
Department of Otorhinolaryngology,
Head and Neck Surgery
Guy's and St Thomas' Hospital NHS
Foundation Trust
London, UK

Rachel Skelly, BSc (Hons)
Advanced Head and Neck Oncology Dietitian
Department of Nutrition and Dietetics
University Hospital Aintree
Liverpool, UK

Andrew C. Swift, ChM, MB, ChB, FRCS, FRCSEd
Consultant Rhinologist and ENT Surgeon
Honorary Consultant,
Alder Hey Children's Hospital and the
Walton Centre for Neurosciences
Department of Otorhinolaryngology,
Head and Neck and Thyroid Surgery
University Hospital Aintree
Liverpool, UK

Bella Talwar, RD, DADP
Clinical Lead Dietitian
Head and Neck Centre
University College London Hospital NHS
Foundation Trust
London, UK

Tim Woolford, MD, FRCS (ORL-HNS)
Consultant Ear, Nose and Throat Surgeon
Department of Otolaryngology, Head and
Neck Surgery
Manchester Royal Infirmary
Manchester, UK;
Honorary Clinical Professor
Edge Hill University
Ormskirk, UK

1 Adenoids

The adenoids are a mass of lymphoid tissue found at the junction of the roof and posterior wall of the nasopharynx. They are a normal structure and part of Waldeyer's ring which includes the palatine and lingual tonsils. Their function includes the production of antibodies and activated white blood cells in response to perceived infectious or other inflammatory threats. The size of the adenoids varies, but in general, they attain their maximum size between the ages of 2 and 7 years, as part of the widespread process of lymphoid hyperplasia that occurs in this age group, and then usually regress in size to become almost negligible by the age of 13 years.

1.1 Pathology

Inflammation, most commonly due to acute viral and bacterial infections, and also allergy and other inflammatory conditions, results in hyperplasia with enlargement and multiplication of the lymphoid follicles. Most of the pathological effects attributed to the adenoids are due to this increase in size. The symptoms caused by hypertrophy result from the obstruction of the nasopharynx and eustachian tube orifices. Persistent bacterial colonisation and biofilms are also contributory factors.

1.2 Clinical Features

1. *Nasal obstruction* leads to mouth breathing, snoring and hyponasal speech. Infants may have difficulty in feeding because they must stop sucking intermittently to take a breath. Nasal discharge, often mucopurulent, and post-nasal drip may develop because of secondary chronic rhinitis and sinusitis. Besides snoring, some children may suffer from episodes of sleep apnoea. The child with the characteristic adenoid facies appearance (an open lip posture, prominent upper incisors, a short upper lip, a thin nose, and a hypoplastic maxilla with a high-arched palate) is rarely seen nowadays because parents and GPs are better informed about the management of obstructive symptoms.

2. *Eustachian tube obstruction* may result in otalgia and deafness due to recurrent bouts of acute otitis media and otitis media with effusion (glue ear).

When there is mild-to-moderate obstruction, the clinical features of adenoid hypertrophy are not always clear-cut. Adenoidal hyperplasia may be incorrectly diagnosed when allergy and rhinitis may be the cause. In most children, examination of the nasopharynx with a paediatric nasopharyngoscope will identify large adenoids.

1.3 Investigations

A rarely required investigation is a lateral soft tissue radiograph. This will give a measure of the absolute size of the adenoids and an assessment of their proportion in relation to the size of the airway.

The most reliable means of assessing the size of the adenoids is examination under general anaesthetic at the time of the surgical procedure. If enlarged adenoids are identified then, with appropriate consent, they can be removed.

1.4 Indications for Adenoidectomy

Adenoidectomy is only indicated if troublesome symptoms can be attributed to abnormal adenoid hypertrophy. The indications for adenoidectomy are as follows:

- Nasal obstruction—especially if associated with significant and persistent mucopurulent rhinorrhoea, suggesting chronic nasal cavity infection.
- Otitis media with effusion (glue ear).
- Recurrent acute otitis media.
- Sleep apnoea—often an adenoidectomy is performed in association with a tonsillectomy. Traditionally, the procedure has been performed by curettage, but suction diathermy and coblation are popular alternative techniques.

A

1.5 Contraindications for Adenoidectomy

- Recent upper or lower respiratory tract infection.
- An uncontrolled bleeding disorder.
- Cleft palate—either overt or sub-mucosal. The adenoids assist in closure of the nasopharynx from the oropharynx during speech and deglutition, and velopharyngeal insufficiency is a rare complication. They should never be removed in a child who has had a cleft palate repair or a congenitally short palate. All children who have a bifid uvula should have a sub-mucous cleft excluded before proceeding with an adenoidectomy.

1.6 Complications

1. Immediate:
   - Anaesthetic complications.
   - Soft palate damage.
   - Persistent haemorrhage.
   - Sub-luxation of the atlanto-axial joint, or other damage to the cervical spine.
2. Intermediate:
   - Secondary haemorrhage.
   - Sub-luxation of the atlanto-occipital joint (secondary to infection).
3. Late:
   - Eustachian tube stenosis.
   - Nasal escape and regurgitation and hypernasal speech (rhinolalia aperta). Hypernasal speech can be a troublesome complication in some children. It often improves with time and speech therapy but may be sufficiently severe to require a pharyngoplasty to correct the problem. It is less likely to occur if children with palatal abnormalities are excluded from operation. Some surgeons advocate removal of the upper part of the adenoid mass leaving a lower ridge of adenoid tissue against which the defective palate may continue to make contact.
   - Persistence of symptoms.

1.7 Haemorrhage

The most serious complication is reactionary haemorrhage. This is treated in the same manner as post-tonsillectomy haemorrhage. The child should be returned to theatre and an attempt made to localise and diathermy the bleeding point with suction diathermy. A post-nasal pack is rarely required because the adenoid bed and any bleeding points can usually be fully visualised either endoscopically, or with palatal retraction and a mirror.

1.8 Signs of Hypovolaemic Shock in Children

Children compensate for a reduction in their circulating blood volume (normally 80–85 mL/kg) with an increase in systemic vascular resistance and heart rate. Their ability to compensate is remarkable, meaning that they can lose up to 30% of their blood volume before becoming hypotensive. Consequently, children decompensate late and rapidly and the clinician must be vigilant for signs of shock to avert a critical situation.

Observe child for the following:

- Tachycardia (age adjusted): Although there may be many confounding causes for a rise in heart rate, for example pain, agitation, fever, etc.
- Tachypnoea (age adjusted): This is a useful and sensitive sign.
- Agitation.
- Signs of impaired organ perfusion: Reduced urine output (usually 0.5–1 mL/kg/h); decreased level of consciousness; delayed perfusion—reduced capillary refill time (> 2 seconds), weak pulses and cool peripheries.
- Hypotension (age adjusted): This is a late sign in children.

1.9 Immediate Management

Confirm the diagnosis of hypovolaemic shock secondary to haemorrhage.

Initial management should follow the 'ABC' approach:

- Call for help!
- **A** Assess airway—ensure airway is patent. If conscious level is decreased, place the child in the recovery position, slightly head down to decrease the risk of aspiration.
- **B** Assess breathing and apply 100% oxygen—respiratory rate, air entry and oxygen saturations. Alert the anaesthetic team in the face of airway compromise and if a return to theatre is anticipated.

- **C** Assess circulation. Gain intravenous (IV) access and take blood for full blood count (FBC), group and save for cross-matching (depending on severity).

1.10 Start Fluid Resuscitation

- A 20 mL/kg bolus of Hartmann's solution—assess physiological response.
- Repeat 20 mL/kg bolus of Hartmann's solution if no response/partial response/initial response followed by deterioration.
- Children who require further fluid resuscitation after these two boluses will require blood as the next resuscitation fluid at an initial dose of 10 mL/kg.
- Institute measures to arrest the bleeding (return to theatre, etc.).

1.11 Follow-Up and Aftercare

In view of the problems with accurate diagnosis, and the potential long-term complications, it is reasonable to review an adenoidectomy child in the outpatient clinic post-operatively.

Further Reading

Lock C, Wilson J, Steen N, et al. North of England and Scotland Study of Tonsillectomy and Adeno-tonsillectomy in Children (NESSTAC): a pragmatic randomised controlled trial with a parallel non-randomised preference study. Health Technol Assess. 2010; 14(13):1–164, iii–iv

MRC Multicentre Otitis Media Study Group. Adjuvant adenoidectomy in persistent bilateral otitis media with effusion: hearing and revision surgery outcomes through 2 years in the TARGET randomised trial. Clin Otolaryngol. 2012; 37(2):107–116

Robb P. The adenoids and adenoidectomy Chapter 26, Volume 2. Scott Browns Otolaryngology, Head and Neck Surgery. 8th edition. CRC Press, 2018

Related Topics of Interest

Suppurative otitis media—acute
Otitis media with effusion
Snoring and sleep-related breathing disorder
Tonsillectomy
Tonsil disease

2 Age-Associated Hearing Loss

As with all sensory systems in the human body, there is a progressive degeneration in the auditory system with ageing. Presbyacusis is the term that describes the deterioration of hearing that characterises old age, now replaced by the term 'age-associated hearing loss' (AAHL). It may be defined as a progressive bilateral sensorineural hearing loss of mid-to-late adult life, where all other causes have been excluded. Indeed, the definition of AAHL is somewhat arbitrary; there is no agreed age above which an individual suffers from age-related hearing loss and below which one does not. Almost invariably, databases displaying age-related, average hearing thresholds for either screened or unscreened populations show a marked increase in the rate of progression of the hearing loss once into the sixth decade. It is, therefore, reasonable to attribute high-tone hearing loss in an individual over the age of 50 to age-related changes (in the absence of any alternative explanation).

2.1 Pathophysiology

Both the sensory peripheral (cochlea) and central (neural) components of the auditory system are affected and the deterioration appears to become more rapid with increasing age. Peripheral degeneration is reported to be responsible for at least two-thirds of the clinical features of presbyacusis. A variety of possible mechanisms exist. Cellular degeneration gives rise to a reduction in the numbers of inner and outer hair cells, particularly at the basal end of the cochlea. This can lead to secondary neural degeneration in the spiral ganglion. Circulatory changes such as arteriosclerosis, atrophy of the stria vascularis and microangiopathy can lead to metabolic upset and further cell death. This leads to an elevation of hearing thresholds and a loss of frequency selectivity. Degeneration in the central pathways leads to a reduction in performance in terms of signal processing. The net result in most instances will be a combined sensorineural, rather than an isolated sensory or neural impairment.

2.2 Clinical Features

Moderate hearing impairment (45-dB hearing level averaged over 0.5, 1, 2 and 4 kHz) occurs in 4% of the 51 to 60 age group, and in 18% of those aged 71 to 80. Men and women are both affected, although men tend to have a slightly worse loss for the same age group.

Initially, patients will complain of difficulty in hearing, particularly in the presence of background noise, so that they find conversations difficult to follow. As the hearing loss progresses, they will become aware of not hearing words and sounds. Recruitment is a frequent problem and adds to the distortion. In addition, the problems and consequences of AAHL are compounded in the elderly because of additional degenerative processes in the central nervous system. This can result in a relative loss in neuronal plasticity, a loss of cognitive abilities and other sensory modalities, particularly sight.

Decreasing hearing acuity also correlates with an increased incidence of falls, depression and dementia in the elderly. The feelings of imprisonment and anxiety that result from the consequent social isolation lead to reduced higher cognitive functioning and psychological well-being, which can in turn increase the economic and societal burden of AAHL. Therefore, it is important, as the life expectancy of our population increases, to make the diagnosis and offer treatment early.

In the absence of any other otological pathology, clinical examination is normal.

2.3 Investigations

In the presence of an appropriate history and a symmetrical sensorineural hearing loss on pure-tone audiometry, little further investigation is required. Hearing loss in a young patient, asymmetry on a pure-tone audiogram, unilateral tinnitus or a conductive component to the audiogram may require further investigation.

MRI scanning may be necessary to exclude a cerebellopontine angle tumour, such as a vestibular schwannoma, in any patient thought to be at risk (as suggested by significant asymmetry or persistent unilateral tinnitus). Most departments will have their own guidelines.

The National Institute for Clinical Excellence (NICE) state that an MRI of the internal auditory meati should be considered for adults with sensorineural hearing loss and no localising signs if there is an asymmetry on pure tone audiometry of 15 dB or more at any 2 adjacent test frequencies, using test frequencies of 0.5, 1, 2, 4 and 8 kHz.

Although several different audiological patterns of hearing loss have been described, depending on the pre-dominant histological changes, a sloping high-frequency loss is the commonest pattern found.

2.4 Management

As there is no curative treatment for deafness associated with ageing, the main aims in management are to assess the degree of disability, to provide a hearing aid and to rehabilitate the patient. There is now some evidence that reducing the accumulation of free radicals within the cochlea may reduce the rate of hearing decline. Antioxidants may therefore have a significant role to play in reducing progression of presbyacusis in the future. These include vitamins A, C and E and also magnesium and zinc.

2.4.1 Hearing Aids

Although about 75% of hearing aid users are over the age of 60, only 18% of the elderly with hearing loss have used hearing aids. There are several reasons for this, including denial of hearing impairment, vanity, acoustic feedback, recruitment and difficulty with manipulating the aid. Many elderly patients live alone and therefore do not see the need to wear a hearing aid unless they are socialising or out shopping. They therefore do not get used to the nuances of the aid, which are initially seen as a nuisance, and in turn they become less likely to wear it in situations where they would benefit from using one. In those with neural presbyacusis, poor speech discrimination may limit the benefit of amplification, as may the performance of the aid itself. Some patients have minimal handicap from their hearing difficulty despite a significant loss and therefore do not present themselves to medical services. Binaural aiding has been shown to produce an additional 10-dB signal-to-noise-ratio advantage, and so is recommended. The evidence suggests that digital aids are preferable to analogue. Loop systems offer an additional benefit to hearing aid users and are available in many public places such as churches, concert halls and lecture theatres. Amplified sounds are transmitted by a fitted induction loop and are picked up by the patient's aid when switched to the appropriate receiving position. Obtaining a hearing aid has become straightforward for patients since the introduction of direct referral from general practice to the chosen local hearing aid provider.

2.4.2 Accessory Aids

Practical measures for individuals with a more severe hearing loss include infrared headphones for use with their television, volume-controlled telephones, louder doorbells, often with an alternative alerting system such as a flashing light or vibrating pager system. Hearing dogs can take on such a role as well as providing a valuable source of companionship in the elderly.

2.4.3 Rehabilitation

Some patients may be helped by rehabilitation in the form of lip reading classes or auditory training. The role of rehabilitation and its benefits for the average hearing-impaired individual are not proven. The presence of comorbidities that affect cognition (e.g. dementia) can significantly impact on an individual's ability and readiness to adapt to the use of hearing aids. In these situations, co-operation is required from caregivers and family members to support ear and hearing aid hygiene and assist with insertion of hearing aids. Early provision of hearing aids is likely to shorten the time required for the individual to gain tolerance of aided speech and grasp the benefits of hearing aid technology. This may also reduce the development of the psychosocial comorbidities that can occur with hearing loss. And finally, whether cause or effect, there is a lower prevalence of depression and dementia symptoms in hearing aid users when compared with a similar elderly group of non-users.

2.5 Follow-Up and Aftercare

There is very good evidence of the importance of follow-up and rehabilitative support after fitting to ensure maximum benefit and hearing aid use. In the longer term, access is required for repairs and replacements, which may be dictated by further hearing deterioration with the passage of time. Routine ENT clinical follow-up is not required.

A

Further Reading

Alvarado JC, Fuentes-Santamaría V, Melgar-Rojas P, et al. Synergistic effects of free radical scavengers and cochlear vasodilators: a new otoprotective strategy for age-related hearing loss. Front Aging Neurosci. 2015; 7:86

Baguley DM, Reid E, McCombe AW. Age related sensorineural hearing impairment. In: Gleeson M, ed. Scott-Brown's Otolaryngology, Head and Neck Surgery. 8th ed. London: Hodder Arnold; 2008;3:3539–3547

Ferguson MA, Kitterick PT, Chong LY, Edmondson-Jones M, Barker F, Hoare DJ. Hearing aids for mild to moderate hearing loss in adults. Cochrane Database Syst Rev. 2017; 9:CD012023

NICE guidance for the management of adult hearing loss. https://www.nice.org.uk/guidance/ng98/resources/hearing-loss-in-adults-assessment-and-management-pdf-1837761878725; June 2018. Accessed December 11, 2018

Related Topics of Interest

Evoked response audiometry
Hearing aids
Noise-induced hearing loss
Pure-tone audiometry

3 Anaesthesia—General

General anaesthesia (GA) for ear, nose and throat (ENT) surgery accounts for about 5% of anaesthetic practice in the United Kingdom. While many of the operations are straightforward from the anaesthetist's point of view, others may present significant challenges. The nature of the pathology found in ENT patients may make airway management and intubation difficult. In many cases, specific consideration will be needed as to how best to provide optimal surgical conditions and access to the 'shared airway', while maintaining safe and effective anaesthetic conditions. This requires communication and cooperation between the surgeon and the anaesthetist so that each understands the concerns, aims and objectives of the other and a mutually acceptable plan of action can be agreed.

3.1 Techniques for General Anaesthesia

General anaesthesia can be classified according to whether ventilation is spontaneous or controlled.

- **Spontaneous ventilation:** The patient is permitted to continue breathing spontaneously throughout the operation. This technique is commonly employed when there is no need to intubate the patient to facilitate surgery, for example during grommet insertion, removal of simple skin lesions under GA and other simple surgery. The patient is rendered unconscious before a laryngeal mask airway is inserted to maintain airway patency.
- **Controlled ventilation:** Positive pressure ventilation is applied to the airway to oxygenate the patient. Controlled ventilation is commonly used following tracheal intubation which, in adults, usually follows the administration of a neuromuscular blocking drug, which relaxes the muscles and renders the patient paralysed. Tracheal intubation (either oral or nasal) is chosen to manage the airway for a host of different reasons depending on the situation, for example a cuffed tracheal tube provides protection against airway soiling; it provides a more 'secure airway' which is less susceptible to being dislodged or moved during surgery; it allows for more reliable delivery of positive pressure ventilation with negligible leakage of anaesthetic gases.

Induction, maintenance and emergence describe the inevitable sequence of all general anaesthetics.

3.2 Induction of Anaesthesia

Propofol is the drug most commonly used to induce anaesthesia. It is presented as a white lipid emulsion for intravenous administration and its effects are dose dependent; at low plasma concentrations, it causes sedation, which becomes deeper with increasing plasma concentrations until consciousness is lost entirely.

Induction of anaesthesia may be achieved using other hypnotic agents, which might be chosen in place of propofol because of a specific desirable characteristic. For example, ketamine may be useful in the hypotensive patient.

'Gas induction' of anaesthesia is done when a patient inhales a mixture of oxygen/air or oxygen/nitrous oxide and sevoflurane which is a volatile anaesthetic agent (see later). Gas induction is most commonly, although not exclusively, used in children who are resistant to having an intravenous cannula sited.

3.3 Neuromuscular Blocking Drugs

If tracheal intubation is required, it is commonplace to give a neuromuscular blocking drug (NMBD) (muscle relaxant) to cause abduction of the vocal cords and allow placement of the endotracheal tube (ETT). Various drugs are available for this purpose and the anaesthetist chooses according to the desirable properties and side effects of each drug, patient factors and the clinical situation. ▶ Table 3.1 lists a few examples.

The effects of a full intubating dose of atracurium, rocuronium or vecuronium last for approximately 30 minutes. It is generally not possible to reverse profound neuromuscular blockade by administering neostigmine, the anticholinesterase which is traditionally used as a 'reversal' agent. Instead, sufficient time must pass to allow the concentration of the NMBD to fall at the neuromuscular junction. Once a sufficient number of receptors are left unoccupied by the NMBD, it is possible to reverse its effects by giving neostigmine. Neostigmine increases the

▶ **Table 3.1** Neuromuscular blocking drugs

Drug name	Mechanism of action	Pros	Cons
Suxamethonium	Depolarising NMBD Binds and stimulates nicotinic receptors at neuromuscular junction	Rapid onset of action (~ 45 s) provides intubating conditions quickly Traditionally used for rapid sequence induction Rapid offset (~ 3–5 min)	Administration causes uncoordinated contraction of muscles. This can lead to myalgia post-operatively ('sux pains') which can be severe Poor anaphylaxis profile Precipitates malignant hyperpyrexia in susceptible patients Prolonged effect in genetically susceptible individuals ('sux apnoea')
Atracurium	Non-depolarising NMBD Competitive antagonist of acetylcholine at neuromuscular junction	Broken down by Hofmann's degradation, i.e. spontaneous breakdown at body temperature and physiological pH. Does not rely on or hepatic metabolism, so useful in patients with impaired organ function	Causes histamine release which can precipitate bronchospasm in susceptible individuals
Rocuronium	Non-depolarising NMBD Competitive antagonist of acetylcholine at neuromuscular junction	In large doses (1 mg/kg) it has a rapid onset of action (~ 1 min) and can be used for rapid sequence induction Effects can be reversed by sugammadex, but this drug is expensive	Anecdotally, has a higher anaphylaxis profile than other neuromuscular blockers
Vecuronium	Non-depolarising NMBD Competitive antagonist of acetylcholine at neuromuscular junction	Minimal effects on cardiovascular system Effects can be reversed by suggamadex	Presented as powder for reconstitution before use

Abbreviation: NMBD, neuromuscular blocking drug.

availability of acetylcholine at the neuromuscular junction. The acetylcholine can then bind to the available receptors at the junction and facilitate muscle contraction once again. There are ways around this; for example, the anaesthetist might choose to give a smaller dose of muscle relaxant to begin with. Sugammadex binds to and inactivates rocuronium and vecuronium molecules to reverse their effects. It is, however, expensive enough for many departments to restrict its use.

3.4 Maintenance of Anaesthesia

Anaesthesia is most commonly maintained using inhalational anaesthesia. Volatile anaesthetic vapours are stored in 'vaporisers' which are attached to the anaesthetic machine. Oxygen + air,

or oxygen + nitrous oxide, flow through the vaporising chamber where they are mixed with the volatile agent. The mixture is subsequently delivered to the patient via the anaesthetic breathing system. The anaesthetist controls the amount of volatile agent delivered to the patient as a percentage of the total volume of gas delivered, and the depth of anaesthesia increases in a dose-dependent fashion. Commonly used volatile agents are listed below. Again, each might be chosen because of the specific advantages it has to offer:

- **Sevoflurane** (yellow vaporiser): Faster onset and offset of action than isoflurane, not irritant to the airways and so can be used for gas induction.
- **Isoflurazne** (purple vaporiser): Slower onset and offset than sevoflurane, irritates the airways and so less suitable for gas induction. Cheaper than sevoflurane.

- **Desflurane** (blue vaporiser): Very fast onset and offset of action, irritant to the airways and so unsuitable for gas induction, useful when rapid emergence is desirable, for example in morbidly obese patients and those with sleep apnoea.

Anaesthesia can also be maintained using total intravenous anaesthesia (TIVA). This usually consists of a continuous infusion of propofol and remifentanil (a very short-acting analgesic drug). Each agent is delivered by an infusion pump and controlled by pharmacological drug algorithms based on the individual patient demographics. This would be used in cases such as those at risk of malignant hyperthermia from inhalational anaesthesia.

3.5 Emergence

To reverse the patient at the end of surgery, the anaesthetist needs to discontinue any inhalational agents, reverse any residual neuromuscular block, and most importantly, provide timely and adequate analgesia appropriate to the surgical situation. It is obviously important not to be giving 'top-up' doses of NMBDs just prior to reversal and communication with the surgeon is needed to prevent this. Care of the airway at reversal is important and referred to in the next section.

3.6 Special Anaesthetic Considerations

3.6.1 Airway Assessment

Airway assessment forms part of the standard anaesthetic pre-operative assessment. Anaesthetic teaching relies on simple 'bedside tests' (e.g. the Mallampati score, range of movement of neck flexion/extension, mouth opening, etc.). However, their predictive accuracy is poor. If a patient has had surgery before, his or her previous anaesthetic notes can provide invaluable information about any difficulties encountered and how these were resolved.

3.6.2 Anticipated Difficult Intubation

Securing the airway in patients for certain types of ENT surgery might prove especially challenging, for example those with tumours obstructing/

encroaching on the airway, following surgery or radiotherapy to the head and neck which has caused deformity/restricted neck movement or mouth opening, abscesses restricting mouth opening, inhaled foreign bodies or conditions causing airway soiling such as posttonsillectomy bleeding. When managing these high-risk patients, clear communication between the surgeon and the anaesthetist is vital. Information should be sought and shared, for example radiological imaging, nasendoscopy findings, clinical drawings or photographs of the airway/tumour morphology, and a clear, stepwise management plan agreed upon and communicated to the whole theatre team. More recent emphasis has been placed on the objective of decreasing the risk of hypoxia during difficult intubations either by continuous oxygen delivery by nasal catheters during laryngoscopy or the application of high-flow ventilatory exchange systems ('Thrive'). The final common pathway of any airway plan might be emergency surgical airway creation, and so the anaesthetist may request that the ENT surgeon be present in theatre, scrubbed and ready to perform an emergency tracheostomy should attempts at oral/nasal intubation fail. In a small number of cases, it may be decided that it is safest to secure the airway by performing an elective awake surgical tracheostomy.

3.7 Hypotensive Anaesthesia

In the past, it was fashionable to induce severe hypotension during anaesthesia to improve the surgical field by rendering it bloodless. This has fallen out of favour, however, because of the risk of critically reducing cerebral perfusion resulting in permanent brain injury. When it is considered necessary, however, there may be an agreement to induce modest hypotension, targeting a mean blood pressure appropriate for each individual patient. This can usually be achieved by controlling depth of anaesthesia, remifentanil infusion, postural adjustments (i.e. slight head-up tilt), adjusting ventilatory parameters, appropriate use of NMBDs, use of specific hypotensive agents, for example β-blockers, etc.

3.8 Recovery from Anaesthesia

The Royal College of Anaesthetists National Audit Project 4 conclusively demonstrated that planning for emergence and extubation was often poor and anaesthetists frequently failed to give due consideration to this perilous time. As a result, airway problems were often more serious in the postoperative period than at induction of anaesthesia.

A strategy for emergence and extubation should be made for every patient. If there is concern that this might be a particularly high-risk time for the patient, then a plan should be made and discussed with the whole team ahead of time, in the same way as for anticipated difficult intubation. Reverting to normal breathing with pharyngolaryngeal competency is not necessarily straightforward either when recovery is slow or incomplete (i.e. anaesthetic factors) or when the surgery has interfered with normal airway function. The anaesthetist may choose to lengthen the time to wakefulness by extubating the tracheal tube and replacing it with a laryngeal mask airway (LMA). The LMA is generally better tolerated and can be left in place till the patient is more awake.

Injury of the recurrent laryngeal nerve may lead to airway problems following extubation. This should always be considered following surgery to the neck, and thyroid surgery in particular because of the anatomy of the nerves in relation to the thyroid gland. Unilateral nerve injury may not cause any airway embarrassment, but bilateral nerve injury can result in adduction of the vocal cords causing total airway obstruction. This might only become apparent once the ETT is removed and may necessitate emergency reintubation. It may then be necessary to perform a tracheostomy, even if the nerve injury has the potential for recovery.

Post-operative bleeding, either in or around the airway, can lead to airway distortion and airway edema which can be rapid in onset. These complications can be exacerbated by coughing or retching, which cause a rise in intracranial and intrathoracic pressure by the Valsalva effect, by hypertension, which can result from pain and anxiety, and posture, particularly lying flat. Uncontrolled bleeding should be managed actively and if doubt exists as to its cause, nasoendoscopy should be considered. If the airway is in danger, appropriate and timely action should be taken to secure it before the clinical situation deteriorates further. If there is bleeding into the neck which is causing airway obstruction, it may be necessary to remove sutures/staples and evacuate any haematoma. While this may immediately improve airway distortion, it should be remembered that laryngeal oedema may also be a factor causing

airway compromise. Consequently, early reintubation should be considered. It may be necessary to use an ETT smaller than that used for the original intubation.

3.9 Special Considerations

1. Laser surgery

   Laser surgery to the airway has increased in popularity in the last decade. Lasers are hazardous because they make use of concentrated, non-divergent, high-intensity energy. When using lasers in the airway, operators must always remain alert to the rare, but significant, risk of airway fires. Risks should be minimised by the following:
   - The use of a laser-resistant ETT, which has two inflation cuffs (so that airway protection is maintained one of the cuffs should be punctured).
   - Inflating the cuffs with saline, rather than air, which might ignite if hit by the laser.
   - Packing the throat with wet gauze.
   - Air should be used in the oxygen mix rather than nitrous oxide, which is more flammable.
   - Keeping the fraction of inspired oxygen below 25%, while the laser is in use, if the patient can tolerate this.

   Should a fire occur, the surgeon should switch off the laser and flood the surgical field with water to cool the tissues. Oxygen delivery should be suspended till the fire is out. A badly damaged or melting tracheal tube may need to be removed. Once the fire is out, oxygen should be reintroduced and anaesthesia reestablished, by face mask if necessary. Examination of the airway with a rigid bronchoscope, reintubation and bronchoscopy with lavage may all be indicated. If damage is severe, a tracheostomy might be necessary.

2. 'Tubeless' anaesthesia

   For certain procedures, the surgeon may request 'tubeless' anaesthesia. There are various ways that the anaesthetist can facilitate this:
   - **Use of low-frequency jet ventilation (LFJV):** The jet ventilation device (e.g. Sander's injector or Manujet) is attached to a side port of the rigid bronchoscope used by the surgeon. The anaesthetist intermittently jets high-flow oxygen down the scope at a rate of 8 to 10 per minute. As the high-flow oxygen jets

through the scope, air is entrained, increasing the tidal volume. Anaesthesia is usually maintained using TIVA. LFJV has the disadvantage of requiring surgical pauses while the jet of gas is delivered because there is movement of the pharynx/larynx during gas delivery as a result of the high pressure.

- **High-frequency jet ventilation (HFJV):** This limits distortion of the airway during gas delivery. High-frequency ventilators deliver jets at a rate of 1 to 10 Hz via a very thin, non-distensible catheter, which is placed above or into the trachea. Airway resection or end-to-end anastomosis can be achieved around this small-lumen catheter.

With either form of jetting, it is essential that there is an exit for the gases used else intrathoracic pressure will build up and lead to pneumothoraces. HFJV machines incorporate pressure monitors, but for the manual situation, diligent clinical surveillance is mandatory.

Further Reading

Arné J, Descoins P, Fusciardi J, et al. Preoperative assessment for difficult intubation in general and ENT surgery: predictive value of a clinical multivariate risk index. Br J Anaesth. 1998; 80(2):140–146

Patel A, Nouraei SAR. Transnasal humidified rapid-insufflation ventilatory exchange (THRIVE): a physiological method of increasing apnoea time in patients with difficult airways. Anaesthesia. 2015; 70(3):323–329

http://www.rcoa.ac.uk/system/files/CSQ-NAP4-ES.pdf. Executive Summary of National Audit Project 4, Royal College of Anaesthetists. Accessed July 28, 2017

Related Topics of Interest

Anaesthesia—local
Anaesthesia—sedation

4 Anaesthesia—Local

The use of local and 'regional' anaesthesia, where local anaesthetic (LA) is infiltrated around a specific nerve to produce numbness in the region it supplies, is gaining popularity in anaesthesia because patients can enjoy the benefits of pain-free surgery without being exposed to the risks of general anaesthesia. While the scope for regional anaesthesia is fairly limited in the field of ENT, soaking of the nasal mucosa in Moffat's solution (which contains the local anaesthetic agent, cocaine), infiltration of skin with local anaesthetic agents to facilitate the removal of 'lumps and bumps' and infiltrating the surgical site with local anaesthetic to provide post-operative analgesia are all commonplace. For this reason, a working knowledge of commonly used local anaesthetic agents is useful to the ENT surgeon. Despite their relatively good safety profile, fatalities have resulted from LA overdose, so all doctors administering these drugs must be aware of the signs and symptoms of toxicity and how to manage it.

The Association of Anaesthetists of Great Britain and Ireland (AAGBI) advises that standard monitoring (blood pressure, electrocardiography [ECG] and pulse oximetry) should be employed when administering LA. Consideration should be given, when appropriate, to inserting an intravenous cannula, to allow for treatment of any LA toxicity that might occur.

4.1 Local Anaesthetic Agents

Pharmacologically, local anaesthetics can be classified into ester and amide types. Esters have an increased likelihood of precipitating hypersensitivity reactions when compared with amides (▶ Table 4.1).

Maximum dosages are adjusted for lean body weight as described by Specialists in Obesity and Bariatric Anaesthesia (SOBAUK) with up to a maximum of 100 kg for males and 70 kg for females.

4.2 Mechanism of Action

Local anaesthetic drugs enter the nerve fibre and bind to sodium channels located on the internal surface of the membrane. Once bound, they inhibit the movement of sodium across the membrane and so prevent the propagation of the nerve impulse. LAs bind more avidly to sodium channels that are open or inactivated and so preferentially affect nerves that have a rapid discharge rate. This means sensory nerve fibres are more susceptible than motor nerves, because they fire at a higher frequency.

In order to pass through cell membranes, any drug must be in its unionised form. The degree of ionisation of any drug depends on its pKa (drugs with a lower pKa—close to pH 7.4—will have a higher unionised fraction than those with a higher pKa) and the pH of the local environment. For this reason,

▶ Table 4.1 Types of local anaesthetics

Amide			Ester		
Name	Max. dose	Duration of action	Name	Max. dose	Duration of action
Lignocaine	3 mg/kg plain 7 mg/kg + adrenaline	1.5 h plain 4 h + adrenaline	Cocaine	3 mg/kg	5–90 min
Bupivacaine	2 mg/kg plain 2.5 mg/kg + adrenaline	4 h plain 8 h + adrenaline			
Levobupivacaine	2.5 mg/kg	4–6 h plain 8–12 h + adrenaline			
Ropivacaine	3.5 mg/kg	3 h plain 6 h + adrenaline			
Prilocaine	5 mg/kg (plain) 7 mg/kg + adrenaline	1.5 h plain 6 h + adrenaline			

LAs are less effective at producing satisfactory operating conditions in infected areas, such as abscesses, because the reduction in pH in these areas results in a higher proportion of ionised drug, making it unable to cross into the nerve cells to exert its effect.

Certain other drugs can be mixed with LA solution to produce a desired effect, for example adding sodium bicarbonate solution will speed up onset of action, by increasing environmental pH and so increasing the fraction of unionised drug; adding adrenaline to the solution causes local vasoconstriction, thereby decreasing washout of the LA and so extending its duration of action. Adrenaline is contraindicated in sites supplied by end arteries (digits and appendages) and should be used with caution in patients with ischaemic heart disease, hypertension and cardiac arrhythmias. The anaesthetist should always be informed that LA is about to be injected so that any immediate adverse events can be observed and drug administration stopped.

4.3 Features of Specific Agents

1. *Lignocaine (Xylocaine)*
   Lignocaine has an immediate onset of action. It is typically presented as a 1% (10 mg/mL) or 2% (20 mg/mL) solution for injection. It is a mild vasodilator and is often given mixed with adrenaline. It is also available as a spray (4 or 10% formulation) and ointments (2–5%) and as a spray is pre-mixed with the vasoconstrictor phenylephrine as 'cophenlycaine'. This is useful for preparing the nostril for endoscopy.

2. *Bupivacaine (Marcaine)*
   Bupivacaine is a vasodilating amide with a slower onset (takes up to 20 minutes for the block to develop) and longer duration of action than lignocaine. It is useful for regional techniques and postoperative analgesia. It tends to produce more motor block than lignocaine. At toxic levels, the drug binds avidly to cardiac sodium channels and so cardiac events tend to be resistant to treatment.

3. *Levobupivacaine (Chirocaine)*
   Levobupivacaine is the single levoisomer of bupivacaine and is less cardiotoxic than the parent drug, bupivacaine. The sensory block lasts longer than that of bupivacaine.

4. *Ropivacaine (Naropin)*
   Ropivacaine is a single isomer of bupivacaine. Ropivacaine is less cardiotoxic than either bupivacaine or levobupivacaine and is also more selective for sensory nerves, producing less motor block.

5. *Prilocaine (Citanest)*
   Prilocaine has no vasodilating effect and lower systemic toxicity. Metabolism to o-toluidine may cause methaemoglobinaemia in susceptible patients. Prilocaine is a component of EMLA skin cream (2.5% lignocaine with 2.5% prilocaine).

6. *Cocaine*
   Cocaine is used as a constituent of Moffat's solution to cause vasoconstriction and anaesthesia of the nasal mucosa. In addition to its LA effect, it inhibits the re-uptake of noradrenaline, serotonin and dopamine resulting in greater concentrations of these neurotransmitters in the brain causing predictable consequences: increase in heart rate and blood pressure, which can precipitate myocardial infarction in those with ischaemic heart disease, euphoria, hallucinations and disinhibition.

7. *Tetracaine*
   Tetracaine is available as a 4% gel and is used only topically on intact skin in preparation for intravenous cannulation. It should not be used on inflamed or infected skin.

4.4 Local Anaesthetic Toxicity

Local anaesthetic toxicity is a rare but potentially fatal complication. Several factors may contribute to the development of LA toxicity including the drug used, the site of injection and rate of entry into the circulation and peak plasma concentration. In addition, the physiological state of the patient will affect drug toxicity, with hypoxia, hypercarbia and acidosis all potentiating cardiac toxicity.

4.4.1 Signs of Toxicity

Clinical signs will increase in severity with increasing plasma concentration:

- Light-headedness.
- Tinnitus.

A

- Perioral tingling and tongue numbness.
- Visual disturbance.
- Agitation.
- Muscular twitching.

4.4.2 Signs of Severe Toxicity

- Sudden alteration in mental status, severe agitation, loss of consciousness.
- Tonic–clonic convulsions.
- Cardiovascular collapse: sinus bradycardia, heart block, asystole or ventricular tachyarrhythmia.

4.4.3 Management

- Stop injecting LA.
- Call for help—crash call if appropriate.
- Make a rapid but thorough assessment of airway, breathing and circulation.
- Open. airway and administer 100% oxygen.
- Confirm or establish intravenous access.
- Correct physiological abnormalities.
- Begin advanced life support if indicated.
- Administer Intralipid according to guidelines.

Treatment of local anaesthetic toxicity is with 20% lipid emulsion (Intralipid) which can be found on the cardiac arrest trolley, along with the dosing guidelines. Initial dose is 1.5 mL/kg over 1 minute, followed by an infusion of 15 mL/kg/h. If after 5 minutes, cardiovascular instability persists, the initial bolus should be repeated up to twice more (making three boluses in total) and the infusion rate should be doubled to 30 mL/kg/h. The total dose of Intralipid should not exceed 12 mg/kg. Recovery from LA-induced cardiac arrest may take over 1 hour.

4.5 Allergic Reactions

Amide local anaesthetic drugs have an extremely low incidence of allergic reactions. Patients will often report allergy to LA following its use for dental procedures. This should prompt further questioning, because they usually report tachycardia or chest tightness following administration. These symptoms do not represent allergy to the lignocaine used, but a normal physiological response to the adrenaline in the mixture. Hypersensitivity and cross-hypersensitivity are not uncommon with ester local anaesthetics.

Further Reading

The SOBA Single Sheet Guideline. http://www.sobauk.co.uk/downloads/single-sheet-guideline. Accessed July 31, 2017
AAGBI Safety Guideline: Management of Severe Local Anaesthetic Toxicity. https://www.aagbi.org/sites/default/files/la_toxicity_2010_0.pdf. Accessed September 4, 2017

Related Topics of Interest

Anaesthesia—general
Anaesthesia—sedation

5 Anaesthesia—Sedation

Procedural sedation and analgesia (PSA) is used in ENT surgery to reduce pain and anxiety and to provide amnesia for surgical procedures. PSA involves the administration of sedatives or dissociative agents, with or without analgesics, to induce an altered state of consciousness that allows the patient to tolerate painful or unpleasant procedures while preserving cardiorespiratory function.

5.1 Depth of Sedation

Four levels of sedation are defined by The American Society of Anesthesiologists (ASA).

1. **Minimal sedation:** A drug-induced state during which the patient responds normally to verbal commands. Cognitive function and physical co-ordination may be impaired, but airway reflexes, ventilatory and cardiovascular functions are unaffected.
2. **Moderate sedation:** A state where a purposeful response to verbal commands either alone (conscious sedation), or accompanied by light tactile stimulation, is maintained. The airway is normally unaffected and spontaneous ventilation is adequate.
3. **Deep sedation:** A state where the patient cannot easily be aroused but responds purposefully to repeated or painful stimulation. It may be accompanied by clinically significant ventilatory depression. The patient may require assistance to maintain a patent airway, and may require positive pressure ventilation.
4. **General anaesthesia:** A controlled state of unconsciousness accompanied by a loss of protective reflexes, including loss of the ability to maintain a patent airway or to respond purposefully to physical stimulation or verbal command.

5.2 Use of PSA in ENT Surgery

Where possible, PSA may be considered in patients unfit for general anaesthesia (GA), for patients who express a preference for it, and for procedures when patient co-operation is useful, for example vocal cord medialisation. When considering this technique, it is imperative to evaluate the surgeon's operative needs and to select the patients carefully. PSA will not be suitable for some, nor provide adequate operating conditions for many ENT procedures.

Middle ear surgery: Tympanoplasty, mastoidectomy, myringotomy, grommet insertion and cochlear implantation can be performed under local anaesthesia and sedation. Under local anaesthesia, many patients experience discomfort including a sense of noise, anxiety, dizziness, backache, claustrophobia or earache. Sedation may help alleviate some of these symptoms.

Nasal surgery: Functional endoscopic sinus surgery, septoplasty, balloon dilation of frontal sinus duct, dacryocystectomy and reduction of fractured nasal bones can all be successfully performed under local anaesthesia with sedation using various intravenous sedatives and/or analgesics.

Head and neck surgery: Excision of head and neck skin lesions, lip lesions, oral, oropharyngeal lesions and laryngeal procedures might lend themselves to PSA.

5.3 Pre-Operative Assessment

The very young and old, frail, morbidly obese, those with obstructive sleep apnoea (OSA), pulmonary and cardiac disease, and patients with significant kidney or liver disease are, amongst others, at higher risk of complications when receiving sedation. These patients may be best served by an anaesthetist administering their PSA. Patients should be carefully assessed for the presence of predictors of difficult bag-mask-ventilation, for example dysmorphic facial features, the presence of a beard, significant cachexia, morbid obesity, history of snoring or limited neck extension. Again, it may be prudent for an anaesthetist to manage these patients. Any patient receiving anything more than minimal sedation should be fasted to reduce the risk of aspiration of stomach contents into the airway. Fasting guidelines for general anaesthesia should be followed.

5.4 Patient Consent

For elective procedures, information about the procedure and intended level of sedation should be explained to the patient well in advance, along with an explanation of all material risks and

A

alternative management options (see Chapter 14, Consent and Capacity). The information should emphasise that during sedation patient is likely to be aware, and may have a recall, but that the intention is to improve comfort and reduce anxiety. On the day of procedure, it should be stressed that sedation is not GA and sedation should be described again from patient's perspective using terminology given in the NAP5 report on accidental awareness under general anaesthesia (AAGA). The rate of reports of AAGA following sedation was as high as after GA. These represent failure of communication between the anaesthetist and patient.

5.5 Monitoring

Ventilation, not just oxygenation, should be the focus of monitoring during PSA. Adequate ventilation ensures airway patency and continued respiratory effort. A pulse oximeter poorly reflects hypoventilation when supplemental oxygen is provided. A well-saturated patient receiving oxygen under sedation may in fact be profoundly hypoventilating with loss of airway reflexes. Ventilation must therefore be monitored by an alternative means. The most accurate method for monitoring ventilation is capnography. Capnography provides early detection of hypoventilation when supplemental oxygen is provided. For moderate or deep sedation, the Association of Anaesthetists of Great Britain and Ireland (AAGBI) recommend the use of continuous waveform capnography. The minimum standards of monitoring for patients receiving sedation are pulse oximetry, non-invasive blood pressure (BP) and electrocardiography (ECG).

Sedation should take place within a specifically designated area, for example a procedure room or theatre. Emergency equipment including full resuscitation equipment, continuous high-flow oxygen delivery and intubation equipment should be immediately available. Oxygen, for example via nasal cannulae, should always be administered from the start of sedation until readiness for discharge following PSA.

5.6 Pharmacological Agents Used for Sedation

The appropriate choice of pharmacological agents for PSA will depend on the nature of the procedure, the planned level of sedation, training and familiarity of the sedation practitioner with potential pharmacological agents, patient factors and the local environment.

1. Entonox

   Entonox is a gaseous 1:1 mixture of nitrous oxide and oxygen usually administered from cylinders containing pre-mixed gas and delivered via a demand valve. It has a rapid onset (30 seconds) and short duration of action (1 minute). It is used as a sedative and minor analgesic for simple procedures, which are mild to moderately painful. Side effects include nausea, vomiting, disinhibition and drowsiness. Nitrous oxide rapidly diffuses from the blood into closed air spaces causing volume expansion and pressure effects (e.g. increasing middle ear pressure). It is therefore contraindicated in middle ear surgery, where there is suspected head injury, and in sinus disease.

2. Benzodiazepines

   Midazolam is the most widely used benzodiazepine for conscious and deep sedation due to its relatively short half-life (1–4 hours) and rapid onset of action (onset 1–5 minutes, peak effect in 12–15 minutes) when given intravenously. After an initial bolus of 1 to 2 mg, it is usually titrated to effect using 0.5-mg boluses. It can also be given orally, buccally and intranasally. It has sedative, anxiolytic, powerful amnesic and anticonvulsant properties. Side effects include respiratory depression, hypotension and paradoxical excitement. Paradoxical excitement occurs in 1 to 2% of patients who receive benzodiazepines. Risk factors include alcoholism, extremes of age and psychiatric comorbidity. It usually manifests as excessive talking, violent movement and emotional release making completion of the procedure difficult. If this occurs, sedation with benzodiazepines should be stopped. Failure to diagnose the patient with paradoxical excitement may lead to uptitration of the sedative dose, creating a vicious cycle. Flumazenil will terminate this condition without reversing amnesia.

   The Department of Health has identified harm due to overdose with high-strength midazolam (5 mg/mL) during conscious sedation as one of the top 10 never events for 2012/2013. The National Patient Safety Agency's rapid response report in 2008, 'Reducing the risk of overdose with midazolam injection in adults', recommends use of low-strength midazolam (1 mg/mL), assessing fully the risk in its use in elderly and ensuring the availability of flumazenil.

3. Propofol
Propofol is a short-acting hypnotic. It has a quick onset and offset time, although the latter is context sensitive. Propofol provides no analgesia but has anti-emetic properties. In some patients, it can cause pain on injection. The dose is titrated to the desired effect as it causes sedation at low dose, through profound unconsciousness at higher plasma concentrations. Propofol causes dose-dependent respiratory depression (progressing to complete apnoea) as well as profound dose-dependent systemic vasodilation and consequently, a fall in blood pressure. Propofol should only be administered by those able to manage its side effects.

4. Opioids
Fentanyl, alfentanil and remifentanil are commonly used short-acting opioids. Many of the properties of these drugs are similar to morphine; however, they are all much more potent, for example alfentanil is 10 times more potent and fentanyl 80 times. Fentanyl is a commonly used analgesic for PSA, usually in combination with midazolam. In addition to their analgesic properties, opioids cause dose-dependent respiratory depression and must be used with caution. Again, these potent drugs should only be given by those able to manage their side effects.

5. Ketamine
Ketamine is a dissociative anaesthetic and profound analgesic that produces a trance-like cataleptic state due to dissociation between the limbic and cortical systems. Ketamine does not cause hypotension and the upper airway reflexes remain intact, but they cannot be assumed to be protective. For this reason, it is a very useful drug and is often used in pre-hospital care and by the military in the field. Ketamine has proved to be extremely safe drug according to a systematic review involving 70,000 patients and has level A evidence for its use in children and level C evidence for use in adults. Side effects include tachycardia, hypertension, laryngospasm, hypersalivation, increased muscle tone, nausea, vomiting,

increased intracranial and intraocular pressure and emergence phenomenon. Ketamine is well known to cause vivid hallucinations and delirium on emergence in some patients. These side effects can be reduced by the co-administration of a benzodiazepine.

5.7 Adverse Events under PSA

Adverse events occur because sedation is a continuum from the fully conscious state to the unconscious, when all the protective reflexes are lost. Safe performance of PSA rests on anticipation of problems and prompt skilled intervention. Research and audit have identified continued avoidable morbidity and mortality from sedation. The single most common recurring theme is the lack of formal training and prompt recognition /treatment of sedation-related complications. The Academy of Medical Royal Colleges (AoMRC) publication has laid down fundamental standards for safe sedation procedures and supported formal competency-based training for health care professionals. The International Sedation Task Force (ISTF) of the World Society of Intravenous Anaesthesia (World SIVA) has produced an adverse event reporting tool to standardise the reporting and tracking of adverse events during procedural sedation. The SIVA tool can be easily adapted for electronic use. Use of the SIVA tool is on the rise and has been shown to set a benchmark for further studies.

5.8 Reversal of Sedation

Respiratory adverse events usually manifest either as hypoventilation or airway obstruction. Hypoventilation occurs either from airway obstruction or centrally from chemical sedation. Airway obstruction commonly occurs due to collapse of the oropharyngeal soft tissues, pooling of secretions or laryngospasm. It is commonly seen in the elderly, obese and patients with a history of sleep apnoea.

Early detection of hypoventilation is essential to prevent desaturation leading to more aggressive interventions. Use a stepwise approach to restore ventilation—stop or slow the drug, re-position the patient and perform chin lift or jaw thrust. If hypoventilation persists, suction of the oropharynx, insertion of a nasopharyngeal airway,

A

bag-mask-ventilation, and/or use of reversal agents will be needed.

Cardiovascular adverse events are uncommon. Hypotension can occur with use of potent sedatives such as propofol, especially in high-risk groups such as the elderly and patients with existing cardiac disease.

Nausea and vomiting can occur following PSA in susceptible patients and is more commonly seen with ketamine. Vomiting that occurs when airway reflexes are compromised may result in pulmonary aspiration.

The benzodiazepine and opioid antagonists, flumazenil and naloxone are usually reserved for emergency use.

Flumazenil reverses the effects of benzodiazepines. Its half-life is shorter than that of the benzodiazepines and so sustained reversal may require multiple doses as well as careful observation to prevent recurrence of the sedated state. The National Patient Safety Agency's (NPSA) rapid response report in 2008 on 'reducing risk of overdose with midazolam injection in adults' recommends use of flumazenil to be regularly audited as a marker of excessive dosage of midazolam. Its use is relatively contraindicated in patients with known seizure disorder and known benzodiazepine dependence.

Naloxone is a competitive antagonist at the opioid receptor and it rapidly reverses the effects of opioids. In the absence of opioids, it has no action. It should be recognised that while the undesirable effects of opioids will be reversed by naloxone, for example respiratory depression, unconsciousness, it will also reverse the desirable analgesic effects. When given intravenously, naloxone is effective within 2 minutes and lasts up to 1 hour. The half-life of naloxone is shorter than that of morphine and so, as with flumazenil, sustained reversal may require multiple doses and careful observation for recurrence of sedation.

5.9 Recovery and Discharge Following PSA

Following the procedure, full monitoring should be continued until the patient meets the criteria for safe discharge. These are return to baseline level of consciousness; normal vital signs; uncompromised respiratory effort and appropriate relief from pain, nausea and vomiting. The patient should receive verbal and written instructions before discharge and be provided with contact details should they have any concerns. A reliable person should be present at the patient's home to provide support and supervision for the following 24 hours.

Further Reading

Association of Anaesthetists of Great Britain and Ireland. Recommendations for standards of monitoring during anaesthesia and recovery 2015. Anaesthesia. 2016; 71:85–93. http://onlinelibrary.wiley.com/doi/10.1111/nae.13316/full. Accessed September 5, 2017

Continuum of depth of sedation: definition of general anaesthesia and level of sedation/analgesia. American Society of Anesthesiologists, Main site. http://www.asahq.org/search?q=sedaion#q=sedation&sort=relevancy. Published 2014. Accessed August 8, 2017

Goksu S, Arik H, Demiryurek S, Mumbuc S, Oner U, Demiryurek AT. Effects of dexmedetomidine infusion in patients undergoing functional endoscopic sinus surgery under local anaesthesia. Eur J Anaesthesiol. 2008; 25(1):22–28

Safe sedation practice for healthcare procedures: standards and guidance. http://www.aomrc.org.uk/wpcontent/uploads/2016/05/Safe_Sedation_Practice_1213.pdf. Published 2013. Accessed August 8, 2017

Related Topics of Interest

Anaesthesia—local
Anaesthesia—general

6 Audit, Quality Improvement and Clinical Governance

6.1 Overview

The aims of clinical audit and quality improvement projects are to improve the quality of care given to patients, and to ensure their safety. This is why it is recommended that clinicians undertake such projects in different aspects of their practice. Audit may be based on clinical or non-clinical areas.

6.2 Clinical Governance

Audit and quality improvement form one of the seven pillars of clinical governance. Clinical governance is an umbrella term encompassing a range of activities through which NHS organisations continually ensure and try to improve the quality and safety of care they offer their patients. The seven pillars are:

1. *Clinical effectiveness and research*—'to ensure the right thing is happening to the right person at the right time in the right place'— this is achieved by developing protocols and guidelines or by adopting national guidance for practice, and by applying an evidence-based approach to treating patients.
2. *Audit and quality improvement*—see later.
3. *Risk management*—by having robust systems in place to monitor and reduce patient and staff hazards, and to learn from mistakes and near misses.
4. *Patient and public experience and involvement*— through patient feedback, complaints and Board of Governors' meetings.
5. *Information governance*—ensuring the use of patient data is kept confidential, accurate and up to date.
6. *Training and education*—providing appraisals and access to relevant courses and conferences for staff to keep their knowledge and skills up to date.
7. *Staffing and staff management*—strategies to ensure the workforce is appropriately maintained and sufficiently skilled.

6.3 Clinical Audit

Clinical audit is a process by which clinical activity is measured and compared against a specific quality or safety standard. Published guidelines or complication rates are often used as this standard. There are specific steps in conducting a clinical audit:

1. Identify a problem or process.
2. Define criteria and standards.
3. Observe practice (data collection).
4. Compare with standard.
5. Implement a change.
6. Re-audit.

Undertaken locally within an individual institution, clinical audits can help to benchmark current performance and highlight areas which are meeting standards, and areas which require improvement. Essentially, it is a form of monitoring exercise within the clinical governance framework, which is why it is considered so important. The statistics generated from the audit process can act as quantifiable evidence to encourage a change in practice to improve underperforming areas. After a period has passed to allow changes to be implemented, practice can be re-observed to see if performance has improved. Re-evaluating or 're-auditing' the data following these changes is often referred to as 'completing the audit cycle'.

As one of the requirements of an audit is that there is a specific standard to be measured against, projects are usually undertaken in the context of a particular aspect of treatment delivery, treatment complication rates, or investigation pickup or request rates.

The exact time for each step of the audit process really depends on the nature of the aspect of practice being audited, and how long it takes within an individual department or institution to reasonably implement any changes that were initially suggested.

6.4 Audit and Research

Sometimes, a review of clinical activity is undertaken in which there is no available standard to measure against. Instead, the review may be undertaken to define a standard. Strictly speaking, since there is no initial standard, this exercise could be regarded as a form of pseudo-research.

A

6.5 Quality Improvement

Quality improvement projects, in contrast to clinical audit, do not require an established standard for comparison. This also means they are not strictly limited to direct clinical care and therefore can be undertaken on any aspect of a patient's clinical pathway. Even holistic aspects of health care, for example the availability of refreshments in an A&E waiting area, can be evaluated through a quality improvement project.

The structure of a quality improvement projects is based on a 'plan, do, study and act (PDSA) cycle'. The steps vaguely echo that of a clinical audit cycle:

Plan   Define an aim or objective for changing (improving) an area of practice and plan data collection to aid satisfying those objectives.
Do   Implement the change.
Study   Assess the data before and after the change and reflect upon the impact of the change.
Act   Identify modifications for the next cycle.

Quality improvement projects aim to be a safe and less disruptive way to implement changes in health care practice. It is recommended that such projects are carefully planned and undertaken on a small-scale basis so that teams can learn from these results and make any necessary adaptations with the ultimate potential to then be able to make the changes on a large-scale basis (otherwise referred to as 'full implementation'). Furthermore, several small-scale changes can be implemented at the same time with several simultaneous PDSA cycles to test out different changes for the same outcome. Through repeated PDSA cycles and adaptations of any proposed changes, teams can be more certain that changes implemented on a large-scale basis will be successful in generating measurable improvements.

6.6 Patient-Related Outcome Measures

A significant theme of a white paper published in 2010 proposing new directions for the NHS, reinforced the concept of increasing patient choice and involvement in their care. Patient-reported outcome measures (PROMs) have become a source of feedback as given by patients to indicate the quality of care delivered to them. The data is collected by measuring a patients' health status or quality of life through short, self-completed, usually condition-specific questionnaires undertaken before and after receiving a treatment. The results of such comparative data serve as valuable information that feeds directly into the clinical effectiveness, audit and patient involvement pillars of clinical governance.

Officially PROMs were adopted by the NHS for joint replacement procedures in orthopaedics, but in the specialty of otolaryngology PROMs have also become increasingly useful for the purposes of audit and quality outcome research. Examples include the following measures:

• The "Glasgow benefit plot" for middle ear surgery (one of the oldest measures in ENT)
• T-14 tool for paediatric tonsillectomy
• Sino-nasal Outcome Test-22 (SNOT-22) questionnaire
• Voice Handicap Inventory (VHI)
• Tinnitus Handicap Inventory (THI)

6.7 National UK Audits and Surgical Outcome Data

In the past few years, as part of the medical appraisal, licencing and revalidation process, and to make clinical (surgical) standards more uniform, there has been an expectation that wherever there is a national audit that covers a clinician's scope of practice, he/she will contribute cases to it. The process started with cardiac surgery and was also intended to provide reassurance to the public regarding standards of care.

Specific national audits relevant to otolaryngology include but are not limited to:

• *Head and Neck Cancer Audit*—Previously known as DAHNO (Data for Head and Neck Oncology), this has been replaced by HANA (Head and Neck Audit). DAHNO was commissioned by the NHS and produced an annual clinical outcome report from a large database comprising data from all UK trusts since 2004. These audits aim to address national variances in the patient pathway from referral to treatment, to try and improve outcomes for head and neck cancer patients and establish consensus recommendations.

• *British Association of Endocrine and Thyroid Surgeons (BAETS)*—Thyroid surgery is one of the few selected procedures where consultant level outcomes are to be made available for public access. Details of individual named surgeons'

A

case-loads and complication rates are included in the data.

- *Epistaxis*—The ENT trainees' research collaborative group (INTEGRATE) have begun undertaking national trainee-led audits. Their first national audit in 2017 has helped to establish national consensus standards for the management of acute epistaxis and has proven that useful, large scale multi-centre data can be collected in an effective manner. Further projects are planned in the future.

- *Tonsillectomy*—This national prospective audit published in 2005 from consenting patients who underwent tonsillectomy in the United Kingdom found that 'hot' tonsillectomy techniques carried a higher risk of post-operative haemorrhage compared to the use of 'cold steel'. The results of this audit have inevitably influenced surgeons' choice of dissection and haemostasis techniques and have provided a national average rate which most individual units continue to audit their rates of haemorrhage against.

- *Tracheostomy*—The National Confidential Enquiry into Patient Clinical Outcome and Death (NCEPOD) is an organisation that carries out surveys into different aspects of patient care. Their work is commissioned by the NHS and their reports are made public. In 2014, NCEPOD published a report of patients who underwent a tracheostomy in the United Kingdom. Alongside the National Tracheostomy Safety Project in 2012, the report produced recommendations to ensure a minimum standard of safety of procedures surrounding insertion, tube care, multi-disciplinary team management and the complications and outcomes of tracheostomy. Many institutions in the United Kingdom base their tracheostomy care policies on the recommendations from this document.

In general, treatment outcome data from national audits serve as a useful tool to provide insight for hospitals and national comparators for individual surgeons, which in turn help to maintain and improve local standards of care for patients. Publicly available data such as surgical outcomes, particularly where individual surgeons are named, can on one hand reassure patients that their surgeon is experienced and participates in a process of professional audit and practice analysis, as well as allowing the patient to have knowledge

of how their surgeon's complication rates compare with other specialists in the same field. However, on the other hand, patients may use this data to specifically select a surgeon to be treated by or seek referral to, which is not the desired purpose of this information. Another concern of the use of national audits is that clinicians may avoid treating high-risk patients to maintain apparent better outcomes. So far, there has been no evidence of this occurring in practice.

6.8 Benefits of Audit and Quality Improvement

Both audit and quality improvement ultimately aim to improve patient care. They can also help to improve processes and departmental activity, thus improving departmental efficiency. It can also offer opportunities for clinicians and other health care professionals to learn about new areas outside of their normal working environment and create opportunities to collaborate with other departments within and outside their institution.

6.9 Some Pitfalls of Audit and Quality Improvement Projects

Whilst audit and quality improvements may seem laudable, they are subject to some general issues:

- Although often effective at a local level, the changes in process and practice are not always directly transferable between Trusts or different units. Therefore, a change that might have been effective in one unit may result in a different outcome, or may be impractical, in a different hospital. National audits attempt to provide recommendations that can be adopted in a more widespread manner. However, even these are not always practical at a local level and thus are often considered as guidelines rather than strict policies.
- The data used for such processes are often sought retrospectively instead of being collected prospectively. Therefore, discrepancies and missing data may be discovered which may affect the end results.
- Some projects have the potential to link under-performance with specific members of a working team, or the criticism of certain

A

practices or departments. Whilst this is an important exercise, it can lead to tension or resistance within teams to change, particularly if individuals feel personally targeted.

To overcome potential problems with audit and quality improvement projects, those involved should be encouraged to remember the primary focus is to ensure patient care is a consistently high standard for both quality and safety.

Further Reading

ACT Academy for NHS Improvement. Quality, Service Improvement and Redesign Tools: Plan, Do, Study, Act (PDSA) cycles and the model for improvement. Available at: https://improvement.nhs.uk/documents/2142/plan-do-study-act.pdf. Accessed August 14, 2018

General Medical Council. The Good medical practice framework for appraisal and revalidation. 2013. Available at: www.gmc-uk.org/-/media/registration-and-licensing/the_good_medical_practice_framework_for_appraisal_and_revalidation_55937137.pdf. Accessed August 14, 2018

British Association of Endocrine and Thyroid Surgeons. Available at: https://www.baets.org.uk/audit/

ENT UK. Available at: https://www.entuk.org/clinical-outcomes-0

National Tracheostomy Safety Project. Available at: http://www.tracheostomy.org.uk/

INTEGRATE (The National ENT Trainee Research Network). National ENT Trainee Research Network. The British Rhinological Society multidisciplinary consensus recommendations on the hospital management of epistaxis. J Laryngol Otol 2017;131(12):1142–1156

Nelson EC, Eftimovska E, Lind C, Hager A, Wasson JH, Lindblad S. Patient reported outcome measures in practice. BMJ 2015;350:g7818

NHS England. Patient Reported Outcome Measures (PROMs). Available at: www.england.nhs.uk/statistics/statistical-work-areas/ proms/. Accessed August 21, 2018

Limb C, Fowler A, Gundogan B, Koshy K, Agha R. How to conduct a clinical audit and quality improvement project. Int J Surg Oncol (N Y) 2017;2(6):e24

Lowe D, van der Meulen J, Cromwell D, et al. Key messages from the National Prospective Tonsillectomy Audit. Laryngoscope 2007;117(4):717–724

The Royal College of Surgeons of England. Good Surgical Practice. 2014. Available at: www.rcseng.ac.uk/-/media/files/rcs/standards-and-research/gsp/gsp-2014-web.pdf. Accessed August 14, 2018

Wilkinson K, Freeth H, Kelly K. 'On the right trach?' A review of the care received by patients who undergo tracheostomy. Br J Hosp Med (Lond) 2015;76(3):163–165

Related Topic of Interest

Evidence-based medicine

7 Barotrauma

Barotrauma implies damage to the body structures due to changes in atmospheric pressure. A number of air-containing body structures can be affected, such as the gut, lungs and sinuses, but it is the ear that most frequently suffers pathological consequences. Barotrauma commonly occurs in flying and diving and also less frequently during hyperbaric oxygen treatment.

7.1 Physics

To understand barotrauma, it is important to remember Boyle's law, which states that as the ambient pressure increases, the volume of a gas decreases. It is given by the formula:

PV = k

where P is pressure, V is volume and k is a constant for the gas in question.

From a diving perspective, this is illustrated in the ▶Table 7.1. Thus, it can be seen that the greatest change in volume occurs within the first 10 m of a dive.

This pressure and volume relationship accounts for most of the problems of barotrauma. However, with diving there is an additional problem. Nitrogen, which makes up approximately 80% of the volume of inspired air, and is metabolically inert, is absorbed by the tissues in a manner that is proportional to depth and duration of the dive. As the diver ascends, nitrogen finds its way out of the tissues and back into the bloodstream, before being exhaled through the lungs. However, if the rate of ascent is too quick, the nitrogen will come out of solution as gas bubbles in the tissues. This condition is decompression sickness, or colloquially 'the bends', from the characteristic stooping posture of affected caisson workers in whom it was originally identified.

▶ **Table 7.1** Boyle's law

Depth (m)	Pressure (atmospheres)	(kPa)	'Bubble' volume
0 (surface)	1	101	100%
10	2	202	50%
20	3	303	33%
30	4	404	25%
40	5	505	20%

7.2 Clinical Effects

7.2.1 External Ear

The external ear is rarely affected by pressure change. However, there is the rare condition of 'reverse- or external ear squeeze' which occurs, usually only when diving, when a pocket of air becomes trapped in the external ear canal, usually due to wax build up or a tight-fitting diving hood. If the eustachian tube is functioning normally, then middle ear pressure will increase with descent while the pressure in the ear canal will fall, leading to an outward bulging of the tympanic membrane. The main symptom is pain, but if the pressure gradient is extreme, then perforation can result.

7.2.2 Middle Ear

The middle ear is by far the commonest site affected by barotrauma. Problems tend to occur more frequently on descent for divers and almost exclusively so for flyers.

The middle ear space is a closed air space that opens via the eustachian tube. When ascending, the ambient pressure falls, the air in the middle ear expands and passively escapes through the eustachian tube. With descent, the ambient pressure, specifically in the external ear canal and nasopharynx, will rise. Pressure equalisation occurs when the eustachian tube opens and ambient pressure air from the nasopharynx is able to enter. If eustachian tube function is compromised, for whatever reason, this process fails to occur. Once a certain pressure differential has been reached (13 kPa, equivalent to a water depth of 1.3 m), the eustachian tube becomes locked and cannot open to equalise. The initial symptom is pain due to indrawing of the tympanic membrane, but if the reduced pressure persists for any length of time, inflammatory changes will occur and include mucosal hyperaemia, mucosal swelling and the development of a middle ear effusion, or even bleeding, which will cause hearing loss in addition to the pain. If the pressure change is sufficiently large and/or rapid, a tympanic membrane perforation can result.

Predicting normal eustachian tube function is not as simple as it might appear; self-reported ability to equalise and a normal tympanogram

B

have no significant predictive ability. A combination of the Toynbee test (pinched nose and swallow) and Bluestone's nine-step eustachian tube test (a series of tympanometry measurements at various middle ear pressures) seems to have much more validity.

Prevention is all about optimising eustachian tube function. The most simple and useful advice is not to sleep during aircraft descent, and to encourage eating and drinking, and therefore eustachian tube opening, especially in children. Alternative strategies include the use of topical decongestants although such studies as exist have suggested that oral decongestants (pseudoephedrine) are more effective. Coexistent rhinitis should be properly controlled prior to flying or diving. The use of short-acting topical decongestants is discouraged in divers as the effect may wear off during the dive and then leave the subject with compromised eustachian tube function and trapped air in the middle ear space. This is another cause of 'reverse ear squeeze', described earlier in the external ear.

For divers, if failure of equalisation and pain occurs, the advice is to stop, ascend a little and try again to equalise. If this is not possible, the dive should be aborted. If an individual persists despite such warning signs, a perforation may occur leading to a sudden influx of water, and the creation of a cold water caloric. The subsequent acute vertigo, and frequently associated vomiting, can be fatal in such a situation. Compromised eustachian tube function is the reason why divers are advised not to proceed if they have a current upper respiratory tract infection (URTI).

The management of established middle ear barotrauma is essentially expectant with additional management to try and improve eustachian tube function; topical and even systemic steroids may be required to reduce inflammation, and decongestants to reduce swelling. If there is evidence of a developing otitis media, antibiotics may be required. In exceptional cases where a middle ear effusion persists beyond 6 weeks, a ventilation tube may be required with or without examination of the post-nasal space. The majority of tympanic membrane perforations heal spontaneously.

Finally, for frequent fliers with significant eustachian tube problems and regular episodes of barotrauma, the insertion of ventilation tubes can be life changing.

7.2.3 Inner Ear

The inner ear is much less commonly affected by barotrauma than the middle ear, but when it is, the effects have a much greater chance of being permanent.

Probably the commonest cause of damage to the inner ear is as a result of a forced Valsalva manoeuvre. If the middle ear pressure is negative compared to atmospheric pressure (meaning that inner ear fluid pressure will be higher than middle ear pressure too), the tympanic membrane will be indrawn which will act on the ossicular chain and depress the stapes footplate, leading to a compensatory bulging of the round window membrane which is already exaggerated due to the lower middle ear pressure.

The forced Valsalva raises intracranial and cerebrospinal fluid (CSF) pressures. The raised CSF pressure is transmitted via the cochlear and vestibular aqueducts to the inner ear, which is already at a relatively raised pressure, as described earlier. At best this can lead to inner ear microhaemorrhages, at worst, a rupture of (usually) the round window membrane and a perilymph fistula. In between there can be labyrinthine membrane tears.

Haemorrhages tend to cause mild vestibular symptoms and a sensorineural hearing loss. Full recovery is the norm.

Labyrinthine membrane tears cause symptoms that mimic a Ménière's attack. Although vestibular symptoms usually recover, the hearing loss may be permanent. Perilymph fistula from labyrinthine membrane rupture leads to hearing loss, tinnitus, a sense of pressure and dizziness. While relatively easy to propose as a possible diagnosis, it is notoriously difficult to confirm. A thorough dive history and a close temporal association to a forced Valsalva are useful in making the diagnosis. A history of disequilibrium made worse by actions that raise intracranial pressure is highly suggestive of inner ear barotrauma. Please see the Chapter 31, Fistula for more information.

If the hearing loss and associated symptoms are relatively mild, a conservative management approach is probably most effective. This includes bed rest, with elevation of the head, and the avoidance of coughing and straining to keep intracranial and CSF pressures low. Steroids are often given empirically, as are adenosine and vitamin B supplements.

With more severe symptoms, or in a milder case where symptoms and signs show deterioration despite appropriate conservative treatment, an exploratory tympanotomy is warranted. In general, recommended advice seems to be that the worse the symptoms, the earlier surgical exploration should be undertaken, although most authorities would wait a few days before exploring the affected ear to allow a conservative approach a chance of success. Any identified leak should be patched with a tissue plug, and if no leak is identified, then both round and oval windows should be 'plugged'. Most series show that the majority of vestibular symptoms respond well to such surgery (87%) although the effect on the hearing loss is much less predictable, with only 40% showing improvement.

Further Reading

Kozuka M, Nakashima T, Fukuta S, Yanagita N. Inner ear disorders due to pressure change. Clin Otolaryngol Allied Sci. 1997; 22(2):106–110

Spira A. Diving and marine medicine review part II: diving diseases. J Travel Med. 1999; 6(3):180–198

Toynton SC. Otitic barotrauma. In: Watkinson JC, Clarke RW, eds. Scott-Brown's Otorhinolaryngology and Head and Neck Surgery. 8th ed. London: CRC Press. 2018; 1099–1140

Related Topics of Interest

Fistula
Ménière's disease

B

8 Caloric Tests

8.1 Physiology

The semicircular canals are paired sensory structures responsible for the detection of angular acceleration. Each canal possesses a dilation at one end called the ampulla. Within the ampulla exists a saddle-shaped crista upon which sits a gelatinous cupula; the membranous canal is filled with endolymph. The inertia of the endolymphatic fluid with head movement means that there is a relative difference in the velocity of the canal and the fluid. This results in fluid being forced through the gap between crista and cupula and a deflection of the stereocilia. In turn, this causes either an increase or decrease in the resting tonic discharge, depending on the direction of deflection. The two labyrinths work in conjunction so that an increase in neural signals from one canal will be associated with a decreased discharge rate from the corresponding canal on the opposite side. As the three canals are mutually at right angles, complex three-dimensional movement information is provided.

8.2 Background

The caloric response can be used to test the integrity of this part of the balance system. It was first described by Robert Barany in 1906, for which he was awarded a Nobel prize in 1914. He postulated that altering the temperature of the endolymph sets up thermally induced convection currents. This fluid movement leads to stimulation of the stereocilia and consequent nystagmus and vertigo. Caloric testing was further refined in 1942 by Fitzgerald and Hallpike when they described a standardised bithermal caloric test, which remains an essential vestibular investigation to this day.

It has become apparent in recent years that thermal convection currents are not the only component in the caloric response. Positional alterations and the presence of a caloric response in microgravity have led to suggestions that a direct thermal effect on the sensory organs may account for as much as one-third of the response, although this in no way reduces the value of the test.

8.3 Procedure

The classic bithermal caloric utilises water at 30 and 44°C, kept at these temperatures in two heated tanks about 1 m above the test couch. The patient reclines on the couch at 30 degrees above the horizontal so as to bring the lateral semicircular canal into the vertical position. After checking that the external canals are clear of wax and debris and that the tympanic membranes are intact, cold water (30°C) is run into the left ear, via a siphon tube and 14-gauge cannula, for 40 seconds. A stopwatch is used to time the period from the start of this manoeuvre to the point at which the nystagmus stops with the patient fixating on a point on the ceiling. This procedure is repeated for the right ear and then for both ears with the warm water (44°C). Five minutes is usually left between each stimulus to allow for normalisation of the temperature in the ear.

Several variations on this basic theme exist. Very cold water (4°C) can be used as a single-temperature screening test and is used as part of the battery of testing for brainstem death. In patients with perforated eardrums, or other significant middle ear pathology, air may be used to supply the thermal stimulus, or water circulated through a closed system (typically at 50 and 24°C). This is not quite so reliable, or effective as standard water irrigation. Further refinements can be added using Frenzel's glasses to remove optic fixation or measuring the nystagmus electrically (electronystagmography). In this case, the slow-phase velocity (SPV) of the nystagmus is measured.

Normally, optic fixation will suppress the nystagmus, such that it will reappear and persist for typically 20 to 60 seconds once optic fixation (and therefore vestibulo-ocular reflex [VOR] suppression) is removed. In those individuals who are frequently exposed to significant vestibular stimulation and who have developed a strong ability to use optic fixation to suppress their nystagmus (fighter pilots, ballet dancers, acrobats, etc.) they may show a shortened duration of nystagmus with optic fixation, but normal total duration without optic fixation. An alternative technique is to perform the procedure without optic fixation, but then introduce it during the test for 10 to 20 seconds. A normal response would be a reduction in the speed of the slow phase of the nystagmus at least 50%.

8.4 Interpretation

By definition, the direction of the nystagmus is described by its fast phase. Cold stimulation leads to nystagmus with the fast phase to the opposite side, while warm stimulation leads to nystagmus with the fast phase to the same side. This is easily remembered by the mnemonic COWS (cold opposite, warm same).

There are three parameters measured by caloric testing: canal paresis or weakness, directional preponderance and fixation index/fixation suppression.

Various formulae exist, based on the recorded times (or SPV) for each part of the standard caloric test, to predict the degree of vestibular activity. The results are given as a percentage figure.

Canal paresis is calculated using Jongkees' formula:

$$CP = \frac{(RC + RW) - (LC + LW)}{RC + RW + LC + LW} \times 100$$

Directional pre-ponderance is as follows:

$$DP = \frac{(RW + LC) - (LW + RC)}{RW + RC + LW + LC} \times 100$$

The most common abnormalities found are *canal paresis* or *directional pre-ponderance* (or a combination of the two). By the nature of the test a canal paresis or directional pre-ponderance must be greater than 15 to 20% to be considered clinically significant.

- Unilateral canal paresis denotes that the response of one side to hot and cold stimuli is reduced or absent compared with the opposite side. This finding invariably implies a lesion of the peripheral vestibular system (e.g. horizontal canal or vestibular nerve on that side). Exceptions to this include patients with lesions at the vestibular nerve root, entry zone of the brainstem (e.g. multiple sclerosis or lateral brainstem infarction), in which there is central pathology and a canal paresis.
- Bilateral canal paresis may be found after aminoglycoside toxicity or meningitis.
- A directional pre-ponderance denotes a non-specific enhancement of nystagmus in one specific direction. It suggests pathology but is usually non-localising (may arise from any part of the peripheral or central vestibular system). It may be localising with some peripheral lesions, when directional pre-ponderance is usually directed away from the diseased ear.
- A failure to suppress caloric-induced nystagmus with visual fixation is invariably a sign of central vestibular system dysfunction.

8.5 Clinical Indications

Caloric testing forms the cornerstone of investigation for any vestibular pathology and is therefore useful in all patients with vertigo. It is the only 'balance' test that can assess each ear independently.

Further Reading

Bronstein AM. Evaluation of balance. In: Michael Gleeson, ed. Scott-Brown's Otorhinolaryngology and Head and Neck Surgery. 7th ed. London: Hodder Arnold; 2008:3:3727–3728

Katx J, ed. Handbook of Clinical Audiology. 7th ed. Philadelphia, Baltimore, New York: Wolters Kluwer; 2015

Stahle J. Controversies on the caloric response. From Bárány's theory to studies in microgravity. Acta Otolaryngol 1990;109(3–4):162–167

Related Topics of Interest

Vestibular schwannoma
Vertigo
Labyrinthitis
Vestibular function tests

C

9 Cervical Lymphadenopathy

Cervical lymphadenopathy is enlargement of, and implies disease involving, the cervical lymph nodes. The commonest causes are infection, inflammation and metastatic neoplasia. Patients with cervical lymphadenopathy present with a lump or several lumps in the neck. It is a common clinical problem and a favourite subject in examinations. Details regarding other neck lumps are found elsewhere (see Chapter 54, Neck Swellings). The remainder of the chapter is confined to cervical lymph node diseases and to the problem of neck node metastases. The causes of cervical lymphadenopathy are summarised as follows:

Infection	a. Acute (commonest): Viral or bacterial upper respiratory tract infection, acute oral and dental pathology, tonsillitis, infectious mononucleosis, Kawasaki's disease in children.
	b. Chronic: Tuberculosis, atypical mycobacterial infection, actinomycosis, toxoplasmosis, brucellosis, HIV, cat scratch disease, periodontal disease.
Inflammatory	Sarcoidosis, systemic lupus erythematosus (SLE).
Neoplastic	Lymphoma, metastases from head and neck primary, metastases from distant sites (e.g. lung, upper gastrointestinal tract, breast), skin cancer metastases.

9.1 Clinical Features

Most patients should present to secondary care via a rapid access referral to a dedicated Neck Lump Clinic. A thorough focused history and past medical history are extremely helpful. Most patients will have reactive lymphadenopathy. There may be a history of intermittent lymph node enlargement/regression which can occur in, not only reactive nodes, but also in lymphoma. Foreign travel and ethnicity may be suggestive. Systemic symptoms including loss of appetite and weight, and night sweats occur in lymphoma when there is a high volume of disease, but can also occur in inflammatory conditions and the menopause. In conjunction with the history a careful examination of the upper aerodigestive tract, ears, head and neck skin (don't forget the scalp) will reveal the most likely diagnosis in most cases. The site, size and number of nodes should be recorded. The position of the nodes may point towards the eventual diagnosis. Enlarged upper neck nodes are usually from a head and neck source, parotid nodes are often enlarged in skin tumours, occipital nodes from scalp skin inflammation, supraclavicular nodes may be from gastric carcinoma (Troisier's sign/Virchow's node), and other sites below the clavicle (e.g. lung, breast, prostate). Generalised lymphadenopathy could suggest a lymphoma or an infection/inflammatory process.

9.2 Investigations

Specific investigations will be dictated by the differential diagnosis.

- Fine-needle aspiration (FNA) biopsy is probably the single most useful diagnostic procedure. False-negative and, very rarely, false-positive results can occur with FNA cytology, so the information must always be used in conjunction with the clinical findings.
- An ultrasound scan may delineate impalpable nodes and confirm the ultrasonic characteristics of the node. Normal lymph nodes are a size less than 1 cm (or 1.5 cm for the jugulodigastric node), oval shaped, have well-defined borders and a well-preserved fatty hilum. Pathological nodes tend to be enlarged, with a round shape, indistinct borders, an infiltrated hilum and increased vascularity (see Chapter 40, Imaging in Head and Neck Surgery). Ultrasound (US) is also useful in directing FNA biopsy. It has been shown in several studies that US-guided FNA biopsy will give more accurate results than non-guided biopsies.
- Patients in whom there is clinical suspicion of an upper aerodigestive tract cancer should have a computed tomography (CT) or magnetic resonance imaging (MRI) scan of the head and neck. A CT scan of the chest and upper abdomen to exclude metastases or a synchronous primary would also be mandatory in this event. Patients who have a lymphoma should have staging CT scans of the neck, chest, abdomen and pelvis. Patients who present with a primary of unknown origin should have an MRI of the head

and neck and a positron emission tomography–computed tomography scan (PET-CT).

- Blood tests will be directed by the suspected cause. Antibody assays and serology are useful if HIV, cat scratch disease, toxoplasmosis or brucellosis are suspected.

9.3 Infection

9.3.1 Tuberculosis

Cervical lymphadenopathy is the most common head and neck manifestation of *Mycobacterium tuberculosis* infection. Most patients do not have a history of recent contact with the disease, but some may have visited epidemic areas. Half of them will have systemic symptoms. The nodes tend to be tender and the overlying skin may be inflamed with occasional sinus formation. US will often show multiple matted nodes. FNA cytology may reveal mycobacteria. A chest X-ray (CXR) and intra-cutaneous tuberculin test (Mantoux) complete the diagnosis. Incisional biopsy should be avoided as it may lead to a discharging sinus. Immediate anti-tuberculous chemotherapy with isoniazid, rifampicin and ethambutol is the usual regime. Neck dissection with excision of soft tissue and skin may be required.

9.3.2 Atypical Mycobacterial Infection

More commonly seen in children and caused by *Mycobacterium avium* complex and occasionally by *Mycobacterium scrofulaceum* and *Mycobacterium haemophilum*. The diagnosis is suggested by a negative tuberculin test. It usually manifests as lymphadenitis in the submandibular region. Suspicion of atypical mycobacterial aetiology of cervicofacial lymphadenitis should warrant surgical excision of all affected lymph nodes. Medical therapy with antibiotics is inferior to surgery. Incision and drainage should not be done as there is a high probability of recurrence and chronic sinus tract formation with discharge. Adjuvant antibiotics are not proven to improve outcome of this disease.

9.3.3 Toxoplasmosis

This is a parasitic infection with *Toxoplasma gondii* whose main reservoir is in cats, but transmission usually occurs from raw or under-cooked meat and unclean vegetables. Patients have cervical nodes with fever and malaise, and the diagnosis is confirmed by serology. Treatment is not usually indicated as it is self-limiting, but pyrimethamine or clindamycin have been used.

9.3.4 Cat Scratch Disease

This is an infection caused by *Bartonella henselae* acquired by exposure to an infected kitten or cat. Patients present with neck nodes and associated fever and arthralgia. A history of cat scratch should alert the possibility of the diagnosis. Diagnosis may be made from serological testing or from polymerase chain reaction (PCR) of a biopsy specimen. Serology consists of indirect fluorescence assay (IFA) and enzyme-linked immunoassay (ELISA) testing to detect serum antibodies to *B. henselae*, a titre above 1:64 suggesting recent infection. Paired acute and convalescent sera, taken 6 weeks apart, and showing a fourfold increase in titres, are confirmatory. PCR requires a biopsy specimen (which is rarely necessary), but it can differentiate *Bartonella* species, sub-species and strains. It is not readily available. Many infections resolve without intervention, but azithromycin and ciprofloxacin have been advocated.

9.3.5 Actinomycosis

Oral cavity anaerobes cause infection in the neck, usually following surgery or trauma to the mouth. It presents as a slow-growing anterior cervical triangle mass, or an abscess with sinus tracts to the skin. It can mimic tuberculosis (TB) or malignancy. The organisms form characteristic colonies known as sulphur granules, which may be apparent on FNA cytology. Treatment is with a 2-month course of penicillin and removal of any carious teeth.

9.4 Inflammation

There are many causes of inflammatory cervical lymphadenopathy including unusual conditions such as Kikuchi's, Castleman's and Rosai–Dorfman disease. However, two of the more common causes are detailed below.

9.4.1 Sarcoidosis

This multi-system chronic inflammatory condition is characterised by the formation of non-caseating, epithelioid granulomata at various sites in the body. It largely affects patients in their 20s to

C

C

40s, but cases do appear infrequently in younger and older patients. Many patients will be asymptomatic, but some will present with fever, fatigue and lassitude. It has a predilection for the lungs, but also the skin (erythema nodosum), the eyes (uveitis), central nervous system (CNS) (Bell's palsy), joints (arthritis) and often causes hypercalcemia. From an ENT perspective, it can cause sinonasal problems, salivary gland swelling (Heerfordt's syndrome is bilateral parotid involvement, anterior uveitis, fever and facial palsy) and commonly, cervical lymphadenopathy. Diagnosis is usually reached by a CXR showing lung disease, a high calcium level, elevated angiotensin-converting enzyme (ACE) level, caseating granuloma on biopsy, and a negative tuberculin test. Treatment is with steroids and symptomatic.

9.4.2 Systemic Lupus Erythematosus

SLE is an autoimmune disease. Symptoms vary but include painful and swollen joints, fever, chest pain and hair loss. ENT manifestations include cervical lymphadenopathy, recurrent mouth ulceration, motility disorders of the oesophagus and a red rash which is most commonly on the face. Often there are periods of illness, called flares, and periods of remission when there are few symptoms. The cause is not entirely clear and it is diagnosed most commonly by anti-nuclear antibodies on serology. There is no cure for SLE. Treatments may include non-steroidal anti-inflammatory drugs (NSAIDs), corticosteroids, immunosuppressants, hydroxychloroquine and methotrexate.

9.5 Neoplastic

9.5.1 Primary Lymphoma

The head and neck region is a common presenting site for lymphomatous lymphadenopathy. Lymphoma affects a wide age range. The nodes are often multiple, large and rubbery in consistency. Diagnosis may be suspected from FNA results, but confirmation requires a formal biopsy, either incisional or excisional, for formal tissue typing. Further management is usually undertaken by a haemato-oncologist and early liaison with them is essential. The patients are usually staged with an MRI or CT scan of the neck and CT of the chest, abdomen and pelvis or may undergo a PET-CT scan.

9.5.2 Metastatic Neck Nodes

- Squamous cell carcinoma (SCC) in a neck node may be metastatic from the upper aerodigestive tract (head and neck primary) or the skin.
- The salivary gland tumours which commonly metastasise are carcinoma ex pleomorphic salivary adenoma, high-grade mucoepidermoid and SCC.
- Papillary carcinoma of the thyroid also has a propensity to present with nodal disease.
- The carcinoma may also be from non–head and neck sites, usually the lung, upper gastrointestinal tract, breast or prostate.

A primary carcinoma arising in the upper aerodigestive tract may metastasise to the lymph nodes of the neck. Cervical node status is one of the most important prognostic factors in the head and neck cancer patient. In a patient with positive nodal disease, the usual expected survival rate for any specific primary tumour can be reduced by up to one-half. Therefore, control of regional metastatic disease constitutes a significant part of the management of head and neck cancer.

Anatomy

There are approximately 150 lymph nodes on each side of the neck and they are divided into superficial and deep groups. Most descriptions of cervical lymphadenopathy begin with which triangle of the neck the nodes are positioned. The anterior triangle is bounded by the mandible, anterior aspect of sternocleidomastoid, and the midline. The posterior triangle is bounded by the sternocleidomastoid, the trapezius muscle and the clavicle (▶ Fig. 9.1). The lymph nodes are usually described within the seven levels of the neck (▶ Fig. 9.2).

The following definitions are recommended for the boundaries of cervical lymph node groups:

- Level I (submental and submandibular nodes)
  Consists of the submental (level IA) nodes—within the triangular boundary of anterior belly of digastric and the hyoid bone—and submandibular lymph nodes (level IB)—within the triangle bounded by the anterior belly of the digastric, the hyoid bone, the posterior belly of digastric and the body of the mandible.

- Level II (upper jugular)
  Consists of lymph nodes located around the upper third of the internal jugular vein and

C

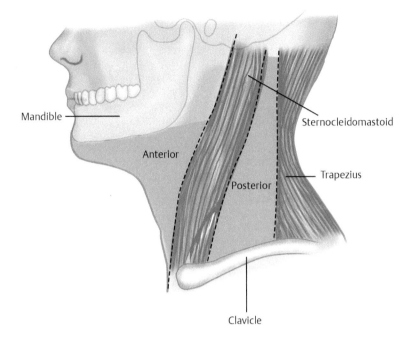

Fig. 9.1 Triangles of the neck.

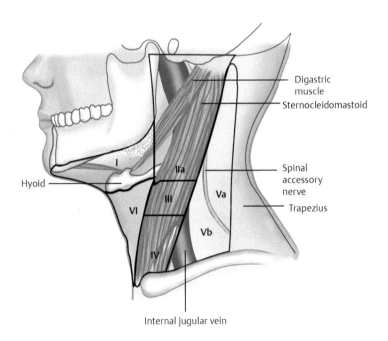

Fig. 9.2 Lymph node levels.

adjacent spinal accessory nerve extending from the skull base above to the level of the inferior border of the hyoid bone below. Sub-level IIA nodes are located anterior medial to the vertical plane defined by the accessory nerve and level IIB nodes are located posterior lateral to the accessory nerve.

- Level III (mid-jugular)
  Consists of lymph nodes around the middle of the internal jugular vein extending from the inferior border of the hyoid bone above to the inferior border of the cricoid below.

- Level IV (lower jugular)
  Consists of lymph nodes located around the lower third of the internal jugular vein extending from the inferior border of the cricoid above to the clavicle inferiorly.

- Level V (posterior triangle)
  Consists of the posterior triangle nodes which are located between the posterior border of the sternocleidomastoid muscle and the anterior border of the trapezius. The supraclavicular nodes are also included in this group. Sub-level VA includes the accessory nerve nodes, whereas sub-level VB includes the nodes following the transverse cervical vessels and the supraclavicular nodes.

- Level VI (anterior compartment group)
  Includes the pretracheal and paratracheal and pre-cricoid (delphian) node and the perithyroidal nodes and nodes along the recurrent laryngeal nerves. The superior boundary is the hyoid bone, the inferior boundary is the suprasternal notch and the lateral boundaries are the common carotid arteries.

- Level VII (superior mediastinal group)
  Pretracheal, paratracheal and oesophageal nodes extending from the suprasternal notch superiorly and up to the innominate artery inferiorly.

Knowledge of the first echelon draining lymph nodes for various primary anatomical sites can be useful:

Level I   Oral cavity, oropharynx.
Level II   Oral cavity, oropharynx, larynx, nose, hypopharynx, parotid, nasopharynx.
Level III Oral cavity, oropharynx, larynx, hypopharynx, thyroid, nasopharynx.
Level IV   Larynx, thyroid, hypopharynx, oesophagus.

Level V   Nasopharynx, hypopharynx, thyroid, oropharynx.
Level VI   Thyroid, larynx, hypopharynx, cervical oesophagus.

Most tumours will metastasise in a predictable manner to certain nodal groups, but it should be remembered that tumours can metastasise to more remote sites (i.e., nasopharyngeal cancers to level V, tongue cancers to level IV) and that the pattern of spread will be disrupted by previous surgery or radiotherapy.

9.6 Staging

The staging system is that proposed by the 8th edition of the International Union against Cancer (UICC) and the American Joint Committee (AJC) for Cancer Staging. It has altered from previous versions to consider the importance of extranodal extension.

N   Regional lymph nodes.
NX   Regional lymph nodes cannot be assessed.
N0   No regional lymph node metastasis.
N1   Metastasis in a single ipsilateral lymph node, 3 cm or less in greatest dimension without extranodal extension.
N2   Metastasis is described as the following:
N2a   Metastasis in a single ipsilateral lymph node, more than 3 cm but not more than 6 cm in greatest dimension without extranodal extension.
N2b   Metastasis in multiple ipsilateral lymph nodes, none more than 6 cm in greatest dimension, without extranodal extension.
N2c   Metastasis in bilateral or contralateral lymph nodes, none more than 6 cm in greatest dimension, without extranodal extension.
N3a   Metastasis in a lymph node more than 6 cm in greatest dimension without extranodal extension.
N3b   Metastasis in a single or multiple lymph nodes with clinical extranodal extension.

Although this system is useful, it has several inherent problems. Clinicians will fail to agree on the presence of a palpable lymph node in as many as 70% of cases. In addition, it is generally acknowledged that the number of lymph nodes involved, the lymph node level and the presence of extracapsular spread (ECS) are the most important prognostic parameters in metastatic disease of the neck.

Nearly all patients will have had a diagnostic US-guided FNA biopsy, but for staging purposes a CT or MRI scan is mandatory. Sentinel node biopsy has been advocated in oral cavity cancer to identify and excise the first echelon nodes using radioscintigraphy, which are then tested for occult disease.

9.7 Treatment

Treatment of cervical lymph nodes is either pro-phylactic (in the clinically negative neck) or therapeutic (in the clinically positive neck). The modality chosen is usually the same as that used for the primary tumour. The surgical treatment of malignant neck nodes is by some form of neck dissection (ND). Conventional and three-dimen-sional conformal radiotherapy (RT) have now been superseded by intensity-modulated radiotherapy (IMRT) which has been shown to have a reduced risk of xerostomia. There is now an increasing use of concomitant chemotherapy (CR) in advanced nodal disease.

Rupture of the lymph node capsule by tumour (ECS) is a bad prognostic sign. Fifty percent of nodes with a diameter greater than 3 cm exhibit this. Post-operative RT or CR to the neck following neck dissection is mandatory in the presence of ECS and positive surgical margins.

N0   The argument supporting treatment is that some lymph nodes may be invaded by tumour and still be impalpable (occult nodes). Risk factors for occult nodes are the site (oral cavity, nasopharynx, oropharynx and supraglottic larynx), the size and his-tological grade of the primary tumour. It has been shown that elective neck dissection reduces the risk of disease-spe-cific death compared with observation. Selective neck dissection (SND) is as effec-tive as modified radical neck dissection (MRND) for controlling regional disease in N0 neck for all primary sites. Prophylactic SND neck has now been advocated in the patient who has a primary tumour with a high incidence (> 15–20%) of occult nodes. This, in fact, includes almost all primary sites except for T1 and T2 glot-tic cancers and T1 oral cavity. Elective

neck irradiation is as effective as elective neck dissection in controlling occult neck disease. If observation is planned for the N0 neck, it should be supplemented with regular US to facilitate early detection.

N1   It is generally accepted that lymph nodes of less than 3-cm diameter can be treated by single-modality therapy. The risk of occult nodal metastases in other appar-ently uninvolved levels of the neck is high. Level V is least likely to be involved with only 3 to 7% of patients having radical neck dissection (RND) having positive nodes in level V. SND is the usual surgical option as it confers control rates comparable to MRND. As approximately 50% of clinically N1 necks are upstaged after pathological assessment, many patients subsequently require post-operative RT. Control rates following RT alone are best in patients with nodes less than 2 cm in size.

N2–N3 If the primary modality is surgery, a MRND has equivalent rates of disease control and less morbidity than a RND. Post-operative RT has been shown to increase regional control particularly in the presence of adverse features (two or more nodes, ECS, positive margins, T3/T4 primary, perineural or vascular invasion). It has been shown that there is improved control with post-operative CR in the presence of ECS and involved surgical margins. If the primary site is suitable for non-surgical treatment, it can be treated with the neck at the same time by chemo-radiotherapy. The PET Neck phase III trial confirmed that there is no role for a planned neck dissection after primary CR. The current recommendation is that the patient undergoes a PET-CT between 10 and 12 weeks following CR, with neck dissection being offered to those who show incomplete or equivocal response of their nodal disease. Complete responders need no further intervention.

9.8 Primary of Unknown Origin

This is defined as a SCC presenting in a lymph node in the neck with no primary index site identified (occult primary). A careful search will usually reveal the primary tumour in the skin or mucosal surfaces of the head and neck, or rarely, in an area below the clavicles, such as the lungs. It is important to search thoroughly for the primary tumour with a focused history and endoscopy in clinic. The high-risk sites are:

- Ipsilateral tonsil.
- Base of tongue.
- Nasopharynx.
- Pyriform fossa.

If there is no obvious or highly suspicious lesion on outpatient assessment, then the patient should be regarded as having an unknown primary and should be evaluated further, this clinical entity being known as a 'clinical!' unknown primary.

9.8.1 Investigations

- These patients by definition have already undergone FNA biopsy to diagnose the presence of SCC. Some may have undergone a core biopsy. Immunohistochemical techniques may not be able to suggest the tumour origin, but can exclude sites, for example by the use of lung or thyroid markers. More specific investigations such as identification of Epstein–Barr virus (EBV) may correlate highly with a nasopharyngeal site. Human papillomavirus (HPV) is a significant aetiological factor in oropharyngeal cancer and so the identification of HPV16 and 18 in a lymph node sample would be strongly suggestive of an oropharyngeal origin. P16 positivity is highly predictive of HPV overexpression and may be used as a surrogate marker to indicate HPV status.
- An MRI scan may show the presence of an occult primary but the investigation of choice is a PET-CT fusion scan.
- Following each of the clinical and radiological assessments, it is necessary to carry out pan-endoscopy of the upper aerodigestive tract under general anaesthesia. Imaging may have identified a potential primary site for a targeted biopsy, but if not, each of the sub-sites of the head and neck should be examined under direct vision and by use of straight and angled endoscopes. Endoscopy with Narrow Band Imaging (NBI) can be useful. NBI relies on the principle of depth of penetration of light, with narrow band blue light having a short wavelength penetrating into the mucosa and highlighting the superficial vasculature.

A blue filter is designed to correspond to the peak absorption spectrum of haemoglobin and this enhances the image of capillary vessels on the surface mucosa. So superficial mucosal lesions that would be missed by regular white light endoscopy are identified. Palpation of oral cavity and tongue base should also be carried out.

- PET-CT imaging, in conjunction with pan-endoscopy and directed biopsy as appropriate, offers the greatest chance of identifying the occult primary tumour. Bilateral tonsillectomy and tongue base (lingual tonsil) mucosectomy, by transoral laser or robotic approach, are also advised. If each of these investigations is negative, then this should be regarded as a 'true' unknown primary and the treatment considered as such.

9.8.2 Treatment

The treatment of an occult mucosal primary is based on the treatment of nodal disease with known primary cancer site. Surgery on its own may be sufficient treatment for N1 necks demonstrating no ECS, but in all other scenarios, it needs to be supplemented by adjuvant radiotherapy with or without chemotherapy. For N2 and N3 disease a combination of neck dissection and radiotherapy, or initial chemoradiotherapy followed by planned neck dissection if a complete response is not evident on imaging. Both of these approaches appear to be equally effective. Patients who have neck dissection and radiation therapy to both sides of the neck and the mucosal surfaces have better neck and local control than those who do not have such extensive treatment. However, this does not seem to translate into prolonged survival. There is no conclusive evidence to support total mucosal irradiation in routine use as there is significant acute toxicity and chronic morbidity, mainly xerostomia with its associated complications and effects on quality of life. IMRT is an improvement as it enables delivery of different doses during total mucosal irradiation, and thus potentially reduces treatment-related toxicity, but even this is contentious.

9.8.3 Prognosis

The rate of emergence of the primary tumour is approximately 3% per year, which is equivalent to the development of second carcinomas in the head and neck, lung and oesophagus. The prognosis varies from a 30 to 70% 5-year survival. The prognosis depends on N stage and position of the node. Supraclavicular nodes have the worse prognosis, probably because many of these represent distant metastases from non–head and neck sites (e.g. lung or stomach).

9.9 Palliative Therapy

Patients with inoperable neck nodes that have fungated through the skin can be treated with local dressings of Kaltocarb and topical metronidazole. These will help prevent colonisation by anaerobes and alleviate the odour from tissue necrosis. Death by carotid artery rupture will usually ensue. The patient should always be treated with appropriate doses of opiate analgesia and anti-emetics. It is imperative that there is adequate social support and that the patient's family doctor is aware of the situation if the patient is to be cared for in the community.

Further Reading

Grégoire V, Ang K, Budach W, et al. Delineation of the neck node levels for head and neck tumors: a 2013 update. DAHANCA, EORTC, HKNPCSG, NCIC CTG, NCRI, RTOG, TROG consensus guidelines. Radiother Oncol. 2014; 110(1):172–181

Jones AS, Cook JA, Phillips DE, Roland NR. Squamous carcinoma presenting as an enlarged cervical lymph node. Cancer. 1993; 72(5):1756–1761

Jones AS, Roland NJ, Field JK, Phillips DE. The level of cervical lymph node metastases: their prognostic relevance and relationship with head and neck squamous carcinoma primary sites. Clin Otolaryngol Allied Sci. 1994; 19(1):63–69

Mehanna H, Rahman J, Mcconkey CC, et al. PET-NECK—a multi-centre randomized phase III controlled trial (RCT) comparing PETCT guided active surveillance with planned neck dissection (ND) for locally advanced (N2/N3) nodal metastases (LANM) in patients with head and neck squamous cell cancer (HNSCC) treated with primary radical chemoradiotherapy (CRT). Health Technol Assess. 2017; 21(17):1–122

Strojan P, Ferlito A, Medina JE, et al. Contemporary management of lymph node metastases from an unknown primary to the neck: I. A review of diagnostic approaches. Head Neck. 2013; 35(1):123–132

Related Topics of Interest

Neck swellings
Neck dissection

10 Cholesteatoma

Cholesteatoma is a collection of 'bad skin' (migrating keratinising squamous epithelium) trapped within the middle ear or mastoid. It is a common and potentially dangerous condition. The incidence is approximately 10 cases per 100,000 population per annum. Between 7 and 10% of people diagnosed with cholesteatoma will develop a cholesteatoma in the other ear.

10.1 Pathophysiology

The single most important fact about the skin of the eardrum is that it migrates from the centre of the drum outward along the external ear canal, carrying keratin and wax debris with it. Therefore, the ear canal is self-cleaning. The skin of the ear canal is the only squamous epithelium that migrates in health. In disease, this skin can migrate into the middle ear and form a progressively enlarging 'cyst of skin' that destroys the tissue it comes up against. This may arise from problems in childhood when the eustachian tube fails to function normally and results in negative pressures behind the eardrum. The normal atmospheric pressure in the ear canal then pushes the eardrum to retract into the middle ear as a 'retraction pocket'. This is usually in the more flaccid, pars flacida, in the attic of the eardrum and made easier if middle ear infections have damaged and thinned the membrane so that it loses its resilience. At first the eardrum skin is able to migrate out of the shallow pocket, but if the pocket becomes too deep, then the skin is unable to flow around the edge of the pocket and the surface layers of dead skin begin to accumulate and a cholesteatoma forms. Published evidence not only suggests that 16% of retraction pockets develop into a cholesteatoma, but also that surgery (either with ventilating tubes, fascial tympanoplasty or cartilage tympanoplasty) does not alter the progression of those pockets that will become cholesteatoma.

Skin can also be implanted or can migrate around the rim of a perforation or pocket in the thicker more ridgid pars tensa and cause a cholesteatoma. Skin may also be implanted at surgery, for example, grommet insertion. It is also thought possible that little feet of skin can migrate inward through the layers of the tympanic membrane and even that middle ear mucosa can metaplase to become squamous. Cholesteatoma can also be congenital, arising from epithelial cell rests in the forming middle ear that usually disappeares at 17 weeks of gestation. Congenital cholesteatomas obstruct the eustachian tube or surround the ossicles, causing a conductive hearing loss. They can be seen as a pearly white mass medial to a normal tympanic membrane. They usually present between the ages of 6 months and 5 years, behind an intact tympanic membrane, but they can sometimes present in adulthood.

The accumulation of dead skin forces the underlying live skin cells to expand so that layer upon layer of dead cells accumulate and are surrounded by a very thin layer of still living and actively growing eardrum skin. The pocket fills with epithelial debris, which in turn becomes infected and further expands under tension. As it enlarges, the cholesteatoma erodes the structures it encounters including bone. The outermost layer of the cholesteatoma, the basal layer of the skin, is metabolically active, producing proteolytic enzymes that are locally destructive, eroding adjacent bone. This damages the ossicles as well as exposes the inner ear, the facial nerve and the meninges of the brain. Deafness can be due to damage in the bones in the middle ear but can also be due to erosion of the inner ear (labyrinth), which is usually associated with dizziness, because of damage to the vestibular apparatus. The cholesteatoma most commonly erodes the lateral semicircular canal in its lateral or anterior aspects and a fistula sign becomes positive. Pressing air into the air canal causes the eyes to move in response. The pressure in the ear canal is directly transferred into the inner ear via the fistula in the lateral semicircular canal, and this movement of fluid simulates a head rotation. The vestibular ocular reflex then moves the eyes to stabilise the visual field in response to this false movement of the head. As there is no head movement, the eyes move to one side.

The facial nerve runs through the middle ear and invasion of this by cholesteatoma can cause a facial palsy. Superior to the middle ear is the brain and invasion of this by the cholesteatoma can lead to brain abcesses, meningitis and venous thrombosis which can cause major neurological conditions including epilepsy and death. The incidence of these complications is not well determined. It is often quoted as 1 to 2% per annum in untreated cholesteatoma, though it is more likely to be about 1 in 200 lifetime risk. Interestingly, as yet, there is no evidence that treatment alters this.

The contents of the cholesteatoma have no blood supply and it becomes easily infected by any bacteria that happen to be around, causing infected foul-smelling pus to be discharged.

10.2 Clinical Features

The patient complains of deafness and/or this foul-smelling discharge. There may be earache. On examination, the principal signs are an attic crust in the pars flacida area, a marginal perforation or a pocket of invading keratin debris. The keratin dries and turns brown looking like wax. The erosion of bone can lead to reactive polyp formation as the underlying bare bone becomes osteitic. Marginal granulations and polyps protruding from the middle ear cleft indicate osteitis and underlying cholesteatoma. Along with the deafness or discharge the patient may present with pain, dizziness, facial nerve weakness or an intracranial infection.

The diagnosis requires clear visualisation of the tympanic membrane to identify the characteristic appearance of a cholesteatoma.

10.3 Investigations

- *PTA*: Typical findings are a mild-to-moderate conductive loss, but there can be any kind of loss or no loss at all.
- *Imaging:* Many surgeons advocate computed tomography (CT) scanning of the temporal bone to elucidate the cholesteatoma. This is sometimes seen as a cavity in the mastoid, or occasionally as a dependent mass in the attic with erosion of the scutum (the shield-like bone above the pars flacida of the eardrum). The extent of cholesteatoma can be estimated on the scan and likewise the status of the ossicles and any erosion into the inner ear or cranial cavity. The position of the facial nerve canal can be seen and its relationship with the cholesteatoma visualised. Magnetic resonance imaging (MRI) or more specifically diffusion-weighted MRI can be used to detect cholesteatoma but is generally reserved

for the detection of recurrence of cholesteatoma after a canal wall up mastoidectomy.
- *Biopsy:* It is only required if malignancy is suspected.

10.4 Grading Systems

There are grading systems used to define the extent of cholesteatoma. In Europe, the approved grading is based on the Japanese Otology Association system that has had some prognostic validation for recurrence of disease. Basically in both, the tympanomastoid space is divided into four sections: protympanum (P), tympanic cavity (T), attic (A) and mastoid (M). Four stages are defined:

- Stage I: cholesteatoma localised in one site.
- Stage II: cholesteatoma involving two or more sites.
- Stage III: cholesteatoma with extracranial complications and/or intratemporal pathological conditions.
- Stage IV: cholesteatoma with intracranial complications.

10.5 Treatment

Treatment is usually surgical and aims to make the ear safe. Conservative treatment such as repeated microsuction can be used. It is often reserved for use in the elderly and infirm or as a temporising means prior to surgery.

The risk of residual disease after corrective surgery varies from 5 to 30%. The success of such surgery is highly dependent on the extent of disease and the type of surgery undertaken.

According to the world literature, 30% of canal wall up operations, 17% of canal wall down operations and 5% of canal wall reconstruction operations fail to cure the cholesteatoma. The failure rate increases with time and is worse in children, possibly reaching 50%.

Further Reading

Anderson J, Cayé-Thomasen P, Tos M. A comparison of cartilage palisades and fascia in tympanoplasty after surgery for sinus or tensa retraction cholesteatoma in children. Otol Neurotol. 2004; 25(6):856–863

Nankivell PC, Pothier DD. Surgery for tympanic membrane retraction pockets. Cochrane Database Syst Rev 2010(7):CD007943

Nunez DA, Browning GG. Risks of developing an otogenic intracranial abscess. J Laryngol Otol. 1990; 104(6):468–472

C

Tono T, Sakagami M, Kojima H, et al. Staging and classification criteria for middle ear cholesteatoma proposed by the Japan Otological Society. Auris Nasus Larynx. 2017; 44(2):135–140

Yung M, Tono T, Olszewska E, et al. EAONO/JOS Joint Consensus Statements on the Definitions, Classification and Staging of Middle Ear Cholesteatoma. J Int Adv Otol. 2017; 13(1):1–8

C

Related Topics of Interest

Mastoid surgery

Tympanoplasty

11 Clinical Assessment of Hearing

11.1 Use of Clinical Tests

It is surprising how often a clinical assessment of hearing is omitted from the routine examination of the otology patient. Voice tests and tuning fork tests are the two main methods, but often only the Weber and Rinne tuning fork tests are performed.

Clinical tests can be used to test the following:

- Identify a hearing impairment.
- Determine the nature of a hearing loss (conductive or sensorineural).
- Grade the severity.
- Detect feigning or a non-organic hearing loss.

The main reason that clinical tests of auditory function are overlooked is that they have largely been superseded by more sensitive and reliable audiometric tests. However, audiometry on occasions may be inaccurate or unavailable. Furthermore, exaggerated thresholds may be missed if suspicion is not aroused by clinical testing. Proponents of clinical testing suggest that audiometry may be unnecessary if the hearing is normal or the results would not influence the management.

11.2 Masking

Masking is as important in clinical testing as it is in audiometric testing. The non-test ear should always be masked when clinically testing by air conduction, and, in theory, always when performing tuning fork tests, though this is not always practicable. There are two techniques in common use.

1. The tragal rub. Occlusion of the auditory canal by putting finger pressure on the tragus with a rubbing motion is the easiest method. Using this technique, speech will be attenuated by approximately 50 dB. There is a risk of under-masking if the sound level of speech arriving at the test ear is greater than 70 dB(A) so a Bárány noise box should be used when testing an ear with a severe or profound impairment or when testing bone conduction with tuning forks.

2. The Bárány noise box. This box produces a broadband noise from a clockwork-driven source. The maximum sound output varies

from approximately 90 dB(A) when a box is held at right angles to the ear and 100 dB(A) when held over the ear. These levels are sufficient to mask the non-test ear in all practical circumstances, but the main problem is cross-masking of the test ear. It should be used when a tragal rub does not provide adequate masking.

11.3 Voice Tests

Difficulties in standardising the technique and variability of the stimulus provided by the examiner have led to criticisms of this test. The easiest and best method of performing monaural free-field voice testing is by using a whispered voice, conversational voice, and then loud voice at 60 cm and then 15 cm. It is usual to start by testing the better hearing ear when there is one. The non-test ear is masked by a tragal rub unless a loud voice is required (use the Bárány noise box). The patient is asked to repeat as accurately as possible what the examiner says. Bisyllable words (e.g. bluebell and cowboy), numbers (e.g. 54, 37 and 63), or combinations of numbers and letters (e.g. 4 B 7) can be used depending on the patient's age and understanding. The examiner starts by using a whispered voice 60 cm away from the patient, which is the furthest away that is possible when masking the non-test ear (obviously limited by the length of the clinician's arm!). The sound level is increased in steps from a whispered voice at 60 cm, to a whispered voice at 15 cm, to a conversational voice at 60 cm, to a conversational voice at 15 cm, to a loud voice at 60 cm, and finally to a loud voice at 15 cm. The test finishes as soon as the patient repeats 50% of the words correctly at any one voice and distance level.

If a patient can hear a whispered voice 60 cm away from the ear, the pure-tone thresholds are likely to be less than 30 dB (normal hearing). Patients who can hear a whisper at 15 cm or a conversational voice at 60 or 15 cm are likely to have thresholds in the range of 30 to 70 dB hearing level (HL) (mild/moderate impairment). Those patients who can only hear a loud voice are likely to have thresholds greater than 70 dB HL (severe/profound impairment).

C

11.4 Tuning Forks

Tuning forks for audiological use are modified to include a finger grip on the stem and an expansion at the base of the stem to allow application to the skull. Ideally, a 512- or 256-Hz tuning fork should be used. The duration of the stimulus decreases with increasing frequency, and it is difficult to activate forks with a frequency higher than 512 Hz sufficiently for them to be heard by those with a moderate or severe impairment. Forks with a frequency lower than 256 Hz can make it difficult for the patient to distinguish between hearing the sound and feeling it by vibration. A tuning fork should be set in vibration by a firm strike one-third of the way from the free end of the prong against a firm but elastic object (e.g. elbow or patella). This should produce a relatively pure tone with minimal overtones. It can then be presented by either air or bone conduction. For air conduction it should be held with its acoustic axis (a line joining two points near the tips of the two prongs) in line with and 2 to 3 cm from the external meatus. For bone conduction, the base plate should be placed firmly on the skull, either mastoid process or vertex depending on the test. Although the tuning fork can theoretically be placed at any point on the skull for bone conduction, some points may give less reliable results.

A variety of tuning fork tests were developed to test absolute hearing thresholds (compared with the examiner), to differentiate real from feigned hearing loss, conductive from sensorineural, and cochlear from retrocochlear hearing loss. With the advent of newer and more sensitive forms of investigation, many of these tests are no longer in everyday use, but knowledge of their existence and rationale is useful.

The tests are based on two main principles:

1. The inner ear is normally twice as sensitive to sound conducted by air as to that conducted by bone.
2. In the presence of a purely conductive hearing loss, the affected ear is subject to less environmental noise, making it more sensitive to bone-conducted sound.

No single test is diagnostic but all can provide useful information when taken in context. Unfortunately, tuning fork tests are unreliable in children.

11.5 Weber's Test

This test is based on the principle that a conductive loss causes a relative improvement in the ability to hear a bone-conducted sound and the test is of most value in a unilateral hearing loss. The tuning fork is struck and placed on the vertex. The vertex is used as opposed to the forehead as the reliability of the test is thus improved from 72 to 86%.

If a conductive loss of 10 dB or more exists, the sound should be heard in the affected ear. If a sensorineural hearing loss is present, the sound will generally be heard in the normal or better ear. In the normal subject or some subjects with a long-standing sensorineural hearing loss, the sound will be heard in the midline.

11.6 Rinne's Test

This test examines each ear individually and is again based on the principle of improved bone conduction perception with a conductive loss. It can be performed in one of the two ways. The subject can be asked to compare either the loudness of the tuning fork when presented by air conduction and bone conduction (placed on the ipsilateral mastoid process) or the duration of the sound when presented by both air and bone conduction. The normal response is to hear the sound as louder and longer with air conduction and is referred to as a Rinne positive. A positive response will also occur with a sensorineural hearing loss. A negative response (Rinne negative) will occur if there is a conductive loss of greater than 20 dB or if there is a severe sensorineural hearing loss. The former is referred to as a true-negative Rinne and the latter as a false negative. The two can be distinguished by using a Bárány sound box, in which case the false negative will become positive as the contralateral, minimally attenuated, bone conduction is masked.

11.7 Bing's Test

This test is similar to the Rinne and is based on the improvement in bone conduction perception in the normal subject when the external auditory meatus is occluded. The tuning fork is struck and placed on the subject's mastoid process. After the subject acknowledges hearing the sound, the ipsilateral meatus is occluded by the examiner's finger and the subject is asked if this makes the sound louder or quieter. Occluding the external auditory canal will block out ambient noise and prevent some of the bone conduction sound, which has emanated into the external auditory canal, from escaping. If the sound becomes louder, the response is positive (and normal). If the sound does not change or becomes quieter, the response is negative, and usually indicates a conductive loss of 10 dB or more.

11.8 Stenger's Test

This test is used to differentiate a real from a feigned hearing loss and is based on the principle that, if two pure tones of equal intensity are presented to both ears at once, the sound will appear to originate in the midline. If the intensity of one side is increased, the sound will appear to originate from that side alone. In practice, the test is commenced by asking the subject to close his or her eyes to help concentrate on the sound. The tester works behind the subject. First a tuning fork is placed 15 cm from the good ear; the subject confirms hearing the sound. A tuning fork is then positioned 5 cm from the bad ear; the subject will deny hearing it. Finally, unknown to the subject, two tuning forks are used simultaneously: one

5 cm from the bad ear and other 15 cm from the good ear. If the hearing loss is real, the subject will hear the sound in the good ear and report this. If the hearing loss is feigned, the subject will hear the sound loudest in the bad ear. Unaware that there is a previously audible sound present at the good ear, the subject will deny hearing anything and this suggests the diagnosis.

Further Reading

Browning GG. Clinical Otology and Audiology. London: Butterworths; 1986:23–37

Committee for the consideration of hearing tests. Report of the committee for the consideration of hearing tests. J Laryngol Otol. 1933; 48:22–48

Golabek W, Stephens SDG. Some tuning fork tests revisited. Clin Otolaryngol Allied Sci. 1979; 4(6):421–430

Hearing loss (Assessment of) - Diagnosis - Approach - Best Practice.bestpractice.bmj.com/best-practice/monograph/434/diagnosis.html. Accessed February 2017

Related Topics of Interest

Examination of the ear
Pure-tone audiometry
Impedance audiometry
Speech audiometry
Non-organic hearing loss

12 Cochlear Implants

Cochlear implantation has evolved to become a safe and reliable means of providing auditory rehabilitation in both adults and children with severe or profound hearing loss.

12.1 Indications and Goals of Cochlear Implantation Programmes

The device aims to provide perception of sound by attempting to emulate the transducer function of the cochlea, thereby stimulating residual auditory neural tissue. In appropriately selected individuals, the original premise that cochlear implantation would allow recognition of environmental sound and serve as an adjunct to lip reading has been realised. In reality, many individuals have derived greater benefit through cochlear implantation including the ability to understand speech with little or no lip reading, ability to use the phone, and enjoyment of music.

12.2 History

The first report of cochlear implantation was from Djourno and colleagues in 1957 who described the insertion of a device into two totally deaf individuals. Paralleled by developments in pacemaker technology, this stimulated considerable interest in the 1960s and 1970s amongst several investigators: the House group in Los Angeles (United States), Michelson and colleagues in San Francisco (United States), Clark and colleagues in Melbourne, (Australia), Hochmair–Desoyer's team in Austria, and Chouard and colleagues in France. Not surprisingly, many of the original and current commercially available devices bear their origins in these pioneering research programmes. 3M and Clarion devices from California, United States (Advanced Bionics); Nucleus (Cochlear) devices from Australia (Cochlear), and Med-El devices from Austria.

The success of these early implant programmes generated considerable interest in the United Kingdom; the first single channel device was implanted in London by Fraser in 1984 with the first multichannel device being inserted by Ramsden in Manchester in 1988. Initially, implant programmes in the United Kingdom were funded through research and charitable sources, but the MRC report by Summerfield and Marshall (1995) based on a multicentre pilot study, in effect procured central funding for cochlear implantation.

12.3 Implant Design

Current cochlear implants consist of two parts: an external component and a surgically implanted internal component. The external part comprises a microphone, speech processor, and transmitter coil. The microphone unit is hooked behind the ear in a manner not dissimilar to a conventional behind-the-ear hearing aid. Sound received by the microphone is converted into electrical energy, which is conveyed to the speech processor. This body-worn component utilises various speech strategies (see later) and sends the processed signal to the transmitting coil which is held on the scalp behind the ear by a magnet in the coil and the implanted part of the device. The transmitter coil transfers the processed information to the internal implanted receiver–stimulator package by transcutaneous induction. From the receiver–stimulator package, information is conveyed to the electrode array which is implanted within the cochlea; the current hypothesis is that the implanted electrodes stimulate the spiral ganglion cells of the auditory nerve directly. Depending on the manufacturer, the number of active electrodes varies from 12 to 24 (multichannel devices). Modified electrode arrays are available for use in the partially ossified cochlea; compressed arrays carrying a smaller number of electrodes or double electrode arrays for insertion into the basal and middle cochlear turns independently. The implanted component of the device needs to be constructed from biocompatible materials with high tensile strength and resistance to corrosion. The electrodes themselves are made of a platinum–iridium alloy housed in silicone with either a ceramic or silicone casing for the receiver package. At the time of writing, the cost of the implant hardware in the United Kingdom is around £20,000.

12.4 Speech Coding Strategies

A speech signal has two main components: spectral (pitch) information and temporal (loudness and change in loudness) information. Various speech coding strategies have evolved over the last 20 years in an attempt to emulate and present this information to the auditory nerve. The original strategies based on extracting vowel and fundamental formant information are now obsolete. Current devices digitise the input and utilise bandpass filters to divide the signal into frequency-specific components. This information is presented in a pulsatile waveform to the individual channels of the electrode array. This reduces cross-interaction between channels thereby enhancing spectral information. By stimulating a smaller number of the available electrodes with the signal components that have the highest amplitude, the overall rate of stimulation increases, enhancing temporal information. The implementation of the principles of the speech strategies differs between manufacturers and continues to evolve. In terms of outcomes, the current strategies for multichannel implantation from the different manufacturers are all capable of providing comparable results.

12.5 Neural Plasticity

This is the ability of the central nervous system to be programmed to learn a task. In cochlear implantation, two components are of paramount importance: changes in the brainstem auditory nuclei and the auditory cortex in response to sound and also the neural plasticity of speech articulation. Auditory plasticity, and with it the ability to listen, is lost by the age of 8 years while the ability to develop good speech articulation only occurs if speech sounds are heard by the age of 3 years. On this basis, hearing-impaired individuals are classified as post-lingual (speech acquired before becoming deaf) or pre-lingual (become deaf before acquiring speech). In addition, a third group comprises those children who lose their hearing around the time of speech development (peri-lingual). Post-lingual adults and children may be considered for implantation. In pre- and peri-lingual children, the timing of cochlear implantation is critical taking into account the issues of neural plasticity.

12.6 Candidacy

The process of selecting appropriate individuals for implantation is of critical importance for a successful outcome and is a task that involves all the members of the multidisciplinary implant team.

The selection criteria continue to evolve and may be considered under the following headings:

1. **Age:** There is no upper age limit as long as the potential recipient is in good health. The initial controversy surrounding implantation in children has abated and implantation is regularly undertaken in selected children below the age of 12 months.

2. **Cause of the deafness:** Within the cochlea, different aetiologies have a greater or lesser effect on the spiral ganglion cell population. In addition, secondary changes in the cochlea such as fibrosis and ossification (such as after meningitis) need to be recognised as surgery may require a cochlear drill-out or use of a modified electrode array as described above.

3. **Duration of severe or profound deafness:** In post-lingually deafened adults, the duration of severe or profound deafness is recognised as a prognostic indicator with respect to outcome, with those individuals deafened for more than 20 years tending to fare less well. Cochlear implantation in profoundly deaf pre-lingual adolescents and adults was previously thought to be futile, yet increasing evidence has been provided detailing the overall benefit in these 'non-traditional' cochlear implant users. With regards to children and adolescents, the relationship between the onset of deafness and speech development is of critical importance.

4. **Audiometric assessment:** Selected individuals that derive little or no benefit from a trial of conventional hearing aids may be considered for cochlear implantation. In children, particularly those with congenital deafness, electrical response audiometry is utilised to confirm the presence of a profound hearing loss and to act as a guide as to which ear to implant. According to NICE guidance in the United Kingdom, cochlear implantation is considered for individuals who hear only sounds louder than 90 dB HL at frequencies of 2 and 4 kHz without acoustic hearing aids. Adequate benefit from acoustic hearing aids is defined as a score of 50% or greater on Bamford–Kowal–Bench (BKB) sentence testing at a sound intensity of 70 dB SPL (adults) or speech, language and listening skills appropriate to age, developmental stage and cognitive ability (children).

C

Bilateral simultaneous cochlear implantation is advocated in children or adults who suffer from blindness. For some implant candidates residual low-frequency hearing may be present. Selection of a thinner implant electrodes in combination with meticulous 'soft surgical' technique has been shown to result in so-called 'hearing preservation' post-operatively. This allows both electric and acoustic stimuli to be heard within the same ear.

5. **Vestibular assessment:** Loss of vestibular function may accompany the hearing loss, particularly after meningitis. Central compensation occurs more readily in children than adults and the latter will require a caloric test to establish the presence or absence of labyrinthine function. If implantation is to be undertaken in the ear with better or only vestibular function, then appropriate preoperative counselling needs to be discussed with the patient.

6. **Otological examination:** Active chronic suppurative otitis media remains a contraindication to implantation. Surgery to render the ear disease free must be undertaken as a prelude to insertion of the device. This is usually staged with obliteration and blind-sac closure of an open mastoid cavity if present. At the time of implantation, the tympanomastoid cleft can be evaluated for the presence of any infection or cholesteatoma and surgery can proceed if the ear is disease free.

7. **General medical history:** The principle of assessment of the patient's general health prior to elective surgery under general anaesthesia applies as for any other planned otological surgery. In the presence of cardiovascular or respiratory disease, a decision has to be reached in terms of the risks of surgery against the benefits of implantation.

8. **Radiological assessment:** This is a mandatory part of the evaluation process. Imaging aims to first establish the presence of a normal cochlea (not always the case in congenital deafness) and to establish cochlear patency. In selected cases, both CT and MRI will be required in order to fully assess the feasibility of inserting the electrode array, yet for many patients MRI may be sufficient. In addition, appropriate radiology gives information about the internal auditory meatus (the narrow meatus with normal facial function may only contain a facial nerve) and provides general information about the temporal bone anatomy such as pneumatisation, soft tissue opacification of the tympanomastoid cleft and the anatomy of the jugular bulb. Radiology may also demonstrate the aetiology in idiopathic cases such as the large vestibular aqueduct syndrome or previously undiagnosed cochlear otosclerosis.

CT scanning may fail to demonstrate cochlear fibrosis and therefore in post-meningitic deafness T2-weighted MRI is the investigation of choice. This may also be considered the case in deafness due to otosclerosis, autoimmune hearing loss, and labyrinthitis due to causes other than meningitis. More recently, the senior author has routinely utilised cone beam CT scanning pre- and post-implantation as the radiation dose is substantially less than conventional CT; the resolution and detail is superior and there is substantially less metal artefact from the implanted electrode array.

9. **Psychological profile and expectations:** The expectations of the potential adult recipient need to be realistic; the implant does not restore hearing in the natural sense and the patient needs to understand this. In addition, the individual needs to be motivated for the intensive rehabilitation that will be required to maximise the potential from the device. In children, the expectations and motivation of the immediate family are also of critical importance. In particular, rehabilitation requires numerous visits to the implant centre possibly over several years and the family needs to commit itself and the child to this process.

12.7 Surgery

Surgery is usually undertaken under general anaesthesia after informed consent with particular reference to the facial nerve and chorda tympani. The authors routinely use a facial nerve monitor and parenteral antibiotics are given at the start of surgery with two further doses post-operatively. A modified post-aural incision is used and the musculoperiosteal flap is usually raised separately. A cortical mastoidectomy with undermined margins is undertaken and an area defined to secure the receiver–stimulator package. This may be in the form of a 'periosteal' pocket or drilled bed in the skull. The facial recess is approached via a posterior tympanotomy preserving a bridge of bone between the tympanotomy and the fossa incudis. The tympanotomy should allow visualisation of the incudostapedial joint and the round window niche.

Some surgeons prefer to enter the basal turn via the round window itself or an opening into the scala tympani is made just anteroinferior to the round window niche (cochleostomy). For the cochleostomy, an attempt is made to initially preserve the endosteum of the scala tympani and to open into the basal turn with a needle rather than the drill, thereby reducing the risk of trauma to the spiral lamina and remaining neural elements. The electrode array is then guided into the cochlea. The receiver package is then secured in its bed either with ties or bone cement. The proximal electrode array lies under the undermined margins and may also be secured with ties, clips, or bone cement. A muscle plug is used to seal the cochleotomy and the posterior tympanotomy conferring further stability. The wound is closed in the conventional manner and a mastoid dressing and pressure bandage applied for 24 hours. A plain Stenver's view X-ray or cone beam CT scan is undertaken to confirm the position of the electrode array in the cochlea.

12.8 Rehabilitation

The initial 'switch on' of the device usually occurs after about 4 weeks when all the post-operative scalp swelling has settled and the wound is fully healed. For several weeks after this, an intensive programme of auditory and speech training takes place with fine tuning of the speech processing map for the particular individual. In children, considerable support from their teachers is required with close cooperation between the implant team and the educationalists. The rehabilitation process continues for several months for adults and years for children. The full benefit of the implant is not usually realised for at least 6 months and may take 12 to 18 months when the learning curve flattens and the recipient adjusts to the new auditory stimulus.

12.9 Outcomes

Numerous tests have been developed to evaluate the outcome of implantation in a given individual.

In adults, open-set tests are commonly used. Such tests assess the ability to distinguish speech without any contextual clues or lip reading. The majority of adults report identification of environmental sound and a marked improvement in their lip reading skills. A sizeable proportion is able to track speech without lip reading and a smaller number can, in ideal conditions, converse almost normally or use the telephone, particularly when listening to familiar voices. The outcomes in children are dependent on their language status at the time that the hearing was lost and to a degree on the age at implantation. In one series, almost all the post-lingually deafened children developed open-set listening with good speech intelligibility. Of the pre-lingually deafened children, around one-half developed open-set listening with good or average speech intelligibility. It is not surprising, therefore, to see children implanted at the age of 2 or 3 years entering mainstream education at the age of 5 or 6 years.

12.10 Complications

1. **Surgical complications:** Surgical complications in cochlear implantation are in fact relatively uncommon. This is probably because surgeons undertaking this type of work already have a considerable otological experience and international implant workshops are readily available for those embarking on this type of surgery. Injury to the facial nerve is rare while chorda tympani trauma is probably under-reported. Damage to the electrode array and electrode misplacement have been reported in most large series. One of the most serious complications is ischaemia or sepsis in the scalp flap with loss of flap viability around the receiver package. This situation is difficult to salvage and may result in device extrusion and subsequent need to remove the device. With experience and meticulous attention to incision placement and soft-tissue handling, major scalp complications can be avoided.

2. **Device complications:** Device malfunction is categorised as a *soft failure* if there is deviation from the specification without total loss of function (such as an electrode fault that can be programmed out) or as a *hard failure* if the implant ceases to function, necessitating reimplantation. Such events have been reported by all the implant manufacturers and tend to occur early in the life of the device. With continuing research and development, device failure has

become less common and by way of example, the cumulative survival for devices from one of the manufacturers is greater than 98% after 5 years.

3. **Non-auditory stimulation:** Undesirable effects of electrical stimulation of the inner ear include pain in the ear, scalp or throat, intrusive tinnitus and facial nerve stimulation. All are uncommon and the offending electrode or electrodes can usually be programmed out. Facial nerve stimulation is a particular feature in those individuals deafened by otosclerosis or temporal bone fractures and it is postulated that the fracture line or otospongiotic focus allows current escape and stimulation of the intralabyrinthine segment of the facial nerve.

12.11 Future Developments

Cochlear implantation is a fertile area for research and development both by implant teams and the manufacturers. Current clinic studies include bilateral implantation, implantation in marginal hearing aid users, cochlear implantation in patients with bilateral vestibular schwannomas and evaluation of music perception. Hardware developments include modiolus hugging electrode arrays, magnetless coupling mechanisms and refinements in speech processing strategies. The ultimate goal is the totally implantable device.

Further Reading

Santa Maria PL, Gluth MB, Yuan Y, Atlas MD, Blevins NH. Hearing preservation surgery for cochlear implantation: a meta-analysis. Otol Neurotol. 2014;35(10):e256-269

Gibson WPR. Cochlear implants. In: Booth JB, ed. Scott-Brown's Otolaryngology. Oxford: Butterworth Heinemann; 1997:1–25

Related Topics of Interest

Pure-tone audiometry
Speech audiometry
Hearing loss-acquired
Paediatric hearing assessment
Hearing aids

13　Congenital Hearing Disorders

Congenital hearing impairment (CHI) is defined as a hearing impairment which is present at birth, usually manifest at birth but may manifest later. There are many disorders accounting for such hearing impairment. They may be conductive, sensorineural or mixed. It is important to diagnose congenital hearing losses as soon as possible as early intervention and rehabilitation may lead to a more successful outcome in terms of the child's communication, speech and language and, indeed, overall development.

13.1　Epidemiology

Permanent congenital hearing impairment (PCHI) on both ears has an incidence of 1.06 per 1,000. It must be borne in mind that the screening process identifies children who are having a measurable hearing loss only. It does not pick up the PCHI group where the hearing loss is congenital but late onset or progressive. In other words, in these children, the aetiology is present at birth but manifests late.

Of the PCHI group, 50% are genetic, 25% nongenetic and 25% idiopathic. Of the genetic subgroup, the majority 70% are non-syndromic; and of these, the majority (75–85%) are autosomal recessive. The commonest (50% of cases) is DFNB1 Connexin 26/30 mutation (▶ Fig. 13.1).

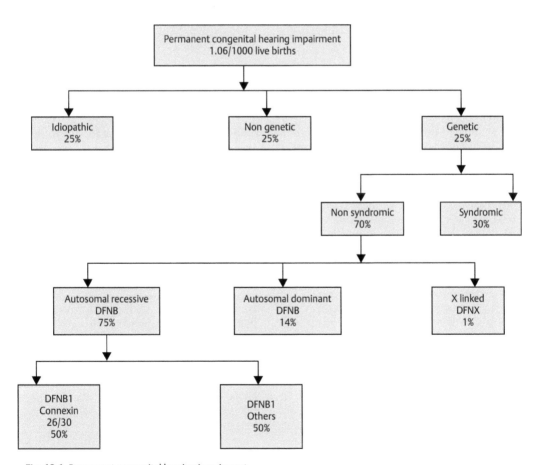

Fig. 13.1 Permanent congenital hearing impairment.

13.2 Pathophysiology of Congenital Hearing Impairment

In order to understand the pathophysiology of CHI, it is important to appreciate peripheral ear physiology. While problems in the structure of the ear all the way from the pinna to the auditory nerve easily explain the hearing loss due to a breach in the onwards transmission and transduction of the acoustic signal, there are numerous proteins and enzymes vital for normal cochlear and nerve function. Mutations which can either be sporadic and de novo or inherited lead to dysfunction.

13.3 Aetiology of Congenital Hearing Impairment

So far, as many as 427 clinical syndromes and 170 chromosomal anomalies have been identified with CHI. Many syndromes can now be mapped to a specific chromosome. Some syndromes are non-genetic or not hereditary.

13.4 Non-Syndromic Genetic Hearing Impairment

Non-syndromic hearing losses are characterised by involvement of the hearing mechanism only, typically sparing other organs. They can be pre- or post-lingual, predominantly sensorineural losses. Dominant inheritance usually results in the latter while the recessive pattern usually results in the former. X-linked inheritance may result in both or a mixed loss.

In addition, there is a group of genetic hearing losses which are a result of mutations in the mitochondria.

The autosomal dominant pattern dubbed DFNA is characterised by marked heterogeneity and often cannot be mapped to a single locus which generates markedly variable hearing losses which can affect certain frequencies only and are late onset and post-lingual; however, DFNA 3, 6, 8, 12 and 19 are pre-lingual. The intensity is usually mild-to-moderate hearing impairment. About 70 loci have been identified and mapped. A cookie bite audiogram may be observed in 30% cases and conductive and unilateral hearing losses have been reported.

The autosomal recessive pattern, on the other hand, is characterised by less heterogeneity and can be mapped to a single locus. Hearing loss may be predictable and is pre-lingual except in the case of DFNB8 which is post-lingual. These mutations are designated as DFNB. They may present with profound sensorineural hearing loss. The commonest gene mutation is Connexin 26/30 which encodes for gap junction proteins GJB2 and GJB6 in the stria vascularis and supporting cells. It is the commonest genetic cause for hearing loss which affects maintenance of the endocochlear potential and structural integrity of the outer hair cell (OHC).

The X-linked inheritance includes DFNX 1, 2, 3, 4 and 6 which are usually post-lingual except DFNX2 and X3 which lead to the X-linked gusher syndrome characterised by a mixed loss. It is a rare but important cause of pre-lingual deafness in children.

The mitochondrial mutations are usually maternally inherited and are responsible for non–dose-dependent aminoglycoside ototoxicity in A1555 del AG.

13.5 Syndromic Genetic Hearing Impairment

In this group of hearing loss, other organs in the body are often affected along with the hearing apparatus; the constellation of extra-auditory and auditory features together make up a syndrome. These are usually genetic and some of them can be mapped to chromosomes, for example, the branchiootorenal syndrome can be mapped to 8q and Pendred's syndrome to 7q. The hearing losses encountered range from purely conductive to sensorineural. Most syndromes present with an associated learning disability. The genetic syndromes with an associated craniofacial deformity can cause prolonged otitis media with effusion (OME) due to eustachian tube dysfunction.

The autosomal dominant craniosynostosis syndromes include Apert's, Crouzon's, Pfeiffer's, and Saethre–Chotzen, with an incidence of 1 in 60,000. They present with abnormalities in the craniofacial skeleton, digital defects, varying degrees of auricular dysplasias and mainly conductive hearing losses with ossicular deformities.

Other autosomal dominant syndromes are the Waardenburg syndrome with heterochromia and white forelock, Goldenhar's syndrome with unilateral maxillary hypoplasia, the branchiooto-renal syndrome affecting the neck, the ear and the renal systems, the Stickler syndrome and the Treacher Collins syndrome with varying degrees of craniofacial dysplasias. The hearing loss types vary due to middle and inner ear problems.

Autosomal recessive syndromes with sensori-neural hearing loss include Usher's syndrome with retinitis pigmentosa, Pendred's syndrome with goitre and enlarged vestibular aqueducts, Refsum's disease with phytanic acid accumulation due to peroxisome deficiency; Cockayne syndrome with neurodegenerative problems due to cortical white matter changes, Alstrom's syndrome with central obesity, retinal dystrophy, and endocrine defi-ciencies and the Jervell and Lange–Nielsen (JLN) syndrome with cardiac conduction abnormalities. Note that some of these syndromes may not pres-ent with an obvious skeletal deformity.

The X-linked genetic syndromes are Alport's with glomerulonephritis, Mohr–Tranebjaerg's with dystonia, the fragile X syndrome with devel-opmental delay and cognitive immaturity and Norrie's syndrome with phthisis bulbi and late-onset progressive sensorineural hearing loss.

Mitochondrial mutations lead to syndromes like mitochondrial encephalopathy, lactic acidosis and stroke (MELAS) and maternally inherited diabetes and deafness (MIDD), which present with hearing loss. Genetic metabolic conditions like hypothyroid-ism and mucopolysaccharidosis can result in a PCHI.

There are some sporadic genetic syndromes which can cause a PCHI of the conductive or the sensorineural type. These include coloboma iris, heart defects, choanal atresia, retardation of growth, gonadal problems and ear abnormalities (CHARGE), Klippel–Feil with vertebral and scapular dystrophy, the lentigines, electrocardiography (ECG) defects, ocular hypertelorism, pulmonary stenosis, abnormalities of the genitals, retardation and deafness (LEOPARD) syndrome and the osteogenesis imperfecta group with stapedial fixation and blue sclera.

Chromosomal addition/deletion syndromes causing PCHI leading to mixed hearing losses can be observed in trisomy 21, 18, and 13, Turner's XO and Noonan's and Di George's 22q 11 deletion. Theoretically, many combinations of chromosomal mutations can produce a PCHI and the possibilities are vast.

13.6 Structural Defects in the Auditory System

A syndrome, genetic or otherwise, may result in a dysplastic auditory system. Therefore, varying degrees of pinna and external auditory canal apla-sias/dysplasias can lead to PCHI. These external ear deformities often mirror middle ear integrity and, in addition, ossicular dysplasias from fixation to discontinuity may result.

Cochlear dysplasias are theoretically numerous. There may be isolated abnormalities of the bony cochlea or the membranous cochlea or both, and in varying degrees. Commonly encountered in clin-ical practice are the Mondini dysplasia with less than two turns in the cochlea, Bing–Siebenmann dysplasia with abnormal membranous labyrinth and the cochleosaccular dysplasias (Scheibe's dysplasia). An extreme variety is the Michel deformity with complete agenesis of the labyrinth.

Vestibulocochlear nerve dysplasias present with PCHI and importantly are often associated with vestibular dysplasias.

Enlarged vestibular aqueduct is a relatively common labyrinthine dysplasia. The child presents with varying degrees of hearing losses including mixed losses due to a third window effect and may be associated with a goitre in 30%: Pendred's syndrome. The condition needs to be diagnosed quickly as the parents must be told as early as possible as minor head trauma may lead to a worsening of the hearing loss.

13.7 Non-Genetic Syndromic/ Non-Syndromic Permanent Congenital Hearing Impairment

Any assault in utero may generate a PCHI. The first trimester is crucial. Maternal infections, for example, chicken pox, herpes, human immunodefi-ciency virus (HIV), cytomegalovirus (CMV), rubella and *Streptococcus* are damaging to the ear, as are substance misuse or drugs (including therapeutic drugs, e.g., phenytoin) especially alcohol-causing fetal alcohol syndrome. These manifest as varying degrees of hearing loss from mild to severe which can be conductive, sensorineural or mixed.

Near-term and perinatal pathologies like prematurity, hypoxia, hyperbilirubinemia can also generate PCHI as well as birth trauma. Some of these present with skeletal and other abnormalities due to the assault of the offending agent on the child's development.

CMV deserves special mention as it is the commonest infection responsible for PCHI.

13.8 Auditory Neuropathy Spectrum Disorder

Auditory neuropathy spectrum disorder (ANSD) is a condition characterised by abnormal auditory brainstem responses in the presence of normal cochlear function as measured by emissions and cochlear microphonic testing. It can be genetic with a mutation in otoferlin and inherited in dominant fashion. Risk factors include prematurity, hypoxia and hyperbilirubinemia. Behavioural thresholds may be normal although it can be picked up by screening. The children develop processing problems which in turn generate speech, language and communication difficulties.

13.9 Idiopathic Permanent Congenital Hearing Impairment

This is a PCHI where no cause, despite extensive investigations, is found. They present a management challenge as the natural history of the condition is not known nor if it could be inherited. About 25% of PCHI is idiopathic. Regular monitoring for optimal and timely intervention and prognosticating vulnerability of the cochlea by sophisticated otoacoustic emission studies may need to be performed.

13.10 Unilateral and Mild Hearing Losses

These losses may still generate significant central processing problems and a reduction in the listening abilities of the children. Some of the syndromes described above can lead to a unilateral hearing loss (e.g., CMV, Goldenhar's, Waardenburg's) and the autosomal dominant, non-syndromic group, due to their heterogeneity, can cause a mild hearing loss.

13.11 The Vestibular System in Permanent Congenital Hearing Impairment

At least a third of PCHI will present with vestibular weaknesses that lead to delayed motor development, hypotonia and overreliance on visual sensors. Some non-syndromic losses and many syndromic losses have concomitant vestibular hypofunction, for example, CHARGE, JLN and Usher's syndrome. While managing a child with PCHI, the vestibular system should also be assessed.

13.12 Diagnosis and Management of Congenital Hearing Impairment

The first step of managing PCHI is diagnosing the hearing loss by age-appropriate hearing test (see Chapter 74, Paediatric Hearing Assessment), followed by prescription fitting of hearing aids. If the loss is profound, cochlear implantation may be initiated after a trial with hearing aids.

Simultaneously, a thorough etiological work-up is crucial for prognosis and further management. This entails a full history and clinical examination which may lead to a syndrome diagnosis. Imaging to visualise structural integrity of the peripheral audiological system, CMV tests and Connexin 26/30 tests along with a detailed ophthalmological assessment are some of the first-line investigations necessary, with a reasonable diagnostic yield. The vestibular system needs to be included in the examination which may narrow down the aetiology further.

At around 8 months postpartum, behavioural, age-appropriate audiometry is required to fine tune management and regular monitoring instituted thereafter. Vestibular rehabilitation is occasionally required. A multidisciplinary team, with representatives from paediatrics, genetics, sensory services, speech and language therapy, and in older children, occasionally, mental health services in addition to the audiovestibular physician and the otologist, should look after the child. It cannot be emphasised enough that managing a PCHI has to be holistic with many specialists working together to achieve the very best outcomes.

Further Reading

Nishio SY, Hattori M, Moteki H, et al. Gene expression profiles of the cochlea and vestibular end organs: localization and function of genes causing deafness. Ann Otol Rhinol Laryngol. 2015; 124(Suppl 1):6S–48S

Toriello HV, Smith SD. Hereditary Hearing Loss and its Syndromes. 3rd ed. Oxford University Press; 2013

Related Topics of Interest

Paediatric hearing assessment
Perilymph and labyrinthine fistula
Vestibular function tests
Evoked response audiometry
Otoacoustic emissions

C

14 Consent and Capacity

14.1 Consent

Before embarking on the management of a competent patient, it is a legal and ethical requirement that the doctor must gain the patient's informed consent. No matter how well meaning, any doctor who touches a competent patient without adequately informed consent may be found guilty of an offence, the so-called tort of negligence. Respect for the principle of autonomy and self-determination underlies the process of consent and so the reductive act of simply getting the patient to 'sign the consent form' is not sufficient. Rather, gaining consent is a process that begins at the first meeting of doctor and patient and should encourage the two-way exchange of information until a suitable management plan is agreed.

To be legally valid, consent must be informed. This means that the patients must understand their options, including the option for no treatment. They must be apprised of the intended benefits and inherent risks of any proposed course of action. It is the doctor's duty to ensure that the patient understands the relevant information and this means that its delivery will need to be tailored according to each individual patient.

Consent need not always be written; verbal or implied consent are both valid. For example, if a person verbally agrees to nasendoscopy and sits still for the procedure, the doctor may continue in good faith. However, although *written* consent is not a legal requirement for all medical interventions, it does provide supporting evidence of the discussion and decision-making process.

The General Medical Council (GMC) advises that *written* consent should be taken in case of the following:

1. The investigation or treatment is complex or involves significant risks.
2. There may be significant consequences for the patient's employment, or social or personal life.
3. Providing clinical care is not the primary purpose of the investigation or treatment.
4. The treatment is part of a research programme or is an innovative treatment designed specifically for the patient's benefit.

14.2 Capacity

A patient must have capacity to give valid consent. Unfortunately, there is no standardised test to ascertain capacity and its assessment is largely subjective. The assessment process described in *Re C* is widely accepted and so a patient is deemed to have capacity if he or she can:

1. Understand and retain the treatment information (they only need to be able to retain this information for long enough to use it to make a decision).
2. Believe that the information provided is true.
3. Weigh the information in the balance and use it to make a decision.
4. Communicate this decision.

Capacity is not an, 'all-or-nothing' state and so a patient's ability to make a choice may depend on how complex the factors involved in the decision are. Simple choices with minimal consequences may be reached by those who have limited ability for complex analysis, while increasingly complicated decisions associated with greater risks demand ever-increasing degrees of capacity. A person who has capacity has the right of absolute autonomy over his or her body and may refuse investigation or treatment even if this might seem illogical or result in dire consequences.

Assessing a patient's capacity can be a daunting task as the implications can be significant. A useful tool to help with this task is the Mental Capacity Act (MCA) and MHA Decision Pathways smartphone app produced by the ethics committee at Imperial College Healthcare NHS Trust. The app is free to download and leads the clinician, stepwise, through the process of assessment.

14.3 Patients Who Lack Capacity

14.3.1 Minors

For patients under 16 years of age, consent to treatment must be given on their behalf by the adult with parental responsibility. However, a minor may be deemed to have capacity if he or she is able to comply with the four-step process described above. Children who meet this standard are often referred to as being 'Gillick competent'. This term originates from the case of *Gillick v West Norfolk and Wisbech* in which Lord Scarman's reasoning formed the basis of the test of capacity in children:

'As a matter of Law the parental right to determine whether or not their minor child below the age of sixteen will have medical treatment terminates if and when the child achieves sufficient understanding and intelligence to understand fully what is proposed.'

Despite this clear legal principle, it is prudent to gain consent for treatment from the responsible adult, in addition to that of a 'Gillick competent' child.

Notwithstanding the legal and ethical theorising, children who have tried to refuse lifesaving treatment have, without exception, been deemed to lack the necessary capacity to make this decision by the courts, even when the child's argument against treatment appears compelling, rational and considered. In reality, it seems children may give their consent to treatment, but may not refuse lifesaving treatment thought to be in their best interests.

14.4 Adults without Capacity

Decision making on behalf of adults who lack capacity is governed by The Mental Capacity Act (MCA) 2005. Amongst other things, this legislation specifies the following:

1. Capacity must be assumed in those of 16 years or older, until proven otherwise.
2. Everything possible must be done to maximise the patient's capacity and enable him or her to make an informed decision; for example, the information presented should be tailored to his or her level of understanding.
3. If the individual lacks capacity, decisions must be made on his or her behalf by the medical team responsible for his or her care. These decisions must be in his or her best interests. The Act specifies that 'best interests' decisions should not be restricted to medical matters but should also consider all other welfare issues.
4. Before losing capacity, a patient may appoint a trusted person with his or her lasting power of attorney. This attorney has the power to make decisions in the patient's best interests including those concerning finance and health. The attorney is not allowed to refuse life-sustaining treatment unless given specific instructions to do so, in writing, by the patient. These powers

come into effect when the patient loses capacity and are rescinded should his or her capacity return.

5. Advance decisions have been granted to legal authority so long as they are executed correctly. They may dictate which treatments are acceptable in various situations but cannot insist on treatment being given in all circumstances.

14.5 Best Interests

It is worth emphasising that when a medical professional decides on behalf of an incapacitated patient, he or she must not restrict his or her deliberations only to medical best interests but must consider, 'medical, emotional and all other welfare issues'. In addition, the law is clear that when making these decisions a doctor should not restrict himself or herself to making a 'substituted judgement', that is, simply guessing what the patient would have decided for himself or herself. Rather, the opinions and wishes of the patient should be 'added to the balance sheet of factors' used to make the decision but should not necessarily constitute the final decision. The concept of best interests' decision making has been criticised by some who say the task is impossible.

14.6 Consent and Jehovah's Witnesses

Jehovah's Witnesses (JW) are Christians whose origins date back to the late 1800s. They are of particular interest to the medical profession because they believe that certain verses in the scriptures forbid them to receive blood products (Genesis 9:3–4, Leviticus 17:11–12, and Acts 15:28–29).

As stated above, a competent adult has the absolute right to refuse medical treatment even if this decision appears irrational or even dangerous. Hence, an adult JW, or anyone else for that matter, has the right to refuse the transfusion of blood products even if this might result in their death.

When taking consent from a JW prior to surgery, it is essential that the doctor discusses and documents the risks of surgery honestly and candidly, with particular respect to blood loss. JWs are usually very well informed and the surgeon must clarify and document which products and measures (e.g., cell salvage), if any, are acceptable to the patient as this may vary between individuals. This list should be clearly documented and countersigned and dated by the patient. Many trusts have a specific consent form for JWs.

14.7 Children of Jehovah's Witnesses

Parents who follow the JW religion may not prevent their children receiving blood products if they are deemed to be in the child's best interests. Obviously, the decision to transfuse must not be taken lightly and in a non–life-threatening situation advice should be taken from trust solicitors if disagreement arises. The trust will apply for a 'Special Issue Order' from the High Court to allow the treatment to go ahead. In a life-threatening situation, the child must be transfused even in the face of parental refusal.

Doctors have the right to refuse to treat JWs electively if they feel unable to comply with the patient's refusal of blood products, but must refer the patient to a colleague who is happy to manage them. In an emergency, however, a doctor must treat the patient with every means possible, short of transfusion. A doctor who transfuses a patient against his or her wishes may later be found guilty of battery and assault.

14.8 Standards of Disclosure

A doctor who treats a patient without valid consent may be found guilty of negligence (see later), but how much information should be disclosed to allow a patient to make an informed choice?

In May 2015, the case of *Montgomery* was heard before the U.K. Supreme Court. The judgement in *Montgomery* brings the law into line with the standards laid out by the GMC in their guidance on Consent. The judges agreed that a patient should be warned of any 'material risk' inherent in the procedure and went on to expand:

'The test of materiality is whether a reasonable person in the patient's position would be likely to attach significance to the risk, or the doctor should reasonably be aware that the particular patient would be likely to attach significance to it'.

They also stated unambiguously:

'The assessment of risk cannot be reduced to percentages'.

This sets a very high bar and means that the doctor must take time to learn about his or her patients' lifestyle, values and concerns so that they understand which risks will be material to each patient and can tailor the provision of information accordingly.

The judges in Montgomery also stated explicitly the following:

- Doctors must not *'bombard patients with information'* for fear of omitting a pertinent risk, as this serves to promote confusion and not autonomy.
- Doctors must discuss all treatment options with the patient, including the option of no treatment.
- Doctors may recommend a particular treatment but may not pressurise the patient into accepting their advice.

They also confirmed that there are three exceptional situations in which nondisclosure is acceptable:

- When the patient expresses a fixed desire not to know the risks.
- When discussing risks posing a serious threat to the patient's health. This threat must be beyond merely causing distress.
- In 'circumstances of necessity' where urgent treatment is needed but the patient lacks capacity to give consent.

14.9 The Statutory Duty of Candour

Doctors have always had a professional duty to inform and apologise to patients when mistakes have been made, but in November 2014, the Statutory Duty of Candour was imposed. This legislation makes it a legal duty to inform a patient (or his or her representative) whenever a patient safety incident occurs which results in death or severe, moderate harm or prolonged psychological harm. As is so often the case, no definition of what constitutes these harms has been offered and it is not yet clear when the duty must be invoked.

The statutory duty applies to organisations, not to individuals, but the Care Quality Commission (CQC) makes it clear that staff must cooperate and ensure that this duty is met. Doctors, who are responsible for the patients' care and used to having candid discussions with patients are most likely to be expected to lead these discussions on behalf of the organisation.

Only time will tell how this new legislation will be enacted and how Trusts will interpret and administer it.

Further Reading

General Medical Council. Good Medical Practice: Consent guidance expressions of consent. http://www.gmc-uk.org/guidance/ethical_guidance/consent_guidance_expressions_of_consent.asp. Accessed June 19, 2018

Re C (Adult: refusal of medical treatment) [1994] 1 WLR 290

Gillick v West Norfolk and Wisbech Area Health Authority [1985] 3 All ER 402. (1)

Re M (Child: refusal of medical treatment) [1999] 2 FLR 1097

Re W (a minor: medical treatment) [1993] Fam 64

Re A (Medical Treatment: male sterilization) [2000] 1 FCR 193

Re G (TJ) [2010] EWHC 3005 (COP)

Montgomery v Lanarkshire Health Board [2015] UKSC 11, [2015] All ER(D) 113 (Mar)

Bolam v Friern Hospital Management Committee (1957) 2 All ER 118

Bolitho v City Hackney Health Authority (1998) AC 232

Related Topic of Interest

Medicolegal aspects of ENT

15 Cosmetic Surgery

Perception of cosmetic medical and surgical interventions has evolved significantly over time. In 1935, Gillies stated, 'The operations for removal of eyelid wrinkles, cheek folds and fat in the neck are justifiable if the patients are chosen with honest discrimination'. Now aesthetic medical and surgical interventions are considered as norm. This chapter seeks to cover medical options including neuromodulators and injectable fillers and surgical options for facial rejuvenation: brow/forehead lift, blepharoplasty, rhytidectomy (face and neck lift) and otoplasty. The list is by no means exhaustive, as other available tools in the aesthetic surgeon's armamentarium (▶Table 15.1) such as dermabrasion, chemical peels and laser treatments for facial rejuvenation are beyond the scope of this chapter.

15.1 Biology of Ageing

Facial ageing is a three-dimensional process that results in devolumisation and descent, which are affected by intrinsic and extrinsic factors. Intrinsic ageing includes atrophy of facial skin and subcutaneous fat, and volume changes in the facial skeleton. The skin loses elasticity and capacity to retain moisture resulting in dryness and sagging. Laxity of retaining ligaments of the face results in descent. Remodelling of the craniofacial skeleton leads to changes in facial dimensions and relative proportions. There is rotation and reduction in height of the maxilla, along with contraction of the bony skeleton. The orbital width on the other hand increases. The combination of above factors ultimately accounts for jowl formation, sagging and rhytids. The primary extrinsic factor for ageing is sun exposure resulting in photoageing, and smoking accelerates this process.

15.2 Non-Surgical Treatment

15.2.1 Botulinum Toxins

Botulinum toxin exists as many preparations, including Botox (Allergan), Xeomin (incobotulinumtoxinA: Merz pharmaceuticals) and Dysport (abobotulinumtoxinA; Azzalure). It is a protein produced by the anaerobic gram-positive bacterium, *Clostridium botulinum*. Botox type A is the most clinically relevant of the seven serotypes (A–G). It works by causing flaccid paralysis of the muscle by inhibiting acetylcholine release at the neuromuscular junction. The weakened and relaxed muscle reduces the amount of unwanted lines of facial expression. Botox is used in various regions of the head and neck for aesthetic and functional reasons (▶Fig. 15.1).

15.2.2 Fillers

Fillers are 'products used to improve appearance and don't impart any health benefits' as defined by the Food and Drug Administration (FDA). They are considered as medical devices and may be referred to by trade names. They may be temporary, for example, hyaluronic acid, semi-permanent, for example, Sculptra (poly-L-lactic acid) or permanent, for example, polymethyl methacrylate. The use of permanent fillers is discouraged due to the adverse results that often require surgical intervention for removal, while hyaluronic acid fillers

▶ **Table 15.1** Guidelines and strategies for facial rejuvenation (combination of treatments should be considered to optimise results)

Patient concerns	Structural change	Treatment option
Superficial wrinkles, skin colour changes, telangiectasia, etc.	Mainly superficial dermal	Laser, IPL, chemical peels, medicated skin care programmes
Mimetic wrinkles with or without volume loss	Deep dermal, subcutaneous	Botulinum toxins, fillers, free fat transfers, direct muscle excision, etc.
Folds (nasojugal, nasolabial, jowls, neck)	Skin laxity, ligamentous laxity, soft tissue atrophy with volume loss, gravity, etc.	Surgery—face lift, neck lift, brow and forehead lift, blepharoplasty, etc.—based on location
Folds, volume loss—malar, chin, etc.	Skeletal loss	Implants, bone grafts, etc.

Abbreviation: IPL, intense pulsed light.

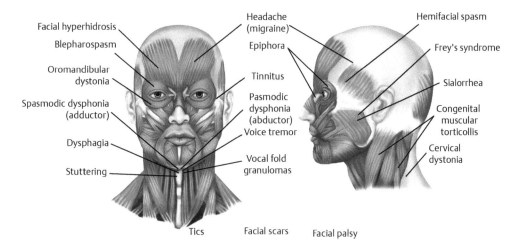

Fig. 15.1 Botox indications.

may be removed with hyaluronidase. Viscosity of products varies with higher viscosity products being used for volumisation versus fine wrinkle treatment with low-viscosity products.

15.2.3 Complications

Botulinum toxin has limited adverse effects that may include swelling, bruising, asymmetric muscle paralysis and headaches. Filler complications include swelling, bruising, infection, 'Tyndall effect' (superficial injection resulting in a blue hue) lumpiness and nodules. The most feared complications are skin necrosis and blindness as a result of embolisation following inadvertent intra-vascular injection in the melolabial and peri-ocular or glabella regions, respectively.

15.3 Forehead and Brow Lift

The aim is to elevate the hairy brow to the bony supra-orbital rim, reduce width of the forehead if required, and reduce the upper eyelid skin excess. It should be considered before upper lid blepharoplasty surgery.

15.3.1 Anatomy

The layers may be remembered by the mnemonic **SCALP**: **S**kin, sub**C**utaneous tissue, galea **A**poneurosis, **L**oose areolar tissue and **P**ericranium. The frontalis is contained within the galea. The

periosteum is continuous with the temporalis fascia at the temporal line and leads to a fascial condensation at superior orbital rim with the orbital septum known as the arcus marginalis.

15.3.2 Surgical Techniques

Various approaches are available for forehead and brow lifts.

- Endoscopic brow lift utilises small incisions within the hair-bearing area using standard 0-degree endoscopes and stack system. The procedure carries the risk of frontal neurovascular bundle injury. This approach should be used judiciously in high hairlines and male pattern baldness.
- In coronal lifts, the incision is made above the hairline with a dissection plane between the perichondrium and galea. It should not be used in high hairline or male pattern baldness patients. This technique is not effective for correction of brow asymmetry and there is a risk of raising the hairline.
- A pretrichial lift at the hairline can be utilised with a high hairline but can result in anaesthesia posterior to the incision.
- The midforehead lift may be utilised effectively in patients with high hairlines and prominent forehead rhytids, particularly men. Sensation may be preserved with subcutaneous dissection. It may leave a prominent scar and does not address the lateral brow or upper forehead.

C

- The direct brow lift is particularly useful for unilateral brow ptosis. The scar is minimised by bevelling the blade parallel with the hair follicles and judicious use of diathermy as in any other hair-bearing area incision to minimise alopecia.
- A transblepharoplasty brow lift may be undertaken via an upper blepharoplasty incision, concealed within the skin crease. Risks include inadvertent injury to the supraorbital nerve causing numbness.

15.4 Blepharoplasty

15.4.1 Anatomy

The orbital septum is a fibrous condensation deep to orbicularis oculi which is continuous with the periosteum and lower lid capsulopalpebral fascia and separates the orbit into anterior and posterior compartments. Whitnall's ligament is a dense fibrous connective tissue that serves as a fulcrum for the levator muscle. The upper lid has two fat pads, central and a paler nasal pad with a lateral lacrimal gland while the lower lid has three fat pads. The inferior oblique courses between the medial and central compartments. Care should be taken to avoid injury to this muscle during fat pad removal to avoid diplopia. Outside the orbit exist further fat compartments. The retro-orbicularis oculi fat (ROOF) lies within the preseptal fat compartment beneath the brow. The suborbital orbicularis oculi fat (SOOF) is a continuation of the malar fat pad and lies immediately inferior to the orbital rim. A significant nasojugal groove indicates atrophy or SOOF fat prolapse in which case fat transposition is required.

15.4.2 Indications

- Dermatochalasis: It is an acquired skin excess, frequently from actinic damage that thins eyelid skin resulting in orbital fat prolapse and ptosis.
- Blepharochalasis: It is characterised by lid oedema resulting in tissue breakdown and orbital fat prolapse.
- Pseudoherniation: Pseudoherniation of orbital fat through a weak orbital septum or orbicularis hypertrophy may result in bagginess.
- Blepharoptosis: It is a result of levator muscle malfunction causing a droopy eyelid.

15.4.3 Pre-Operative Evaluation

History: Any history of thyroid disorders, allergic dermatitis, bleeding disorders, and ophthalmic disorders, for example, dry eyes should be carefully noted. Previous facial cosmetic surgery should also be noted. Motivation factors for surgery and preoperative photos should be undertaken.

Examination: Ophthalmic examination should identify any pre-operative visual or globe abnormalities including assessing Bell's phenomenon with forced lid opening to observe upward rotation of the globe. Schirmer's test may be used to exclude a dry eye. The brow position should be assessed to see if the patient would benefit from a brow lift prior to blepharoplasty. Evaluation of skin type and redundancy, muscle hypertrophy and lacrimal gland ptosis should be undertaken. The degree of ptosis is determined by measuring the margin reflex distance (MRD-1 and MRD-2). Levator function may be assessed by measuring the upper lid margin from upward to downward gaze which should be at least 12 mm. Any lagophthalmos or lateral hooding should be noted.

The inferior orbital sulcus should be less than 5 to 6 mm from the inferior lid margin. Evaluate fat herniation by asking the patient to look superiorly. Palpate the inferior orbital rim. Lid distraction tests lower lid laxity to see if tightening is required. If the lower lid is displaced anteriorly by more than 10 mm or settles slowly, then the patient is likely to have ectropion or scleral show and would benefit from lid tightening. Lid retraction is undertaken by displacing the lower lid inferiorly to see if the puncta moves by more than 3 mm indicating a lax canthal tendon, which may be addressed with a canthopexy.

15.4.4 Surgical Techniques

- **Upper eyelid blepharoplasty:** The upper lid is addressed after the brow and before the lower lid. Mark the estimated upper lid skin to be removed. Leave at least 20 mm of skin. Pinch the excess skin with forceps with the patient in an upright position. This should move the eyelashes without the lid margin. Avoid extending the incision beyond the medial canthus to prevent a webbed scar. Intra-operatively, the lid should leave 1 to 2 mm lagophthalmos. Lateral hooding can be addressed by extending the incision lateral to the orbital rim, which may be extended more superiorly in women. A strip of orbicularis oculi may be removed with the heavy lid for better definition. The orbital septum is opened to access the pseudoherniated fat, which is clamped and excised. Lacrimal gland ptosis may be treated by plication to the periosteum.

- **Lower eyelid blepharoplasty:** The two approaches are subciliary and transconjunctival. The former approach is most common, which allows for easier independent modification of skin and muscle. It leaves an external scar with the risk of vertical eyelid retraction. The transconjunctival approach has no visible scar and avoids lid retraction. It may be used effectively in patients with excessive fat herniation with little skin redundancy.

Post-operative care involves cold compresses, head elevation and rest from strenuous physical activity. Complications include mila, subconjunctival ecchymosis, haematoma, lagophthalmos, ectropion, scleral show, ptosis, pseudo epicanthal folds, epiphora, dry eyes, diplopia, chemosis, persistent fat pocket and most significantly blindness. This latter complication is very rare, and is associated with retrobulbar haematoma, which is more likely after lower lid blepharoplasty. Treatment involves urgent lateral canthotomy.

15.5 Rhytidectomy

The aim of the procedure is to rejuvenate the face for a more youthful look. The areas addressed mainly include jowls and midface (hollowed cheeks).

15.5.1 Anatomy

Beneath the skin and subcutaneous tissue lies the superficial muscular aponeurotic system (SMAS), which was first described by Mitz and Peyronie in 1976. The SMAS is continuous with the platysma, superficial temporal fascia and numerous mimetic muscles of the face. It is adherent to the parotidomasseteric fascia and lies superficial to the parotid fascia, facial nerve and facial artery.

The temporal and marginal mandibular branches are most at risk during surgery. The temporal branch may be located using Pitanguy's line running from 0.5 cm below the tragus to 1.5 cm above the lateral eyebrow. At a point midway between the two latter

landmarks, over the zygomatic arch, the nerve penetrates the deep temporal fascia into the superficial temporal fascia. It is at this point that the nerve is most at risk of injury. The marginal mandibular branch is 1 cm below the angle of the mandible after exiting the parotid. It lies deep to the platysma within the submandibular fascia and superficial to the facial vein. The main sensory nerve that is encountered is the great auricular nerve at the anterior edge of sternomastoid, which is superficial as the skin is adherent to the sternocleidomastoid fascia with diminishing platysma in this region.

The ligaments attach the skin to the skeleton and fascia. The zygomatic ligament attaches the zygomaticomaxillary suture to the overlying skin and the mandibular ligament attaches the anterior mandible to the parasymphyseal skin. The parotid ligament attaches to overlying skin while the masseter ligament supports the medial cheek over the body of the mandible. It is weakness of this latter ligament that contributes to jowl formation.

15.5.2 Pre-Operative Evaluation

History: The routine pre-operative history should identify contraindications to surgery such as connective tissue disorders, uncontrolled diabetes, any condition that increases bleeding risk directly or via required anticoagulation and psychosocial disorders. Careful note should be made of smoking and weight loss, as a pre-operative stable weight is preferable.

Examination: Ideal candidates for surgery are aged 40 to 60, with a good bony framework, strong cheek bones and chin, normal hyoid position and without excessive subcutaneous fat. Evaluate the midface, as a fuller midface without a deep melolabial fold is more favourable. The jaw and neck will complete the examination to look for jowl formation and loss of cervicomental angle or low submandibular gland position. The latter may become more prominent following rhytidectomy and some surgeons will elect to reduce the submandibular glands as a result. Screen for any pre-malignant skin conditions and take pre-operative photos.

15.5.3 Surgical Techniques

The incision extends from the temporal region down to the pre-auricular region and may be

C

behind the tragus in females but should be anterior in males to avoid changing the facial hair line. It then extends postauricular and over the mastoid back into the hairline. When below the hairline, care should be taken to remain below the follicles to prevent alopecia. However, a more superficial dissection may be required over the great auricular nerve. If inadvertently transected, recognition should prompt intra-operative reanastomosis to preserve long-term sensory function and prevent neuroma formation. A separate incision may be made in the submental region to undertake neck liposuction. There are also further options for concurrent laser treatment or fat transfer.

The techniques include skin-only lift (not recommended by the authors), minimal access cranial suspension (MACS) lift, SMAS lift, Sub-SMAS technique, deep plane lift and sub-periosteal lift. Sub-SMAS is practiced by majority of surgeons, to correct the jowls.

The sub-periosteal technique can be used to correct ptosis of the forehead, peri-orbital areas, glabella and malar regions. It, however, won't correct redundant skin in the cheek and cervical regions and can cause prolonged facial oedema.

Various multi-plane and mini-lift variations have been developed with a mixture of the previously mentioned advantages and disadvantages. The mini-lift incision may lack a temporal or postauricular component and have many names such as S-lift, short scar, and MACS lift. These approaches have reduced surgical time and risk, with a quicker recovery time. The limited access procedure reduces the view of relevant anatomy and makes skin redraping more challenging.

The neck is addressed at the same time as the face. Liposuction may be undertaken in the submental and submandibular regions between the anterior borders of sternocleidomastoid. The platysma may be plicated in midline and a lateral wedge excision may be undertaken at or below the hyoid to recreate a sharper cervicomental angle.

The main complications include haematoma and nerve injury. While weakness of the temporal or marginal mandibular branches may be observed, midfacial weakness should be explored as this is likely to represent buccal or zygomatic transection. Early exploration and primary repair are the best chance for return of spontaneous movement. Flap necrosis is more likely with smokers, diabetics and excessive wound tension. Other complications such as hypertrophic scar, incision irregularities,

earlobe, submental deformities, and more rarely infection or parotid injury can occur. Meticulous haemostasis and careful planning of skin redraping under minimal tension without overaggressive liposuction will minimise these complications.

15.6 Otoplasty

The aim is to achieve aesthetic result as popularised by McDowell which has the following criteria: all upper third ear protrusion must be corrected; the helix of both ears should be seen beyond the antihelix from the front view; the helix should have a smooth and regular line throughout; the postauricular sulcus should not be markedly decreased or distorted; the helix to mastoid distance should fall in the normal range of 10 to 12 mm in the upper third, 16 to 18 mm in the middle third, and 20 to 22 mm in the lower third; the position of the lateral ear border to the head should match within 3 mm at any point between the two ears.

15.6.1 Anatomy

The key anatomical anomalies that create a prominent pinna include loss of the antihelix, the depth of the conchal bowl and lobule prominence. The two features may occur in isolation or together.

15.6.2 Pre-Operative Evaluation

History: Any history of bullying is particularly relevant. The optimal age of correction is at 5 to 6 years prior to escalation of bullying while still allowing the ear to be almost at adult size.

Examination: Assess the subunits of the ear including the abnormalities of the subunits creating the protrusion. Check for any pre-operative asymmetry. Measure the helix to mastoid distances at the apex of the helix, the external auditory canal and the lobule. Pre-operative photos should be taken including an anterior full-face, posterior full-head, and lateral close-up views of the auricles.

15.6.3 Surgical Techniques

- Nonsurgical moulding techniques, for example, EarBuddies may be used in newborn infants with all subunits present in a dysmorphic auricle in the first year while the cartilage may be amenable to sculpting with splints.

- Minimal invasive techniques involving the use of implants, for example, Earfold have been developed recently and are inserted under local anaesthetic. The main advantages are demonstration of the expected correction preoperatively; avoid the use of a head bandage, and the operative and recovery time is reduced significantly. Incisionless otoplasty was developed in 1995 by Fritsch, as a percutaneous suture technique. This is geometrically similar to the Mustarde and Furnas techniques as described later. However, the suture entry and exit points correspond with each other in a percutaneous fashion.

- Surgical techniques may be either suturing or cartilage splitting. Mustarde sutures involve horizontal mattress sutures that recreate the antihelix. This is useful for paediatric cases and minimises the risk of haematoma. It is more challenging for adults with stiffer cartilage and does have the risk of suture extrusion. In isolation, this technique will not address the conchal bowl or lobule. Cartilage splitting or scoring technique involves longitudinal incision in the auricular cartilage along the axis of the new antihelix. This can be used with stiffer adult cartilage to good effect but does carry a higher risk of haematoma. The potential long-term cosmetic deformity can be more difficult to correct. Combinations of suturing and scoring, such as the Farrior technique, involve removing wedges of cartilage to support the mattress sutures. The conchal cartilage may be either addressed with Furnas' setback sutures securing the conchal bowl to the mastoid periosteum or with removal of the excess cartilage.

Complications may occur early or late in the post-operative period. Early complications include haematoma and wound infection. Haematomas usually occur in the first 24 to 48 hours and should be drained urgently if it occurs. The initial cardinal symptom is excessive pain felt beneath the head bandage. Wound infection may occur after 3 to 5 days and antibiotics should cover *Staphylococcus* and *Pseudomonas*. Late complications include asymmetry, suture extrusion, keloid scars and telephone or reverse telephone deformity depending on under- or over-correction of the superior and inferior poles of the auricle, respectively.

Further Reading

Hilinski JM, Toriumi DM. The ageing face. In: Gleeson M, Browning G, Burton M, et al, eds. Scott-Brown's Otorhinolaryngology Head and Neck Surgery. Great Britain, GB: Hodder Arnold; 2008:3068–3076

Joseph AW, Desai SC. Otoplasty. In: Desai SC, ed. Facial Plastic and Reconstructive Surgery: Clinical Reference Guide. San Diego, CA: Plural Publishing; 2017:541–550

Leatherbarrow B. Blepharoplasty. In: Gleeson M, Browning G, Burton M, et al, eds. Scott-Brown's Otorhinolaryngology Head and Neck Surgery. Great Britain, GB: Hodder Arnold; 2008:3048–3067

Loyo M, Lee LN, Kontis TC. Injectable fillers of the face. In: Papel ID, ed. Facial Plastic and Reconstructive Surgery. New York, NY: Thieme; 2016:264–281

Mandavia R, Dessouky O, Dhar V, D'Souza A. The use of botulinum toxin in otorhinolaryngology: an updated review. Clin Otolaryngol. 2014; 39(4):203–209

Perkins SW, Waters HH. Rhytidectomy. In: Papel ID, ed. Facial Plastic and Reconstructive Surgery. New York, NY: Thieme; 2016:139–158

Quatela VC, Antunes MB. Endoscopic forehead and midface lift. In: Papel ID, ed. Facial Plastic and Reconstructive Surgery. New York, NY: Thieme; 2016:159–174

Zoumalan RA, Goodman JF, Tanna NT, Arden RL, Golub JS, Pasha R. Reconstructive and facial plastic surgery. In: Pasha R, Golub JS, eds. Otolayngology Head and Neck Surgery: Clinical Reference Guide. San Diego, CA: Plural Publishing; 2014:435–518

Related Topics of Interest

Rhinoplasty
Reconstructive surgery

16 Cough

Cough is one of the most common symptoms to present to primary and secondary care physicians. Chronic cough can be a difficult condition to treat, and the cough can have a significant impact on a patient's quality of life. They may also complain of other laryngeal symptoms including dysphonia. Often when these patients have been seen by ear, nose and throat (ENT) specialists in the past, the cough has been attributed to laryngopharyngeal reflux and post-nasal drip. However, more recently chronic cough has been thought to be caused by hypersensitivity of the afferent nerves of the airways. There are a number of potential causes and differentials that need to be investigated. It is now recommended that these patients are treated with a multi-disciplinary approach, with input from ENT, respiratory, speech and language therapists and physiotherapist.

16.1 Cough Reflex

Cough is a reflex action to clear the lower airways by an involuntary expiration against a closed glottis. This protective reflex has a complex pathway. It starts with stimulation of an afferent sensory limb with cough receptors lining the pharynx, larynx and airways. The afferent fibres then travel along the vagus nerve to the cough centre, which is located in the medulla of the brainstem. The reflex arc continues from the brain stem via efferent fibres that pass along the vagus, phrenic and spinal motor nerves to the muscles of the larynx, pharynx, diaphragm and abdominal wall.

There are three main afferent receptors in the airway:

1. Rapidly adapting receptors that respond to mechanical stimuli.
2. Slowly adapting receptors that respond to chemical stimuli.
3. C-fibres that respond to chemical stimuli.

The receptors in the larynx respond to both mechanical and chemical stimuli. In chronic cough, the cough reflex leads to neuroplasticity resulting in peripheral and central sensitisation. This results in an over-sensitive cough reflex, which maintains the chronic cough and known as *chronic cough hypersensitivity syndrome* and *laryngeal hypersensitivity*.

16.2 Aetiology

An acute cough is defined as being present for less than 3 weeks and most commonly occurs following an upper respiratory tract infection of viral origin. A chronic cough continues for more than 8 weeks and can be due to a number of different causes. The patients referred to ENT have normally already had some investigations in primary care and/or by the respiratory physicians. Patients with normal chest imaging, non-smokers and no underlying respiratory condition are often referred to ENT to exclude any other causes of cough.

16.2.1 Differential Diagnosis

The differential diagnosis of chronic cough caused by an ENT condition:

- Laryngopharyngeal reflux.
- Post-nasal drip.
- Chronic rhinosinusitis.
- Laryngeal hypersensitivity.
- Laryngeal dysfunction.
- Allergic response.
- Airway stenosis.

There are many other causes for cough not listed above such as compression from an enlarged thyroid mass, pharyngeal pouch, oesophageal dysmotility, oesophageal webs and strictures, neuro-laryngological disorders, vasculitidies and cranial nerve palsies—all of which may present to ENT. However, there will be other signs and symptoms attributed to them and they are unlikely to have a chronic cough on its own.

16.3 Clinical Assessment

Clinical assessment entails taking a focussed history, clinical examination of the neck, mouth, oropharynx and flexible nasopharyngolaryngoscopy.

16.3.1 History

- The symptom history should focus on when the cough started and if there were any initial causes such as a viral infection. In particular, are there any triggers, for example strong smells or change in atmosphere? Is the cough more severe at different times of the day or night? Are there are any associated laryngology symptoms such as voice disturbance, swallowing problems, sore throat, globus sensation and laryngospasms? The history should also include nasal symptoms including nasal obstruction, post-nasal drip, history of rhinosinusitis and polyposis. Patients should also be asked about any weight loss, reflux or indigestion symptoms, regurgitation of foods and the red flag symptoms for head and neck malignancy such as referred otalgia. A respiratory systemic enquiry should be taken to include any history of shortness of breath, noisy breathing, productive cough, type of sputum, fevers, sweats and haemoptysis.

- Past medical history should include asking about any associated respiratory conditions such as asthma, any prior head and neck surgery (including investigations for thyroid conditions).
- Medication history is also required to ask of any medications including anti-hypertensives such as angiotensin-converting enzyme (ACE) inhibitors that can cause cough and any oral inhalers or nasal sprays that may aggravate a cough.
- Social history should include smoking history, working environment and voice usage.

16.3.2 Examination

A full ENT and head and neck examination is required. Oral examination should assess for any oral pathology, enlarged tonsils and post-nasal drip. Nasal examination is performed to assess nasal obstruction, signs of nasal polyps and rhinosinusitis. Neck examination should check for any masses and enlarged thyroid gland.

Laryngoscopy is required to assess the mobility of the vocal folds, including any paradoxical vocal cord movement, lesions on the vocal cords, granulomas, signs of infection (such as candidiasis) and inspection of the subglottis to look for stenosis. Signs of laryngopharyngeal reflux on laryngoscopy can be measured using the reflux finding score (▶ Table 16.1). A reflux finding score of more than 12 is suggestive of reflux.

16.3.3 Investigations

Patients with other respiratory symptoms such as shortness of breath or productive sputum will require further investigations. These may have

▶ Table 16.1 Reflux finding score

Sign on laryngoscopy	Score
Pseudosulcus (infraglottic oedema)	Absent = 0 Present = 2
Ventricular obliteration	Partial = 2 Complete = 4
Erythema, hyperaemia	Arytenoids = 2 Diffuse = 4
Vocal fold oedema	Mild = 1 Moderate = 2 Severe = 3 Polypoid = 4
Diffuse laryngeal oedema	Mild = 1 Moderate = 2 Severe = 3 Obstructing = 4
Posterior commissure hypertrophy	Absent = 0 Present = 2
Granuloma/granulation tissue	Absent = 0 Present = 2
Thick endo-laryngeal mucous	Absent = 0 Present = 2

been performed by respiratory physicians and normally include chest imaging (chest X-ray, high-resolution computed tomography (CT) scan of the chest, respiratory function tests (spirometry, flow-volume loops), eosinophilia testing and bronchoscopy.

Further imaging of the sinuses and neck can be useful depending on the history and clinical findings. Allergy testing such as serum allergy tests and skin prick testing may also be helpful.

There are a host of investigations for laryngopharyngeal reflux, which include oesophageal pH manometry, gastroscopy, transnasal oesophagoscopy, oropharyngeal pH monitoring and salivary pepsin test. There are also patient questionnaires, such as the reflux symptom index with a score of greater than 5 being suggestive of laryngopharyngeal reflux.

16.3.4 Management

The treatment of cough requires a multidisciplinary team approach with input from respiratory physicians, gastroenterology, speech and language therapist and physiotherapist. The development of specialist cough clinics has helped to diagnose and treat cough in the most effective way.

C

Laryngopharyngeal reflux

There are a number of treatments for laryngopharyngeal reflux. Lifestyle change is important and an explanation or advice sheet should be given. This should include which food and drink to avoid, the benefit of a food diary, avoiding eating large meals close to bedtime and foods that relax the lower oesophageal sphincter (such as caffeine). Medication regimes for reflux include a course of proton pump inhibitors, which when taken on an empty stomach will reduce the amount of acid produced. Antacids and those with a high alginate content taken after food can also be helpful. Further investigations for gastro-oesophageal reflux disease may find other causes for reflux (such as hiatus hernia) and may require treatment from gastroenterology and upper gastro-intestinal surgeons.

Rhinosinusitis

Although post-nasal drip is unlikely to be the main cause for the cough, treatment of an underlying nasal condition may help to reduce some of the nasal symptoms. Treatment for chronic rhinosinusitis (with or without polyps), vasomotor rhinitis and allergic rhinitis could have some improvement on the larynx and airway. Management includes good nasal hygiene, saline sinus rinses, steaming, topical nasal medications (such as nasal steroids) and endoscopic sinus surgery.

16.3.5 Medications

Prior to starting any new medications for cough, the current medication should be reviewed. ACE inhibitors should be changed to an alternative anti-hypertensive even if predating the cough. The inhalers used for any respiratory condition and the technique should be assessed. Some inhalers will leave less residue on the larynx and the use of spacers, regular mouthwash and gargles can prevent local infection and irritation.

There are a variety of over-the-counter antitussive medications. However, the majority have shown little evidence of being effective. Codeine has long been used as a cough suppressant, but is associated with adverse effects. Other pharmacological treatments aim at desensitising the airway, similar to the treatment of facial pain. Medications such as gabapentin, pregabalin and amitriptyline have all been used.

16.4 Speech and Language Therapy and Physiotherapy

There are a number of techniques that speech and language therapists can use to improve chronic cough. Treatments involve improving vocal hygiene and decreasing muscle tension may reduce laryngeal sensitivity. Psychotherapy and relaxation methods can be helpful to break the cycle of chronic throat clearing and coughing. Educating the patient on steaming and the importance of increasing hydration will prevent the airways drying out and becoming more irritable. Patients with dysphonia, increased muscle tension, laryngospasm and paradoxical vocal cord movement will all benefit from therapy. However, changing a patient's behaviour is challenging and requires a patient who is compliant and motivated.

There is crossover between the techniques used by speech and language therapists and physiotherapists. Physiotherapy such as breathing techniques and improved posture can all be beneficial in reducing the symptoms of cough.

Further Reading

Morice AH, McGarvey L, Pavord I; British Thoracic Society Cough Guideline Group. Recommendations for the management of cough in adults. Thorax. 2006; 61(Suppl 1):i1–i24

Ryan NM, Gibson PG, Gibson PG, Fowler SJ. Recent additions in the treatment of cough. J Thorac Dis. 2014; 6(Suppl 7):S739–S747

Hull JH, Backer V, Gibson PG, Fowler SJ. Laryngeal dysfunction: assessment and management for the clinician. Am J Respir Crit Care Med. 2016; 194(9):1062–1072

Chamberlain Mitchell SA, Garrod R, Clark L, et al. Physiotherapy, and speech and language therapy intervention for patients with refractory chronic cough: a multicentre randomised control trial. Thorax. 2017; 72(2):129–136

Related Topics of Interest

Globus pharyngeus
Rhinosinusitis–chronic without nasal polyps
Rhinosinusitis–chronic (with nasal polyps)
Hypopharyngeal carcinoma
Speech and swallow rehabilitation following head and neck surgery
Speech and language therapy for benign voice disorders

17 Day Case ENT Surgery

A day case patient is one who has a planned admission, operation and discharge on the same day. Anaesthesia is modified to allow rapid recovery and to minimise post-operative pain, nausea, and vomiting. Pre-admission planning and protocol-driven, nurse-led discharge allow a day unit to run efficiently. The option of day case surgery is largely governed by the unit facilities, the type of surgery and patient factors.

17.1 Introduction

Day surgery is continually evolving. In recent years, the complexity of procedures suitable for day case surgery has increased. Protocols devised with the local anaesthetic department have allowed many patients with a range of comorbidities to have day surgery. The pre-operative preparation should determine a patient's fitness to undergo day surgery. Such surgery tends to be determined by age, American Society of Anesthesiologists (ASA) status and body mass index (BMI). Acute conditions or patients on a target pathway can be treated effectively as day cases too. It is recommended that each unit has a clinical lead to develop local policies, guidelines and clinical governance. Detailed advice leaflets should be available as should a robust discharge protocol and effective audit.

17.2 Definition

An ear, nose, throat (ENT) surgical day case patient is one who has a planned admission for operation and discharge on the same day. The definition of 'same day' is not as obvious as one might think. In the United Kingdom, it is defined as the same calendar day. In the United States, it is defined by a 24-hour window such as being admitted after 7:30 a.m. on day 1 and discharged by 7:00 a.m. the next day. In the United Kingdom, this would be defined as a 1-day stay, but the problem then arises, if a hospital has a 24-hour staffed day unit and the patient stays overnight on that unit and not in an inpatient bed, as how to define the stay. Most would simply define it as a 1-day stay on a day unit. There may be financial implications for this, because in the U.K. clinical commissioning groups pay an enhanced tariff for many procedures performed as a day case. The corollary of this is that hospitals need to have agreements with the local commissioning groups as to what stay provides an enhanced tariff before deciding on whether investing in a 23-hour 'day unit' is financially viable.

17.3 The Day Case Unit

The patient may be admitted into either a self-contained day surgery unit with its own admission suites, wards, theatres and recovery area. Less desirably, a day case ward is used with patients transferred to a main theatre. Stand-alone day case units, sited away from a major hospital, have become reasonably common in the United Kingdom. Facilities for recovery are required. Full admission procedures and records are required, which therefore excludes those operations and procedures undertaken in the outpatient or accident and emergency department.

17.4 Surgical Factors

Previously, this chapter listed procedures suitable for day case surgery, but very few ENT operations now would routinely require an inpatient bed. Major whead and neck surgery, including anterior and lateral skull base surgery would fit into this small group. A sensible approach might be to have day case surgery as a default option for surgery so that the surgeon would then, in effect, be asking if there is any reason why surgery cannot be performed as a day case.

Operations taking more than an hour, such as mastoid surgery, which were previously thought to be too long for day case surgery, are now suitable, particularly if there is an experienced, competent anaesthetist (who might, e.g., use remifentanil for major ear surgery to allow a controlled hypotensive anaesthetic and rapid recovery). A notable procedure which was being performed as a day case procedure in some centres and which is now deemed *not* suitable following a British Association of Endocrine and Thyroid Surgeons (BAETS) position statement is thyroid lobectomy.

Examples of procedures suitable to be performed as a day case are as follows:

- Rhinology—submucous diathermy (SMD), inferior turbinoplasty, septoplasty, septorhinoplasty,

D

functional endoscopic sinus surgery (FESS), dacryocystorhinostomy.

- Otology—grommets, myringoplasty, mastoidectomy, stapedectomy, ossiculoplasty.
- Head and neck—panendoscopy and biopsy, microlaryngoscopy and biopsy of T1 and most T2 patients (but *not* those requiring an awake intubation and debulking of large-volume tumours or when there is pre-operative stertor or stridor), cord medialisation, neck lump excision, skin cancer excision.
- Paediatrics—grommets, adenoidectomy, endoscopy, tonsillectomy.

Examples of procedures not suitable to be performed as a day case are as follows:

- Rhinology—inferior turbinate excision, anterior skull base surgery.
- Otology—petrosectomy, labyrinthectomy, vestibular schwannoma surgery.
- Head and neck—thyroid lobectomy, total thyroidectomy, parathyroidectomy, panendoscopy and biopsy of T3 and T4 laryngeal and pharyngeal tumours or any endoscopy where there is pre-operative stertor/stridor due to tumour, tonsillectomy in adults with sleep apnoea, major head and neck surgery such as laryngectomy, selective neck dissection, and any surgery involving microvascular free tissue transfer or myocutaneous flaps.
- Paediatrics—tonsillectomy for sleep apnoea, angiofibroma surgery.

An important factor which determines the percentage of surgery that can be performed as a day case is the unit's opening and closing time. The ideal is to have a unit open 24 hour a day so that patients can have a 23-hour admission if required but are still day cases from a tariff perspective. This would apply to patients having afternoon mastoid or thyroid surgery, for example, when a 7- or even 10-p.m. closure might lead to either inappropriate early discharge or the need for an overnight bed.

17.5 Patient Factors

- An adult must be available to supervise the patient during the evening and first night.
- A telephone must be accessible so that the hospital can be contacted in an emergency. The home should be within a 20-minute drive of

the hospital if the patient is at risk of a primary haemorrhage, for example, after tonsillectomy, adenoidectomy or submucosal diathermy.

- The patient must be taken home by an adult in a car or taxi on discharge.
- No mechanical device should be used or cooking undertaken, and legal documents should not be signed during the first 24-hour post-operative period, when alcohol is also forbidden.
- Driving is not advised within 48 hours of a general anaesthetic.

Fitness for surgery should be determined by the patient's health as determined by a pre-operative assessment. At this assessment, inclusion and exclusion criteria as agreed with the local anaesthetic department are used to determine if the patient is suitable. The patient's BMI should be used as one factor in an overall fitness assessment but should not be used as a single criterion to determine fitness for surgery.

17.6 ASA Classification

The ASA classification of physical status is important. Most patients are of ASA 1 or ASA 2 status (no illness or mild-to-moderate systemic illness) with class 3 and 4 generally excluded unless they are minor procedures performed under local anaesthetic +/- sedation.

- Class 1: The patient has no organic, physiological, biochemical or psychiatric disturbance and the pathological process for which surgery is to be performed is localised.
- Class 2: Mild-to-moderate systemic disturbance caused either by the condition to be treated surgically or other pathophysiological processes, for example, non–insulin-dependent diabetes mellitus or essential hypertension.
- Class 3: Severe systemic disturbance from any cause or causes, for example, complicated or severe diabetes, combinations of heart disease and respiratory disease or others that impair normal functions severely.
- Class 4: Extreme systemic disorders, for example, patients who are in an extremely poor physical state such as those with cardiac decompensation, severe trauma with irreparable damage, complete intestinal obstruction of long duration in a patient who is already debilitated.

17.7 Children

Special facilities for children are required. They should have their own designated ward away from adult patients, with its own play area and parental waiting area. A pre-admission visit allows familiarisation. The ideal is to have a children-only operating list as part of a children's day unit, so that children are not recovered in an area with adult patients. Most district general hospitals will have a locally agreed compromise such as a designated area of recovery for children who are away from adult patients. The children's area should be staffed by paediatric trained nurses.

17.8 Benefits of Day Surgery

For patients:
  Reduced disruption to life.
  Early mobilisation.
  Less psychological preparation required.
  Anaesthetic administered allows rapid recovery.
For hospitals:
  Lower costs.
  Reduced inpatient theatre workload.
  Increased efficiency.

Aside from the financial cost of building and staffing such units, which should be offset by increased efficiency (the time between finishing a case and starting the next should be reduced compared to an inpatient list), the main potential disadvantage is the risk that a patient might have an unsafe discharge. This might be because patients have not fully recovered from anaesthesia or have not been adequately assessed post-operatively. Strong governance and leadership supporting decisions to admit planned day case patients who are deemed not fit for discharge are essential.

Further Reading

Quemby DJ, Stocker ME. Day surgery development and practice: key factors for a successful pathway. Contin Educ Anaesth Crit Care Pain. 2014; 14(6):256–261

Related Topics of Interest

Anaesthesia—general
Anaesthesia—local
Anaesthesia—sedation

D

18 Drooling

'Drooling' (Sialorrhoea), or overspill of saliva is physiological condition in children until they develop good oral muscle control, typically at the age of 4 or 5 years. Before that, saliva may dribble onto the chin and neck, in some cases causing eczematous chin reactions. In children with poor neuromuscular function—typically children with cerebral palsy—salivary overspill may persist into later childhood and adult life, causing distress for parent and child. 'Sialorrhoea' is a misnomer as these children produce normal quantities of saliva; the problem is with salivary clearance. They will often have a poor swallow, and some will have aspiration and airway problems.

18.1 Management

Many children and parents manage the situation without medical intervention. The child usually improves as he or she gets older and voluntary muscle control improves as the child learns to focus on his or her swallowing. The drooling is often worse when the child is intensely focused on an activity—for example, a computer screen. In severe cases, several changes of clothes a day are needed and the child and parents become distressed and seek intervention. A multidisciplinary approach works best as often paediatricians, neurologists, and speech and language therapists (SALT) may have much to contribute.

18.2 Treatment Options

- Conservative management, with watchful waiting as the child develops, is appropriate in many cases.
- Anti-cholinergic agents to dry secretions—hyoscine patches, bezopine, and oral glycopyrrolate—are often used under the supervision of a paediatrician.
- Physical therapies—under the supervision of a SALT with a special interest in this condition—can help train children to improve salivary clearance.

- A variety of intra-oral devices have been used with some success.
- Botulinus toxin (Botox) injections into the salivary glands (usually the submandibular glands but in some cases the parotid, often under ultrasound guidance) are offered by some surgeons.

18.3 Surgery

The role of adenotonsillectomy is uncertain, but if the tonsils and adenoids are very large and obstructing the swallow, adenotonsillectomy can bring about considerable benefit. Surgery of the salivary glands is a last resort.

Various techniques, including the following, have been tried:

- Ligation of the parotid ducts (rarely done nowadays).
- Transposition of the submandibular ducts, re-routing them to the tonsillar fossa.
- Exceptionally, removal of the submandibular glands.

Each of these techniques has its complications, including dry mouth—with adverse effects on dentition—late obstruction of the transposed or ligated ducts, and ranula formation.

Further Reading

Gleeson M. Salivary gland disorders in childhood. In: Clarke RW, ed. Pediatric Otolaryngology: Practical Clinical Management. Stuttgart: Thieme; 2017:355–363

Walshe M, Smith M, Pennington L. Interventions for drooling in children with cerebral palsy. Cochrane Database Syst Rev. 2012; 11:CD008624

Related Topics of Interest

Paediatric genetic syndromes and associations
Paediatric airway problems

19 Epiglottitis

Acute epiglottitis is an uncommon but dangerous bacterial infection of the supraglottis, but pre-dominantly the loose connective tissue of the epiglottis. An 8-year review of cases in the United States from 1998 to 2006 showed a mortality rate, from an average of about 4,000 cases per year, of about 1%.

19.1 Hib Vaccine

The *Haemophilus influenzae* type B (Hib) conjugate vaccine is a biosynthetic vaccine. Antibodies against the polysaccharide capsule of *H. influenzae*, namely polyribosylribitol phosphate (PRP), provide immunity against *H. influenzae* infection and so it was initially thought that purified PRP would be an excellent vaccine and this was introduced in the 1980s. In practice, purified PRP stimulated a poor immune response due to the recognition of PRP by B cells but not T cells. It was recognised that when PRP was linked with a highly immunogenic protein carrier, a much stronger immune response occurred due to T and B cells recognising the covalent PRP. This conjugated vaccine has been given in the United Kingdom since 1992, as part of the childhood vaccination programme. It is given as a 1:5 vaccine (also includes diphtheria, tetanus, whooping cough and polio) at 2, 3, and 4 months and then at 12 months as a 2:1 vaccine with Men C. Its introduction has seen more than a 90% reduction in the incidence of meningitis, pneumonia and epiglottitis as well as a reduction in acute otitis media.

19.2 Epidemiology

Prior to the introduction of the Hib vaccine as purified PRP in the 1980s and as the conjugate vaccine in the 1990s, epiglottitis was usually seen in children, particularly between the ages of 3 and 5, but also affecting adults. For example, in Sweden in 1987 prior to the introduction of the Hib conjugate vaccine the incidence was 20.9 per 100,000 in children aged up to 5 years but fell to 0.9 per 100,000 by 1996 after the Hib vaccination was introduced in 1992. The incidence has continued to fall as take up levels have increased. In Denmark, where immunisation is compulsory, the incidence has fallen in children to 0.2 cases per 100,000.

In adults, the incidence in developed nations has remained constant at 1 to 2 cases per 100,000, presumably because Hib is routinely offered only to children.

19.3 Aetiology

Hib remains the most common organism despite the Hib vaccination programme, probably because of non-uptake in some children or a poor immune response to the vaccine in others. In adults, Hib continues to be the commonest organism to cause epiglottitis because of waning immunity in younger adults who have been vaccinated and because older adults will not have been immunised. *Streptococcus pyogenes*, *Streptococcus pneumoniae* and *Staphylococcus aureus* have also been isolated, particularly in adults. It is uncertain why the infection has a predilection for the epiglottis. In children under the age of 3 years *H. influenzae* tends to cause meningitis. It has been suggested that previous contact with *H. influenzae* in early childhood may later be followed by a type III Arthus hypersensitivity reaction which may account for the rapid onset of epiglottitis.

19.4 Clinical Features

The disease may present at any time of the year but is more common in winter. Initially, the child usually complains of a sore throat and pain when swallowing. Inflammation and oedema of the supraglottis will rapidly progress to cause muffling of the voice and respiratory obstruction. Inspiratory stridor then occurs. A critically ill, breathless child may then present to the casualty department having a toxic, flushed appearance and a high temperature (38–40°C). The child will usually be desperate to sit up and lean forward to aid breathing. This, and the associated pain on swallowing, will cause dribbling of saliva. The provisional diagnosis is made on the history and examination. Nothing that may acutely further distress the child should be allowed. Therefore, the parents should always be present and the doctors quietly reassuring. No attempt to depress the tongue, draw blood, or perform flexible laryngoscopy should be undertaken as distress may precipitate laryngospasm.

E

19.5 Investigations

Maintenance of the patient's airway is the primary consideration, and all investigations should be delayed until this is secure. If the child presents quite early in the disease and there is no stridor, a lateral soft tissue neck radiograph may be undertaken to confirm a swollen epiglottis, but it is important the child has priority and does not have to wait in a queue (the clinician in charge must personally communicate this to the radiologist). The taking of a radiograph should never be done if there are already signs of respiratory difficulty. Furthermore, no child should be sent for a radiograph without the continuous presence of someone skilled in paediatric intubation.

19.6 Treatment

The first requirement of treatment is to safeguard the airway. An experienced paediatric anaesthetist and otolaryngologist should be in attendance. The child will be in an upright position, leaning forward to maximally facilitate breathing. Lying a child flat may result in airway obstruction. Intravenous access is not attempted and the child should be moved to a quiet induction area with adjacent operating facilities. A gentle inhalation induction using sevoflurane and oxygen is preferred. The oxygen saturation is closely monitored with pulse oximetry. A parent should be present and at all times the child is talked to and reassured. When the child is asleep, the parent is shown from the room. Direct laryngoscopy should be performed to establish the diagnosis and to pass an endotracheal tube. Oedematous aryepiglottic folds and a cherry-red epiglottis are characteristic signs of the disease. An appropriately sized orotracheal tube is inserted to immediately restore the airway. This can then be replaced with a nasotracheal tube as they are more readily tolerated and more securely fixed, but not at the risk of losing a precarious airway. There may be difficulty establishing an endotracheal airway, and if intubation fails, a rigid bronchoscope should be inserted immediately and subsequently replaced with an endotracheal tube. Rarely, a cricothyroidotomy or tracheostomy may be necessary.

Once an airway has been established, culture swabs are taken from the epiglottis and a blood culture is performed. An intravenous line is inserted for fluid replacement and antibiotic therapy. The current drugs of choice for epiglottitis are ceftriaxone or cefotaxime, both third-generation cephalosporins, because about 30% of *Haemophilus* strains are resistant to ampicillin. For a patient allergic to cephalosporins, clindamycin and vancomycin may be given. Intravenous steroids should be considered. A nasogastric tube should be inserted for feeding. The sedated child is transferred to a paediatric intensive care unit for rehydration, antibiotics and humidified inspired gases.

19.7 Follow-Up and Aftercare

There is usually a prompt response to treatment with fluid replacement, antibiotics and possibly steroids. As the epiglottic oedema settles, an increasing leak around the endotracheal tube should be seen. Once the child is afebrile and appears well, extubation can be considered. This is usually possible after about 48 hours.

Further Reading

Guldfred LA, Lyhne D, Becker BC. Acute epiglottitis: epidemiology, clinical presentation, management and outcome. J Laryngol Otol. 2008; 122(8):818–823

Tibballs J, Watson T. Symptoms and signs differentiating croup and epiglottitis. J Paediatr Child Health. 2011; 47(3):77–82

Related Topics of Interest

Paediatric airway problems
Paediatric endoscopy

20 Epistaxis

There are three key points to remember regarding epistaxis:

1. Epistaxis is common and usually arises from Little's area.
2. Endoscopic sphenopalatine artery (SPA) ligation will resolve most non-traumatic spontaneous epistaxis, if not resolved by conservative measures.
3. Traumatic epistaxis may be due to nasal trauma involving the vomer and the superior portion of the nasal septum which is supplied by a branch of the anterior ethmoidal artery (AEA). Ligation of both the AEA and SPA may therefore be required in traumatic epistaxis.

20.1 Aetiology

1. Local causes:
   - Iatrogenic. Probably the commonest cause as every endonasal surgical procedure including turbinate surgery will cause some epistaxis. Medical treatment with nasal steroids is another common iatrogenic cause, by virtue of mucosal irritation.
   - Traumatic (fractures, foreign body, nose picking).
   - Inflammatory (rhinitis, particularly from an upper respiratory tract infection [URTI] or allergic rhinitis, sinusitis).
   - Neoplastic (benign, such as a pyogenic granuloma of the septum and juvenile angiofibroma, a wide range of malignancy of the nose, sinuses and nasopharynx).
   - Environmental (high altitude, air conditioning).
   - Endocrine (menstruation, pregnancy).
   - Idiopathic.

2. General causes:
   - Anticoagulants (warfarin, aspirin, clopidogrel and apixaban).
   - Diseases of the blood (haemophilia, leukaemia).
   - Hereditary haemorrhagic telangiectasia (Osler–Weber–Rendu disease).
   - Hypertension.
   - Raised venous pressure, for example, due to paroxysms of coughing (as in chronic obstructive pulmonary disease [COPD] or whooping cough).

20.2 Blood Vessels Involved

The upper parts of the nose are supplied by branches from the internal carotid artery (anterior and posterior ethmoidal arteries which are branches of the ophthalmic artery) and the rest from branches of the external carotid artery, namely, the greater palatine (from the maxillary artery), the sphenopalatine (terminal branch of the maxillary artery), and the septal branch of the superior labial (a branch of the facial artery). Little's area (Kiesselbach's plexus) is the commonest site of bleeding. It is named after James Little, an American surgeon, who in 1879 described an area 'about half an inch from the middle of the column (septum)" as a common site for epistaxis. It was Kiesselbach (a German otolaryngologist practicing in Erlangen) who published a paper in 1884 pointing out that at Little's area four arteries anastomose to form a vascular plexus. These arteries are the anterior ethmoidal, sphenopalatine, greater palatine and the septal branch of the superior labial artery. Woodruff, in 1949 described a venous plexus within the posterior part of the inferior meatus (Woodruff's plexus) as a possible source of posterior epistaxis. McGarry showed there are vessels at this site, but there is no evidence the site is a cause of epistaxis.

20.3 Sites Affected

Little's area is the commonest site of epistaxis but the majority are minor and are ignored by the patient or treated in primary care. Its frequency is due to multiple factors; it is a site prone to trauma from nose picking and wiping, Little's area is prone to drying if the anterior septum is deviated, which leads to irritation and then trauma. It is a site with a vascular plexus so will bleed easily if traumatised.

Studies have looked at the site of an epistaxis in patients coming to A&E and assessed by an ear, nose and throat (ENT) registrar. Only a third had a Little's bleeding source, 40% had a posterior septal bleeding source, and the remainder were on the lateral nasal wall, often from within the middle meatus.

E

20.4 Clinical Assessment

Assess the patient for signs of shock, gain intravenous access and decide if immediate resuscitation, including intravenous fluid infusion is necessary. Investigations should include a full blood count (FBC) (check haemoglobin [Hb], white cell count, and platelets), clotting studies, and blood for group and save, if necessary. It is important that nursing support is available. Protect the patient's clothing and your own with an apron, and wear gloves. Take a full history and on examination try to identify a specific bleeding point. If the bleeding is profuse, then the use of Moffet's solution, as a spray or soaked cotton wool patties, or co-phenylcaine spray (lignocaine 5% with phenylephrine), applied to the affected nostril should be considered. The patient should be sitting forward with elbows on thighs and fingers pinching the soft part of the nose while looking down with the mouth open. In this position, the head remains above the heart, so this will reduce venous pressure. Blood draining posteriorly in the nose will then drip out of the mouth. Pressure on the nostrils can be supplemented with ice cold packs over the nose and sucking ice cubes both of which have been shown to reduce nasal blood supply.

20.5 Management

The aims are to arrest the epistaxis and to treat the underlying cause. Once the epistaxis is controlled, the anterior nares should be inspected by means of anterior rhinoscopy after gently microsuctioning away any clot. If no bleeding point is identified, then a flexible or rigid endoscope should be used to inspect the posterior nares. The former is more comfortable and with practice or an assistant holding the tip, it can be used to electrocauterise the posterior bleeding points.

Silver nitrate cautery or bipolar electrocoagulation should be used to an identifiable bleeding point. The latter is more reliable if available, but care should be taken not to burn the septal cartilage as this might cause a septal necrosis and perforation. If Little's area has been cauterised, then the area should be kept moist and infection prevented by using a nasal antibiotic, nasal cream or gel until the cauterised area has healed (usually around a fortnight).

Anterior nasal packing should be considered if a bleeding point is not identified. Gel-coated packs with balloons (such as Rapid Rhino Epistaxis balloons) or absorbable nasal dressing (such as meropore, NasoPore) are the least traumatic, but if not available, bismuth iodoform paraffin paste (BIPP) can be considered.

Tranexamic acid is an underused treatment adjunct. This medication slows the resolution of clot.

Calm reassurance coupled with sedation (intravenous [IV] diazepam) will reduce the patient's anxiety. If nasal packing is required, systemic antibiotics should be given to prevent otitis media from eustachian tube blockage and sinusitis. Examination under general anaesthetic may become necessary if the above measures fail or should the patient rebleed once a nasal dressing has been removed. This may allow identification of the bleeding point and electrocautery or if no definite source is identified, SPA ligation.

20.6 Surgical Intervention

Endoscopic SPA cauterisation/clipping. This was first described by Budovitch and Saetti in 1992. Occasionally, a septoplasty is needed for access. The maxillary artery in the pterygopalatine fossa (which lies behind the posterior wall of the maxillary sinus) becomes the SPA as it enters the nose through the sphenopalatine foramen within the posterior aspect of the middle meatus. Its position is quite reliable in that it lies about 5 mm anterosuperior to the posterior insertion of the middle turbinate within the middle meatus. To find the artery, do the following:

1. Raise a mucosal flap on the lateral nasal wall within the posterior part of the middle meatus starting just anterior to the posterior wall of the maxillary sinus. An experienced endoscopic surgeon can usually raise a mucosal flap and find the artery without entering the maxillary sinus.
2. To determine where the posteromedial wall of the maxillary sinus is, use a Freer's elevator to palpate the lateral nasal wall within the middle meatus, beyond the uncinate process but below the bulla ethmoidalis. The wall here, corresponding to the medial wall of the maxillary sinus, consists of eggshell thin bone, often deficient in places, and is springy. As one travels more posteriorly, this springiness is replaced by the hard bone of the posterior maxillary sinus wall as it curves anteromedially.

3. Here, a vertical incision is made onto hard bone, within the middle meatus, curving slightly posteriorly beneath the posterior insertion of the middle turbinate, without entering the maxillary sinus.
4. For a less experienced surgeon, or if the surgeon is presented with tricky anatomy, it is best to enter the posterior aspect of the maxillary sinus from the middle meatus. This will then allow a view of the posterior wall of the maxillary sinus so that the surgeon can then be sure of his/her landmarks. To do this, simply make the middle meatal incision 5 mm more anterior to that described above, but still keeping below the bulla ethmoidalis and of course beyond the uncinate process.
5. A mucosal flap is then raised posterosuperiorly, 10 to 15 mm in height with the lower margin of the flap being the posterior insertion of the middle turbinate. Usually about 5 mm above this posterior insertion, one will find a small projection of bone, the crista ethmoidalis. The SPA and its branches lie posterior and occasionally inferior to the crista.

Bipolar diathermy or clipping with titanium Ligaclips can be used to occlude the vessel. Further epistaxis may be due to re-canalisation of the artery, particularly if bipolar diathermy is used, or from having missed a branch of the SPA proximal to the cauterised/clipped trunk. Repeat bipolar diathermy of the SPA and perhaps also the AEA is then indicated. Bilateral SPA ligation for unilateral epistaxis may very occasionally be indicated for recurrent epistaxis despite SPA ligation. Epistaxis is theoretically possible from a contralateral source due to a limited collateral blood supply.

Ligation or clipping of the maxillary artery in the pterygomaxillary fossa. Very occasionally, there is need to locate and clip the maxillary artery in the pterygopalatine fossa, for example, if there is a lateral nasal wall mass engulfing the SPA. A transnasal endoscopic approach is now preferred to a Caldwell–Luc approach. A large middle meatal antrostomy is fashioned to expose the maxillary antrum and allow a view of the posterior wall of the maxillary sinus. Mucosa over the posterior wall is scrapped away and a window of bone in the posterior wall of the maxillary sinus is removed with Kerrison's punch forceps. Periosteum is exposed by removing this window of bone and is incised to expose fat within the pterygopalatine

fossa. The fat is gently separated to allow the artery and its branches to be identified. Each tortuous branch is clipped in turn.

Anterior ethmoidal artery clipping is required for uncontrollable bleeding from the upper part of the nose medial to the middle turbinate or from the frontal recess. The former arises from a fracture of the vomer due to nasal trauma, the latter from iatrogenic injury during endoscopic sinus surgery (ESS). The approach to the AEA is via a medial orbital incision with lateral displacement of the upper orbital contents. The artery is surrounded by periosteum about 2.5 cm deep to the orbital rim just above the level of the medial canthus and is readily controlled by clipping. Remember the 24–12–6 rule: the average distance from the orbital rim to the AEA is 24 mm; from the AEA to the posterior ethmoidal artery (PEA) is 12 mm; and the distance from the PEA to the optic nerve is 6 mm.

External carotid artery ligation in the neck may need to be performed if maxillary artery clipping is unsuccessful. It is best to ligate the artery as high in the neck as possible, ideally above the facial artery, as this will result in a greater reduction of SPA blood pressure.

Embolisation of vessels under radiographical control with gel sponge or beads is advocated in some centres where there is a radiologist with a special interest in embolisation. Retrograde embolisation of the internal carotid artery (ICA) causing a cerebrovascular accident or unilateral blindness are potential risks, however.

20.7 Hereditary Haemorrhagic Telangiectasia

A specific problem in the management of epistaxis (and favourite examination topic) includes hereditary haemorrhagic telangiectasia (HHT) or Osler–Weber–Rendu disease. This is an autosomal dominant disorder and is the first identified disease caused by defects in a transforming growth factor-β (TGF-β) superfamily receptor. There is loss of the muscularis layer and disturbance of the elastic lamina of both venous and arterial vessels. The four clinical diagnostic criteria are epistaxis, telangiectasia, visceral lesions and a first-degree relative with HHT.

It manifests with mucocutaneous telangiectases and arteriovenous malformations which can

E

affect the nose (epistaxis is the most common presentation), mouth, and particularly the tongue, lung, liver, spleen, urinary tract, gastrointestinal tract, conjunctiva, trunk, arms and fingers.

Treatment is symptomatic. For the nose, KTP laser ablation, septodermoplasty, and Young's procedure (complete anterior nasal occlusion from the raising of medial and lateral anterior nasal skin flaps) are surgical options. Tamoxifen (an antioestrogen) and bevacizumab (a monoclonal antibody that inhibits vascular endothelial growth factor) are possible medical treatments.

Further Reading

Alderman C, Corlett J, Cullis J. The treatment of recurrent epistaxis due to hereditary haemorrhagic telangiectasia with intranasal bevacizumab. Br J Haematol. 2013; 162(4):547–548

Traboulsi H, Alam E, Hadi U. Changing trends in the management of epistaxis. Int J Otolaryngol. 2015; 2015:263987

Related Topics of Interest

Examination of the nose

Rhinosinusitis—appropriate terminology

E

21 Eponyms in ENT

Alexander dysplasia	The least severe type of inner ear dysplasia. The cochlear duct and basal turn of the cochlea are usually the only structures affected, resulting in a high-frequency hearing loss.
Alport syndrome	Syndrome that consists of haematuria with progressive renal failure (usually starting in the mid-teens), progressive sensorineural hearing loss and retinal flecks. There is a defect in type IV collagen and the symmetrical high frequency sensorineural hearing loss is primarily due to a loss of hair cells. Eighty percent inherited in an X-linked recessive pattern, but there is also autosomal dominant and autosomal recessive inheritance.
Apert syndrome	Crouzon's with syndactyly. A rare autosomal dominant craniofacial disorder.
Arnold's nerve	The auricular branch of the vagus. It arises from the jugular ganglion, passes through the temporal bone via the mastoid canaliculus and exits the skull through the tympanomastoid fissure. It supplies the skin of the posterior external canal and posterior auricle.
Barre-Lieou syndrome	Consisting of sharp pain beginning in the neck and radiating up to the occiput and then forward. It is most common in patients between 40 and 60 years of age. Pain is usually on one side and aggravated by certain movements of the head. Sensory disturbances, including vertigo, tinnitus and cloudy vision, may accompany the pain. The cause is not known. It is also known as *cervical migraine*.
Barrett oesophagitis	Replacement of the squamous epithelium of the distal oesophagus by columnar epithelium, similar to that which lines the stomach. The most common cause is chronic gastroesophageal reflux, and 2% to 5% of cases may progress to adenocarcinoma.
Bartholin duct	The major duct of the sublingual gland. It is formed by the confluence of several of the more anterior small sublingual ducts (ducts of Rivinus) and empties into either the submandibular duct on directly into the floor of mouth at the plica sublingualis.
Battle sign	Ecchymosis over the mastoid process. It is indicative of a temporal bone or posterior fossa fracture.
Behçet syndrome	Classically, a symptom complex consisting of oral ulcers, genital ulcers and iritis. The oral lesions can be extensive and may be the initial manifestation of the disease. It is seen most frequently in young adults in Japan and in Mediterranean countries. The cause is unknown; both viral and immune-complex aetiologies have been proposed.
Bezold abscess	A subperiosteal abscess of the temporal bone, most commonly found in the region just anterior to the mastoid tip. The cause is usually a mastoiditis with extravasation through the inner bony table into the digastric fossa.
Bing–Siebenmann dysplasia	Complete membranous labyrinthine dysplasia.
Boerhaave syndrome	Spontaneous rupture of the oesophagus, usually due to severe vomiting.
Bogorad syndrome	Profuse lacrimation during eating. It is usually the result of faulty regeneration of autonomic nerves after facial trauma, with parasympathetic fibres originally intended for the salivary glands going to the lacrimal gland instead. It is also known as *syndrome of crocodile tears*.
Bonnet syndrome	A combination of tic douloureux and Horner syndrome.
Bowen disease	(i.e. cutaneous SCC in situ). A variant of squamous cell cancer characterized by a full-thickness dysplasia of the epidermis. It is by definition non-invasive, but it can progress to invasive carcinoma. It appears as a red, scaly patch in sun-exposed areas and it can be confused with psoriasis.
Brown sign	Blanching of a red or blue mass in the tympanic membrane when air pressure is applied by pneumo-otoscopy. It is indicative of a glomus tympanicum tumour.

E

Brown vertical retraction syndrome	A congenital or acquired pseudo paresis of the inferior oblique muscle, whereby the eye cannot be elevated beyond mid-gaze. The congenital form is thought to be due to a congenitally shortened superior oblique tendon, whereas the acquired syndrome may be due to either recent trauma (e.g. orbital fracture with entrapment) or previous trauma with formation of adhesions.
Broyle's ligament	Anterior commissure ligament of the larynx.
Brunner abscess	Abscess of the posterior floor of the mouth.
Burckhardt dermatitis	An eruption of the external ear. It consists of red papules and vesicles that appear after exposure to sunlight. The rash usually resolves spontaneously.
Carhart notch	Raymond Thomas Carhart in 1950. One of the pioneers of audiology and also first to use the term '*air-bone gap*'. An artefactual loss of bone conduction sensitivity that is greatest at 2 kHz. Most commonly associated with otosclerosis but can occur with otitis media with effusion (OME) and ossicular chain fixation. It is thought to be due to the fact that when bone conduction is tested, a proportion of the sound energy causes the ossicles to vibrate and resonate. The bone conduction threshold improves on correction of the conductive defect.
Churg–Strauss syndrome	Now known as eosinophilic granulomatosis with polyangiitis (EGPA), is an autoimmune condition that causes vasculitis of small and medium-sized blood vessels in persons with a history of airway allergic hypersensitivity. It usually manifests in three stages: allergic, eosinophilic and vasculitic.
Chvostek sign	A facial twitch obtained by tapping the facial nerve in front of the tragus. It can be indicative of hypocalcaemia.
Cogan syndrome	Typically, a sudden onset of interstitial keratitis and vestibuloauditory symptoms, usually in young persons but sometimes in the elderly. Patients report blurring of vision, orbital pain, vertigo and tinnitus. The symptoms may progress quickly to blindness and deafness, followed by resolution and later relapse. Treatment currently consists of steroids.
Cowden syndrome	A rare autosomal dominant inherited disorder whose primary ears, nose and throat manifestation are hamartomas of the skin and mucous membranes. Patients with this disease also may have thyroid goitres or adenomas, gastrointestinal polyps and fibrocystic breast disease. They are at increased risk for malignancies in all of these areas, particularly breast cancer. *Increased risk of follicular thyroid carcinoma.*
Crouzon syndrome	Named after Octave Crouzon, a French physician. Craniofacial dysostosis affecting the skull and the first branchial arch (precursor of the maxilla and mandible). This autosomal dominant syndrome is caused by a mutation in the fibroblast growth factor receptor. Characterized by hypertelorism, exophthalmos, a hypoplastic mandible and downward-sloping palpebral fissures.
Curtius syndrome	Hypertrophy of an entire side of the body or of a single part. When it occurs in the face, it is known as *congenital hemifacial hypertrophy*.
Dandy syndrome	Oscillopsia caused by bilateral loss of vestibular function, usually as the result of bilateral labyrinthectomy.
Darier disease (keratosis follicularis)	Multiple erythematous, crusted papules distributed over the face and body. These may be particularly troublesome in the external ear canal. White, ragged papules also may be present in the oral cavity.
Dejean syndrome	Characterized by exophthalmos, diplopia, superior maxillary pain and numbness along the route of the trigeminal nerve. It is classically caused by a nasal tumour that traverses the pterygopalatine fossa and invades the floor of the orbit.
De Quervain's thyroiditis	Fritz de Quervain, 1904, Swiss surgeon from Basel. He also suggested iodised salt for endemic goitre. Subacute granulomatous thyroiditis. Most common cause for painful thyroid. Initial hyperthyroidism followed sometimes by transient hypothyroidism and then return to euthyroid state.

E

DiGeorge syndrome	Now known as 22q11.2 deletion syndrome. CATCH-22 (= cardiac defects, abnormal facies, thymic hypoplasia, cleft palate and hypocalcaemia resulting from 22q11.2 deletions). An autosomal dominant defective development of the third and fourth pharyngeal pouches, most frequently manifesting as partial or total agenesis of the thymus (and therefore immune deficiency due to lack of T cells) and parathyroids. Abnormal development of the heart, aortic arch, mandible, external ear and philtrum also may be present. The most common presenting sign is hypocalcaemia in the neonatal period.
Eagle syndrome	Elongation of the styloid process or ossification of the stylohyoid ligament, causing recurrent nonspecific throat discomfort, foreign body sensation, dysphagia or facial pain. Surgical shortening of the styloid process can be effective.
Epstein pearls	Multiple small white nodules on the palate and oral mucosa of newborns. Histologically, they are composed of concentric layers of keratin. No treatment is needed because they disappear spontaneously within a few months.
Escherich sign	Protrusion of the lips elicited by percussion of the inner surface of the lips or tongue. It is seen in hypocalcaemia.
Fordyce disease	A developmental anomaly characterized by enlarged, ectopic sebaceous glands (Fordyce spots) in the oral mucosa. These glands appear as numerous small yellowish white granules.
Frey syndrome	Lucia Frey, 1923, Polish neurologist. Died in the Holocaust. Also known as *auriculotemporal syndrome*. Following parotid surgery, parasympathetic fibres from the auriculotemporal nerve grow into the severed axonal sheaths of sympathetic nerve fibres which innervate the sweat glands. Acetylcholine is the common neurotransmitter. Thus, when a stimulus for salivary flow occurs, sweating of the skin overlying the parotid bed also occurs.
Furstenberg test	Enlargement of a nasal encephalocele on compression of the internal jugular veins.
Garcin syndrome	Consists of motor and sensory deficits involving cranial nerves III through XI. Garcin syndrome can be caused by basilar skull fracture with haemorrhage, basal meningitis, cavernous sinus thrombosis or tumours of the parapharyngeal space. It is also known as *hemipolyneuropathy*.
Gardner syndrome	A subtype of familial adenomatous polyposis. Characterized first usually by multiple osteomas that develop in the skull and facial bones, including the mandible. It is an autosomal-dominant disease; other symptoms include multiple epidermoid cysts of the skin, papillary thyroid cancer and polyposis of the colon and rectum. There is a tendency for these polyps to become malignant.
Goldenhar syndrome	Named after Maurice Goldenhar, a Belgian-American ophthalmologist. Also known as oculo-auriculo-vertebral (OAV) syndrome, it is characterized by underdevelopment of the mandible, external ear, orbit, facial muscles and hemivertebrae of the vertebral column. It is a form of hemifacial microsomia.
Gorlin syndrome	Nevoid basal cell carcinoma syndrome (NBCCS). Autosomal dominant condition that can cause unusual facial appearances and a predisposition for basal cell carcinoma with multiple keratocytic odontogenic tumours.
Gradenigo syndrome	Count Giuseppe Gradenigo, an Italian otolaryngologist. Otorrhoea, pain in the distribution of the ophthalmic branch of the trigeminal nerve and abducens nerve palsy. Originally caused by an extradural abscess involving the petrous bone, this syndrome is now more commonly caused by a tumour at the petrous apex, such as a cholesteatoma, meningioma or other tumour. It is also known as *petrous apex syndrome*.
Griesinger sign	Pain, redness and swelling of the tip of the mastoid, indicative of thrombophlebitis of the sigmoid sinus with involvement of the mastoid emissary veins.
Grisel's syndrome	Non-traumatic subluxation of the atlanto-axial joint caused by inflammation of the adjacent tissues. This is a rare disease that usually affects children. The condition often follows soft-tissue inflammation in the neck such as in cases of upper respiratory tract infections, peritonsillar or retropharyngeal abscesses. Post-operative inflammation after certain procedures such as adenoidectomy can also lead to this condition in susceptible individuals such as those with Down's syndrome.

E

Hashimoto's thyroiditis	Described by Hakaru Hashimoto, a Japanese physician, whilst studying in Germany at the University of Gottingen. Returned to Japan at the start of World War I and died of typhoid. Also known as chronic lymphocytic thyroiditis. An autoimmune disease where auto-antibodies to thyroid peroxidase, thyroglobulin and thyroid-stimulating hormone (TSH) are usually present. It is the most common cause of primary hypothyroidism in North America.
Hennebert sign	In the presence of a normal tympanic membrane, changes in pneumatic pressure produce nystagmus (positive fistula test). The nystagmus is more marked on application of negative pressure. This sign is present with congenital syphilis and is believed to be due to an excessively mobile footplate or to be caused by motion of the saccule mediated by fibrosis between the footplate and the saccule.
Hitselberger sign	Loss of sensation in the postero-superior part of external auditory meatus. May be caused by a vestibular schwannoma.
Hollander syndrome	A rare syndrome in which congenital deafness (presumably due to cochlear abnormalities) is linked to the appearance of a goitre in the third decade of life. Thyroid function tests are normal, but biopsy of thyroid tissue shows a partial defect in thyroxine biosynthesis.
Horner syndrome	Johann Horner, Swiss ophthalmologist. Characterized by (mild) ptosis, miosis (constricted pupil) and anhidrosis due to damage of cervical sympathetic nerves.
Horton neuralgia	An autonomic nervous system disorder also known as cluster headache. Patients have unilateral headaches centred behind or close to the eye, along with ipsilateral nasal congestion, suffusion of the eye, and increased lacrimation. Attacks may occur daily for several weeks, then disappear for months or years until another series (cluster) begins.
Hutchinson teeth	Characterized by small and widely spaced teeth (especially the upper incisors) with notches on their biting surfaces. Only permanent, rather than deciduous, teeth are affected. It is a characteristic sign of congenital syphilis.
Jacobson's nerve	The tympanic branch of the glossopharyngeal nerve (cranial nerve IX). It supplies sensory fibres to the mucosa of the middle ear; running with it are preganglionic parasympathetic fibres that leave the middle ear as the lesser superficial petrosal nerve to eventually innervate the parotid. These fibres are cut in an attempt to relieve the gustatory sweating seen in Frey syndrome.
Jacod syndrome	Consists of progressive ophthalmoplegia, usually starting with paralysis of the oculomotor nerve. This is accompanied or followed by hypesthesia in the distribution of the ophthalmic branch of the trigeminal nerve, exophthalmos and finally involvement of the optic nerve itself. It is caused by a middle cranial fossa tumour that compresses the nerves near the apex of the orbit. It is also called *orbital apex syndrome*.
Jervell and Lange-Nielsen syndrome (JLNS)	First described by Anton Jervell and Fred Lange-Nielsen in 1957. A type of long QT syndrome, associated with severe, bilateral sensorineural hearing loss (i.e. always have electrocardiogram (ECG) for paediatric cochlear implants). *Autosomal recessive*.
Kallmann syndrome	Consists of hypogonadism secondary to lack of gonadotropins, and anosmia due to agenesis of the olfactory bulbs. It is dominant with variable penetrance. The male-to-female ratio is 3:1.
Kartagener's syndrome	Manes Kartagener in 1933. An autosomal recessive primary ciliary dyskinesia with situs inversus. (bronchiectasis, chronic sinusitis and situs inversus).
Kiesselbach's plexus or area	Named after Wilhelm Kiesselbach (1839–1902) a German otolaryngologist. A region in the anteroinferior part of the nasal septum where four arteries anastomose to form a vascular plexus of that name. The arteries are: • Anterior ethmoidal artery (from the ophthalmic artery). • Sphenopalatine artery (terminal branch of the maxillary artery). • Greater palatine artery (from the maxillary artery). • Septal branch of the superior labial artery (from the facial artery). It also has been referred to as Little's area after James L. Little, an American surgeon, who first described the area in 1879.

E

Koplik spots	Pale round spots on the oral mucosa and conjunctiva that are seen in the beginning stages of measles.
Körner's septum	A remnant of the petrosquamous suture line, which may persist as a plate of bone separating the superficial (squamous) group of mastoid air cells from the deeper (petrous) cells.
Langer lines	Tension lines in the skin.
Lemierre's syndrome	André Lemierre, in 1936. French bacteriologist (also known as postanginal septicaemia). Refers to thrombophlebitis of the internal jugular vein. It most often develops as a complication of a bacterial sore throat infection (e.g. *Fusobacterium necrophorum*) in young, otherwise healthy adults. The thrombophlebitis is a serious condition and may lead to further systemic complications such as bacteraemia or septic emboli.
Lermoyez syndrome	Characterized by attacks of tinnitus and deafness followed by a bout of vertigo that surprisingly relieves the vestibuloacoustic symptoms. It is similar to Ménière's disease. The symptoms in Lermoyez syndrome tend to occur in younger patients than Ménière's disease does, and unlike the latter, gradually resolve over time with no permanent hearing loss.
Lhermitte's sign	Jean Lhermitte, French neurologist in 1924. Sign usually attributed to multiple sclerosis but also a rare complication of radiotherapy to the head and neck region, causing myelopathy of the spinal cord. Symptoms consist of transient electrical sensation running down the spine and limbs upon neck flexion.
Lillie–Crowe test	Used to diagnose unilateral lateral sinus occlusion. Digital compression of the opposite internal jugular vein causes the retinal veins to dilate because the major venous outflow tracts on both sides are now blocked.
Ludwig's angina	German physician, Wilhelm Friedrich von Ludwig who first described this condition in 1836. *ankhon* = Greek for strangle. A rapidly spreading infection of the submandibular, sublingual and submental spaces. It produces swelling and elevation of the tongue and a brawny induration of the floor of the mouth. It is a diffuse infection, with little or no abscess formation. Its major danger is airway obstruction, and patients may require a tracheostomy until the swelling subsides. The cause of Ludwig angina is usually an odontogenic infection, with streptococci, bacteroides and oral anaerobes being the most common pathogens. Treatment is by antibiotics and drainage of any area of fluctuance.
Maffucci syndrome	Characterized by cavernous haemangiomas of the head and neck. Affected patients also have multiple endochondromas, with shortening of the involved bones. Twenty to 40% of patients have malignant degeneration of one or more endochondromas into chondrosarcoma.
Marjolin ulcer	A squamous cell carcinoma that arises at the site of an old burn scar, often 20 to 40 years after the initial burn. It is often locally aggressive and metastasizes early.
Meckel's cartilage	The embryonic cartilage from which the mandible, incus and malleus are derived. (First branchial arch.)
Meckel's cave	A diverticulum of dura and arachnoidea encephali mater that lies on the anterolateral surface of the petrous ridge in the middle cranial fossa and contains the trigeminal ganglion.
Melkersson–Rosenthal syndrome	Characterized by manifestations in childhood or early adolescence as recurring attacks of unilateral or bilateral facial paralysis with concomitant swelling of the lips and tongue. Affected patients also have a fissured tongue that becomes more prominent with age. It is an autosomal-dominant disease with variable penetrance. The cause is unknown.
Ménière's syndrome	In 1861, Prosper Ménière gave a presentation to the French Academy of Medicine describing a series of patients who experienced episodic vertigo and hearing loss. Ménière's syndrome is characterised by episodic vertigo, sensorineural hearing loss and tinnitus. A sensation of aural fullness commonly accompanies this classical triad of symptoms.
Michel aplasia	Complete labyrinthine aplasia. Middle ear structures may be absent. The external ear and canal are usually normal in appearance.

E

Mikulicz cells	Named after Johann von Mikulicz, a Polish professor of surgery. Large vacuolated histiocytes containing phagocytised bacteria, characteristic of rhinoscleroma.
Mikulicz disease	Bilateral, recurrent inflammatory enlargement of the lacrimal and salivary glands. When due to a manifestation of some other systemic disease, such as lymphocytosis or tuberculosis, it is known as Mikulicz syndrome. Pathology shows a diffuse lymphocytic infiltrate.
Möbius syndrome	Congenital facial paralysis (usually bilateral) with paralysis of the abducens nerve and sometimes other oculomotor nerves. Pathologically the few cases studied have usually shown hypoplasia of the involved brainstem nuclei.
Mondini dysplasia	A cochlea with incomplete partitioning and a reduced number of turns, an enlarged vestibular aqueduct and a dilated vestibule. Sensorineural hearing loss may present in childhood and can be associated with minor head trauma. There is also a predisposition to perilymph fistulae and meningitis.
Sinus of Morgagni	A defect between the upper edge of the superior constrictor muscle and the buccopharyngeal fascia through which the eustachian tube passes.
Nager syndrome	Characterized by facies similar to those seen with Treacher Collins syndrome. Affected patients also present with preaxial upper limb defects, microtia, atresia of the external auditory canals and malformation of the ossicles. Conductive and mixed hearing losses may occur. The inheritance pattern has not been determined, because most cases are sporadic. Also known as *acrofacial dysostosis*.
Oliver sign	A pulling sensation felt in the larynx and trachea due to an aortic arch aneurysm. It is most evident when the head is extended.
Ondine's curse	Named after the myth of Ondine, a water nymph who had an unfaithful mortal lover. He swore to her that his 'every waking breath would be a testimony of [his] love', and upon witnessing his adultery, she cursed that if he should fall asleep, he would forget to breathe. Eventually, he fell asleep from sheer exhaustion, and his breathing stopped. Failure of respiratory drive, especially during sleep. Congenital central hypoventilation syndrome (CCHS). Treatment is tracheostomy with mechanical ventilation at night, although bilateral phrenic pacing has been used successfully in some patients.
Orphan Annie-eye nuclei	Large nuclei which appear empty. Typically seen in papillary thyroid carcinoma but also seen in autoimmune thyroid disease and polymorphous low-grade adenocarcinoma. Named after a comic strip character popular in the 1930s, Little Orphan Annie, who was depicted with vacant circles for eyes.
Ortner syndrome	A rare cause of hoarseness in infants with congenital cardiac disease. Compression of the left recurrent laryngeal nerve between the aorta and a dilated pulmonary artery results in paralysis of the left vocal cord.
Osler–Weber–Rendu disease	Hereditary haemorrhagic telangiectasia, characterized by punctate telangiectasias usually developing around puberty and commonly seen in the oral and nasal mucosa and tongue. Patients commonly present with epistaxis and may have visceral arteriovenous malformations (AVMs). Autosomal dominant inheritance.
Pancoast tumour	Henry Pancoast, American radiologist. Pulmonary sulcus tumour of pulmonary apex. Usually non-small cell carcinoma.
Pancoast syndrome	Shoulder pain radiating down the distribution of the ulnar nerve of the arm, caused by local extension of a tumour in the apex of the lung that eventually invades the brachial plexus. Horner syndrome, indicating involvement of the cervical sympathetic chain, also may be present.
Passavant ridge	A horizontal mucosal fold across the posterior pharynx that is the point of contact by the soft palate when the nasopharynx is closed during the act of swallowing. Whether this is an active or passive fold is still unresolved.

E

Pendred syndrome	An autosomal-recessive syndrome consisting of a bilateral congenital sensorineural hearing loss, enlarged vestibular aqueducts and the appearance of a goitre years later in mid-childhood. T4 levels are usually low to absent, and a perchlorate test is diagnostic. The hearing loss is non-reversible.
Peutz–Jeghers syndrome	An autosomal-dominant disorder whose two main components are benign polyps of the intestinal tract and mucocutaneous melanotic macules. The latter bring these patients to the attention of the otolaryngologist and may appear at any time from infancy to adulthood. The macules are most common around the facial orifices (perioral, perinasal and periorbital) and on the buccal mucosa. This syndrome is not to be confused with Gardner syndrome, in which the intestinal polyps tend to become malignant.
Pfeiffer syndrome	Named after Rudolf Arthur Pfeiffer. An autosomal dominant craniosynostosis with abnormalities of the hands and feet. Associated with mutations in fibroblast growth factor receptor.
Pierre Robin sequence	Named after a French dental surgeon. Consists of micrognathia (relative) glossoptosis and cleft palate. There is no sex predilection. The cause is believed to be arrested intrauterine development; the syndrome may occur as an isolated triad or as part of a larger constellation of defects. Affected infants often present with choking and aspiration, presumably due to the hypoplastic mandible and glossoptosis.
Plummer–Vinson syndrome	The disease is named after two Americans: the physician Henry Stanley Plummer and the surgeon Porter Paisley Vinson. It is occasionally known as Paterson–Kelly or Paterson–Brown-Kelly syndrome in the United Kingdom, after Derek Brown–Kelly and Donald Ross Paterson. Characterized by pale skin, dysphagia, atrophy of the tongue papillae, and sometimes oral leukoplakia or angular cheilitis, found almost exclusively in middle-aged women. This condition is primarily due to an iron-deficiency anaemia, with a deficiency of vitamins and protein apparently also playing a role. The dysphagia is attributed to the formation of an oesophageal web, although how or why the web is formed is unknown. There also may be an increased risk of postcricoid cancer in these patients. Treatment is iron supplementation. It is also known as *sideroblastic dysphagia*.
Prussak's space	The upper tympanic recess, bounded by the pars flaccida laterally, the neck of the malleus medially, the lateral mallear ligament superiorly, and the lateral process of the malleus inferiorly. Because it has only small openings anteriorly and posteriorly, it can be a common site for cholesteatoma.
Raeder syndrome	Characterized by severe unilateral orbital pain with accompanying miosis and ptosis, but not anhidrosis. Paralysis of one or more ocular nerves may be seen. It is also known as incomplete *Horner syndrome.*
Ramsay Hunt syndrome	Herpes zoster oticus. Classically described as a unilateral otalgia and facial paralysis accompanied by a vesicular rash in the external ear. It is caused by a herpetic infection of the cranial nerves. Patients also can have a sensorineural hearing loss, vertigo and tinnitus. There have been some reports of improvement in symptoms following treatment with oral acyclovir.
Rathke's cleft cyst	A benign growth found on the pituitary gland in the brain, specifically a fluid-filled cyst in the posterior portion of the anterior pituitary gland. It occurs when the Rathke's pouch does not develop properly, and ranges in size from 2 to 40 mm in diameter.
Reed–Sternberg cells	Binucleate or multinucleate B cells with prominent nuclei characteristic of Hodgkin's lymphoma.
Riedel's thyroiditis	Bernhard Riedel, a German surgeon, first recognized the disease in 1883. An extremely rare form of chronic thyroiditis in which a fibrotic reaction of unknown aetiology replaces most thyroid tissue and frequently extends out of the thyroid capsule to compress adjacent structures. Patients are usually middle-aged women and may present with a painless neck mass, dysphagia, or hoarseness. Now thought to be a type of immunoglobulin G4 (IgG4) disease.
Ducts of Rivinus	Small salivary ducts that pass directly from the upper border of the sublingual gland to empty into the oral cavity. Also see Bartholin duct.

E

Node of Rouvier	Lateral retropharyngeal node. It is a common target of metastases in nasopharyngeal carcinoma.
Fissures of Santorini	Fissures in the anterior bony external auditory canal leading to the parotid region.
Scarpa's ganglion	Antonio Scarpa, Italian anatomist and surgeon. The ganglion containing the cell bodies of the bipolar cells making up the vestibular nerve. It is located at the lateral end of the internal auditory canal.
Scheibe aplasia	Also known as cochleosaccular dysplasia, it is the most common type of cochlear dysplasia. The bony labyrinth is completely formed, as are the utricle and semicircular canals. The pars inferior (saccule and cochlear duct) are undifferentiated, and the membranous cochlea is malformed.
Sjögren syndrome	All known as sicca syndrome and described in 1933 by Henrik Sjögren, a Swedish ophthalmologist. Defined by the presence of two or more of the following symptoms: dry eyes (keratoconjunctivitis sicca), dry mouth (xerostomia), painless swelling of the parotid glands and polyarthritis. Most frequently seen in middle-aged women, its aetiology is unknown, although an autoimmune cause is suspected.
Sluder neuralgia	Similar to Horton neuralgia (cluster headache) and also known as *sphenopalatine neuralgia*. It is sometimes treated by vidian neurectomy.
Stickler syndrome	It was first studied and characterized by Gunnar B. Stickler in 1965. Hereditary progressive arthro-ophthalmopathy. A group of hereditary conditions affecting collagen. Stickler syndrome is characterized by distinctive facial abnormalities, ocular problems, hearing loss, and joint problems. Some subtypes have an autosomal dominant inheritance pattern while others are autosomal recessive.
Sturge–Weber syndrome	Characterized by a unilateral port-wine stain somewhere within the distribution of the trigeminal nerve. It is apparently a defect of the mesodermal component of blood vessels and is further characterized by angioma of the leptomeninges, orbit, mouth and nasal mucosa. Intracerebral calcifications seen on plain radiographs are diagnostic. Symptoms include seizures, hemiparesis and glaucoma. There is no known treatment.
Tapia's syndrome	Spanish otolaryngologist Antonio Garcia Tapia in 1904. Unilateral extracranial nerves X and XII palsy. It was first described in two bullfighters who were gored in the neck. The syndrome also may be caused by a tumour in the deep lobe of the parotid and has been reported in brachial plexus blocks and post-intubation.
Tolosa–Hunt syndrome	Unilateral retroorbital pain and ophthalmoplegia, which may be either steadily progressive or recurrent. It is thought to be due to inflammation of the cavernous sinus by any of several causes.
Thornwaldt cyst	A cyst that arises from the pharyngeal bursa (pouch of Luschka). Its location is in the midline of the posterior nasopharynx, surrounded by adenoid tissue. It can become infected and present as a nasopharyngeal mass.
Treacher Collins syndrome	Also known as mandibulofacial dysostosis, an autosomal dominant disorder characterized in children by a severely hypoplastic mandible. Infants sometimes require tracheostomy because of lack of anterior support of the tongue. Other features of the syndrome are down-sloping palpebral fissures, defects of the external ear, auditory canal, and ossicles, and occasionally, cleft palate. TCOF1 mutations are the most common cause of the disorder.
Trotter syndrome (sinus of Morgagni syndrome)	May be seen with tumours of the nasopharynx that block the eustachian tube and produce a conductive hearing loss secondary to middle-ear fluid. Other symptoms may be pain in the distribution of the ophthalmic branch of the trigeminal nerve, decreased mobility of the soft palate, and possibly trismus.
Trousseau's sign	Armand Trousseau, a French physician in 1861 described tetany caused by a tourniquet placed around the arm of a patient with hypocalcaemia.

E

Tullio phenomenon	First described in 1929 by the Italian biologist Prof. Pietro Tullio (1881–1941). During his experiments on pigeons, Tullio discovered that by drilling tiny holes in the semicircular canals of his subjects, he could subsequently cause them balance problems when exposed to sound. Said to be present when a loud noise precipitates vertigo. It can be present with congenital syphilis or a perilymph fistula. The tympanic membrane and ossicular chain must be intact with a mobile footplate.
Turner syndrome	Gonadal dysgenesis syndrome. The phenotype is always female, and the karyotype is usually XO. Signs and symptoms include growth retardation, webbed neck, primary amenorrhea, lack of secondary sex characteristics, cardiac abnormalities and ocular problems. Treatment is oestrogen replacement.
Usher syndrome	Described by Charles Usher, a Scottish ophthalmologist in 1914. A leading cause of deaf-blindness. Characterized by a multitude of progressive sensory deficits, including sensorineural hearing loss, retinitis pigmentosa and anosmia. The mechanism is postulated to be degeneration of both central pathways and neuroectodermal tissue at the sensory end-organ. Autosomal recessive.
Vail syndrome	A unilateral, nocturnal pain in the nose, face and eye along with rhinorrhea and symptoms of sinusitis. It is postulated to be due to irritation of the vidian nerve secondary to sphenoid sinusitis. It is also known as *vidian neuralgia*.
Vernet syndrome	Another jugular foramen syndrome with involvement of cranial nerves IX, X and XI. It may be due to trauma, an aneurysm, a tumour, or other conditions.
Vidian nerve	Also called the *nerve of the pterygoid canal*. It is formed by the union of the greater and deep petrosal nerves. It is sometimes sectioned in an attempt to control severe vasomotor rhinitis.
Villaret syndrome	Similar to Vernet syndrome, with the addition of the deficits associated with Horner syndrome, indicating involvement of the cervical sympathetic chain. This syndrome suggests a lesion distal to the jugular foramen, usually in the retrostyloid area.
Waardenburg syndrome	Described by Dutch ophthalmologist Petrus Johannes Waardenburg in 1951. An autosomal dominant group of disorders characterised by sensorineural hearing loss, which may be present at birth or develop later in life, and changes in pigmentation. Other manifestations of the syndrome include hypertelorism (type I Waardenburg), heterochromia iridis and partial albinism which often expressed as a white forelock. Hirshsprung's disease is associated with type IV.
Wallenberg syndrome	Also known as *lateral medullary syndrome or posterior inferior cerebellar artery syndrome*. Characterized by vertigo, nystagmus, nausea and vomiting, Horner syndrome, dysphagia, dysphonia, falling to the side of the lesion, and loss of pain and temperature sense on the ipsilateral face and contralateral side below the neck. It is caused by thrombosis of the posteroinferior cerebellar artery, leading to ischemia of the ipsilateral brainstem.
Weber syndrome	Classic symptoms of damage to the oculomotor nerve at its emergence from the mid-brain, combined with damage to the adjacent pyramidal tract prior to its decussation. In addition, there is ipsilateral paralysis of cranial nerve III and contralateral paralysis of the extremities, face and tongue.
Wildervack (cervico-oculo-acoustic) syndrome	A congenital syndrome seen primarily in females, presenting at birth with a mixed hearing loss, a short, webbed neck with fused cervical vertebrae, and bilateral abducens palsy. It is similar to Klippel Feil syndrome.
Winkler disease	Chondrodermatitis nodularis chronica helicis. A disease of the helix of the ear, seen primarily in men over 40 years of age. It presents as one or more painful nodules. Pathologically, both the skin and the perichondrium are involved. Treatment is surgical excision, with recurrences common.

E

22 Evidence-Based Medicine

22.1 Introduction

Over 20 years ago, Professor David Sackett and his colleagues defined evidence-based medicine (EBM) as the conscientious, explicit and judicious use of current best evidence in making decisions about the care of individual patients. This remains an excellent definition, drawing out all the key aspects of evidence-based practice. It refers to current best evidence and not specifically to evidence from randomised controlled trials (RCTs), or even systematic reviews, despite their premier position in the evidence hierarchy. The critical issues here are that the evidence used should be the best available, and up-to-date.

The process is conscientious, explicit and judicious; each of these is important. Care must be taken in each and every aspect of the use of the evidence, just as an otolaryngologist would with every other element of patient care. The process must be explicit. While not every stage may be outlined explicitly to the patient during a consultation, the practitioner needs to avoid obfuscation and be clear in her or his own mind about how they are weighing the evidence. This must, in particular, include weighing the benefits against any potential harm or cost. 'Judicious' implies careful and sensible judgement—the use of common sense. EBM is not, nor ever has been—'cook book medicine' involving the slavish following of fixed rules. Rather, the practice involves a careful integration of knowledge of the relevant evidence with the patient's own individual characteristics.

Amongst the most important of these are the patient's values and beliefs, and their attitude towards risk and uncertainty. The original definition rightly highlights the care of *individual* patients. Although data from the trials and reviews that underpin evidence-based practice may come from groups of patients, and aggregated data derived therefrom, the evidence from this data is used, by the clinician, for the individual management of their patient. The evidence can only be used to make good decisions when the clinician has a clear understanding of the patient's unique characteristics (how pathophysiological processes are affecting them personally, in their specific context) and their wishes, values and beliefs.

In the 21st century, we have learnt the importance of shared decision making. The original definition of Sackett et al may nowadays be seen to be rather paternalistic. It focuses on the practitioner of EBM making the decisions for, or on behalf of, the patient. A more modern version might be as follows:

'EBM is the conscientious, explicit and judicious use of current best evidence in helping individual patients to make decisions about their care'.

This revised definition emphasises that patients and health professionals work together and share the decision-making process.

22.2 Systematic Reviews and the Evidence Hierarchy

EBM practitioners look for 'best evidence'. The Oxford Centre for Evidence-Based Medicine has developed a hierarchy of different types of evidence. This can help practitioners when they are looking at different types of evidence into, for example, the effects of treatment, diagnostic test accuracy, prognosis, harms and screening. When considering the effectiveness or otherwise of interventions (treatments), the highest level of evidence (level 1) is provided by systematic reviews (or, much less commonly, by an N-of-1 randomised trial). Level 2 evidence can come from a randomised trial or an observational study where the treatment effect is large. ▶ Table 22.1 lists the levels of evidence for therapeutic studies.

Systematic reviews locate, appraise and synthesise evidence from scientific studies using a particular, pre-specified, scientific method. This is in contrast to the more traditional, nonsystematic review articles that have been (and continue to be) published in the literature. It is common nowadays to find articles in journals purporting to be systematic reviews; there is evidence that inclusion of such articles can improve a journal's impact factor. However, the reader should beware. Not all published systematic reviews are of high quality. Many fail to follow a pre-specified plan, or are conducted in such a way that they may be prone to bias.

In order to minimise the chance of bias, and to avoid re-duplication of effort, the authors

▶ **Table 22.1** Levels of evidence for therapeutic studies

Level	Type of evidence
1A	Systematic review (with homogeneity) of RCTs
1B	Individual RCT (with narrow confidence intervals)
1C	All or none study
2A	Systematic review (with homogeneity) of cohort studies
2B	Individual Cohort study (including low quality RCT, e.g. < 80% follow-up)
2C	"Outcomes" research; Ecological studies
3A	Systematic review (with homogeneity) of case-control studies
3B	Individual Case-control study
4	Case series (and poor quality cohort and case-control study
5	Expert opinion without explicit critical appraisal or based on physiology bench research or "first principles"

Source: From the Centre for Evidence-Based Medicine, http://www.cebm.net
Abbreviation: RCT, randomised controlled trial

E

of systematic reviews should write a protocol setting out, before they start, what they plan to do. That protocol should be published and should ideally be lodged with a database such as PROSPERO, an international prospective register of systematic reviews. Cochrane (www.cochrane.org) is an independent, global, not-for-profit, charitable organisation, originally established in 1993, that publishes high-quality systematic reviews electronically in the Cochrane Library (www.cochranelibrary.com). These reviews have been described as setting the 'gold standard' for systematic reviews. All Cochrane reviews are based on protocols that have previously been published in the library.

The protocol for a systematic review sets out the specific clinical question that the authors are asking. In the case of a review of treatment, it describes the sort of **p**atients (participants) that the authors are interested in, what **i**ntervention or treatment the review evaluates, what **c**omparator and, very importantly, what **o**utcomes are of interest to the authors. These four elements— **P**articipants, **I**ntervention, **C**omparator, and **O**utcomes—constitute the 'PICO'. Asking the right question—getting the right PICO—is a critical stage in the systematic review process. It is especially important that systematic reviews look at the right outcomes. These should be the outcomes that are most important to patients, their families and practitioners, and are not necessarily those that have been most frequently evaluated by

researchers. It is always tempting to measure things that can most easily be measured, but the authors of systematic reviews are encouraged to take a step back and ask themselves: Which outcomes are most important to patients and how best can these be measured? Ideally, this is done without prior knowledge of the outcomes that have in fact been evaluated in previous studies. In reality, most authors have some awareness of these as they have a pre-existing interest in trials in this area.

The clinical question posed by the authors of a systematic review may be very broad or very narrow. An example of a very broad question might be 'interventions for patients with sleep apnoea'. Such a title implies that the authors might include studies that have evaluated adults and children, with sleep apnoea diagnosed in any way (or even simply suspected on clinical grounds). Also, that all possible interventions would be of interest: surgery (of any sort), medication, continuous positive airway pressure (CPAP), devices, etc. It says nothing about the outcomes of interest.

At the other extreme, a very much narrower title would be CPAP to improve cognition in young children (≤ 10) with sleep apnoea proven using polysomnography. This is a much narrower group of participants (children ≤ 10 with polysomnography-proven sleep apnoea) and a single intervention (CPAP) and a single outcome (cognition). As detailed as this title might appear, there are still some uncertainties that would need to be spelt out in the protocol. What does 'polysomnography-proven sleep apnoea' really mean? What specific diagnostic criteria would need to be present? What type of CPAP are we interested in? Used for how long? How is 'cognition' to be measured, over what period, and at what time points?

It should be clear to the reader that if a question is too focussed, it is less likely that the authors of the review will find studies that address the issues in question. Even if one or more studies are identified, will the results of the ensuing review be applicable to the sorts of patients most people see in their clinics? But conversely, if the question is too broad, other problems arise. Is it then sensible to combine the studies in a single review? As we will see below, if a systematic review includes a meta-analysis, the assumption is that the set of studies being synthesised by meta-analysis are evaluating a common treatment effect. This is unlikely to be the case with a heterogeneous set of trials including a wide variety of participants and interventions.

The protocol also specifies the type of studies that the review will evaluate. Many systematic reviews are reviews of RCTs. However, it is possible to do systematic reviews of non-randomised or observational studies. Many novice reviewers believe that it will be easier to do a systematic review of non-randomised studies than of RCTs. This is not usually the case. Cochrane, and in general the broader scholarly community preparing systematic reviews, has invested much effort in honing the techniques required to 'locate' and 'appraise' RCTs. For a systematic review to be comprehensive, and hence for it to be of the highest quality, it is imperative that all trials that merit inclusion are located and assessed. Considerable efforts have been made over the last 20 years to identify *all* RCTs that have been undertaken (whether published or not) and to encourage prospective registration of trials now being undertaken. The Cochrane Library includes the Cochrane Central Register of Controlled Trials (CENTRAL). This brings together the specialist registers of randomised and quasi-randomised controlled trials from each of the over 50, subject-specific, Cochrane Review Groups. This is a unique and rich resource for those seeking records of RCTs. Searches for non-randomised studies are more difficult to undertake and will not necessarily identify all the studies that might reasonably be included in a systematic review.

Similarly, there are established, published, evaluated methods for 'appraising' RCTs. These evaluate the 'risk of bias' of the identified studies. The assessment of risk of bias in non-randomised studies is less well developed and these studies are invariably, inherently, at greater risk of such biases than RCTs. Full details of the methods of the systematic review in general and risk of bias assessment in particular are beyond the scope of this chapter, but the Cochrane Handbook provides comprehensive guidance on undertaking a high-quality systematic review. The handbook also explains why the 'risk of bias' of a study included in a review is more important than the 'quality' of a study. It is easy to confuse these two notions but the distinction is important. There are many situations where an RCT may have been done to as high a quality as possible, but there remains a risk of bias. A simple example is a situation where blinding of participants or those who provide the intervention or assess the outcomes is not possible. Here we have a high-quality trial, but there is still a risk of bias. Conversely, a trial may have been undertaken and reported and it is not clear to the reader of a report whether some of the features of a high-quality trial are present or not (e.g., there may be no report of a sample size calculation). This may therefore be thought of as a low-quality trial. However, nonetheless, the trial may have clearly been conducted in such a way that the risk of bias is low.

The word 'quality' will often appear in a systematic review, in a different context. That is, in an assessment not of the quality of a study but the quality of evidence for a particular *outcome*. The 'Grading of Recommendations Assessment, Development and Evaluation (GRADE) approach provides a system for rating quality of evidence and strength of recommendations that is explicit, comprehensive, transparent and pragmatic and is increasingly being adopted by organisations worldwide'. This approach has been widely adopted and is used in Cochrane reviews as a way of conveying to users the strength of evidence, or certainty, of the findings of the review.

22.3 Meta-Analysis

Having located and appraised the trials relevant to the question posed in a systematic review, it *may* be appropriate to undertake a meta-analysis. Such an analysis is not an obligatory part of a review.

It is perfectly acceptable to present the results of individual trials that the review has identified, separately, and in a narrative fashion on some occasions. This may be the only possibility when, for example, different studies have measured different outcomes or measured the same outcomes in different ways.

The results of studies should *only* be combined mathematically in an analysis if it is sensible to do so. The data from the trials being combined in this way must be measuring the same phenomenon or effect, in the same way. That is, the method of measurement must be the same in the individual trials or at the very least it must be possible to extract data from the individual studies that allow the reviewer to produce comparable data from the individual studies.

It may be helpful to consider an 'ideal' meta-analysis. Imagine a large, multicentre RCT conducted across, say, four centres. The inclusion criteria for the trial are the same at all centres, and the intervention is the same. All centres measure the same outcomes in the same way. In this case, the aggregated results, from the four individual centres, could be meta-analysed in the sure and certain knowledge that the conditions for a meta-analysis had been met. In reality, the individual patient data, rather than aggregated data, would be available and would be combined. The key thing about this example is the similarity between the data from all four centres, even though each contributed different, individual patients. There is no doubt that the centres were each measuring the same thing and that the four 'point estimates' (the mean effect for each centre) were estimating the mean of all the patients combined across all four centres, and that in turn this was an estimate of the 'population mean,' the hypothetical population of *all* patients with these characteristics subjected to this treatment.

Now, consider four different trials, in different countries, but with only trivial differences between the inclusion criteria and the intervention. Might it be reasonable to combine the results from each of these in a meta-analysis? Probably, if the differences were indeed only trivial. However, what if the differences were non-trivial? In one trial, the participants were, on average, slightly older. In another, they were significantly sicker. Can these studies be combined? This is where the clinical expertise of members of the systematic review team becomes critical. There are *often* non-trivial differences between studies included in a systematic review, potentially in terms of all elements of the PICO, but especially important here are the participants and the intervention. Clinical expertise will decide whether it is sensible to combine studies.

Sometimes it is deemed appropriate *a priori* (in the protocol) to specify that studies with similar characteristics *will* be combined, but that specific subgroup analyses will be performed. This is because it is anticipated that specific characteristics may affect the nature or extent of any treatment effect (they may be so-called 'effect modifiers'). For example, it might be expected that patients with 'serious' disease may respond differently from those with 'mild or moderate' disease. A carefully conducted subgroup analysis can explore this.

Whether a subgroup analysis is specified in advance, it is always important to look critically at the result of combining data from studies in a meta-analysis, and to seek to identify any 'heterogeneity'. Simply by visually examining the forest plot that is part of a meta-analysis, it may be clear that the scatter of results (the variation between the results of individual studies) is more than might be expected by chance alone (recall that in the idealised meta-analysis described above, nobody would expect all the results from each of the four centres to be exactly the same; some variability is bound to occur). It is also possible to conduct a statistical test to assess this. This is the I^2 test. The test asks the question: Can the amount of variability between the results of different studies in this analysis be accounted for by chance alone? If the answer is yes, heterogeneity is low (and the I^2 value—given as a percentage—is also zero or low). If heterogeneity is high, the reviewer needs to ask themselves why this is the case. One possibility is that there are significant differences between the studies included in the meta-analysis and to undertake such an analysis is therefore inappropriate.

22.4 Results

When interpreting the results of a systematic review and meta-analysis, there are many important issues, but two deserve special mention. Firstly, 'absence of evidence' is not the same as 'evidence of absence'. Many reviews will not find

E

evidence of a treatment effect, but this is not the same as 'proving' that something is ineffective and review authors must not make the mistake of saying so.

Secondly, all practitioners and patients must carefully consider, before undertaking a review (or indeed a trial) what—for any specific outcome—would constitute a clinically meaningful difference in whatever measurement was used to assess that outcome. It is all too easy to focus on 'statistically significant' findings, when what is more important is a difference in outcomes that means something to patients.

22.5 Conclusion

In the 21st century, in all areas of life, there is now a focus on an evidence-based approach. This is no longer solely in health care. Professionals and lay people alike need a clear understanding of what this means and how best evidence is sought, appraised, analysed and then integrated with many other important individual and societal factors.

Further Reading

Alderson P. Absence of evidence is not evidence of absence. BMJ. 2004; 328(7438):476–477

Collaboration C. The Cochrane Handbook. http://www.cochrane-handbook.org. Accessed December 18, 2017

Elwyn G, Frosch D, Thomson R, et al. Shared decision making: a model for clinical practice. J Gen Intern Med. 2012; 27(10): 1361–1367

Guyatt GH, Oxman AD, Vist GE, et al; GRADE Working Group. GRADE: an emerging consensus on rating quality of evidence and strength of recommendations. BMJ. 2008; 336(7650): 924–926

Higgins JP, Thompson SG, Deeks JJ, Altman DG. Measuring inconsistency in meta-analyses. BMJ. 2003; 327(7414): 557–560

Howick J, Chalmers I, Glasziou P, et al. The 2011 Oxford CEBM Levels of Evidence (Introductory Document). http://www.cebm.net/index.aspx?o=5653

PROSPERO International prospective register of systematic reviews. https://www.crd.york.ac.uk/prospero/

Sackett DL, Rosenberg WM, Gray JA, Haynes RB, Richardson WS. Evidence based medicine: what it is and what it isn't. BMJ. 1996; 312((7023):71–72

Related Topic of Interest

Literature review and statistics

E

23 Evoked Response Audiometry

In response to sound stimulation, neural electrical potentials are produced by various parts of the auditory system from cochlea to cortex. Evoked response audiometry (ERA) is the technique designed to measure these signals. No conscious response is required from the patient, thus these tests can be considered as more objective measures of the auditory system (there is usually a subjective evaluation of the waveforms obtained but some equipment utilises an objective measure of the probability of the waveform being present). ERA is ideal where patient cooperation is not forthcoming, such as small children, suspected malingering adults, etc.

The evoked potentials may be evoked by an external stimulus (exogenous) where the response is related to the nature of the stimulating signal or by a cognitive response to a signal (endogenous) related more to the psychological significance of that signal.

Other than electrocochleography, these potentials are recorded using scalp electrodes and are, by their nature, of small magnitude. Therefore, efforts need to be made to amplify the signal and reduce the background signal 'noise'.

Signal detection is optimised by appropriate electrode placement with recording electrodes at opposite positions so that a positive potential in one corresponds to an equal and opposite negative potential in the other. Background noise is reduced by having the subject in a quiet, dimly lit room and a comfortable position to avoid distractions and eye, and other muscle, movements. The signal-to-noise ratio is improved by amplification, filtering, removal of random noise (picked up by the ground electrode) and by repetition and averaging.

The amplitudes and latencies (time delay) of the various potentials differ at various parts of the auditory system and this information can be used appropriately for amplifier and filter settings, to allow a more focused analysis of the various potentials.

Furthermore, the nature (click/chirp/tone burst), frequency and volume of the stimulus also affect amplitude and latency. So, for example, louder sounds, by virtue of synchronously stimulating more neural elements, produce shorter latencies and larger amplitudes.

Finally, the majority of measured responses are designated as transient. In other words, the interval between successive stimuli is sufficient to allow the auditory system to return to its resting state before the next signal occurs. However, if the interval between stimuli is shortened so that the response to the previous signal has not died away before the next signal is received, then the resulting response is referred to as a 'steady-state response' (SSR).

There are a number of different measurable responses, shown in ▶ Fig. 23.1, and includes cochlear, brainstem, middle-latency, long-latency and cognitive potentials. Middle-latency potentials, at around 25 ms, lend themselves to SSRs and are the most studied of this phenomena.

E

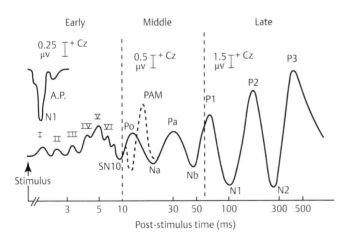

Fig. 23.1 Range of evoked response audiometry (ERA) responses.

The three tests in commonest use are as follows:

1. Electrocochleography.
2. Auditory nerve and brainstem-evoked potentials.
3. Cortical electrical response audiometry.

23.1 Electrocochleography

Electrocochleography (ECochG) aims to measure the signal produced by the cochlea and cochlear nerve in response to acoustic stimulation.

23.2 Technique

The patient lies comfortably in a soundproof room. A ground electrode is attached to the patient's forehead and a reference electrode to the ipsilateral mastoid. The active electrode is usually a transtympanic needle placed on the promontory (tympanic membrane or extratympanic canal electrodes may be used but give a less satisfactory signal) after preparation with local anaesthetic (EMLA). The test signal can be produced using a loudspeaker or headphones (especially if acoustic conditions are less than ideal). Wideband clicks and high-frequency tone bursts are the usual stimulating test signals.

23.3 Physiology

The signal recorded by ECochG is described as a compound action potential (▶Fig. 23.2). It is diphasic at threshold and is made up of three parts: (a) The cochlear microphonic (CM): This signal is produced by the hair cells and resembles the pattern of the basilar membrane vibration. It has no threshold and increases in amplitude with the stimulus intensity. Its polarity follows that of the test signal. (b) The summating potential (SP): This complex potential is derived from a variety of sources but, in essence, is an alteration of the electrical potential baseline (usually negative) in response to a sound stimulus. It is also produced by cochlear hair cells and does not adapt in response to high stimulation rates. (c) The action potential (AP): This is the depolarisation of the cochlear nerve and is similar in many respects to any neural depolarisation. It has a threshold, is independent of signal polarity, and exhibits adaptation.

23.4 Clinical Indications

High-resolution computerised axial tomography and magnetic resonance imaging (MRI) have superseded many older otological investigative techniques and consequently removed many of the indications for EcochG, particularly the search for an acoustic neuroma. In current practice, ECochG is rarely used but may be useful for the following:

1. Threshold testing. ECochG is the most accurate of the electrical response audiometric techniques for threshold testing and can predict to within 5 to 10 dB of the psychoacoustic threshold at 3 to 4 kHz. Unfortunately, it gives little low-frequency information (< 1 kHz) but has the advantage of being a monaural test technique and is relatively resistant to minor muscular contractions which would preclude brainstem response audiometry and is unaffected by general anaesthetic. It is therefore

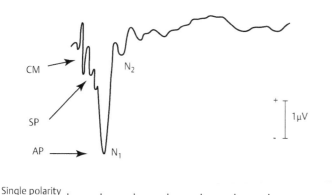

Fig. 23.2 Example of electrocochleography waveform.

particularly useful in very young children or those with neurological disorders.

2. Investigation of suspected Ménière's disease. Typically, there is an increase in the summating potential with a normal action potential in the affected ear.

3. Intra-operative monitoring during surgery around the inner ear and internal meatus.

23.5 Auditory Nerve and Brainstem-Evoked Potentials

Brainstem-evoked response audiometry (BERA), auditory brainstem response (ABR) or auditory brainstem-evoked potentials (ABEPs) record the signals produced in the cochlear nerve and brainstem detected by electrodes placed over the mastoid, forehead and vertex.

23.6 Technique

The patient reclines on a bed or couch to ensure relaxation and less muscle tension. The electrodes are surface electrodes. The active electrode is attached to the vertex (or high on the forehead), the reference electrode to the ipsilateral (test ear) mastoid process and the ground electrode to the contralateral mastoid process. The hardware and test signals used (wideband clicks and high-frequency tone bursts) are identical to those used for EcochG, but the filter and time window settings are altered. The signals are usually presented using headphones to allow monaural testing. As the evoked responses are so small, they are easily masked by other neuromuscular signals. It is therefore important that the patient stays as still as possible and, because of the size, several thousand responses are analysed as opposed to hundreds in ECochG. The results are analysed by measuring the absolute values for various wave latencies and the interwave latencies (I–III, I–V, III–V), and comparing results between the two ears. Age and gender normative data are available, as are correction factors for hearing loss. The accuracy of the I–V latency can be improved by combining ECochG with BERA to aid the detection of wave I.

23.7 Physiology

The signal recorded by this technique is a multiwave complex (▶Fig. 23.3). Seven waves are recognised but the last two, VI and VII, are unreliable and variable in comparison with the preceding five waves. There has been much debate and investigation to try and identify the various wave generators. The current state of understanding is reflected in ▶Table 23.1 which shows typical normative latencies for each wave.

23.8 Clinical Indications

1. Vestibular schwannoma detection was done historically, but this has been superceded by MRI scanning. However, this test remains useful in cases where MRI is contraindicated and can be used in conjunction with high-resolution CT of the internal auditory meatus (IAM)/cerebellopontine angle (CPA) to help exclude acoustic neuroma/vestibular schwannoma.

E

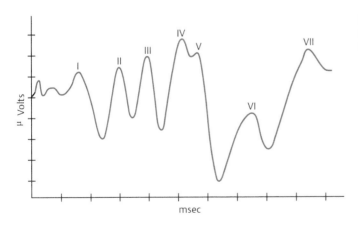

Fig. 23.3 Example of an otoneurological investigation auditory brainstem response (ABR).

2. Threshold testing (▶Fig. 23.4). This is particularly useful in children who have failed neonatal screening with otoacoustic emissions as it is non-invasive, and not influenced by anaesthetic. It is also useful in adult cases who cannot be passively cooperative. Testing with click stimuli can estimate threshold at around 3 to 4 kHz to within approximately 10 dB.
3. Brainstem lesions. BERA can be used to define the site of a brainstem lesion depending on the presence or absence of successive waves, and asymmetrical interwave latencies. Unusual results, such as poor waveform morphology, may indicate multiple sclerosis.
4. Intra-operative testing. The technique may be used as a monitor during tumour surgery designed to preserve hearing. Note that wave

▶ **Table 23.1** Typical normative latencies for each wave

Wave	Site of generation	Latency (ms)
I	Cochlear/lateral cochlear nerve	2.0
II	Medial cochlear nerve/cochlear nucleus	3.0
III	Superior olive/lower pons	4.0
IV	Lateral lemniscus	5.1
V	Lateral lemniscus	5.7

These potentials are very small and rarely reach more than 1 mV (potentials of 10 mV may be obtained in electrocochleography).

V is preserved, but the amplitude decreases and latency increases with reducing stimulus intensity.

23.9 Cortical Electrical Response Audiometry

Cortical electrical response audiometry (CERA), also called the auditory long-latency–evoked potential (ALEP), is a relatively late phenomenon and can be detected as a bi- or triphasic wave commencing after 60 ms and continuing beyond 200 ms (▶Fig. 23.5). The first two waves are thought to be exogenous and related to the stimulus. However, the third wave, occurring after 200 ms, is too late to be considered a primary cortical response and almost certainly represents a secondary, perceptual cortical phenomenon (endogenous); as such its presence can be associated with clinical hearing. Unfortunately, it is strongly influenced by the patient's conscious level and attendance to the stimulus and so is only of value in the cooperative patient. If feasible, it offers excellent frequency specificity.

23.10 Technique

The patient sits comfortably in a chair, and is encouraged to stay still, awake and mentally alert,

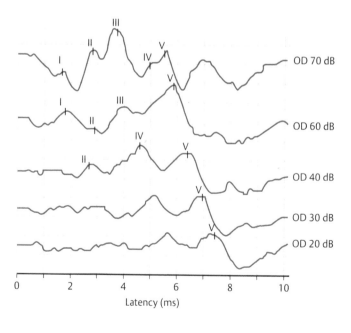

Fig. 23.4 An example of threshold estimation auditory brainstem response (ABR).

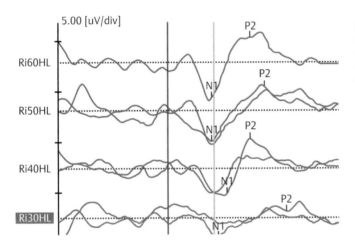

Fig. 23.5 Example of cortical electrical response audiometry (CERA) waveforms—note the N1–P2 amplitude reduces with reducing stimulus levels.

E

as movement and consciousness level can easily influence the response. Surface electrodes are placed with the active on the vertex, reference on either mastoid process and ground on the fore-head. Tone bursts are the preferred test stimuli and are presented by headphones. Fewer than 100 responses need to be sampled to achieve a useful result. Threshold is taken as the point at which the V potential disappears. Peaks N1 and P2 are the most predictable and useful.

23.11 Clinical Indications

1. Threshold testing (▶Fig. 23.5). This can be performed by both air and bone conduction if required. In medicolegal cases, this is often but not exclusively restricted to 1, 2 and 3 kHz or other key diagnostic frequencies required for the given claimant. When the recording conditions are good, the estimated CERA thresholds are usually within 10 dB of true threshold.

2. Central deafness. In rare patients ECochG and BERA are normal but the V potential is absent.

Further Reading

Katx J. Handbook of Clinical Audiology. 7th ed. Philadelphia, Baltimore, New York: Wolters Kluwer; 2015

Weihing J and Leahy N. Evoked measurement of auditory sensitivity. Chapter 52 in Scott-Browns Otolaryngology, Head and Neck Surgery, 8th Edition, Volume 2. Editors in Chief – Watkinson JC & Clarke R. Published by CRC Press, Taylor & Francis group, Boca Raton, London, New York, 2018

Related Topics of Interest

Vestibular schwannoma
Ménière's disease
Noise-induced hearing loss
Non-organic hearing loss
Paediatric hearing assessment

24 Examination of the Ear

There is no doubt that you will be asked to assess an ear in a clinical ear, nose, throat (ENT) examination. Time taken in practising your technique is therefore well spent. It is not just a question of spotting clinical signs or a disease process. The examiner will want to establish that you have an orderly and thorough technique, and that you are able to present your findings accurately and clearly. You will be asked how you would manage the patient, so be thinking about this as you present your examination findings. The common topics will include a patient with hearing impairment, otorrhoea, otalgia, tinnitus, vertigo, facial palsy or a combination of these. A methodical approach will impress the examiners, but a clumsy cluttered technique is likely to depress you and them.

24.1 Method

Be bare below the elbows and make sure that you wash/clean your hands before every patient. This is mandatory in clinical practice and it is imperative you are seen to do so in the clinical examination. Be polite with the patient, make sure that you clearly introduce yourself before starting the examination and explain what it is that you have been asked to do. Ask which is the better hearing ear. Always begin the examination with the better ear and never touch the patient before asking if there is any tenderness. The ear should be examined with an electric powered head light and the ear canal and tympanic membrane with an otoscope or microscope. The patient should be seated sideways to the surgeon, who sits opposite the ear to be examined and reflects light onto it.

24.2 Pinna

Examine the pinna in front and behind for signs of inflammation or skin lesions. The mastoid process should be carefully examined for scars, redness or tenderness. Be particularly careful not to miss a fading post-auricular or endaural scar or a pre-auricular pit/sinus. Note any discharge from the external auditory meatus as well as any inflammation of the skin. Common examination subjects include congenital lesions of the pinna (e.g., microtia, which may be associated with an ossicular chain discontinuity), cauliflower ears, perichondritis and surgical scars.

24.3 External Auditory Canal

To examine the external auditory canal, pull the pinna upward, outward and backward. In infants, owing to non-development of the bony external meatus, the pinna has to be drawn downward and backward. Select a suitably sized speculum for insertion into the external canal. The otoscope should be held in the right hand for examination of the right ear and in the left hand for examination of the left ear. Irrespective of the preferred grip of the otoscope (hold it like a pen or within the hand), there should always be a fulcrum with the little finger (for a pen grip) or index finger (for a hand grip) on the patient's face. This reduces the risk of damage to the patient's ear allowing the otoscope to move with them if there is sudden head movement. Introduce the otoscope speculum just past the hairs of the outer canal, but avoid contact with the sensitive bony part of the canal. Note any inflammation, signs of infection (discharge, spores, granulation tissue) and ask if you may remove wax or debris. A good view of the tympanic membrane should then be possible. Common examination subjects include canal stenosis and exostoses.

24.4 Tympanic Membrane

Look for the prominent lateral process and handle of the malleus. Examine all quadrants of the membrane. The long process of the incus is frequently observed behind and parallel to the handle of the malleus and it is sometimes possible to see it articulate with the head of the stapes.

If there is a perforation, note its position, size and whether it is central or marginal. If you do discover a perforation, then make sure you can describe the middle ear anatomy you see looking through it. For example, the promontory, round window, incudostapedial joint, dehiscent fallopian canal or tympanosclerosis may be visible. If the tympanic membrane is abnormal and the middle ear cleft does not appear to be ventilating normally (i.e., appears retracted, atelectatic, or there is tympanosclerosis), ask if you may use a pneumatic otoscope to assess the mobility of the membrane. Immobility may be due to fluid in the middle ear, a perforation or tympanosclerosis. If the patient has had mastoid surgery, determine the type of cavity, the access to the cavity (meatoplasty size and height of the facial ridge) and decide if the cavity is healthy or not. If clinically indicated, tell the examiner that you would like to perform a fistula test by applying tragal pressure or preferably use the pneumatic otoscope. Look for conjugate deviation of the eyes away from the examined side and then (while maintaining pressure) nystagmus in the direction of the diseased side. Remember to tell the patient what you are doing beforehand if you are performing a pneumatic assessment of the tympanic membrane or performing a fistula test.

24.5 Hearing Tests

Perform free field speech tests by asking the patient to repeat words spoken with a whispered voice, conversational voice and shouted voice at 60 cm from the ear. The non-test ear is masked either by using a Bàràny noise box or by pressing the tragus backward and rubbing it with the index finger so as to produce masking. The patient sits side onto the surgeon so that lip reading is not possible.

Use double-figure numbers or bisyllabic words as the words the patient is asked to repeat should not be easy to guess. The Rinne and Weber tuning fork tests, using a 512 Hz fork, should then be performed to help differentiate between a conductive and sensorineural hearing loss.

24.6 Other Tests

If the patient has eustachian tube dysfunction or a middle ear effusion, nose, the postnasal space and the eustachian tube orifice should be examined to determine if there is nasal or nasopharyngeal pathology such as CRSwNP or a nasopharyngeal tumour. If the patient has otalgia and the ear examination is normal then inspect the whole of the upper aerodigestive tract, the temporomandibular joint and the cervical spine to determine if there is an identifiable cause of referred otalgia. The cranial nerves should be formally examined if there is active ear disease. In a short case, examiners will sometimes stipulate that they are only interested in facial nerve function, and this should always be routinely tested in examination of the ear.

24.7 Summary of Examination of the Ear

- Introduce yourself to the patient.
- Position the patient.
- Ascertain which is the better ear and start with this.
- Inspect the pinna, mastoid and external auditry meatus.
- Pneumatic otoscopic examination of the typanic membrane.
- Fistula test.
- Free field voice tests.
- Tuning fork tests.
- Facial nerve.
- Postnasal space.
- Nose and postnasal space.
- Whole of upper aerodigestive tract, the temporomandibular joint and cervical spine (if patient has referred otalgia).

Related Topics of Interest

Clinical assessment of hearing
External ear conditions
Examination of the nose
Examination of the head and neck

25 Examination of the Head and Neck

There have been substantial transformations to the diagnosis and treatment of head and neck diseases, with technical advances in equipment available and clinical approach, and these are now manifest in modifications of the examination. Examination of the head and neck was often described as an 'examination of the throat'. Throat is a vague term, usually implying the laryngopharynx. Fibreoptic endoscopy has almost completely replaced indirect laryngoscopy with a mirror in all but some developing countries. The scope of head and neck surgery has become far more wide-ranging and encompasses not only pharyngolaryngeal disease, but also salivary gland disease, thyroid disorders and a variety of symptoms which present to 'Target' (otherwise called 2-week cancer wait) clinics.

The symptoms associated with throat disease include hoarseness, dysphagia, odynophagia, sore throat, lump in the throat, (referred) otalgia, cough, lump in the neck and weight loss. Common findings on examination are vocal cord palsy, vocal cord oedema, vocal cord polyps, vocal cord nodules, laryngeal papilloma, occasionally patients with a neoplasm and laryngectomy patients. Patients with metastatic neck nodes may be used in the head and neck clinical examination, but benign problems are commoner subjects, including salivary gland tumours, thyroid nodules and neurovascular lesions (e.g., carotid body tumours). Other than examinations which have simulation, it is more likely that candidates will be given an external sign or lump to evaluate rather than a case that requires endoscopic evaluation.

25.1 Method

The technique outlined in this topic is ideal for a long case but may need to be modified for a short case. Listen carefully to the examiner's instructions and do what is asked. Do not irritate the examiner by examining parts of the patient that have not been mentioned. However, if in doubt, it is better to be thorough.

Be bare below the elbows and make sure that you are seen to have washed your hands prior to engaging with the patient. Introduce yourself and clearly explain to the patient what you have been asked to do and for their permission to proceed. Be polite and have a reassuring demeanour. It may be necessary to wear gloves depending on the examination required (e.g., bimanual examination of the oral cavity) and these will be readily available.

An electric headlight will usually be available and can be used. The surgeon should sit with his or her knees together and the legs to the right side of the patient's. Ask edentulous patients to remove their dentures. Expose the whole of the neck up to and including the clavicles. Remove any neck scarf which may hide a wound or stoma. It is surprising how many times candidates do not follow this simple advice and miss important pathology.

25.2 Oral Cavity

Inspect the lips for perioral lesions. Ask the patient if there is any tenderness in the mouth. Take two metal tongue depressors and insert them to retract the buccal mucosa on each side. Ask the patient to protrude the tongue and move it from side to side and then up to the palate and down. This should allow an inspection of the dorsal and ventral surfaces of the tongue, the tongue's lateral borders, and the floor of the mouth; it also tests hypoglossal nerve function. Pay attention to the retromolar trigone area. The two tongue depressors are then used to examine the buccal mucosa, teeth and alveolar ridges, and the opening of the parotid ducts opposite the upper second molar.

25.3 Oropharynx

Dispense with one of the tongue depressors and use the other to depress the tongue. Check over the palate, the tonsils and the posterior pharyngeal wall. Ask the patient to say 'aah' and check movement of the palate. Remove the tongue depressor and put a glove on. Bimanually, palpate the floor of the mouth overlying the submandibular duct for calculi or masses. Palpate the base of the tongue, as a tumour in this site may not be visible but easily palpable.

25.4 Nasopharynx

Explain to the patient what you are about to do. Some patients are unable to cope with endoscopy because they find it uncomfortable or have an overactive gag reflex. Lidocaine hydrochloride 5% and phenylephrine hydrochloride 0.5% topical solution sprayed into the nose can be used as a local anaesthetic and decongestant. This is usually well tolerated and allows a more thorough inspection and assessment of vocal cord movement. Be sure to tell the patient to avoid food and drink for the next hour. Despite this, there are still some patients who will not tolerate the procedure and may need to be assessed under a general anaesthetic. It is unlikely in a professional postgraduate examination that the patients will have an overactive gag reflex as they are specially selected.

The nasopharynx will usually be examined by using a 2.7-mm 0- or 30-degree rigid or a 3.6-mm flexible nasendoscope. If this is not available, a mirror examination can be used. Warm a post-nasal mirror and pass it through the mouth while gently holding the tongue down with a tongue depressor. Ask the patient to breathe gently through the nose. Whatever method, look carefully for any obvious lesion, but be particularly vigilant on inspection of the laterally placed eustachian tube elevations, above which lie the fossae of Rosenmüller, the usual site of origin of nasopharyngeal carcinoma.

25.5 Examination of the Larynx and Pharynx

Direct inspection of the larynx and pharynx can be provided with use of fibre-optic scopes. Most individuals will tolerate this without anaesthesia, but those who find it uncomfortable or have an overactive gag reflex can be given lidocaine and phenylephrine topical solution sprayed into the nose. The patient should be instructed to avoid food and drink for the next hour. The flexible nasopharyngoscope should be held between the index finger and thumb and inserted into the nose. The middle and ring fingers should rest gently on the patient's nose, as a pivot point and to steady the scope in the event of patient movement. The endoscope is advanced along the floor of the nose to the nasopharynx, which is inspected. The patient is asked to breathe through the nose at this point. This brings forward the soft palate and opens the nasopharyngeal isthmus to allow a view of the oropharynx and larynx distally. The scope is gently guided past the soft palate into the oropharynx. At this juncture, warn the patients that they may feel a tickle in the throat, and ask them to concentrate on keeping their breathing steady, as this may help avoid a gag reflex. A view

of the tongue base, vallecular and lingual surface of the epiglottis can be achieved by asking the patient to protrude the tongue. Inspect the supraglottic larynx, the vocal cords and the posterior pharyngeal wall and the piriform fossa. The piriform fossa can be further examined by asking the patient to blow his or her cheeks out and turning the head to the right and left. Pooling of saliva is known as Jackson's sign. There are many causes of Jackson's sign such as incoordination of the swallow or any cause of hypopharyngeal obstruction such as a pharyngeal pouch, hypopharyngeal/cervical oesophageal malignancy or a post-cricoid web. Ask the patient to vocalise by saying 'eee' and 'aah', assess vocal cord movement and look for evidence of an ulcer or exophytic lesion. The subglottis can be assessed in compliant patients by looking through the cords. Once the examination is over, remove the scope slowly and carefully, as this too can be uncomfortable for the patients, and give them a tissue to clear their nose.

Indirect laryngoscopy is not used in U.K. examinations and used very sparingly in examinations in developing countries as it has been replaced by endoscopic examination. Explain to the patient what you are about to do. Warm a laryngeal mirror and check its temperature on the back of your hand. Ask the patient to protrude the tongue and gently grasp it with a swab held in the left hand. The patient should then be requested to breathe normally through the mouth as the mirror is introduced gently up to the soft palate. If the patient's nose breathes and arches up the tongue, obstructing the view, it is possible to obtain some improvement by asking the patient to quietly make an 'aah' noise breathing in and out. Inspect the base of the tongue, the vallecula and the upper part of the epiglottis. Examine the posterior pharyngeal wall, and then both sides of the epiglottis, the aryepiglottic folds, the pyriform fossae, the arytenoids, the ventricular folds and the vocal cords. Note any inflammation, ulceration or exophytic lesion. The movements of the vocal cords are studied by asking the patient to say 'ee' followed by a deep breath and 'ee' again. Note any abnormal movement or fixation of the cords.

25.6 Examination of the Neck

Check the neck for any obvious skin lesion or ulceration. Be careful not to overlook a fading wound. Check that the patient does not have a stoma. Ask the patient to swallow and watch the larynx move.

E

A thyroid goitre may also be seen moving with the larynx. An enlarged neck mass may be visible; note its position and inform the examiner that you have seen it. Ask the patient to count to 10 out loud and assess the voice. Get the patient to breathe deeply in and out through the mouth and note any stridor.

The neck should be palpated from behind and in an orderly sequence so that no areas are missed. Be gentle. Ask the patient if there is any tenderness. Start at the mastoid bone and palpate down the line of the trapezius muscle and in the posterior triangle down to the clavicle. Feel for supraclavicular and infraclavicular nodes.

Then palpate down the line deep to the anterior border of the sternocleidomastoid muscle for deep cervical nodes. When your fingers reach the suprasternal notch, palpate up the anterior triangle, feeling the trachea, thyroid gland, laryngeal cartilages and hyoid bone. Loss of normal laryngeal crepitus (Trotter's sign) may indicate a postcricoid neoplasm. Feel for submental lymph nodes, submandibular nodes, the parotid gland, preauricular nodes, and finally occipital nodes. If a lump is felt, note its site, size, shape, consistency and fixation to adjacent tissues or skin. If you think a lump is pulsatile or attached to the carotid, auscultate and listen for a bruit. If a lump is palpated in the anterior triangle, see whether it moves on swallowing. If you think a lump is cystic, see if it transilluminates.

If a salivary gland mass is discovered, be sure to examine the oral cavity (check dentition, duct orifices and tongue movement), the oropharynx (medialisation of the tonsil in parapharyngeal tumour) and facial nerve movement. Check the other salivary glands (systemic illness like Sjögren's), head and neck skin (metastases from a skin tumour can go to the parotid) and examine the neck for nodes.

If a thyroid nodule or goitre is identified, examine the neck for nodes, check there is no stridor in large goitres and examine the larynx for vocal cord movement. Pemberton's sign may be elicited by asking the patient to raise his or her arms, a retrosternal goitre will rise and may cause obstruction of the superior vena cava. The patient will become plethoric and respiratory distress will ensue. If a thyroid goitre or nodule is detected, it is important to perform a clinical examination of thyroid function status.

25.7 Summary of Examination of the Throat

- Introduce yourself to the patient.
- Position the patient and expose the neck down to the clavicles.
- Assess speech.
- Examine oral cavity and oropharynx perorally.
- Examine nasopharynx, oropharynx, hypopharynx and larynx with flexible nasopharyngoscope.
- Examination of the neck.

Related Topics of Interest

Examination of the ear
Examination of the nose
Laryngeal carcinoma
Nasopharyngeal tumours
Oral cavity carcinoma
Oropharyngeal carcinoma
Salivary gland neoplasms
Thyroid disease—benign
Thyroid disease—malignant

26 Examination of the Nose

A working diagnosis of nasal disease may be possible after an accurate history has been taken. The essential symptoms are nasal obstruction, sneezing, rhinorrhoea, postnasal drip, headache and facial pain, abnormal sense of smell, epistaxis, snoring and cosmetic deformity. A previous history of trauma or allergy may also be relevant. Nasal disease is common, signs can be elicited quickly, and management of the common diseases makes for good discussion.

Common findings are septal deviation, hypertrophied turbinates, septal perforation and nasal polyps. It is therefore essential that you are familiar with the aetiology, relevant investigations and treatments of these conditions. There may be a combination of signs (e.g., a deviated septum and nasal polyps), so be thorough with your examination.

26.1 Position of the Patient

Be bare below the elbows and make sure that you are seen to wash/clean your hands before seeing each patient. Be polite with the patient, make sure that you clearly introduce yourself before starting the examination and explain what you have been asked to do. Sit opposite the patient, with your knees together and to the right side of the patient's legs. This is more elegant than sitting with your legs astride the patient's.

26.2 External Nose

Examine the nose in relation to the rest of the patient's face. Pay particular attention to the size and shape; the curve or deviation of the bony and cartilaginous dorsum, the width or projection of the tip, the shape of the columella and nares. The thickness of the skin may be relevant if cosmetic surgery is contemplated. Look for swelling, bruising, erythema or for ulceration of the skin. An old examination favourite is a patient with the lupus pernio rash of sarcoid on the nasal or facial skin, with a septal perforation. Turn the patient's head to the left and right to check the profile. Be especially vigilant to look for a fading lateral rhinotomy scar or hidden bicoronal incision wound behind the hairline.

The patency of the nasal airway is assessed by occluding each nostril in turn with the tip of the thumb and asking the patient to gently breathe through the nose or alternatively watching the shiny surface of a tongue depressor held under the nose cloud over as the patient exhales. Cottle's manoeuvre is used to assess obstruction at the nasal valve. The patient's cheek is gently retracted laterally and the patient asked to report whether this improves nasal airflow. Palpate the nose to confirm the position of the nasal bones, skin thickness, and cartilaginous framework. The tip should be palpated to evaluate tip support and lifted with the thumb to obtain a view of the nasal vestibules.

26.3 Nasal Cavity

Anterior rhinoscopy is carried out using a Thudichum speculum. Gently introduce this into the nose remembering that the nasal mucosa is very sensitive. If a lesion is immediately obvious, for example, nasal polyps or a nasal tumour, note the position in relation to the turbinates and septum. Do not assume that they will be the only abnormality; be thorough in the rest of your examination. Assess the mucosa; note its colour, vascularity and crusting. Examine the septum's position in relation to the nasal airways and maxillary crest, noting any deviation to one side or dislocation off the crest. Examine the mucoperichondrium for its colour and vascularity and note any lesions. If there is a perforation of the septum, note its position, size and the presence of any granulation tissue. Examine the lateral nasal wall and evaluate the size and colour of the inferior turbinate.

If a better view is needed, the nasal mucosa can be shrunk using a local anaesthetic/vasoconstrictor spray (lidocaine hydrochloride 5% and phenylephrine hydrochloride 0.5% topical solution). The patient should be warned not to eat or drink following this for approximately 1 hour. Endoscopic examination is essential in clinical practice and technique may be assessed in an examination. A 2.7- or 3.4-mm diameter (0- or 30-degree) rigid endoscope or a flexible nasopharyngoscope may be used. Examiners may have strong views as to which is preferable; some will say the flexible

E

E

scope is more comfortable, others will argue that the rigid scope provides an enhanced view. The procedure is traditionally performed using three passes of the endoscope.

First pass: This pass is along the floor of the nose. The inferior meatus is examined remembering that this is where the nasolacrimal duct drains. The inferior turbinate mucosa is examined. The inferior turbinate size will be reduced because of the decongestant and this will enable progression of the scope towards the nasopharynx. Inspect the posterior end of the septum, the choanae, through which the posterior ends of the inferior turbinates may be visible. In the lateral nasopharyngeal wall, the tubal ridges of the pharyngeal ends of the eustachian tubes can be seen. The fossae of Rosenmüller lie immediately medial to the medial tubal ridge and can be the site of a nasopharyngeal carcinoma.

Second pass: This pass is between the inferior and middle turbinate. The presence of polyps or mucopurulent material should be noted. Accessory ostia may be identified. As the scope advances posterior and medial to the middle turbinate, the sphenoethmoidal recess can be examined and the sphenoid ostium may be seen.

Third pass: The scope is passed lateral to the middle turbinate in the middle meatus. The middle meatus mucosa (oedema, polyps, pus) and the ostiomeatal complex (infundibulum, uncinate and ethmoidal bulla) can be assessed.

26.4 Oral Examination

Inspect and percuss the upper teeth. The floor of the maxillary sinus lies over the alveolar process of the maxilla and the roots of the second premolar and first molar teeth. Assess movement of the soft palate, and if there is a bifid uvula, be aware that this may signify a submucous cleft.

26.5 Neck

Inspect and palpate the neck and look for the presence of lymphadenopathy. The lymphatic drainage from the anterior part of the nose is to the submandibular nodes and upper deep cervical nodes. Drainage from the posterior part is to the middle deep cervical nodes.

26.6 Summary of Examination of the Nose

- Introduce yourself.
- Position the patient.
- Inspect the external nose.
- Examine the nasal tip and vestibule and assess the nasal airways.
- Anterior rhinoscopy with a Thudichum speculum.
- Endoscopic examination using three-pass technique.
- Oral examination.
- Neck.

Related Topics of Interest

Examination of the ear
Examination of the head and neck
Nasal swellings
Nasopharyngeal tumours
Rhinoplasty
Septal perforation

27 Examinations in ENT

An examination system in Otorhinolaryngology has been established in the United Kingdom for many years. The Diploma in Laryngology and Otology (DLO) was introduced in 1923 and preceded the specialty FRCS examinations. The Diploma in Otolaryngology, Head and Neck Surgery (DO-HNS) was instigated in 2003 to replace the DLO, under the auspices of the Royal College of Surgeons of England.

Surgical training has undergone significant change over the last decade and competence became the main focus of assessment. The latter led to the development of a new Intercollegiate FRCS in 2006 and revision of the MRCS in 2008. The current U.K. specialty examinations in ENT are the DO-HNS, the MRCS (ENT), and the FRCS (ORL). All of the U.K. specialist surgical examinations are now fully Intercollegiate between the Royal Colleges of Edinburgh, England, Glasgow and Ireland.

The European Examination Board in Otolaryngology, Head and Neck Surgery (called the European Board of ORL-HNS) was created by the Union of Medical Specialists ORL Section (UEMS-ORL) for countries that did not have a surgical examination system in place. The examination comprises two parts. Part 1 is a 100 question MCQ and only those who have passed Part 1 are eligible for Part 2. Part 2 is an oral examination. The first MCQ took place at the Academy of ORL-HNS in Mannheim in 2009, and the complimentary oral examination took place in Vienna in 2010. Those who have passed their home national board examination and are recognised as specialists in their home country and who pass the European Board examination are allowed to be called 'Fellows of the European Board of ORL-HNS'. Other successful candidates, not yet certified as specialists in their home country, receive a 'Diploma of the European Board of Otolaryngology'.

There are completely separate examination systems around the world that also award a surgical Fellowship qualification such as the FRCSC in Canada, FRACS in Australia and New Zealand, FCS(SA) in South Africa and FCSHK in Hong Kong. Further details of these examinations can be found on their relevant websites.

27.1 Examination Standards

The purpose of any examination system is to set and maintain a pre-determined standard of professional practice. The assessment therefore provides a sense of credibility and reassurance to both patients, the public and other professionals, that a standard of practice has been achieved.

While the standards to be achieved are set by the various examination bodies, in the United Kingdom these have to be accepted and agreed by the General Medical Council.

U.K. Trainees in Otorhinolaryngology are required to have either the MRCS (ENT), the DO-HNS or both in order to apply for a numbered higher surgical training post, commencing at ST3 level. The FRCS (ORL) is an exit examination that should be taken towards the end of training.

The Intercollegiate MRCS (ENT) and DO-HNS examinations both test knowledge to a standard that trainees should have reached 2 to 3 years after qualification, and includes domains such as clinical knowledge, clinical and technical skills, communication and professionalism.

Examiners who partake in the U.K. examinations all have to undergo a selection process after application and once successful, each examiner undergoes a pre-examination training course that also includes Equality and Diversity training.

Candidates should be aware that they are not allowed to memorise or copy examination questions, or pass these on to other parties such as revision courses. Mobile phones or other electronic devices are therefore not allowed in the examination room. Such activity is seen not only as cheating that leads to disqualification from the examination but also a breach of both copyright and probity that could lead to the candidate being reported to the GMC.

27.2 The Intercollegiate MRCS and MRCS (ENT)

The General Surgery MRSC, called the MRCS, is different to the MRCS (ENT) by having the same Part A but a different Part B.

27.3 MRCS

To be eligible, candidates must hold a medical degree accepted by the GMC or Medical Council of Ireland for provisional or full registration. Overseas candidates must hold a medical degree acceptable to the councils of the four colleges. There are two components:

27.3.1 MRCS Part A

This is a General Surgery (including some ENT questions) MCQ section, that comprises two separate MCQ papers with a combination of single best answer (SBA) questions and extended matching questions. The first paper is a 3-hours paper that tests applied basic sciences; the second paper lasts for 2 hours and assesses the principles of surgery in general. To achieve a pass in Part A the candidate is required to demonstrate a minimum level of competence in each of the two papers and to have achieved the pass mark set for the combined total mark from the two papers. Candidates must have passed Part A to be eligible to sit for Part B.

27.3.2 MRCS Part B

This is an objective structured clinical examination (OSCE) that consists of 18 examined stations, each of 9 minutes' duration, with each station carrying a maximum mark of 20 points. The OSCE tests candidates on applied knowledge of anatomy, surgical pathology, applied surgical science and critical care, and applied skills such as clinical and procedural skills, history taking and communication skills in both giving and receiving information. Actors/actresses take on the role of patients for the purpose of this examination.

Candidates are allowed six attempts to pass Part A and four attempts to pass Part B. The GMC has deemed that this must be achieved within 7 years.

Candidates who pass MRCS Part A and MRCS Part B may be awarded the MRCS, an examination required to enter higher non-ENT surgical training such as General Surgery and Neurosurgery. Some CT1 doctors who have General Surgery in their rotation but wish to be ENT surgeons may pass the MRCS then take Part 2 DO-HNS to be awarded MRSC (ENT) too (see further).

27.3.3 MRCS (ENT)

Candidates are expected (but it is not compulsory, see later) to take and pass Part A MRCS before attempting Part 2 DO-HNS.

Candidates who pass Part A MRCS and Part 2 DO-HNS may be awarded the MRCS (ENT).

To be awarded the DO-HNS, candidates must pass the Part 1 DO-HNS which is an ENT MCQ, and pass Part 2 DO-HNS. Parts 1 and 2 can be taken in any order.

It is permissible, however, for candidates to take Part 2 DO-HNS and then attempt MRCS Part A and then to be awarded the MRCS (ENT). It is also permissible for candidates who have the DO-HNS (i.e., have passed Parts 1 and 2 of the DO-HNS) to then attempt the MRCS Part A and if successful, be awarded the MRCS (ENT).

For those candidates who wish to sit both DO-HNS and MRCS, this must be done sequentially; sitting the examinations simultaneously is not permitted.

27.4 The Intercollegiate DO-HNS Examination

This examination is now fully intercollegiate, and is intended to assess aspiring otorhinolaryngologists in training and doctors who practice in another specialty that interacts with otolaryngology, including general practitioners with an interest in the specialty.

There are two components to the examination:

27.4.1 Part 1: An ENT MCQ Paper

This consists of multiple True–False and Extended Matching questions, combined into a single 2-hour paper.

27.4.2 Part 2: An Objective Structured Clinical Examination

The OSCE examination consists of up to 28 active stations and 3 rest stations, each station timed by a bell and lasts for 7 minutes. Several stations are manned by examiners, sometimes with actors, and include history taking, communication skills, clinical examination techniques and consenting for certain procedures.

E

Parts 1 and 2 can be sat in any order but cannot be taken simultaneously. This facilitates candidates with Part A MRCS and Part 2 DO-HNS (and therefore who have already gained the MRCS [ENT]), to sit Part 1 DO-HNS to also achieve the DO-HNS diploma (as they then have both Parts 1 and 2 of the DO-HNS). Part 2 DO-HNS must be taken within 7 years of Part 1.

Candidates eligible to sit the DO-HNS must have a primary medical qualification acceptable to the GMC for provisional/full registration, or to the Council of Ireland, similar to the MRCS regulations.

While not mandatory, it is strongly advised that candidates should have the equivalent of 6 months' full-time experience in ENT prior to applying for the examination.

Candidates with MRCS (ENT) and so by definition have passed DO-HNS Part 2, may then take DO-HNS Part 1 and if successful will then achieve the Intercollegiate Diploma (DO-HNS).

Candidates have a maximum of four attempts at this examination but are still able to go on to have a further four attempts at MRCS Part B.

27.5 The Intercollegiate FRCS (ORL)

27.5.1 Application and Eligibility

Candidates wishing to sit the intercollegiate FRCS (ORL) have to be in specialist training year ST6 or above or have equivalent experience if they are not part of a rotational training scheme. Their application must be accompanied by a completed structured reference from their trainer or programme director stating that they have attained a level of training and experience suitable for the examination. The latter helps prevent doctors who have not reached this level from going through with an examination process that is both expensive, and seen very much as an exit examination that should be taken at the completion of training.

27.5.2 Revision Courses

Most candidates will choose to attend one of the examination training courses that are now well established in the United Kingdom. While these are often helpful, it is important for candidates to know that examiners are not allowed to tutor on such courses. The course may therefore not truly reflect the experience that the candidate will have during the actual examination.

27.5.3 Component Parts

There are two parts to the FRCS (ORL) examination:
Section 1–The written MCQ examination
Section 2–The oral/clinical examination

There are two dates for the FRCS (ORL) examination each year, approximately 6 months apart. Section 1 takes place in January and July and section 2 in April and November.

Section 1 papers are sat at DVLA test centres local to candidates' places of work, while section 2 occurs in various locations within the United Kingdom and Ireland.

27.5.4 Section 1—The Written MCQ Examination

The MCQ examination consists of two separate examination papers that are sat on the same day. One paper consists of 110 SBA questions with a duration of 2 hours. The other paper has 135 extended matching item (EMI) questions with a duration of 2 hours 30 minutes.

The questions that make up the two papers are selected from a large question bank. Each question is specifically coded so that the examination papers can be blueprinted and balanced with regards to the multiple domains that need to be tested. The domains include a wide range of clinical topics as well as professional behaviour and leadership aligned with the GMC's 'Good Medical Practice' guidelines.

Quality Assurance

Individual questions are generally written by a pair of examiners before being quality assured by a separate pair of examiners, prior to entry into the question bank. The performance of each question is statistically monitored at each examination, and poorly performing questions are excluded from the examination prior to marking each paper. This process takes place at the standard setting meeting held shortly after each examination date. This meeting is attended by 12 or more examiners who standard-set the papers by performing a modified

E

E

Angoff procedure in which they assess the degree of predicted difficulty of each question. The pass mark is then calculated, making allowance for the cohort of candidates and the difficulty of the papers, ensuring a degree of consistency between individual examination dates.

Questions that are excluded from the examination are returned to the question writing group for further attention. This whole process aims to maintain examination papers with high quality of questions that test both judgement and higher-order thinking. It also ensures questions are relevant and aligned with current opinion and thinking.

The reproducibility and test reliability of the whole MCQ examination is statistically assessed by the Kuder–Richardson (KR-20) value, that should be greater than 0.7 (range 0.00 to 1.00), but normally achieves a value close to 0.9 for our specialty.

27.5.5 Section 2—The Oral/Clinical Examination

Candidates who are successful at the MCQ examination are invited to attend for section 2.

The section 2 examination includes the following components:

- Oral *viva voce* assessments in head and neck, otology, rhinology and paediatric domains.
- Short case clinical examinations in all of the above domains.
- Communication skills assessment.

The oral viva voce examination questions are all pre-selected by the Board prior to the examination. Each question is then calibrated at the pre-examination meeting attended by all of the examiners. The examiners are reminded to make allowance for the stress and anxiety factors that may affect candidates during the process of the examination.

The oral viva voce examination consists of six individual questions, over a period of 30 minutes, shared between two examiners.

The short case clinical examinations include two individual patients over a period of 20 minutes, with the prime aim of assessing clinical skills and technique.

The communication skills section consists of a 30-minute clinical encounter with an actor/actress who is briefed with a clinical scenario.

Each component is marked by a closed marking scheme ranging from 4 to 8, with 6 being a

pass. Descriptor sheets are utilised to assist the examiner with assigning a suitable mark. The marking system does allow candidates to compensate for low marks in some domains by scoring highly in others. There is a total of 90 marking opportunities in section 2 and the number needed to pass is a total of 540. The highest scoring candidate receives a gold medal at the Royal Society of Medicine, the presentation alternating between the Otology section and the Laryngology and Rhinology section.

Every effort is made to ensure that the process is fair and equitable, and candidates should not be examined by the same pair of examiners on more than one occasion.

The examination process is observed and assessed by three individual examination assessors who are all experienced past examiners. The assessors are selected by the Board and compile a full report that includes all aspects of the examination. As part of this process, each examiner is individually assessed on two separate occasions during the process of the examination.

Candidates are allowed to attempt the examination on four occasions only. The examination is administered entirely by its own Secretariat situated in Hill Place, adjacent to the Royal College of Surgeons of Edinburgh.

27.6 The European Board Examination in Otorhinolaryngology—Head and Neck Surgery

The European Board Examination (EBE) has become a really popular examination that attracts candidates from many European (EU) countries as well as many non-EU countries, and particularly the Middle East and Turkey.

Representatives of the UEMS Section Boards met in Glasgow in 2007 and created a 'Glasgow Declaration' that stated European Board Examinations should be complimentary to existing national examinations. Countries that do not have an examination are encouraged to use the EBE as a quality mark for safe independent practice at the end of specialist training. The examination is specifically aimed at certified specialists or trainees in their last year of training, who should have the support of their training board. Candidates applying for this examination outside of the EU must include a signed surgical log book, full CV and a Government-issued photo ID.

The examination is in two parts:

Part 1: A 3-hour MCQ paper that consists of 100 questions.

Part 2: An oral examination in rhinology, otology and head and neck.

There is a syllabus that covers what candidates can be examined on. Candidates must pass Part 1 in order to proceed to Part 2. The pass mark for Part 1 is set at 60% and 85 to 90% of candidates pass this section. The MCQ section has taken place in various cities, normally aligned with a major conference.

Successful candidates may then proceed to the oral viva voce examination that is always held in November in Vienna at a specific venue that offers suitable facilities. The oral examination is based very much on the style of the Intercollegiate FRCS, with two examiners per table. Each candidate is examined on four questions at each of three tables covering three main domains: rhinology/otology, audiology, balance/head and neck. The domains include paediatric ENT and facial plastics.

The duration of each viva session is 24 minutes. The mean pass rate for candidates is 73%. Those who are already certified become Fellows and the others gain a Diploma of the European Board of ORL-HNS.

The accepted perception is that this examination is at about the equivalent standard of U.K. Membership and Diploma examinations, but does not come to the equivalent standard of the Intercollegiate FRCS examination, and within the United Kingdom it is not accepted as an equivalent qualification to the FRCS in applications for Consultant posts within the UK NHS.

Further Reading

The Glasgow Declaration. 2007: www.old.med.bg.ac.rs/download.php/tempus/glasgow%20Declaration.pdf/269

E

Related Topics of Interest

Examination of the ear
Examination of the head and neck
Examination of the nose

28 External Ear Conditions

28.1 Pinna

The pinna is embryologically formed, from six cartilage hillocks of His, which fuse to form the convoluted shape of the human pinna. It comprises skin over perichondrium on a cartilage skeleton. It acts as a 'funnel' to focus sound waves into the external ear canal; it also has some sound localisation properties as the incident sound wave is distorted by the folds of the pinna in a direction-dependent way.

There are a number of common pathologies affecting the pinna that may be discussed in an examination setting:

28.2 Protruding or Prominent Ears

This is a common occurrence although no formal figures exist for prevalence; many individuals with significant abnormalities will have no complaints while others will have significant complaints from even minor abnormalities. Like all aspects of aesthetics, much of the complaint will relate to the psychology of the patient or his/her parents.

The commonest abnormalities are a poorly developed antihelical fold or an overly developed and prominent, deep conchal bowl.

Many different surgical techniques exist to correct deformity. All rely on exposing and making alterations to the cartilage skeleton. In small babies, with modest deformity, the 'EarBuddies' can be used as a non-surgical alternative. A specially designed 'scaffold' is applied and taped to the baby's pinna for a period of time (weeks to months) which encourages the pinna to grow and adopt the appropriate shape. In adults with poorly developed antihelical folds 'Earfold' nitinol implants are gaining popularity, with the advantage of being inserted under local anaesthetic.

28.3 Trauma

In such a prominent position on the side of the head, the pinna is frequently subject to both blunt and sharp trauma. With such a good blood supply, lacerations heal exceptionally well, even skin flaps which appear to have a very tenuous pedicle.

Exposed or damaged cartilage should be trimmed, and the skin carefully sutured.

After blunt trauma, blood can gather between the cartilage and the perichondrium. This is therefore called a subperichondrial haematoma. As the cartilage derives its nutrient supply from the perichondrium, failure to treat this can lead to cartilage resorption and fibrosis with the consequent 'cauliflower ear' deformity seen frequently in boxers and rugby players.

Small haematomas may be managed by single or serial aspiration under sterile conditions. Larger and more persistent haematomas may require formal incision and drainage, followed by through and through compression sutures (classically over a suitably sized button, or semirigid dressing material) left in place for several days to prevent recurrence.

28.4 Perichondritis

This is an inflammation of the skin and perichondrium of the external ear. It is usually caused by a bacterial infection, secondary to local trauma, such as burns, bites, piercings, aspiration of haematoma or surgical incisions, but it may follow a local infection such as otitis externa. The commonest organisms are *Pseudomonas aeruginosa* or *Staphylococcus aureus*. It is distinguished from relapsing polychondritis by the absence of cartilage involvement elsewhere.

Treatment is usually with appropriate, high-dose antibiotics. Abscess formation will require incision and drainage. Resistant cases may require debridement to remove any devitalised tissues.

28.5 Skin Lesions

The skin of the pinna is not immune to any of the common dermatological problems. However, its exposed position makes it particularly prone to the effects of sun damage, and so skin cancer in the form of both basal cell and squamous cell carcinomas is common. The reader is referred to the Chapters 97 and 98 on skin cancers for further information.

An important differential diagnosis and common pathology on the pinna is chondrodermatitis nodularis helicis. This is thought to be a localised area of damage to the cartilage skeleton, perhaps due to local pressure trauma, or as an inflammatory reaction to cold temperatures that creates an acute inflammatory response in the overlying tissues and skin. It presents as an exquisitely tender, sometimes red, nodule on the ear, usually on a prominent cartilage fold, in contrast to most neoplastic pathologies, which tend to be painless. The patient will often report it is too painful to lie on the affected ear.

Topical steroid and antibiotic creams have been tried, and occlusive dressings, but the most effective treatment keeping the ear warm that may allow the chondritis to become inactive (so advise to wear ear muffs in cold outdoor weather) or formal excisional biopsy, which has the added advantage of excluding a malignant process.

28.6 External Ear Canal

28.6.1 Ear Wax

In all other parts of the body, the superficial keratinised squamous epithelium is constantly shed, usually as a result of friction from clothing or washing. This is not possible in the external ear canal and so it has developed the property of epithelial migration. Squamous epithelium on the tympanic membrane moves radially until it reaches the canal walls, where it turns and moves laterally. When it reaches the hair-bearing cartilaginous portion of the canal, the superficial layer starts to separate. It then mixes with the secretion of the ceruminous and pilosebaceous glands and any collected debris to form what we recognise as ear wax. The ceruminous glands are found in the skin of the outer third of the external acoustic meatus and secrete a liquid material at the base of the hairs. After secretion, evaporation occurs to leave a sticky, waxy substance that is able to trap dirt, squames and microbes.

Wax can be secreted in one of two forms. Wet wax is produced by most Afro-Carribean and Caucasians and is familiar as moist, sticky and honey-coloured. The dry type is commoner in Central and Southeast Asians and tends to be greyer in colour, less sticky, granular and brittle. The gene for wet wax is dominant. Regardless of type, ear wax tends to become drier with age as a result of reduced glandular numbers and activity. Wax is then normally loosened by transmission of movement from the temporomandibular joint from chewing or talking, allowing its passage out of the external auditory meatus. This natural process can be upset by a number of factors and cause wax impaction. Impaction is commoner in males owing to the presence of thicker, coarser hairs in the lateral part of the external auditory canal. Narrow canals, earplugs, zealous use of cotton buds, and even a hearing aid mould may impede the normal flow of wax to the periphery. In some people, no obvious cause is found to account for the impaction and it has been suggested that desquamation of the superficial layer of the meatal epidermis is impaired.

Clinical Features

Impaction of wax can cause a sensation of obstruction, deafness, otalgia, vertigo and coughing (via the auricular branch of the vagus—Arnold's nerve), although wax impaction is a relatively rare cause of hearing loss. Most of these symptoms are improved by removing the wax, which can usually be accomplished by syringing, using a wax hook or microsuction.

Management

Syringing involves the use of a Higginson syringe. It is a potentially dangerous method to remove ear wax because the water pressure delivered to the external ear canal is unregulated and depends on the skill/experience of the operator. It was the single biggest cause of medicolegal claims against GPs and understandably has been superceded by an electric pump irrigation system that delivers body temperature water into the external ear canal at a set pressure to minimise the risk of ear canal or tympanic membrane injury. Both of these methods direct a jet of warm (body temperature) water along the roof or posterior canal wall so that it passes behind the wax and forces it outward. The procedure is often best preceded by a week or two of using a ceruminolytic agent (sodium bicarbonate drops are efficacious, safe and inexpensive). The irrigation system is relatively safe and has greatly reduced the complications that frequently occurred with syringing and include coughing, pain, local trauma, otitis externa and, rarely, tympanic membrane perforation and otitis media. Tympanic membrane trauma may cause acute sensorineural hearing loss and permanent tinnitus.

Contraindications to ear irrigation include frequent previous episodes of otitis externa, a

E

known or suspected perforation, previous tympa-nomastoid surgery and a 'difficult ear', such as a narrow or tortuous ear canal.

In these cases, and for the reasons cited above, removal under direct vision with an operating microscope using microsuction or a wax hook is often a more appropriate and safer alternative.

28.7 Keratosis Obturans

This uncommon condition occurs when there is a failure of the normal process of migration. Keratinocytes and keratin debris collect in the deep part of the external auditory meatus. As with collections of keratin anywhere, this sets up a low-grade inflammatory response. Osteoclast-stimulating mediators are produced, resulting in a resorption of bone and usually a widening of the bony canal. It is sometimes confused with primary cholesteatoma of the external auditory canal, which tends to be a more localised condition.

Clinical Features

Patients usually present with an acute exacerbation of the inflammatory process. Otalgia is usually the dominant feature, although there is usually a conductive hearing loss from the occluded canal. The otoscopic appearances are similar to an acute otitis externa around impacted wax. The keratin takes this appearance because the part in contact with the air oxidises and changes colour.

Management

Removal of the keratin plug is essential to control the inflammatory process. This is often difficult as the patient is usually in considerable pain from external ear canal erosion and a general anaesthetic is sometimes required. Topical antibiotic/steroid combinations are advised to prevent a secondary otitis externa. In the long term, these patients require periodic monitoring and aural toilet.

28.8 Exostoses and Osteomas

Osteomas are uncommon benign tumours of bone usually arising from the tympanosquamous or tympanomastoid suture line. Exostoses, on the other hand, are common. They are hyperostoses of the tympanic bone of the external canal. They appear to be caused by a periosteal reaction from exposure to cold air or more commonly cold water usually from swimming in the sea. In both conditions, although the lumen of the canal may be reduced, they rarely gain sufficient size to cause symptoms. If problems do occur, they are usually caused by large exostoses significantly blocking the ear canal which in turn then impairs the normal process of epithelial migration. In these cases, surgical excision of the exostoses may be indicated. Osteomas can often be removed via a permeatal approach, while exostoses will more often require a formal postaural or endaural approach, to avoid both complications and recurrence.

28.9 Other Conditions

The skin of the ear canal can exhibit the same pathologies as afflict the skin elsewhere on the body. Skin cancer is very rare in the ear canal, but when it occurs, squamous cell carcinoma is the most common (70%).

Further Reading

Robinson P and Hollis S. Exostosis of the external auditory canal. Chapter 80 in Scott-Browns Otolaryngology, Head and Neck Surgery, 8th Edition, Volume 2. Editors in Chief – Watkinson JC & Clarke R. Published by CRC Press, Taylor & Francis group, Boca Raton, London, New York, 2018

Hanger HC, Mulley GP. Cerumen: its fascination and clinical importance: a review. J R Soc Med. 1992; 85(6):346–349

Related Topics of Interest

Examination of the ear
Foreign bodies in ENT
Otitis externa
Medicolegal aspects of ENT

29 Facial Nerve Palsy

A facial nerve palsy is a catastrophic event for a patient. It should be remembered that idiopathic palsy (Bell's palsy) is the commonest type and the majority of these patients have complete facial neve recovery. Early identification of the cause, appropriate treatment to avoid and limit long-term changes, and eye care are the tenets of optimal management.

29.1 Anatomy

The facial nerve is broadly divided into intracranial, intratemporal and extratemporal segments. Anatomy of the intracranial portion of the facial nerve is complex. Briefly, voluntary control is initiated by supranuclear inputs arising from the cerebral cortex projecting to the facial nucleus. Cell bodies of the upper facial motor nerves giving rise to the frontal branch receive bilateral cortical inputs, and neurons to the remainder of the facial nucleus receive contralateral cortical innervation. This explains why supranuclear (central) lesions affecting the facial nerve will not paralyse the forehead on the affected side, resulting in a unilateral facial paralysis with forehead sparing. Spontaneous facial movements are centrally transmitted via the extrapyramidal system, which involves diffuse axonal connections between multiple regions including the basal ganglia, amygdala, hypothalamus and motor cortex. The facial nuclei contain the cell bodies of facial nerve lower motor neurons, which exit the brainstem at the cerebellopontine angle, where it is joined by the nervus intermedius.

Both the facial and vestibulocochlear nerves enter the internal auditory meatus of the temporal bone simultaneously with the facial nerve located superior to the vestibulocochlear nerve. The facial nerve enters the fallopian canal which consists of labyrinthine, tympanic and mastoid segments. The labyrinthine segment is the narrowest segment. The geniculate ganglion resides within the distal part of the labyrinthine segment of the facial nerve. It gives rise to the first branch of the facial nerve— the greater petrosal nerve—which carries visceral motor parasympathetic fibres to the lacrimal gland. Two other branches—external petrosal nerve and lesser petrosal nerve—extend from the geniculate ganglion to provide innervation to the middle meningeal artery (sympathetic) and parotid gland (parasympathetic), respectively. The junction of the labyrinthine and tympanic components of the fallopian canal is formed by an acute angle (genu). The tympanic segment connects with the mastoid segment at the second genu and the facial nerve gives off three branches (stapedius, sensory branch of the facial nerve, chorda tympani) within this region. The chorda tympani is the terminal branch of the nervus intermedius.

The extratemporal component of the facial nerve starts when the facial nerve exits the stylomastoid foramen. It is relatively superficial in children and thus post-auricular incisions must be carefully planned because the trunk of the facial nerve is a subcutaneous structure at this level. However, in adults, the facial nerve is protected laterally by the mastoid tip, tympanic ring and mandibular ramus. After exiting the stylomastoid foramen, the facial nerve gives off motor branches to the posterior belly of digastric, stylohyoid, and the superior auricular, posterior auricular and occipitalis muscles. The facial nerve then travels along a course anterior to the posterior belly of the digastric and lateral to the external carotid artery and styloid process before dividing into its main motor branches (frontal, zygomatic, buccal, marginal mandibular, cervical) at the posterior edge of the parotid gland. The facial nerve trunk is usually identified approximately 1 cm deep and just inferior and medial to the tragal pointer.

The frontal branch is usually situated within the temporoparietal fascia. Therefore, injury to this nerve can be avoided if a subcutaneous plane superficial to the temporoparietal fascia or a deep plane on the surface of the deep temporoparietal fascia or between the superficial and deep layers of the deep temporal fascia was maintained during facelift procedure or parotidectomy. The marginal mandibular branch of the facial nerve, which innervates the depressor anguli oris musculature, is posterior to the facial artery and usually located above the inferior border of the mandible. The buccal branches become superficial as they emerge from the anterior border of the parotid gland lying beneath the superficial musculoaponeurotic system (SMAS).

Communication with the vestibulocochlear nerve occurs within the internal auditory meatus, with the otic ganglion and sympathetic afferents from geniculate ganglion branches, and with the auricular branch of the vagus nerve from a branch of the mastoid segment of the facial nerve. Extracranially, there are communications with the glossopharyngeal, vagus, greater auricular and the auriculotemporal nerves and multiple communications with branches of the trigeminal nerve. These interconnections explain the mastoid, ear, face and neck pain associated with herpes zoster and Bell's palsy, and the referred otalgia, face, occipital, throat, and neck pain which may occur with malignant disease.

29.2 Classification of Nerve Injury

Peripheral nerve injury may be classified in two different methods: the Seddon system and the Sunderland classification. The Seddon system defines three grades of nerve injury: (1) neuropraxia (conduction block due to cessation of axoplasmic flow), (2) axonotmesis (disruption of axons and distal wallerian degeneration), and (3) neurotmesis (disruption of endoneurium, perineurium and epineurium). The Sunderland classification which classifies injury into 5 degrees, is complex but more specific.

Evoked electromyography and maximal stimulation test response neurophysiological studies show that a neuropraxia injury gives normal results and an axonotmesis up to 10% of normal, but more severe injury gives no response. These studies can be used to provide a prognosis and to indicate if recovery is occurring.

29.3 Associated Features

Altered facial nerve function occurs with a variety of conditions and in a variety of forms.

1. *Synkinesis* The voluntary and reflex movement of groups of muscles that normally do not contract together. For example, blinking may be accompanied by movement of the corner of the mouth. This may occur after neurotmesis (or more severe injury) when the axons do not find their correct endoneural sheath. The longer the recovery of facial palsy is delayed, the higher is the incidence of synkinesis.
2. *Hemifacial spasm* This is an intermittent, involuntary spasm of the orbicularis oculi muscle which may spread to include other or all muscles of facial expression. It is thought to be most commonly caused by compression of the nerve by an artery in the posterior fossa. If this is confirmed by a magnetic resonance imaging (MRI) scan and angiography, the cause may be treated medically (e.g., muscle relaxants), Botox injection or surgically. Cerebellopontine angle tumours, Bell's palsy and facial nerve injury may also cause this phenomenon.
3. *Facial myokymia* In this condition, there are multiple fine but asynchronous facial movements often described as a 'bag of worms' appearance. It is associated with brainstem gliomas and multiple sclerosis.
4. *Blepharospasm* This is unilateral or more commonly bilateral involuntary spasmodic eye closure. Injection of botulinum A toxin into the orbicularis oculi may provide temporary relief.
5. *Crocodile tears* Lacrimation with eating can occur because of facial nerve injury in the region of the geniculate ganglion, where regenerating gustatory nerve fibres destined for the parotid gland are misdirected to the myelin sheath within the greater superficial petrosal nerve.

29.4 Severity Grading

There are numerous grading scales developed for facial palsy although none objectively document facial nerve function, track recovery and facilitate communication between health care professional effectively. Nevertheless, the most commonly used system is that of House–Brackmann which grades from I: normal function in all areas, to grade VI: total paralysis. Factors such as symmetry, resting tone and muscular movement at forehead, eye and mouth are used to score the dysfunction.

All ear, nose and throat (ENT) medical staff should grade all new facial palsy patients and follow-ups according to the House–Brackmann grading system. (▶ Table 29.1)

29.5 Causes of Facial Palsy

1. *Bell's palsy (55%)* An acute lower motor neuron facial palsy of unknown aetiology and therefore a diagnosis of exclusion. It is probably a herpes virus–induced immune response that leads to inflammation, swelling and consequent impaired function of the facial nerve.

▶ **Table 29.1** House–Brackmann grading system

Grade	Characteristics
I—Normal	Normal facial function in all areas
II—Mild dysfunction	*Gross* Slight weakness noticeable on close inspection May have slight synkinesis. At rest, normal symmetry and tone *Motion* Forehead: moderate-to-good function Eye: complete closure with effort Mouth: slightly weak with maximum effort
III—Moderate dysfunction	*Gross* Obvious, but not disfiguring difference between the two sides Noticeable, but not severe synkinesis, contracture or hemifacial spasm At rest, normal symmetry and tone *Motion* Forehead: slight-to-moderate movement Eye: complete closure with effort Mouth: slightly weak with maximum effort
IV—Moderately severe dysfunction	*Gross* Obvious weakness and/or disfiguring asymmetry At rest, normal symmetry and tone *Motion* Forehead: none Eye: incomplete closure Mouth: asymmetric with maximum effort
V—Severe dysfunction	*Gross* Only barely perceptible motion At rest, asymmetry *Motion* Forehead: none Eye: incomplete closure Mouth: slight movement
VI—Total paralysis	No movement at all

2. *Ramsay Hunt syndrome (synonym: herpes zoster oticus) (7%)* Caused by herpes zoster virus.
3. *Trauma (19%)* This may be external or iatrogenic. External trauma includes head injuries, temporal bone fracture (transverse fractures more frequently cause facial palsy) or penetrating trauma, usually in the parotid region.
4. *Tumour (6%)* These may arise from the nerve (facial nerve schwannoma), external compression of the nerve (vestibular nerve schwannoma) or invasion of the nerve (most commonly with parotid tumours).
5. *Infection (4%)* A lower motor neuron facial palsy may occur with acute suppurative otitis media (ASOM) (in the 8% who have a dehiscent fallopian canal), chronic suppurative otitis media (CSOM) either with or without cholesteatoma and malignant otitis externa.
6. *Central causes* For example, secondary to multiple sclerosis, gliomas or cerebrovascular accidents.
7. *Other causes* For example, sarcoid, drugs, myasthenia gravis and Guillain–Barré syndrome.

29.6 Clinical Features

In Bell's palsy, the facial nerve palsy is usually of rapid onset and associated with otalgia, altered facial sensation and taste. It recurs in 12%, more commonly on the contralateral side. Severe otalgia with vesicles involving the external ear associated with crusting, external ear canal oedema, a sensorineural hearing loss, tinnitus and vertigo are all common in Ramsay Hunt syndrome. The communications of the facial nerve may allow the face, neck, tongue, palate and buccal mucosa to become involved. It rarely recurs, but only 60% recover to House–Brackmann grade I or II. When trauma has caused the palsy, it is important to know the severity of a palsy as soon as possible after nerve injury as this will influence the management. Facial nerve palsies caused by tumours and infection are discussed elsewhere (see Related Topics of Interest).

29.7 Investigations

A high-resolution computed tomography (CT) or MRI scan to include the petrous temporal bone will exclude cerebellopontine angle tumours as a source of the palsy, sometimes necessary in suspected Bell's palsy as this is a diagnosis of exclusion. It may localise injury in cases due to trauma or chronic suppurative otitis media. An evoked electromyogram (EEMG), in which a stimulating electrode is placed adjacent to the stylomastoid foramen and recording electrodes are placed either on the skin over the facial muscles or through the skin into the muscles, is helpful. This test is used to examine the integrity of the facial nerve. If the EEMG response remains above 10% of normal during the first 10 days after injury, there is an excellent chance of grade I or II recovery (85%). The prognosis overall for those below this level is only a 20% chance of achieving grade I or II recovery, and many surgeons will therefore advocate surgical decompression of the nerve in these circumstances.

29.8 Management

1. *General* Reassurance and explanation are essential for all patients. Eye care is mandatory in order to prevent corneal ulceration and comprises artificial tears, eye closure with tape onto which is applied a light pressure dressing of cotton wool, ointment at night and eye protection when outdoors on windy or hot dry days with an eye pad. In patients with marked symptoms a lateral tarsorrhaphy or the insertion of a gold weight into the upper eyelid may be necessary as a permanent or temporary manoeuvre to ensure adequate eye closure.

   Management of patients with facial palsy is best delivered via multiprofessional teams. Patients with partial recovery will require facial physiotherapy literature, which suggests that the therapeutic use of surface EMG in conjunction with facial physiotherapy can help patients to develop selective muscle control and decreases synkinesis.

2. *Specific*
   a. *Bell's palsy* Based on high-quality randomised controlled trials with a preponderance of benefit (improvement in facial nerve function, faster recovery) over harm (steroid side effects, cost), clinicians should prescribe oral steroids within 72 hours of symptom onset for patients 16 years and older. Caution should be exercised in patients with diabetes, morbid obesity, previous steroid intolerance and psychiatric disorders; pregnant women should be treated on an individualised basis. Current evidence recommends against prescribing oral antivirals without steroids. Surgical decompression is only supported by low-level evidence based on non-randomised case series.

   b. *Ramsay Hunt syndrome* In addition to oral steroids, the commencement of acyclovir 800 mg five times daily for 7 days as early as possible during an attack may reduce the length of the infection and post-herpetic neuralgia. Contemporary literature review suggests that 70% of patients treated with combination steroids and antivirals achieve House–Brackmann grade I or II. Adequate analgesia is essential and splinting the external ear canal with a pope wick expanded with antibiotic/steroid drops will reduce the otalgia.

   c. *Trauma* If a complete lower motor neuron facial palsy is noted immediately after external trauma, this suggests that the nerve has been severed, and expedient exploration is recommended. It is preferable to anastomose the proximal to the distal stump after each has been prepared to present a clean surface. This must be performed without tension on the nerve and should this not be possible after preparation of the stumps, perhaps because significant debridement was necessary or the injury involved a significant length of nerve, then a cable of sural or great auricular nerve is necessary. A partial palsy or a delayed onset of a palsy can be managed conservatively with sequential EEMG monitoring. A course of oral steroids may facilitate reduction inflammation and hasten recovery.

F

d. *Tumour* The facial nerve is usually sacrificed if it has been infiltrated by tumour which cannot therefore be teased off the nerve. A cable graft is indicated in these circumstances.

e. *Infection* The management in these circumstances is discussed elsewhere in the book (see Related Topics of Interest). In summary, a palsy secondary to ASOM should be treated conservatively but that secondary to CSOM requires mastoid exploration to eradicate the underlying disease, although formal decompression of the nerve is probably unnecessary.

29.9 Follow-Up and Aftercare

If no recovery of function has occurred within a year of injury in those with a severe or complete palsy (grade V or VI), facial reanimation procedures, for example, hypoglossal or masseteric facial nerve graft, temporalis muscle sling, or a gold weight for the upper eyelid, may be indicated. Other facial procedures, for example, brow lift, midface lift, may be required as an adjunct to improve cosmetic facial symmetry.

Adequate counselling regarding eye care is essential. Maximum recovery may take 12 months so that no decision regarding permanent facial reanimation procedures should be undertaken until then. All patients should be regularly reviewed by a facial physiotherapist, and if necessary, a clinical psychologist as well for further support.

Further Reading

Bradford CR. Facial reanimation. Curr Opin Otolaryngol Head Neck Surg. 1994;(4):369–374

El-Kashlan H, Kileny P. Outpatient facial nerve evoked electromyography testing. Curr Opin Otolaryngol Head Neck Surg. 1998;(6):334–337

Fattah AY, Gurusinghe AD, Gavilan J, et al; Sir Charles Bell Society. Facial nerve grading instruments: systematic review of the literature and suggestion for uniformity. Plast Reconstr Surg. 2015;135(2):569–579

House JW, Brackmann DE. Facial nerve grading system. Otolaryngol Head Neck Surg. 1985;93(2):146–147

Jowett N, Hadlock TA. An evidence-based approach to facial reanimation. Facial Plast Surg Clin North Am. 2015; 23(3):313–334

Kim L, Byrne PJ. Controversies in contemporary facial reanimation. Facial Plast Surg Clin North Am. 2016; 24(3): 275–297

F

Related Topics of Interest

Suppurative otitis media—acute
Suppurative otitis media—chronic
Cosmetic surgery

30 Fistula

A fistula is an abnormal communication between two epithelial-lined surfaces. It is not to be confused with a sinus, which is a blind ending tract lined with epithelium. Fistulae may be congenital or acquired. Congenital fistulae usually occur as a result of a disorder of embryological development. Acquired fistulae occur as a result of infection, inflammation, malignancy, trauma or they may be iatrogenic.

30.1 Congenital Head and Neck Fistula

An understanding of embryology is required to manage congenital fistulae. They are usually due to a disorder of development of the branchial arch system. They have a range of expression and may present as a simple sinus (blind-ending, epithelial-lined pits), a cystic lump or a fistula with internal and external openings.

The branchial apparatus appears at about the fourth week of foetal development. It consists of six paired arches, separated by clefts externally (ectodermal) and pouches internally (endodermal), and is responsible for the formation of the lateral structures of the face and neck. The persistence of a cleft or pouch alone may lead to a simple sinus opening externally, or internally, respectively. Persistence of both can lead to the development of a fistula with both internal and external openings, joined by a fistula track.

30.1.1 First Branchial Arch Fistula

The first branchial arch is responsible for the formation of the malleus, incus, mandible and maxilla, amongst other structures. The first arch pouch forms the eustachian tube and middle ear, while the dorsal portion of the first arch cleft forms the external auditory meatus; the ventral portion is normally obliterated. When it persists, a first arch fistula will form. Although relatively uncommon (accounting for < 5% of branchial arch fistulae), they tend to be relatively large, have their superior opening in the external auditory canal and their inferior opening in the neck, somewhere between the tragus and the hyoid bone. They have a variable relationship to the facial nerve. Like all such fistulae, they carry a significant risk of infection and so are best excised. A full parotidectomy approach will be required, often after a prior fistulogram.

30.1.2 Second Branchial Arch Fistula

These are the commonest form of such fistula, accounting for approximately 95% of cases. The second branchial arch is responsible for the formation of the stapes, the stylohyoid ligament and the posterior portion of the hyoid bone. The second arch pouch forms the bed of the tonsillar fossa. The second arch also grows and extends inferiorly, over the second, third and fourth branchial clefts, which are normally obliterated. Where this obliteration does not occur, branchial cysts can form. If there is a connection to the skin, then a branchial sinus will form. If, in addition, there is a connection to the second branchial pouch, a fistula will be formed.

Such fistulae usually have a skin opening low in the neck, at the anterior border of the sternomastoid, and an internal opening in the tonsillar fossa. They usually pass between the internal and external carotid arteries.

Investigations usually involve a fistulogram, and may include a contrast computed tomography (CT) or magnetic resonance imaging (MRI) scan. Again, there is a risk of infection with such fistula and so surgical excision is warranted. The surgery will commence with an elliptical incision around the lower cervical opening but may require one or more further incisions, higher in the neck, to allow full visualisation of the fistula and to facilitate safe and complete excision. On rare occasions, an ipsilateral tonsillectomy may also be required.

30.1.3 Third and Fourth Branchial Arch Fistula

These fistulae are much less common than those described above. Where they occur, they tend to have a similar opening in the neck to the second arch fistulae, but the internal opening will be found in the pyriform fossa, or pharynx. Investigation and surgical excision follow the principles described earlier.

30.2 Acquired Fistula

30.2.1 Oroantral Fistula

An oroantral fistula is an abnormal communication between the oral cavity and the maxillary sinus. It can be caused by infection (tuberculosis, syphilis, leprosy), malignant neoplasms, phycomycoses, midline granuloma (a form of lymphoma), developmental clefts and cocaine abuse, but the most common cause of an oroantral fistula is tooth extraction. Maxillary first molars account for 50% of oroantral fistulae caused by extractions. It can occur as a consequence of infection of a bone graft placed during a sinus floor augmentation procedure. (Such procedures are performed through a lateral sinus window, not unlike a Caldwell–Luc approach. The sinus mucosa is elevated and some form of bone graft is placed in the floor of the sinus to create a thicker bony sinus floor to allow for the placement of osseointegrated dental implants).

Management

As always, prevention is better than cure, and so good surgical technique with a tension-free closure at the time of an initial tooth extraction is ideal. Small fistulae (< 5 mm) can usually be managed conservatively, or with simple primary closure after freshening the edges of the defect. Larger defects can be managed in a variety of ways but usually require some form of tissue to fill the defect and facilitate healing. The workhorse flaps in this situation are some form of buccal mucosal, or palatal mucoperiosteal, flap. Additional materials that have found some utility include gold, aluminium, polymethylmethacrylate, and even polyurethane foam.

Such fistulae are often managed by an oral or maxillofacial surgeon. However, any coexisting sinusitis, whether acute or chronic, will also require treatment, on its own merits, in order to encourage fistula healing and closure. This aspect will usually require the involvement of an ear, nose and throat (ENT) surgeon.

30.2.2 Orocutaneous Fistula

An orocutaneous fistula is a pathological communication between the cutaneous surface of the face and neck and the oral cavity. They are not common, but dental infections, salivary gland lesions, neoplasms and developmental lesions can cause orocutaneous fistulae, fistulae of the neck and intraoral fistulae. Chronic dental periapical infections or dentoalveolar abscesses are the most common cause of intraoral and extraoral fistulae. Fascial plane infections, neck space infections and osteomyelitis can cause cutaneous fistulae.

Osteomyelitis is more likely to develop in patients with uncontrolled diabetes and in those who have undergone irradiation following oral cavity or oropharyngeal carcinoma and who develop osteoradionecrosis. This occurs due to irradiation damage to osteocytes and impaired blood supply to the bone. The affected area becomes hypoxic and the bone necrotic. It usually occurs in the mandible, and causes chronic pain, ulceration, pathological fracture and orocutaneous fistula formation.

Prevention of osteoradionecrosis is a pivotal part of treatment planning. All head and neck cancer patients who are to receive radiotherapy should have an orthopantomogram (OPG) and be seen by a restorative dentist prior to therapy. They will ensure maximal oral hygiene and remove any carious teeth.

Treatment of established osteoradionecrosis is controversial. 'Triple therapy' of antibiotic medication (e.g., tetracycline), combined with pentoxifylline and tocopherol treatment are often used. Hyperbaric oxygen therapy has been advocated, but NICE only recommends it in the context of a trial. Surgery will ususally entail excision of the diseased bone, skin and mucosa and reconstruction with a composite flap and microvascular repair (e.g., fibula flap).

30.2.3 Chylous Fistula

The thoracic duct is at risk of damage during division of the lower end of the internal jugular vein during left-sided neck dissection. This is not a true fistula but rather a leak of chyle that finds its way out through the neck wound. If it can be identified at the time of surgery, it should be repaired, by tie, suture or muscle patch. However, in a fasting patient, the oily appearance is not always seen, and it is not until after the patient resumes dietary (oral) intake that the white, milky fluid becomes obvious, usually first seen in a neck drain inserted at the time of surgery.

Small leaks can be managed conservatively with low-fat diets and pressure dressings but unfortunately, high-volume leaks (> 300 mL/d)

F

carry a significant risk of hypoproteinemia and electrolyte loss. Such leaks may require reexploration and formal repair.

30.2.4 Pharyngocutaneous Fistula

A pharyngocutaneous fistula is an abnormal tract joining the pharynx to the skin of the neck. Fistulae are unlikely after closed pharyngeal surgery but may occur following open surgery to the head and neck in which the pharyngeal mucosa has also been damaged. Consequently, laryngectomy is the most commonly associated procedure. Furthermore, in recent years with an increasing focus on, and philosophy for organ preservation, chemoradiotherapy is finding a much greater role as the predominant treatment modality for even quite advanced laryngeal cancer. Consequently, laryngectomy is most frequently performed as a salvage procedure after failure of primary treatment. The risk of pharyngocutaneous fistula is significantly greater in this situation, with rates of 35 to 60% quoted, as compared to 5 to 15% for primary laryngectomy.

Additional risk factors include the following:

- Infection.
- Post-operative haematoma/chylous fistula/seroma.
- Residual neoplastic disease.
- Poor nutritional status/anaemia.
- Poor surgical technique.

30.3 Clinical Features

The patient will frequently develop a low-level pyrexia 3 or 4 days post-operatively, associated with cellulitis around the neck wound. A swinging pyrexia and abscess formation may ensue. Typically, on the seventh day the collection will rupture onto the skin and a fistula will form. At this stage there will be a discharge of mucopus and the patient's general condition will improve. In time, the discharge will become more mucoid and ultimately, saliva alone is discharged. In many cases, spontaneous resolution will occur, usually within 6 weeks. In persistent cases, especially in those having residual tumour or previous radiotherapy, there is the uncommon but ever-present spectre of a carotid blowout. The presence of such a fistula usually delays clinical progress (including speech therapy and functional rehabilitation) and hospital discharge.

30.4 Investigation

The diagnosis will be strongly suspected from the clinical features, especially from a red fluctuant swelling in the neck. After rupture, if the tract is small, the diagnosis may be confirmed by a water-soluble (gastrografin) swallow. With persistent and profuse discharge from a fistula, the urea, electrolytes and serum proteins should be checked regularly and the haemoglobin kept above 10 g/dL. Occasionally, a fistula occurs several days after commencing oral feeding in patients who have had an apparently uncomplicated post-operative course. A gastrografin swallow performed on the 10th to 12th post-operative day will show an anterior sinus in about 15% of patients, and it is this group who is at a significantly higher risk of developing such a fistula. It is suggested that nasogastric feeding be continued in this group for a further week and the gastrografin swallow repeated thereafter. In most cases, the sinus will have resolved, but if not, the process is repeated until healing.

30.5 Management

With the philosophy of prevention in mind, many surgeons will elect to support the neopharyngeal suture line with a pectoralis major muscle flap at the time of a salvage laryngectomy. There is mixed evidence for the benefit of such an undertaking but a number of centres and studies have presented data to show an approximate 50% reduction in their salivary fistula rate.

However, should it occur, a pharyngocutaneous fistula is initially managed conservatively. Nasogastric or gastrostomy feeding continues until the fistula has healed. The wound should be cleaned regularly and absorbent dressings used to avoid maceration of the surrounding skin until all necrotic tissue has separated and healing has started, this initial stage taking 2 or 3 weeks. The fistula may take many weeks to close spontaneously, and if personal and home circumstances are suitable, the patient can be allowed home and reviewed regularly in outpatients. Provided that the fistula continues to reduce in size, no surgical intervention is necessary, although granulation tissue should be biopsied to exclude recurrent disease in cancer patients. If the size does not reduce over any 2-week period after the initial separation stage, a prudent plan would be to endoscope the patient under a general anaesthetic to exclude recurrent disease then to proceed with a repair.

If the fistula opening is less than 1-cm diameter, a local rotation skin flap should be considered in the first instance. These often fail, however, because local tissue is relatively ischaemic either as a result of previous radiotherapy or because of scar tissue formation during healing. If a local flap fails or the defect is too large to consider this, the repair method of choice will depend on the surgeon's experience and microvascular training, and includes the pectoralis major myocutaneous flap, the deltopectoral flap, the radial forearm fasciocutaneous flap, the anterolateral thigh flap, and jejunum used as a tube or as a mucosal patch. Two flaps may be needed because it is important to line both the mucosal and cutaneous surfaces.

30.6 Follow-Up and Aftercare

Patients who have had surgery for a fistula are followed up at the same interval as those who did not develop a fistula, although they are at a higher risk of developing a stenosis at the level of the fistula. This may settle after several dilations, but occasionally the stenosis recurs persistently and frequently so that excision of the affected segment with reconstruction is indicated. Those who have had surgery for benign disease are unlikely to develop a stenosis, but follow-up for a year to exclude a late onset would seem sensible.

Further Reading

Lian TS, Nathan CA. What is the role of flap reconstruction in salvage total laryngectomy? Laryngoscope. 2014; 124(11): 2441–2442

Mizrachi A, Zloczower E, Hilly O, et al. The role of pectoralis major flap in reducing the incidence of pharyngocutaneous fistula following total laryngectomy: a single-centre experience with 102 patients. Clin Otolaryngol. 2016; 41(6):809–812

Related Topics of Interest

F

Hypopharyngeal carcinoma
Laryngectomy
Neck swellings

31 Foreign Bodies in ENT

This chapter covers the problems encountered with a foreign body in the ear, nose and throat (ENT). A button battery foreign body in the ear or upper aerodigestive tract can cause life-threatening and life-changing injury and is an absolute surgical emergency. Sharp or bony throat foreign bodies and irritative bronchial foreign bodies should be removed as an emergency. Patients with a suspected pharyngeal foreign body but normal flexible endoscopy, increasing odynophagia and pain on gentle side-to-side manipulation of the larynx are indications for an examination under anaesthetic.

tissues (it does not occur from leakage from the battery) causing a caustic burn to the tissues in contact with the battery. Therefore, septal perforation, external ear canal skin destruction, tympanic membrane destruction, pharyngeal perforation and oesophageal perforation are all possible with such a foreign body. Tissue destruction has been described within minutes of tissue contact. Its possibility as a foreign body in a patient means it should be regarded as an absolute surgical emergency, and immediate removal of the battery without waiting for a patient to be starved should occur.

31.1 Introduction

Placing a foreign body in one's ear or nose is not the usual practice of a sensible, mentally stable adult, and therefore one tends to see such foreign bodies in children, adults with learning difficulties, or those with mental health problems.

Normally, if the correct environment is created for such patients, they will allow a single attempt at removing the foreign body. An unsuccessful attempt that hurts the patient usually leads to a refusal to allow a second attempt and indeed they may not even allow a second doctor to examine the ear or nose. A correct environment is an uncluttered but child-friendly, warm, quiet treatment room, where the doctor and nurse can be calmly and confidently reassuring.

Nasal and ear foreign bodies are most commonly found in curious young children from the age of about 2 years onwards. Younger children may not have sufficient dexterity to insert an object into their nose or ear and the corollary of this is that such children may need to be discussed with the safeguarding team.

Button batteries as a foreign body in the ear, nose, throat or oesophagus should be highlighted because of the destruction of tissue in contact with the battery that might occur with devastating life-changing and sometimes life-threatening complications. The problem has been known for 30 years but was only recently highlighted with an NHS England safety alert of risk of death or serious harm. A button battery in contact with tissue on both sides of the battery, and even a spent battery, creates an electric current between the terminals. This causes sodium hydroxide to build up in the

31.2 Foreign Bodies in the Nose

The foreign body may be inorganic or organic. Inorganic foreign bodies include buttons, beads, metal, plastic from toys, stones, etc. They are often asymptomatic and may be discovered only accidentally during an examination for an unrelated complaint. Organic foreign bodies include sponge, rubber, paper, wood, peas and nuts. These are irritant and nasal mucosa usually becomes inflamed causing discharge and obstruction. A unilateral nasal discharge in a child should be regarded as being due to a foreign body until proved otherwise. The discharge is initially mucoid, then mucopurulent, and this in turn becomes pungent and sometimes sanguineous. Sinusitis may be a complication. Calcium and magnesium carbonates and phosphates may be deposited around a foreign body to form a rhinolith. Rhinoliths become impacted and usually require removal under a general anaesthetic.

31.2.1 Management

Confirmation of the presence of the foreign body is from the history and examination of the child. The child sits on either a parent's or nurse's knee. The anterior nares are exposed by gentle elevation of the nasal tip with a thumb (the rest of the fingers fanned and resting on the top of the head) and examined with a headlight. Alternatively, an auroscope with a 4.5-mm speculum may give a better view. Many children are cooperative provided they feel safe and reassured and it is possible, in many children, to remove a foreign body without the need for general anaesthesia (GA). Good illumination is essential, and all the instruments required should be to hand. The first effort will be the best and often the only attempt the child will allow. If it fails or if the foreign body is situated posteriorly in the nasal cavity, then a general anaesthetic will be required. It is important therefore that the attempt is made, or is supervised by as senior an ENT surgeon as possible. In very young children, it is reasonable for a parent or nurse (with parental consent) to sit the child on his or her lap with one hand firmly holding the head and the other arm tightly holding the trunk and the child's arms. The child's legs are secured between the adult's legs.

Removal is best accomplished with a wax hook or an old eustachian tube catheter. It is passed point downwards above the foreign body, which is brought to the floor of the nose and raked anteriorly. Cupped forceps or crocodile forceps are preferable for the removal of thin objects, such as buttons or soft organic objects, such as sponge.

In every case, the nasal cavity must be examined afterwards as there may be a second foreign body more posteriorly. The child should be discharged with a supply of Naseptin cream if there is mucosal inflammation or infection.

31.3 Foreign Bodies in the Ear

Ear foreign bodies are more common in school children than toddlers. The objects found may be organic (pieces of paper, rubber from open fit hearing aids in adults, pencil, seeds, peas and beans) or inorganic (beads, buttons, crayons and stones). Inorganic foreign bodies are often asymptomatic, but organic objects may give rise to otitis externa by local irritation of the epithelium of the meatal walls. Discharge and hearing loss from blockage of the external ear canal may occur. One of the commonest foreign bodies in adults is cotton wool from attempting to clean their ears.

31.3.1 Management

A foreign body in the external ear canal is usually easily seen on otoscopy. Removal may appear to be easy, but usually requires the skills and facilities of a specialist. Ill-directed attempts at the removal of foreign bodies by the untrained may lead to complications. Some foreign bodies should only be removed under a general anaesthetic. An example is an impacted large bead that has been inserted or displaced beyond the isthmus. This can be very tricky to remove even under a general anaesthetic.

Objects lying superficial to the external ear canal isthmus may be removed with suction, forceps or a fine hook using an operating microscope. Forceps are useful for soft materials such as paper, cotton wool or sponge but should never be used to remove smooth spherical objects such as beads and stones, as they will tend to push them further down the ear canal. Insects should be killed before syringing by instilling olive oil drops into the ear canal. If a large object has impacted beyond the isthmus, a drop of fibrin glue on the object, applied when slightly tacky and attached to the free end of a cotton bud may allow the object to be extracted.

Once the object is out, the tympanic membrane should be examined to ensure it has not been damaged. If there is a canal trauma or signs of an otitis externa, then antibiotic-steroid eardrops should be prescribed.

31.4 Foreign Bodies in the Pharynx

Sharp and irregular foreign bodies may become impacted in the tonsils, base of tongue, vallecula or pyriform fossae. Small fish bones are the commonest and usually lodge in the tonsil.

31.4.1 Management

The patient, usually an adult, will be able to localise the side and site with reasonable accuracy. A thorough examination of the oropharynx with a headlight and tongue depressor may reveal the offending bone. If a foreign body is not visualised, then flexible nasopharyngoscopy should be performed looking at the base of tongue, vallecula and pyriform fossae. The larynx should be gently manipulated from side to side looking for significant discomfort. Some patients will have no abnormal findings, and a lateral soft tissue radiograph is then indicated. If this too is normal, they should be reassured that their symptoms are likely to be due to a scratch from a foreign body. If the index of suspicion is quite high, then review a day or two later is sensible. If the foreign body sensation has started to wane, then it is probably due to a scratch and if repeat examination is again normal, the patient can be reassured with no further routine follow-up but with instructions to return if the resolution of symptoms does not continue. If swallowing has become more painful and gentle side-to-side manipulation of the larynx is painful,

F

indicating mucosal inflammation, this suggests there may be a pharyngeal foreign body. If flexible nasopharyngolaryngoscopy remains normal, most surgeons would want to perform a rigid endoscopy under GA.

If the flexible nasopharyngolaryngoscopy identifies the foreign body, it is often possible to remove the foreign body under local anaesthetic throat spray. In a patient anaesthetised with lignocaine spray and positioned on a flat bed with the neck and shoulders supported on a pillow, it is possible to pass the blade of a Macintosh laryngoscope into the vallecula to view the tongue base, vallecula and pyriform fossae, and therefore a visualised foreign body in this region can be removed. Some departments use a flexible bronchoscope, with a channel for grasping forceps, to remove a visualised pharyngeal foreign body. Patients who have been anaesthetised with lignocaine spray should be warned not to eat or drink for 2 hours as the laryngopharynx will be relatively insensate.

General anaesthesia is required to remove a foreign body from the pharynx if the patient is young or unable to tolerate the above examination.

31.5 Foreign Bodies in the Oesophagus

The risk of impaction of a foreign body depends on the size, shape and material of the object. The presence of an abnormality in the patient's aerodigestive tract, for example, a stricture, will make impaction more likely. A large bolus of swallowed food may become impacted even in a normal oesophagus. Children, mentally handicapped patients and some psychiatric patients are at risk of swallowing non-food foreign bodies. The commonest objects are coins in children and fish or meat bones in adults. Impaction is commonest at the level of the cricopharyngeus muscle but may also occur at the level where the oesophagus is crossed by the left main bronchus or at the cardia.

31.5.1 Clinical Features

Adults are usually aware of having swallowed something and can localise reasonably accurately the level at which it is impacted. Children and psychiatric patients may not be so reliable. Discomfort or pain in the oesophagus and difficulty in swallowing are the cardinal symptoms. Dysphagia may be total. The foreign body may

cause coughing and excessive salivation. Clinical examination may be normal, but pooling in the pyriform fossae is usually evident. There may be localised tenderness in the neck and crepitus owing to surgical emphysema if there has been an oesophageal perforation.

31.5.2 Management

Lateral and anteroposterior soft tissue radiographs of the neck and chest radiographs are mandatory. Some foreign bodies are easily identified because they are radiopaque. The inexperienced may confuse calcification in the laryngeal cartilages with an opaque foreign body. Widening of the soft tissue postcricoid space or a persistent air bubble in the oesophagus may occur. Widening of this space by more than the width of one vertebral body indicates cellulitis caused by an impacted foreign body. If the foreign body has caused a tear, surgical emphysema will be shown radiologically. A gastrografin swallow (pale yellow, transparent, water-soluble, iodine-based liquid) or Omnipaque 500 swallow (colourless, transparent, water-soluble, iodine-based liquid) can be performed before or after removal of a foreign body if more information is needed to determine whether such a perforation is present.

If the obstruction is due to an impacted soft, non-bony, food bolus, the safest treatment is to admit the patient and give a dose of intravenous hyoscine butylbromide and diazepam. This may allow the oesophagus to relax and permit the passage of the bolus. Some surgeons have suggested drinking a soda (fizzy drink) will encourage this process. The patient should have a barium swallow after bolus removal to determine if there is an identifiable cause for the obstruction such as an oesophageal neoplasm, an oesophageal stricture or an uncoordinated swallow.

If there is an impacted sharp or bony object, the patient requires an oesophagoscopy as an emergency procedure. Using a rigid oesophagoscope, the foreign body is identified and if possible, it is drawn into the end of the scope using forceps. The scope and the foreign body should be withdrawn in unison under direct vision. If there is a mucosal tear, the patient should remain in hospital for 24 hours post-operatively, have antibiotics prescribed, and be nil by mouth for the first 4 hours and only water for the next 4 hours. The pulse, temperature, blood pressure and respiratory rate

F

should be monitored every half hour for the first 4 hours and then hourly for the next 4 hours and the surgeon informed if the patient complains of chest or back pain. The neck should be examined initially every half hour for a couple of hours to determine if there is surgical emphysema. Perforation of the oesophagus should be treated with intravenous antibiotics and nasogastric feeding. Perforation of the thoracic oesophagus should initiate an early liaison and referral to a thoracic surgeon. Surgical repair should be considered depending on the perforation's site and size and the patient's general condition.

31.6 Foreign Bodies in the Trachea and Bronchi

Inhalation of a foreign object is most common in children under the age of 3 years. The event can easily escape a parent's notice. A history of an unexplained choking fit should be sought, particularly if there is an unaccounted for small object with which the child was playing. Adults usually give a clear history of foreign body inhalation. Most inhaled foreign bodies enter the right main bronchus, which is larger and more vertical than the left.

31.6.1 Clinical Features

After the initial inhalation, which causes choking and coughing, and sometimes cyanosis, the foreign body may pass into the trachea. Here, it may initially cause just mild irritation and no more than an intermittent cough or throat clearance. Sometimes there is an inspiratory or a biphasic stridor and sometimes an expiratory wheeze. For this reason, if there is a good history suggestive of inhalation of an object, the child should have a bronchoscopy even if there are no chest symptoms and signs. A foreign body may partly occlude the bronchus and act as a valve so that the partly obstructed lung becomes overinflated. A foreign body which is causing a complete obstruction of a bronchus will produce collapse of that lung segment, followed by consolidation.

Vegetable foreign bodies are particularly dangerous (nuts, pips, vegetables, fruits) as they will cause an intense inflammatory reaction of the bronchial mucosa leading to a pneumonitis.

A chest X-ray is therefore mandatory and may show the foreign body if it is radiopaque or show signs of consolidation, collapse or hyperinflation if it is not.

Radiolucent objects are suspected when there is unexplained atelectasis, obstructive emphysema, mediastinal shift or consolidation of the lung.

31.6.2 Treatment

Bronchoscopy should be performed as soon as possible. A senior ENT surgeon and anaesthetist are required. A variety of bronchoscopes, suction tubes and forceps appropriate to the nature of the foreign body and size of the patient need to be readily available. Flexible fibre-optic bronchoscopy by the chest physicians for adult bronchial foreign bodies is used in some centres. Ventilating Hopkins rod bronchoscopes should be available with young children.

Antibiotics and physiotherapy may be necessary after bronchoscopy if there are signs of pneumonitis.

Further Reading

Figueiredo RR, Azevedo AA, Kós AO, Tomita S. Complications of ENT foreign bodies: a retrospective study. Rev Bras Otorrinolaringol (Engl Ed). 2008; 74(1):7–15

McRae D, Premachandra DJ, Gatland DJ. Button batteries in the ear, nose and cervical esophagus: a destructive foreign body. J Otolaryngol. 1989; 18(6):317–319

Related Topics of Interest

Paediatric airway problems
Paediatric endoscopy

F

32 Functional Endoscopic Sinus Surgery

The endoscopic approach has replaced the external approach as the default approach in sinus surgery for benign disease. It is used in combination with the external approach for most sinonasal malignancies. Although life-threatening and life-changing complications of endoscopic sinus surgery are rare, extensive experience and expertise is necessary in basic endoscopic sinus surgery before training in extended applications is undertaken, usually as part of a rhinology fellowship. The role of balloon sinuplasty in sinus disease has not yet been fully defined, but it is an acceptable alternative technique to endoscopic sinus surgery for blocked ostia of the maxillary, frontal and sphenoid sinuses.

32.1 Principle

Most infections of the sinuses are rhinogenic, that is, disease spreads from the nose to the paranasal sinuses. The anterior ethmoid sinus air cells and clefts are regarded as prechambers of the frontal and maxillary sinuses. Disease of these prechambers may interfere with ventilation and drainage of the frontal and maxillary sinuses and cause acute or chronic mucosal disease. Similarly, disease of the posterior ethmoid sinuses may interfere with ventilation and drainage of the sphenoid sinus.

Endoscopic sinus surgery is minimally invasive surgery, which aims to provide ventilation and drainage of the ethmoid sinuses and the secondarily involved maxillary, frontal and sphenoid sinuses. The emphasis of surgery is to preserve, as far as possible, normal anatomy and mucosa. Mucosal stripping leaves exposed sinus bone, which does not heal with ciliated respiratory epithelium, but with either scar tissue or a low columnar non-ciliated epithelium. Scarring and absence of cilia may lead to an area of mucosa that is not self-cleaning. Mucous dries on this area and this may lead to chronic infection of mucosa and underlying bone. This in turn causes mucosal oedema which can compromise ventilation and drainage. Good surgical technique is therefore paramount.

32.2 Pathophysiology

Mucus produced in the maxillary sinus is transported from the floor of the sinus along the sinus walls, to the natural ostium by mucociliary transport. The frontal and maxillary sinuses communicate with the nose through a complex system of narrow clefts, which allow drainage and ventilation. These clefts are only a few millimetres wide and contain opposing mucosal surfaces lined with ciliated respiratory epithelium. If extensive contact of opposing mucosal surfaces occurs, whatever the cause, the ciliary beat activity may be impeded so that spaces are blocked and do not drain. Common locations for contact areas in the sinuses include the frontal recess, the ethmoidal infundibulum, the turbinate sinus (cleft between the bulla and middle turbinate) and the lateral sinus, which lies above and behind the ethmoid bulla.

Anatomical variations of the middle turbinate, uncinate process and the ethmoid bulla are common. The incidence of these variations is the same in a population with no history of sinus disease and a population with recurrent acute or chronic sinusitis. Therefore, anatomical variations, while of academic interest, are not thought to predispose to sinusitis. Persistent mucosal disease of the ethmoidal infundibulum, frontal recess and posterior ethmoids may predispose patients to recurrent maxillary, frontal sinus and sphenoid sinus infection.

32.3 Indications for Endoscopic Sinus Surgery

- Recurrent acute rhinosinusitis.
- Chronic rhinosinusitis resistant to medical therapy.
- Polypoidal rhinosinopathy resistant to medical therapy.
- Mucoceles.
- Sinus mycosis.
- Adjuvant surgery to allergy treatment.
- Antrochoanal polyps.
- Endoscopic bipolar diathermy for anterior/posterior epistaxis.
- Blockage of the nasolacrimal duct requiring endoscopic dacryocystorhinostomy.
- Endoscopic resection of inverted papilloma.
- Endoscopic ligation/diathermy of the spheno-palatine artery for epistaxis.

Extended applications include the following:

- Endoscopic arrest of cerebrospinal fluid (CSF) rhinorrhoea.

- Endoscopic orbital decompression, most commonly for dysthyroid eye disease.
- Endoscopic drainage of an orbital abscess.
- Endoscopic optic nerve decompression.
- Endoscopic pituitary surgery.
- Endoscopic Draf procedures for frontal sinus disease and laterally based frontal sinus mucoceles often because disease has been contained within the frontal sinus because of anatomical variations (such as a Kuhn cell).
- Endoscopic resection of sinoethmoid and anterior skull base malignancy, combined with an open approach.
- Endoscopic transpituitary surgery to resect clivus tumours such as chordoma.

Extensive experience and expertise is necessary in basic endoscopic sinus surgery before training in extended applications is undertaken, usually as part of a rhinology fellowship. Experience in the setting up and use of image guidance is important for undertaking many of these procedures. Revision cases can be challenging, particularly if primary surgery, performed by inexperienced surgeons, has caused a lack of anatomical landmarks, significant scarring, and narrowing of natural ostia due to mucosal stripping.

32.3.1 Investigations

A high-definition computed tomography (CT) scan of the paranasal sinuses on bone setting is required before undertaking endoscopic sinus surgery (except for the treatment of epistaxis). A common protocol would be a rapid-sequence multislice CT scan with 0.5-mm slice thickness for the frontal recess surgery and 1 mm for the rest of the sinuses. The scan can be reconstructed in any plane, but the coronal slices are usually the most useful. Axial slices allow one to determine the orientation of the internal carotid artery and optic nerve in the region of the posterior ethmoid and sphenoid sinus. A gadolinium-enhanced magnetic resonance imaging (MRI) is indicated if sinonasal malignancy or inverted papilloma is suspected as this will allow one to distinguish solid tumour from retained sinus secretions. An MRI will accurately delineate the extent of anterior skull base tumours extending into the nose.

32.3.2 Surgical Technique

Surgery limited to the anterior ethmoid sinuses may be performed under local anaesthetic with topical vasoconstriction and perhaps sedation, but more extensive surgery, for example, frontal recess surgery and posterior ethmoid surgery usually require a general anaesthetic. Endoscopic sphenopalatine artery ligation, if necessary with a septoplasty, can usually be performed under a local anaesthetic in patients unfit for a general anaesthetic.

The aim of surgery for rhinosinusitis is to re-establish ventilation and drainage of the diseased paranasal sinus group involved as defined by the patient's symptoms and CT scan. Uninvolved sinus groups are not disturbed. Surgery is performed in a stepwise manner from front to back (Messerklinger's technique) or from the sphenoid forward (Wigand's technique).

Through-cutting instruments, which cleanly cut through the mucosa and bone of sinus air cells, prevent avulsion and stripping of mucosa.

The microdebrider cleanly cuts and aspirates tissue. In experienced hands the microdebrider can be used for a complete sphenoethmoidectomy. The microdebrider is an extremely efficient way of removing soft tissue disease, and in particular, polypoid rhinosinopathy, but its detractors claim its usefulness for bone work is not proven as it may cause excessive scarring. It may, in the unwary, cause disastrous orbital injuries by rapidly sucking and debriding the orbital contents (in particular, fat which can cause intraorbital bleeding and blindness, and the medial rectus which will cause a medial rectus palsy and lifelong diplopia) if the lamina papyracea is breached.

Most experienced endoscopic surgeons in the United Kingdom have both through-cutting instruments and the microdebrider to hand during surgery. An endoscopic washer which irrigates the endoscope tip is particularly useful in long cases when repeated removal of the endoscope for tip cleaning may cause trauma and increase the risk of post-operative adhesions and vestibular crusting.

Balloon sinuplasty is a recognised technique to create ventilation of the maxillary, frontal and sphenoid sinuses rather than a formal dissection of the relevant sinuses. The technique has suffered from a lack of good-quality follow-up data although recent studies have suggested quality-of-life improvement that is similar to FESS but a higher price of consumables and setup costs. In another study, 40 patients having balloon sinuplasty were compared to 45 having FESS. The sinuplasty group had a greater percentage of patient-reported acute sinusitis exacerbations, less resolution of thick nasal discharge, and a 10% revision surgery rate

F

compared to none in the FESS group. It is therefore important that surgeons advocating this technique keep outcome data and diligently compare their data to published outcomes of other surgeons.

32.4 Complications

Complications of endoscopic sinus surgery may be life threatening or cause significant long-term morbidity to patients. Complications may be reduced by a thorough understanding of sinus anatomy, study of the CT scan pre-operatively to look for potential pitfalls, extensive cadaver dissection and observation of the surgical technique of experienced surgeons. Attendance at a postgraduate sinus anatomy course that allows cadaveric dissection is of considerable benefit to trainees. The inexperienced surgeon should be closely supervised by an experienced endoscopic sinus surgeon. Many complications occur due to not recognising sinus anatomy, or to working in a poor visibility surgical field, due to intraoperative bleeding.

Major complications are particularly likely to happen once the surgeon has gained some confidence and experience in the technique but has not yet learned the finer points of anatomy, nor learned when to stop during a procedure. If the surgeon is uncertain of the anatomy, or cannot visualise landmarks due to bleeding, then he or she should ask for advice, or if this is not available, then stop the operation. It is much better to complete the surgery with a second-stage procedure than to cause a major complication at the initial procedure.

1. Peri- or intra-operative
   - Anaesthetic reaction.
   - Bleeding.
   - Penetration of the lamina papyracea to cause periorbital bruising and intra-orbital bleeding or a serious orbital injury such as medial rectus trauma or optic nerve injury.
   - CSF leak due to penetration of the anterior skull base. This may also occur when mobilising the middle turbinate medially or laterally due to the attachment of the anterior third of the middle turbinate to the lateral lamina of the lamina cribrosa.
   - Nasolacrimal duct injury.
   - Injury to structures impinging upon the lateral sphenoid sinus wall, namely, the internal carotid artery and optic nerve.

2. Immediate post-operative
   - Intra-orbital bleeding.
   - Epistaxis.

Blindness and diplopia from perioperative complications will only become apparent on patient waking.

3. Early post-operative
   - CSF leak (sometimes an unrecognised intra-operative complication).
   - Intra-cranial infection (meningitis, brain abscess).

4. Late complications
   - Intra-nasal adhesions, particularly within the ethmoidal cavity, between the middle turbinate and septum, or between the lateral nasal wall and nasal septum.
   - Sequelae of peri-operative and early post-operative complications.
   - Recurrent disease.

32.5 Management of Major Complications

1. CSF rhinorrhoea
   A CSF leak is the commonest major complication of endoscopic sinus surgery. If the leak is identified at the time of surgery, then the site of the leak should be confirmed, and the leak arrested. There are many techniques described to arrest the CSF leak, but the commonest methods are to use temporalis fascia, muscle, fat or a combination to plug the defect. A middle turbinate flap or a free turbinate graft may be used to reinforce the repair. Tisseel glue may be used to obtain a good seal with a piece of silastic used to separate the graft from intra-nasal packing. This is left in situ for several days. A lumber drain is usually unnecessary.

2. Intra-orbital bleed
   This is one of the most feared complications of endoscopic sinus surgery and may occur when the anterior ethmoidal artery has been divided during surgery and retracts into the orbit while continuing to bleed. The artery runs through the orbital fat as the ophthalmic artery and exits medially within the orbit collecting a layer of orbital periosteum as it passes through the lamina papyracea to enter the anterior ethmoid just below and behind the frontal sinus ostium.

On most occasions, the anterior ethmoidal artery is merely traumatised and not divided so it does not retract. If it is divided, it may be held within the ethmoid cavity by attachments of mucosa which are running between the artery and the lacrimal bone. It is most likely to happen when the artery is divided when lying within a bony canal running from the orbit to the anterior cranial fossa, as in these circumstances there will be no soft tissue attachments preventing the artery from retracting into the orbit. An intraorbital bleed caused by such an event will cause the eye to rapidly bulge and become tense, and rapid decompression of the orbit is necessary to save the patient's vision.

It has been recommended that a lateral canthotomy be performed, perhaps with division of the orbital septum in the lower lid, to allow the orbital contents to flow laterally and anteriorly and buy the surgeon some time to locate and ligate the anterior ethmoidal artery. However, most surgeons will not have seen nor performed this procedure before and with a patient's vision in immediate danger it is arguably not the time to start. In such circumstances, most advocate an external ethmoid approach to the anterior ethmoidal artery which is cauterised or ligated if located. The lamina papyracea is removed and a formal orbital decompression performed with incision of the orbital periosteum as for dysthyroid eye disease. This will allow orbital fat and soft tissues to herniate into the ethmoids and will also provide drainage for any continued bleeding.

An endoscopic decompression of the orbit is an alternative for the experienced surgeon. The surgeon has already performed an ethmoidectomy and the lamina papyracea is identified and the thin bone removed endoscopically exposing the orbital periosteum which is then incised. This medial endoscopic decompression approach has the disadvantage of great difficulty in identifying the bleeding anterior ethmoid vessel, which will lie very high and posterior within the orbital fat.

32.6 Follow-Up and Aftercare

Epithelialisation of the ethmoid cavity is usually complete within 2 to 4 weeks of surgery. Postoperative saline nasal douching, morning and night, to soften nasal crusts and secretions so they may then be expelled by blowing the nose, is advised. This usually allows the ethmoid cavity to heal and to become crust-free at 2 to 4 weeks' postsurgery obviating the need to remove persisting crusts. Postoperative steroids and antibiotics may be indicated depending on the surgeon's preference and the underlying disease process.

Further Reading

Bizaki AJ, Taulu R, Numminen J, Rautiainen M. Quality of life after endoscopic sinus surgery or balloon sinuplasty: a randomized clinical study. Rhinology. 2014; 52(4):300–305

Bolger WE, Brown CL, Church CA, et al. Safety and outcomes of balloon catheter sinusotomy: a multicenter 24-week analysis in 115 patients. Otolaryngol Head Neck Surg. 2007; 137(1):10–20

Koskinen A, Myller J, Mattila P, et al. Long-term follow-up after ESS and balloon sinuplasty: Comparison of symptom reduction and patient satisfaction. Acta Otolaryngol. 2016; 136(5):532–536

Suzuki S, Yasunaga H, Matsui H, Fushimi K, Kondo K, Yamasoba T. Complication rates after functional endoscopic sinus surgery: analysis of 50,734 Japanese patients. Laryngoscope. 2015; 125(8):1785–1791

Wigand ME. Transnasal ethmoidectomy under endoscopical control. Rhinology. 1981; 19(1):7–15

F

Related Topics of Interest

Rhinitis—allergic
Rhinitis—non-allergic
Rhinosinusitis—appropriate terminology

33 Globus Pharyngeus

Globus pharyngeus is the description of a typical symptom complex, and a diagnosis of exclusion. The symptoms are variably described, but generally are perceived as the sensation of a lump, discomfort, tightness or foreign body in the throat. It is a common reason for ENT clinic referral and the emphasis is primarily on the exclusion of a serious underlying disorder, and secondarily, the identification of underlying contributory factors that can be treated. The priority for most patients is the exclusion of cancer, but it should be remembered globus pharyngeus is very common and throat cancer is very uncommon.

33.1 Clinical Presentation and Assessment in Clinic

Patients can be of any age and of either sex. The complaint is typically of a sensation of a lump in the throat, usually between the sternal notch and thyroid cartilage. The patient might perceive the lump as an irritation, a foreign object stuck in the throat, catarrh stuck in the throat (and maybe as a post-nasal drip), persistent dryness and, or tightness. It is often difficult to define and describe, hence the variety of descriptions. It is usually central but can lateralise.

Initial clinical assessment consists of taking a thorough history, ENT examination and flexible nasopharyngolaryngoscopy.

▶ Table 33.1 summarises the commoner and important possible underlying causes or factors (when there is one that can be identified), and the symptoms and signs that can help to guide the clinician. When an underlying pathology can be identified, then the diagnosis is no longer 'globus pharyngeus' rather that of the underlying pathology.

The first priority is the identification of features that might suggest the possibility of cancer. These are described in ▶ Table 33.1. A key direct question to ask the patient is what happens to the symptom when eating or drinking. Typically in globus pharyngeus, the symptom will improve or even disappear for a time, and tends to be more noticeable when not swallowing or with a 'dry' swallow.

A worsening of symptoms with swallowing should alert the clinician to a physical abnormality, including cancer. Other features that alert the

clinician to a possibility of cancer are noted in ▶ Table 33.1. Note that the absence of a smoking history should not be taken as a reassuring factor, especially in the current era of human papillomavirus (HPV)-driven oropharyngeal cancer.

The second priority is to identify any other specific underlying cause. This includes laryngopharyngeal reflux (LPR). All of the typical LPR symptoms noted in ▶ Table 33.1 can be present when there is no reflux at all, as in cases of a muscle tension disorder. They are therefore very non-specific. The classic endoscopic signs attributable to LPR can also be found, at least to a degree, when there is no LPR. In the absence of classic LPR symptoms and clinical signs, then this diagnosis should be questioned, as it is arguably overdiagnosed in clinical practice.

An underlying neuromuscular motility or tension disorder is probably the most common underlying problem, although this is impossible to diagnose. Disorders of motor function have been demonstrated in globus patients, including elevation of cricopharyngeal sphincter pressure, midoesophageal dysmotility and poor lower oesophageal sphincter relaxation, but there is still debate as to whether these are primary or secondary phenomena. There is also debate as to whether these findings may interrelate with psychological distress. Furthermore, many patients found themselves in the viscous cycle of having the globus symptom, repeatedly throat clearing, which then makes the muscle tension (especially cricopharyngeus muscle tension) worse, leading to a worsening perception of symptoms, further throat clearing, and so on.

33.2 Investigations and Management

The subsequent investigation and management is dependent on the clinic findings. Clearly, in some (a small minority) cases, a specific diagnosis will be made (or at least strongly suspected). In these cases, for example, a cancer, thyroid goitre, arytenoid granuloma, etc., subsequent investigation and management will be directed accordingly.

If there are enough 'red flags' or potentially suspicious features, then a more in-depth investigation of the upper aerodigestive tract is mandated.

▶ **Table 33.1** Identifiable underlying causes of globus pharyngeus symptoms

Type of disorder	Detail	Clinical features/comments
Cancer	Oropharynx Hypopharynx Larynx Upper oesophageal	Soreness/pain, especially worse on swallowing
		Odynophagia
		Food sticking
		Otalgia
		Lateralising symptom
		Progressive symptom development
		Abnormality seen on flexible laryngoscopy
		Lymphadenopathy
Mucosal irritation	Laryngopharyngeal reflux (LPR)	Tickly throat
		Cough
		Worse in morning
		Hoarseness
		Other GORD symptoms
		Sore throat
	Arytenoid granuloma	Cough
		Hoarseness Otalgia Lateralised throat discomfort/soreness
		Endoscopic finding
	Rhinosinusitis/post-nasal drip	Probably overdiagnosed
		Must have clear examination evidence of chronic sinusitis for this to be a possibility
Extrinsic compression	Goitre/thyroid mass	Palpable on examination (unless totally retrosternal) Visible on CT scan
	Osteophyte	Arthritis history Visible on X-ray
Pouch	Pharyngeal pouch	Structural, therefore worse with swallowing Slow swallowing
		Regurgitation Recurrent chest infections Halitosis
Neuromuscular	Cricopharygeal muscle tension Oesophageal motility disorders Vocal cord palsy	May be related to psychological distress, including fear of an underlying cancer
		Causes and is made worse by repeated throat clearing or dry-swallowing Voice change Pooling or vocal cord palsy visible on nasopharyngoscopy
Psychological factors	Probably leads to musculoskeletal disorder	Probably leads to musculoskeletal disorder
		Mental health disorder
		Fear of throat cancer may be stated or understated
Hyposalivation	Drug side effect (anti-cholinergic medications)	Drug history
		Dry mucosa
	Sjögren's syndrome (SS)	Other clinical features of SS

Abbreviation: GORD, gastro-oesophageal reflux disease.

This can take the form of formal panendoscopy under general anaesthesia, or, alternatively, outpatient transnasal oesophagoscopy (TNO).

A barium swallow may be helpful if there is true swallowing dysfunction (i.e., true dysphagia, regurgitation, etc.) and may show a pharyngeal pouch, oesophageal web, stricture or achalasia. Cervical arthritis and impinging osteophytes may be seen. However, a barium swallow is frequently normal and has a low diagnostic yield, and so some observers have questioned its role in the diagnosis of globus pharyngeus.

In the absence of suspicious features, then, the most important intervention is arguably reassurance regarding the lack of suspicion or evidence of a cancer, which is often the patient's main (or only) concern. In cases in which the underlying problem is either one of underlying muscle tension or anxiety, or both, this reassurance may be enough to help resolve the symptoms. However, it is also useful to encourage patients to get out of the habit of recurrent throat clearing and to drink more water, more often, in order to get out of the vicious cycle described earlier.

When there is a suggestion of LPR (▶Table 33.1), then a trial of antireflux treatment is worthwhile. This entails twice-daily proton pump inhibitor (PPI), with or without gaviscon and with or without lifestyle changes. When patients do not have gastro-oesophageal reflux disease (GORD), they are often fairly sceptical about silent LPR and getting them to comply with such measures may be a challenge.

33.3 Follow-Up and Aftercare

In the scenario of the absence of suspicious features, as described earlier, then the next question is whether to discharge the patient. If there are no concerning or potentially concerning symptoms or features, then discharge may be reasonable, particularly with specific guidance given to the patient and GP about returning if there are changes in the symptoms. Otherwise, a review in 6 weeks—3 months may be warranted in order to establish whether there is any progression, emergence of more worrying features, or establish response (if any) to anti-reflux measures. At follow-up, there will be another opportunity to reassess the patient and arrange panendoscopy or TNO, if required or indicated.

Further Reading

Alaani A, Vengala S, Johnston MN. The role of barium swallow in the management of the globus pharyngeus. Eur Arch Otorhinolaryngol. 2007; 264(9):1095–1097

Dumper J, Mechor B, Chau J, Allegretto M. Lansoprazole in globus pharyngeus: double-blind, randomized, placebo-controlled trial. J Otolaryngol Head Neck Surg. 2008; 37(5):657–663

Haft S, Carey RM, Farquhar D, Mirza N. Anticholinergic medication use is associated with globus pharyngeus. J Laryngol Otol. 2016; 130(12):1125–1129

Karkos PD, Wilson JA. The diagnosis and management of globus pharyngeus: our perspective from the United Kingdom. Curr Opin Otolaryngol Head Neck Surg. 2008; 16(6):521–524

Sanyaolu LN, Jemah A, Stew B, Ingrams DR. The role of transnasal oesophagoscopy in the management of globus pharyngeus and non-progressive dysphagia. Ann R Coll Surg Engl. 2016; 98(1):49–52

Related Topics of Interest

Hypopharyngeal carcinoma
Pharyngeal pouch
Cough
Laryngeal carcinoma
Vocal fold paralysis

G

34 Halitosis

Halitosis is common even in fit, healthy individuals and will occur in most patients at some part of the day due to a variety of factors. In most, halitosis is short lived as the cause is immediately recognised and addressed, but in others, further investigation is required. Persistent objective halitosis is usually caused by poor oral hygiene or by volatile sulphur compounds collecting within layers of dead squames on the dorsal surface of the tongue. A range of systemic disease and certain drugs can also cause halitosis so that a detailed history is important. There are some patients with no objective halitosis, who may have visited doctors in many specialties for advice, and continue to complain of bad breath. Such patients may require psychological counselling.

34.1 Classification

The causes of halitosis can be divided into the following:

1. Physiological.
2. Pathological:
   a. Oral cavity.
   b. Extra-oral.
      • Upper aerodigestive tract, gastro-oesophageal and lower respiratory tract.
      • Systemic causes.
3. Drug causes.

About 15% of patients who complain of smelly breath have no detectable malodour (pseudohalitosis). In view of there being no true halitosis, the treatment of such patients consists of counselling and reassurance about their misconception. In this group, some will have had true halitosis that has been successfully treated but they still believe, despite counselling, that they have halitosis. Other patients with pseudohalitosis have never had true halitosis and they too may not respond to counselling. These patients are described as having halitophobia or delusional halitosis.

34.2 Physiological Halitosis

This is usually mild and short lived. It is often present on waking when it is due to a reduction in saliva production at night combined with the drying effects of mouth breathing. Dehydration has similar effects as it will lead to a reduction in saliva production and a dry mouth. This then allows the increased production of volatile sulphur compounds (VSCs) by oral bacteria and gives rise to halitosis. Drinking tea, coffee or alcohol, smoking a pipe or cigarettes and eating certain food such as garlic and raw onion may also cause a physiological halitosis.

34.3 Oral Cavity Pathology

Saliva plays a crucial role in the oral cavity, and is involved in taste, lubrication, water balance and oral hygiene. Saliva acts as a mechanical cleansing agent, its buffers combat acid/alkali excesses and the secreted immunoglobulins have an important anti-infective function. Any prolonged reduction in salivary flow allows an increase in the local bacterial flora. These microorganisms break down proteins with the production of odiferous volatile gases and consequent halitosis as well as leading to an increase in gingivitis, dental caries and periodontal disease, themselves a cause of halitosis. A decrease in saliva production can occur temporarily, for example, during sleep and with anxiety or more permanently from previous radiotherapy if the field involves the oral cavity and pharynx. It is also associated with cardiac and renal failure and some autoimmune conditions (Sjögren's disease).

There may be a predisposition to forming a thick layer of dead squames on the dorsal tongue surface which is exacerbated by other factors such as smoking, poor dental hygiene and dehydration. This layer of squames contains VSCs and is a significant cause of objective halitosis.

Any local inflammatory lesion may become secondarily infected and lead to halitosis. Vincent's disease, also known as Vincent's angina, trench mouth or Vincent infection, is acute necrotising ulcerative gingivitis. It is reasonably common, the main features being painful, bleeding gums, ulceration of the interdental papillae and acute necrotising pharyngitis. It is caused by fusiform bacilli (*Bacillus fusiformis*) and spirochetes (*Borrelia vincentii*).

Poor dentition may allow the trapping of food within or between teeth. A localised osteitis

H

following dental extraction may lead to a dry socket and infection. Oral cavity malignancy, for example, of the tongue and floor of mouth, is associated with necrotic tissue formation and halitosis.

34.4 Extra-Oral Pathology

1. Upper aerodigestive, gastro-oesophageal, and lower respiratory tract causes
   Inflammation and infection of these areas may cause halitosis. Therefore, tonsillitis, quinsy, tonsil debris, tonsilloliths, pharyngitis, acute rhinosinusitis and chronic rhinosinusitis (particularly when due to strep milleri) may all cause halitosis as may pneumonia, bronchiectasis and a lung abscess. Malignancy affecting these areas may also cause halitosis and includes tonsil, tongue base, hypopharyngeal, laryngeal and bronchial malignancy. A pharyngeal pouch may collect debris and gastro-oesophageal reflux disease may cause pharyngolaryngeal inflammation so that both conditions may cause halitosis. Achalasia causes stagnant food debris to collect in the oesophagus as may an oesophageal stricture and malignancy.

2. Systemic causes
   A reduction in food intake during any systemic illness will lead to ketosis and typical ketotic breath. Diabetic ketoacidosis is typified by a sweet acetone smell. Renal failure can lead to uraemia and uraemic breath smells of ammonia. Late liver failure and portal hypertension gives rise to foetor hepaticus, also known as breath of the dead! The breath has a sweet but faecal smell. Dimethyl sulphide is thought by many to be the main contributor. A secondary form of trimethylaminuria is associated with liver failure and it has been suggested that trimethylamine, which has a rotting fish odour in low concentration, ammonia-like in higher concentration, may be a contributor to foetor hepaticus. Trimethylamine is found in the vagina in those with bacterial vaginosis and some texts have become confused and implied bacterial vaginosis is a cause of halitosis, but of course this is incorrect!

3. Drugs
   Drugs can cause halitosis by several mechanisms: they may cause a dry mouth (anticholinergics, diuretics); they may alter the normal oral and pharyngeal flora (antibiotics); or their metabolites may be excreted by the lungs (chloral hydrate, iodine-based medications).

34.5 Clinical Features

Halitosis is usually due to oral cavity causes. It is commonest in those with poor dental hygiene and periodontal disease. There is a natural decline in salivary flow and an increase in dental disease with age. A full history should be taken to establish any possible systemic or drug causes. Clinical examination should establish objective evidence of halitosis. A useful manoeuvre is to ask the patient to breathe through the mouth and the nose separately; if the smell is still present when breathing through the nose, an extra-oral cause should be suspected.

There are presently no objective tests for halitosis.

34.6 Investigations

Investigations should be directed at the suspected cause and might include a chest radiograph and blood tests to exclude systemic disease.

34.7 Management

Management should be directed at the underlying cause and will often fall outside the remit of the ENT surgeon. Those with systemic causes and severe chest disease will require referral to an appropriate physician. Patients with a psychological problem may require referral to a psychologist for counselling or to a psychiatrist. Periodontal disease will require the services of a dental practitioner. Most oral inflammatory conditions will resolve spontaneously but any that persist demand biopsy and subsequent definitive treatment. Pharyngitis, tonsillitis and sinonasal disease can all be treated appropriately by the ENT surgeon.

General advice on adequate dental care and adequate hydration should be given. Anti-microbial mouthwashes such as chlorhexidine may reduce the bacterial load but regular use may cause the teeth to stain. Regular, gentle tongue scraping will remove dead squames from the dorsal surface and reduce the VSC load. In some patients with objective halitosis and little pathology, a lengthy (2–3 months) trial of low-dose antibiotics to alter the local bacterial flora may be helpful. Follow-up and aftercare will be dictated by the underlying cause.

Further Reading

Vali A, Roohafza H, Keshteli AH, et al. Relationship between subjective halitosis and psychological factors. Int Dent J. 2015; 65(3):120–126

Zalewska A, Zatoński M, Jabłonka-Strom A, P, aradowska A, Kawala B, Litwin A. Halitosis—a common medical and social problem. A review on pathology, diagnosis and treatment. Acta Gastroenterol Belg. 2012; 75(3):300–309

Related Topics of Interest

Rhinosinusitis—chronic (with nasal polyps)
Tonsil disease

H

35 Headache and Facial Pain

35.1 Introduction

The head and neck region is a complex area anatomically, and this no less applies to its sensory innervation. Pain in the head and neck region is common. While no formal figures exist to substantiate this, personal experience, clinical anecdote and exposure will leave the reader in no doubt of the validity of this statement. A useful definition of pain was issued in 1986 by the International Association for the Study of Pain, and survives unchanged to date:

An unpleasant sensory and emotional experience associated with actual or potential tissue damage or expressed in terms of such damage.

Most patients will initially manage their pain with simple analgesia, and relevant medicines, based on their self-diagnosis, in the hope that it will settle quickly. If this does not happen, then they may become concerned that the pain is a consequence of some damaging physical process, whether that be infection, inflammation or tumour. At this point, they are likely to seek medical advice, usually from their GP, and if they find no resolution there, specialist referral usually follows. There is often clinical enthusiasm to attribute head and neck pain to some form of organic process without sufficient interrogation. These patients present to numerous specialists, undergo multiple investigations and sometimes unsuccessful surgical procedures before finally receiving appropriate diagnosis and treatment. It is unsurprising that many patients have had symptoms for years and have become disillusioned with the medical profession. Their symptoms are compounded by the inevitable emotional and psychological component that goes with chronic pain. If symptoms have been present for some time, successful pain management will not be achieved without acknowledgement of this fact.

Headaches and facial pain not only pose a frequent clinical scenario and diagnostic dilemma, but a problem in managing patients' perceptions and expectations. As facial pain is a common manifestation of head and neck pain, sinonasal symptoms, whether from simple upper respiratory tract infections (URTIs) or rhinitis are also very common, the two regularly become connected in the patient's mind (and often that of their GP!) and the patient

presents with 'sinus pain'. The ENT surgeon is then asked to address the patient's 'sinusitis'. With this in mind, it is clearly beneficial for the ENT surgeon to have some general knowledge of the causes, features and treatment of headaches and facial pain.

35.2 Clinical Assessment

If facial pain is to be successfully managed, it is essential to spend sufficient time with the patient to elicit a full history. There should be an emphasis on duration of both the problem and the episodes, triggers and associated symptoms. When taking a pain history, the patient will frequently find it difficult to convey the experience of the pain. The patient should be encouraged to use descriptive terms, such as *burning, cramping, throbbing, stabbing* which are of more value in suggesting diagnosis than words that indicate intensity, for example, *sore, agonising, excruciating*.

A full ENT examination should be performed and should include nasal endoscopy. It is preferable to try and avoid unnecessary investigations but, in these patients, scanning may be required to demonstrate the absence of underlying organic pathology.

Pain assessment tools have been developed which may aid the clinician in accurately defining the pain. The McGill Pain Questionnaire attempts to define the qualitative aspects of pain, while the Visual Analogue Scale is the most widely used pain intensity measure.

35.3 Headaches Classification

The International Headache Society has recently (August 2016—ichd-3.org) updated its classification (endorsed by the World Health Organisation) of headaches into three broad groups:

1. Primary headaches.
2. Secondary headaches.
3. Painful cranial neuropathies (neuralgias and facial pain).

35.3.1 Primary Headaches

- Migraine. There are 7 groups, of which migraine with aura and migraine without aura are the commonest and 20 subgroups.

- Tension-type headache. These are frequent and infrequent episodic tension headache, chronic tension headache and probable tension headache.
- Trigeminal autonomic cephalalgias. These include cluster headache and paroxysmal hemicrania.
- Other primary headaches. These include primary stabbing headache, primary cough headache, primary exertional headache, primary headache associated with sexual activity, hypnic headache, primary thunderclap headache, hemicrania continua and new daily persistent headache.

35.3.2 Secondary Headaches

- Trauma or injury to the head and/or neck. These include acute or chronic post-traumatic headache attributed to mild, moderate or severe head injury; acute and chronic headache from whiplash; headache from epidural and subdural haematoma; acute and chronic post-craniotomy headache.
- Cranial or cervical vascular disorder. These disorders include ischaemic stroke and transient ischaemic attack; intra-cerebral or sub-arachnoid haemorrhage; unruptured vascular malformations such as arteriovenous malformation cavernous angioma, dural arteriovenous fistula; headache from arteritis such as giant cell arteritis; carotid or vertebral artery pain such as from arterial dissection, post-endarterectomy, post-angiography and post-angioplasty.
- Non-vascular intra-vascular disorders. These disorders include high intra-cranial pressure from hydrocephalus or idiopathic intra-cranial hypertension, low intra-cranial pressure from a lumbar puncture or idiopathic headache from non-infectious inflammatory disease such as neurosarcoidosis or aseptic meningitis, from an intra-cranial neoplasm (can cause raised intra-cranial pressure, carcinomatous meningitis, lymphocytic hypophysitis or primarily from the tumour itself), from an intra-thecal injection, from an epileptic seizure, from Chiari malformation type 1.
- Substance abuse or its withdrawal. Substances include alcohol, cocaine, cannabis, medication such as analgesia overuse, opioid overuse, triptan overuse. Withdrawal from caffeine, opiates and estrogen may cause headaches.

- Infection. This includes intra-cranial infection such as meningitis, encephalitis, brain abscess and subdural empyema; systemic infection including bacterial and viral and retroviral (HIV) infection.
- Disorder of haemostasis. These include headaches attributed to hypoxia and/or hypercapnia (such as high-altitude headache, diving headache and sleep apnoea headache), from hypothyroidism and fasting, cardiac cephalalgia, from dialysis, headache from arterial hypertension including pre-eclampsia and eclampsia.
- Disorder of cranium, neck, eyes, ears, nose, sinuses, teeth, mouth or other facial or cervical structures. Disorders of the neck include cervicogenic headache, retropharyngeal/posterior cervical tendonitis and craniocervical dystonia; eye disorders include acute glaucoma, refractive errors, heterotropia and ocular inflammatory disorders; other facial disorders include pain (otalgia, temporal and facial pain) from disorders of the temporomandibular joint.
- Cranial neuralgias, nerve trunk pain and deafferentation pain. The neuralgias are trigeminal, glossopharyngeal, superior laryngeal, nervus intermedius, nasociliary, supraorbital, postherpetic, occipital neuralgia and optic neuritis.
- Psychiatric disorder such as from somatisation disorder and psychotic disorder.

35.3.3 Painful Cranial Neuropathies, Other Facial Pains and Other Headaches

- Painful cranial neuropathies and other facial pains. These are ocular diabetic neuropathy, persistent idiopathic facial pain (the International Headache Society's preferred term for atypical facial pain), burning mouth syndrome, Tolosa–Hunt syndrome (unilateral headache, orbital pain, ocular palsies).
- Other headache disorders not elsewhere classified.

It is beyond the scope of this chapter to cover all the various categories of headache, but it is worth reviewing some of the commoner pathologies.

35.4 Migraine

The prevalence of migraine headache in the general population is said to be 10 to 15%. Onset of

H

symptoms is usually between puberty and the fifth decade. It is commoner in women and there is often a family history. Only about 10% of migraine headaches exhibit the classical signs of aura (most commonly a visual phenomenon, but may take the form of dysaesthesia in the ipsilateral limb or face, or as a mood change), which precedes the headache by 10 to 60 minutes. The characteristic feature of migraine is its throbbing nature, which is usually unilateral in onset, but which may spread to involve the whole head and face and is accompanied by some degree of photo and phonophobia and nausea. It lasts for 4 to 72 hours and the sufferer is free of pain between attacks. Precipitating factors include psychological stress, sleep deprivation, endocrine changes (such as menstruation) and dietary triggers (especially tyramine-containing foods and irregular meals). The aetiology is not fully understood, although there is undoubtedly a vascular component. A rise in cerebral blood flow in the occipitoparietal cortex precedes the headache, and this is followed by a 25% reduction in flow spreading forward from the occipital region. These changes seem to account for the symptoms of aura. The headache itself is probably due to the dilation of cranial non-cerebral vessels. Experimental studies in animals suggest that the trigeminovascular system is the final common pathway where the migraine headache is generated.

Treatment can consist of symptomatic relief with simple analgesics and anti-emetics. An impending attack may be aborted with an ergotamine preparation taken orally or by inhaler. Also available are the triptan family of drugs, such as sumatriptan, a cranioselective 5-HT1 agonist, which is effective at any stage of an attack when given. Prophylaxis consists largely in avoiding precipitating factors. Drugs such as β-blockers, pizotifen, diltiazem, methysergide and cyproheptadine have all been used in an attempt to stabilise the cranial circulation.

35.5 Myofascial Headache

Myofascial headache is also called 'tension headache'. This is described as a deep, dull, aching, pressure-like pain which may be uni- or bilateral, and of gradual or sudden onset. There are no neurological abnormalities. Myofascial pain is usually associated with trigger points in the muscle and its surrounding fascia, which refer either locally or to a distant site which is usually unrelated to any dermatomes or myotomes. Trigger points are palpable as tender bands within the muscle which, when pressed, will either reproduce the patient's pain or refer it to a characteristic reference zone. Trigger points are thought to arise following muscle trauma, either as a single event or a repeated microtrauma, such as poor posture or teeth grinding. Certain muscles appear to be particularly prone to developing trigger points, including sternomastoid, temporalis, pterygoid, trapezius and neck strap muscles. Pain is often referred forward from the occipital region to the temple, forehead, orbit or ear.

Treatment consists of restoring normal function to the affected muscles by gentle stretching and mobilisation. To permit this it is helpful to reduce discomfort in the muscle body with cooling spray, ice, local anaesthetic injection or acupuncture needling of trigger points. The assistance of physiotherapists may be useful. If the pain has remained undiagnosed for some time, it is common for a degree of pain behaviour to develop. In this situation, psychological therapy may be required, coupled with such techniques as deep relaxation and counselling to improve the patient's insight into the condition. Adequate hydration, avoiding alcohol and improving posture are important. Chronic tension headache does not respond well to analgesics and the most effective medication may be amitriptyline or venlafaxine as a second-line treatment. Tension headaches and migraine may be related and may coexist.

35.6 Cluster Headache

This is a rare but important cause of unilateral facial pain. It takes its title from the grouping together of attacks into clusters, consisting of 1 to 8 headaches per day for 3 to 12 weeks. Symptom-free periods of 3 to 18 months separate the clusters. Diagnosis is sometimes confused with trigeminal neuralgia (TGN). A careful history will reveal clear differences from TGN by duration of attacks, associated symptoms and temporal profile. Age of onset is between 20 and 40 years and there is a male–female ratio of 7:1. The pain is deep and throbbing and is extremely severe. It may appear at the same time each day during a cluster and may wake the subject from sleep. There are always associated autonomic phenomena such as nasal congestion, injected conjunctivae and facial sweating. Each attack lasts for 15 minutes to 3 hours.

Symptom relief during an attack may be achieved with oxygen, which causes transient cerebral vasoconstriction, ergotamine subcutaneously or by inhaler or sphenopalatine ganglion block with intranasal local anaesthetic. Sumatriptan given by sub-cutaneous injection may relieve an attack. For prophylaxis, drugs such as prednisolone in a reducing dose, methysergide (long-term use may cause retroperitoneal fibrosis) and calcium channel blockers (e.g., verapamil) have all met with some success.

35.7 Trigeminal Neuralgia

The principal sensory nerve to the face and head is the trigeminal nerve. TGN, also called *tic douloureux*, is an agonisingly painful condition which usually affects 50 to 70 year olds, although it has been described outside these age limits. It affects men and women equally. In the first half of the last (20th) century, before effective remedies were widely available, it was associated with a high incidence of suicide.

Diagnosis must demonstrate three elements:

1. Pain occurs within one or more divisions of the trigeminal nerve.
2. Pain is described as a brief intense electric shock or knife-like sensation.
3. Pain is elicited by normally innocuous stimulation of a trigger zone.

The mandibular division (III) is the most commonly affected, followed by the maxillary (II) and ophthalmic (I) divisions. The pain can induce spasms of the facial muscles on the affected side (hence *tic*). Bilateral symptoms are rare. It is believed to be caused by local demyelination of the trigeminal root entry zone, most usually by a small, tortuous artery or vein in the posterior cranial fossa. Magnetic resonance imaging (MRI) of sufficiently high resolution may demonstrate such a vessel, and may also help to exclude other causes of these symptoms such as multiple sclerosis, acoustic neuroma, base of skull tumours and vascular anomalies such as aneurysms and vertebrobasilar atherosclerosis.

Treatment should start with an anti-convulsant. Carbamazepine (100–400 mg tds) is the most widely used drug, although other anti-convulsants such as clonazepam and phenytoin have been used. Gabapentin (100–300 mg tds) has had promising results in treating neuropathic pain and has been awarded a product licence for this indication. Side effects may be problematic, especially in the elderly patient. Alternatively, destructive lesions to the gasserian ganglion with alcohol or glycerol injection, or radiofrequency diathermy are usually effective, although patients must be warned that symptom relief will be accompanied by sensory loss to the affected part of the face. Pain often returns 6 months to 5 years after such treatment, necessitating a repeat procedure.

If a vascular loop has been demonstrated by MRI, decompression of the nerve root via a posterior fossa craniotomy has a high chance of prolonged symptom relief. However, surgery of this nature carries significant morbidity, especially in the elderly, and less invasive treatments are to be preferred.

35.8 Other Neuralgias

Although less common, other cranial nerves may give rise to neuralgia whose manifestation is similar to TGN. Glossopharyngeal neuralgia (GPN) is characterised by stabs of pain in the ear, base of tongue, tonsillar fossa or beneath the angle of the mandible. Triggers include talking, swallowing and coughing. Adequate pain relief is important, as malnutrition due to inability to swallow is a distinct possibility. Neuralgia of the nervus intermedius is felt deeply in the ear, lasting for seconds or minutes, with a trigger zone in the posterior wall of the auditory canal. As with TGN, an aberrant vascular loop may be demonstrated near the nerve's origin. It has been suggested that GPN may be associated with an unusually long styloid process, or calcification in the stylohyoid ligament, irritating the nerve (Eagle's syndrome). Local anaesthetic and steroid injections around the styloid process, and surgical removal of the elongated process have both been tried with mixed success.

35.9 Midfacial Segment Pain

This probably represents a variant of tension-type headache and is common in ENT clinics. The pain is felt in a 'butterfly distribution' starting from the nasion or nasal bridge and extending laterally around the eyes and into the cheeks. It is often described as a pressure sensation and there may be associated frontal or occipital headache. Patients seem to respond well to amitriptyline or tension headache treatments.

H

35.10 Atypical Facial Pain

This is the pain that does not easily fit into any other diagnostic grouping. It is often described in dramatic terms and is variable and inconsistent. It is a diagnosis of exclusion. Many of these patients have extensive records and other pain syndromes. Treatment is challenging and involves use of larger doses of amitriptyline, gabapentin or pregabalin, and is likely to require psychological or pain clinic support.

35.11 Acute Herpes Zoster

Most individuals acquire varicella zoster virus during childhood infection with chicken pox. The virus may lie dormant in the dorsal root ganglia of peripheral nerves for many years until opportunistically reactivating, causing an anti-dromic infection along the nerve. Infection is commoner in the aged and the immunocompromised. It presents with itching, pain, dysaesthesia and paraesthesia along the course of the affected nerve, followed a few days later by cutaneous vesicular eruptions. These form scabs within a week or so and heal within a month, though this may take longer in the immunocompromised patient. For reasons which are not understood, the ophthalmic division of the trigeminal nerve and the fourth to tenth thoracic nerves are more commonly affected than others.

Treatment of acute zoster consists of pain relief and in accelerating the resolution of skin lesions. Analgesics and acyclovir should be given systemically and as a cream as early in the condition as possible in order to allow more rapid recovery and to minimise the incidence of postherpetic neuralgia. Early treatment with tricyclic anti-depressants has also been recommended, both as an analgesic for the acute condition (vide infra).

35.12 Postherpetic Neuralgia

This is neuralgia after an acute episode of herpes zoster infection and affecting the area of distribution of the zoster attack. The incidence is reported as being up to 50% following acute infection. It is more likely to develop in elderly patients, and two studies indicate that women are affected more than men in a ratio of 3:2. The pain experienced is usually burning, but occasionally throbbing or stabbing. There is often a sensory deficit and allodynia (pain caused by a normally innocuous stimulus) to light touch is often a feature. It is thought that this phenomenon is caused by alteration of the modulating effect of large-diameter sensory nerves (proprioception) at the dorsal root entry zone (i.e., the pain gate is held wide open) following viral damage during the acute infection. The ability of nerve fibres to repair themselves diminishes with age, which may account for the increased incidence of PHN with advancing years.

Treatment of burning pain and dysaesthesia is best achieved with tricyclic anti-depressants such as amitriptyline in the lowest effective dose, since the incidence of dose-related side effects is high in the elderly. The mechanism of action of these drugs is unknown, although they undoubtedly influence neurotransmitter systems high in the central nervous system (CNS). Gabapentin and valproate may help lancinating pain and techniques such as transcutaneous electrical nerve stimulation (TENS) and acupuncture may also be of value. Also available is a topical preparation of capsaicin, extracted from chilli peppers, which acts by depleting substance P levels (an important neurotransmitter in pain fibres). It is most effective in treating burning pain.

35.13 Summary

Sinonasal disease is an uncommon cause of significant facial pain and headache. A thorough history and examination, with judicious investigations is necessary to uncover the underlying diagnosis, and avoid inappropriate and unnecessary treatment.

Further Reading

Kamani T, Jones NS. 12 minute consultation: evidence based management of a patient with facial pain. Clin Otolaryngol. 2012; 37(3):207–212

Bhalla R and Woolford T. Diagnosis and Management of Facial Pain. Chapter 112 in Scott-Browns Otolaryngology, Head and Neck Surgery, 8th Edition, Volume 2. Editors in Chief – Watkinson JC & Clarke R. Published by CRC Press, Taylor & Francis group, Boca Raton, London, New York, 2018

Related Topics of Interest

Rhinosinusitis—complications
Functional endoscopic sinus surgery
Otalgia

36   Hearing Aids

It is estimated that there are 4 million people with hearing loss in the United Kingdom who could benefit from wearing hearing aids, but they don't. There are many different types of hearing aids. Familiarity with these types allows a clinician to work as a team with audiologist to advise and help patients use the correct aid for their circumstance. Hearing aids augment hearing, but in patients with a sensorineural hearing loss will not return hearing to normal. Other forms of rehabilitation, such as hearing therapy, may further benefit such patients.

According to a survey by Action on Hearing Loss, the earlier hearing aids are used, the more the patient will benefit from them. Quality of life improves because these patients no longer feel isolated. In particular, their social interactions improve as they can understand and therefore contribute to conversations as well as benefiting from being able to hear better on the telephone, television and social media.

A hearing aid is any device that amplifies sound or assists the hearing-impaired individual, but in the present context it will be taken to mean an electroacoustic device used to amplify sounds. Cochlear implants are described in a separate chapter (Chapter 12).

36.1 Design

It is important to be familiar with the basic design of a hearing aid as many patients attending the ENT department have them. You might be asked to describe one in an examination. The basic components of any hearing aid are a receiver (microphone and/or induction coil), an amplifier/processor, a sound transmitter (earphone, bone conductor) and a power source (primary cell). There are two types of signal processing systems: analogue and, the most currently used nowadays, digital.

1. Analogue systems

   These systems are rarely used as hearing aids but there might be some long-term hearing-impaired patients who will not get on with digital aids or might need a body-worn type hearing aid. In analogue systems, an acoustic signal, which is a constantly varying sound pressure wave, is converted to its electrical analogue at the microphone stage of the hearing aid circuit.

2. Digital systems

   Digital hearing aids are the current default hearing aids provided by the NHS and private sectors. They were introduced in 1996 and continue to be upgraded.

   Digital systems work on frequency channels and bands. Frequency channels are a range of frequencies that are created by a digital filter or series of digital filters within a hearing aid. Most of the signal processing functions operate on a channel-by-channel basis. These functions are expansion (amplification), compression, digital noise reduction, feedback suppression and directionality (direction of sound). Multiple channels provide selective amplification and improve feedback suppression, digital noise reduction and speech discrimination in quiet and background noise. Multiple channels may equalise the loudness of several people who might be contributing to conversation. Frequency bands are the number of adjustment 'switches' provided in the programming software to obtain manipulation.

   Digital hearing aids have directional microphones whose function is to enhance the signal-to-noise ratio by detection of clearer sound from the front of the listener and reduced sound from other directions. The microphone has two inlet ports: sound coming from behind hits the front port later than the rear port (external delay), and sound entering the rear port is delayed by a low-pass filter (internal delay). Directional microphones are more useful in the presence of 'wordy' sound and work best in those wearing an occlusive mould.

   Environmental noise suppression is digitally managed by splitting the sound into various frequency channels. In each channel, the aid gives a predominant signal to either noise or speech, depending on the shape of the sound envelope. The aid analyses fluctuations in signal amplitude. Speech produces slow- and large-amplitude fluctuations, while noise produces fast- and small-amplitude fluctuations.

   In some hearing aids, output sound can feed back into the microphone causing acoustic feedback. Digital systems can reduce this feedback by phase reversal (feedback frequencies are reversed in phase and played back when feedback is detected) and frequency clipping (gain

H

cut). In addition, they reduce audibility of internally generated sounds or environmental soft sounds which will not benefit the patient. This is called expansion or microphone noise reduction.

Recent digital aid innovations include wireless facilities such as Bluetooth synchronising programme and volume changing. There is also the possibility of attaching the aid to a small ear-level receiver that attaches to a hearing aid. The teacher will wear a transmitter microphone that transmits via Bluetooth, sound to the ear-level receiver, and then into the hearing aid. Such a device can improve the ability to hear the teacher and so help students of all ages.

36.2 Types of Aid

1. *Behind-the-ear (BTE) aids* The body of the aid sits behind the wearer's ear and is normally connected by a hollow plastic tube to an ear mould, which allows sound passage to the ear. There are three main groups of BTE aids available on the NHS, the 10, 30 and 50 series, with the power of the aids increasing correspondingly. Within each series are several models with differing patterns of frequency response. All contain an induction coil which can be used with telephones, televisions and in theatres and cinemas fitted with induction loops, to bypass much of the unwanted background noise. There are also very many similar models available in the private sector from the various commercial manufacturers.

2. *In-the-ear (ITE), in-the-canal (ITC) or completely-in-the-canal (CIC) aids* These commonly available commercial aids have an external shell, made usually of acrylic, and conforms to the shape of the wearer's conchal bowl (ITE) or outer external ear canal (ITC) or wholly within the canal (CIC). These aids have their working parts in the ear mould.

They are less obtrusive than the standard BTE aids but are expensive and occasionally prone to feedback problems due to the proximity of microphone and 'speaker'.

3. *Body-worn (BW) aids* These aids are usually worn with a strap around the neck and the body of the aid on the patient's chest. By virtue of their size, they can be made very powerful, and the distance between microphone and earphone means that, even with high amplification, feedback is rarely a problem. They are, however, prone to picking up the sounds of rustling clothes and are rather cumbersome. There are two series available on the NHS: BW 60 and BW 80.

4. *Bone conduction devices* (▶ Fig. 36.1) These are very similar to the standard body-worn aid but feed their output to a bone conductor rather than an earphone. They are indicated in the event of conductive or mixed hearing loss when use of a conventional air-conduction hearing aid is impossible, contraindicated or ineffective. The most common situations include chronic meatal discharge (chronic otitis externa and otitis media), ear canal stenosis or canal atresia. The ENT UK 2010 position paper on bone conduction devices states that because of the benefits of bone-anchored hearing aids over conventional bone conduction hearing aids, the latter have, on the whole, been replaced by the former.

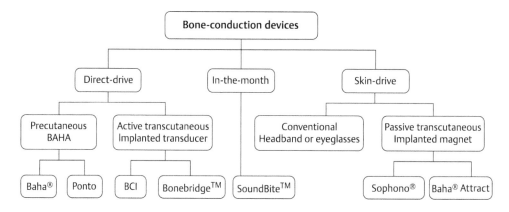

Fig. 36.1 Bone conduction devices and their applications.

Conventional bone conduction aids require a transducer, placed on the opposite side of the head, usually on the mastoid, to be held in place by a soft band or tight steel band. The latter is rarely used nowadays as may cause problems with pressure effects (especially in children). The sound processor clips onto a plastic disc. They use transcutaneous conduction, so they are not recommended for long-term use. They are particularly useful for children less than 30 months of age.

Single-sided hearing impairment is now an indication for bone conduction aiding as binaural hearing is necessary for speech discrimination in background noise and for accurate localisation of sound.

36.3 Direct-Drive or Osseointegrated Hearing Aids

There are two devices in clinical use, both relying on the transmission of mechanical vibrations to the skull bone.

a. In the bone-anchored hearing device (BAHD), a percutaneous titanium abutment is fixed to a titanium screw implanted in the mastoid by minimally invasive dissection. A vibrator is then mounted directly onto the abutment, which is fed either from a microphone and circuit in a small box with the vibrator or from a body-worn hearing aid (for higher output power).

b. The Xomed Audiant bone conductor consists of an encased rare earth magnet implanted completely under the skin and fixed into bone with a titanium screw. Externally, another magnet serves to hold its surrounding induction coil in place over the implanted magnet. By passing electric currents (derived from what is essentially a hearing aid) through the induction coil, an electromagnetic field is set up that causes the implanted magnet, and hence the skull, to vibrate.

In addition to the above indications for bone conduction aiding, the clinical criteria for implantation is as follows:

• Permanent bilateral conductive or mixed hearing loss.
• Bilateral conductive or mixed hearing loss where one ear works better than the other. Patients must have tried conventional air-conduction aids without reasonable subjective benefit.

• Unilateral conductive hearing loss with an ear canal stenosis that is unlikely to benefit from meatoplasty; or who have had revision surgery and failed to tolerate an air-conduction aid.
• Profound unilateral sensorineural hearing loss.
• Bilateral conductive hearing loss due to ossicular disease not appropriate for surgical correction or unable to be aided by an air-conduction aid.

The audiological criteria should be a conductive or mixed hearing loss with a bone conduction pure-tone average for 0.5-, 1-, 2- and 3-kHz frequencies of at least 45 dB HL for the Devino or BP 100, 55 dB for the Intenso and 70 dB for Cordelle II (body processor). The air-conduction pure-tone average should not be better than 40 dB (for adults), and a maximum speech discrimination score greater than 60% when using a phonetically balanced word list.

c. The Soundbridge or implantable middle ear aid converts sound from the microphone of the audio processor into mechanical vibrations. These signals are transmitted through the skin to the implanted part under the skin which transmits the signals to the floating mass transducer (FMT). The signal is then converted into mechanical vibrations onto a coil that is attached to the patient's incus. The FMT is 2.3-mm long, 1.8-mm wide, and it vibrates at 0.1 µm (= 0.0001 mm). It reduces feedback and produces a more natural, clearer sound. However, NHS availability is dependent on local clinical commissioning policy.

The criteria for implantation will include mild-to-severe sensorineural hearing loss (55-dB loss maximum at 500 Hz) with an air–bone gap less than 10 dB and non-progressive hearing loss. The patient should be unable to wear BTE, ITE, or CIC due to chronic ear canal conditions (see earlier). In addition, the patient's speech understanding should present a score of 50% or better on a monosyllabic word test at 65 dB SPL in free field using hearing aids at the most comfortable listening (MCL) level with headphones. Suitable candidates should have normal middle ear anatomy and function as shown by acoustic reflex test results and no retrocochlear or central pathology.

d. The SoundBite system consists of an easy to insert and remove in-the-mouth (ITM) hearing device. It fits around either the upper left or right back teeth. A microphone unit is worn

H

behind the ear and transmits wirelessly to the ITM device. The mouthpiece converts the signal to vibrations which, by transmitting sound through the teeth and mandibles, stimulate both cochleae.

e. Spectacle aids These involve modification of standard spectacle frames to incorporate a hearing aid. They can then be used in a number of ways: as a standard hearing aid, as a bone conductor or for contralateral routing of signal (CROS). In this last variation, sound is picked up from the side of the head with poor hearing and fed to the contralateral side, which has better hearing. Bluetooth CROS aids are available for those who do not want to or need to wear spectacles.

36.4 Other Considerations

Many factors will influence the choice of hearing aid. The actual degree and nature of the hearing loss will dictate the amplification characteristics. The cause of the deafness will influence the type of aid chosen, as will vanity and available finance. It is important to establish the patient's requirements and to remember that an aid will not cure the underlying disease.

1. Type
   A spectacle-type aid is useful for those people who regularly wear glasses as they are relatively inconspicuous. They are often chosen when there is one very impaired hearing ear and a requirement for contralateral signal routing. A bone conduction aid is ideal in those cases where a hearing loss exists in association with active outer ear or middle ear inflammatory pathology. A body-worn aid is useful for anyone with a profound hearing loss. For most NHS patients, an ear-level aid will be found to be suitable.

2. Ear moulds
   Several modifications can be made to the ear moulds. These may be made for both auditory and medical reasons. Venting the mould will reduce the low-frequency response. In patients prone to otitis externa, it is useful to ventilate or even skeletonise the mould to provide aeration. Unfortunately, feedback becomes more likely with a high-power aid or if the mould is vented. A slim BTE aid can be connected to thin tubing attached to a silicone cup as the chosen mould in an 'open-fit' hearing aid.

3. Some digital hearing aids can be adjusted using a remote control for volume and programme. These are ideal for patients with fluctuating hearing and/or tinnitus (i.e., those with Ménière's disease).

4. General
   Although it is preferable to provide binaural aids in cases of bilateral hearing loss, this is still sometimes difficult to achieve or is inappropriate. Which ear to aid will then depend on a number of factors, including patient preference, available dynamic range and discrimination scores in each ear. The presence of an active inflammatory process in either ear might hinder the decision to aid. Medical factors such as manual dexterity relating to arthritis, strokes, amputations, etc. also have a bearing.

36.5 Follow-Up and Aftercare

NHS England and the Department of Health published the 'Action Plan on Hearing Loss' guidance in March 2015. It encourages and promotes change across all levels of public service and identifies hearing needs for children and adults. After the initial fitting, a period of support and rehabilitation is essential to allow the patient to gain confidence and achieve useful function with the hearing aid. Subsequent attendance for servicing and repairs will also be required and should be made available.

Further Reading

Hearing loss in adults: assessment and management in development [GID-CGWAVE0833] Published: 21 June 2018

Hill OBE, Holton K, Regan C. Action Plan on Hearing Loss. NHS England and the Department of Health. https://www.england.nhs.uk/wp-content/uploads/2015/03/act-plan-hearing-loss-upd.pdf. Accessed December 14, 2018

NHS Commissioning Board Clinical Commissioning Policy: Bone Anchored Hearing Aids, NHS Commissioning Group-April 2013

Related Topics of Interest

Cochlear implants
Noise-induced hearing loss
Age-associated hearing loss
Otosclerosis
Pure-tone audiometry
Speech audiometry

H

37 Hearing Loss—Acquired

37.1 Introduction

Acquired hearing loss affects over 11 million people in the United Kingdom with this figure set to rise to 15.6 million by 2035 (Action on Hearing Loss). Nine hundred thousand currently have severe or profound hearing loss. It is associated with significant social isolation and, in the elderly, with cognitive decline. There are therefore significant societal implications from hearing loss.

This chapter will summarise the most common causes of acquired hearing loss and discuss the current options available for hearing rehabilitation.

37.2 Investigation

Diagnosis of hearing loss is usually made using psychoacoustic techniques. Pure-tone audiometry is in widespread use and can differentiate conductive from sensorineural hearing loss. It does not, however, provide a measure of functional hearing and word (e.g., Arthur Boothroyd words) or sentence testing (e.g., Bamford Kowal Bench [BKB] or City University of New York [CUNY] Sentences) that may be used to provide additional information on functional hearing. This is important as patients often complain of distortion of hearing as well as an inability to hear adequately and it is only functional tests of hearing that will identify those with distortion. Hearing aids only amplify the existing hearing and the benefits of aiding in those with distorted hearing may be limited.

Objective measures of hearing loss may also be used in some circumstances especially to identify malingerers. These include brainstem-evoked response audiometry (BSER) and cortical-evoked response audiometry (CERA). Tympanometry has a role in confirming the presence of a tympanic membrane perforation or middle ear effusion. Otoacoustic emissions may also be helpful in differentiating neural from sensory loss and is helpful in the diagnosis of auditory neuropathy. It is also the screening test used in neonatal hearing screening.

Cross-sectional imaging has an important role to play in some patients. High-resolution computed tomography (CT) may be helpful in the investigation of conductive hearing losses. It can identify ossicular discontinuity and otosclerosis and allows assessment of the extent of cholesteatomatous disease. Magnetic resonance imaging (MRI) is also helpful in certain situations, mainly for the exclusion of intra-cranial causes of sensorineural hearing loss such as vestibular schwannoma.

37.3 Aetiology

Causes of acquired hearing loss can be divided into conductive and sensorineural. Conductive hearing loss results from impairment of the passage of sound from the external environment to the cochlea. This can result from disease of the external ear, tympanic membrane or middle ear. Sensorineural hearing loss results from disease of the cochlea, cochlear nerve or central auditory pathways. ▶Table 37.1 summarises the most common causes of acquired conductive hearing loss. ▶Table 37.2 summarises the most common causes of acquired sensorineural hearing loss.

37.4 Conductive Hearing Loss

Many forms of conductive hearing loss can be addressed with surgery to the ossicular chain although traditional hearing aids and implantable bone conduction hearing aids may also be options.

37.5 External Auditory Canal

- *Foreign bodies and wax* are usually easily removed with microsuction. Syringing has fallen out of fashion in recent years mainly because of the risk of perforation and trauma to the external ear canal.

▶ Table 37.1 Most common causes of acquired conductive hearing loss

External ear canal	Wax
	Foreign bodies
	Stenosing otitis externa
	Exostoses and osteomas
Tympanic membrane	Perforation
Ossicular chain	Fixation, e.g., otosclerosis
	Erosion, e.g., cholesteatoma
	Subluxation and fracture, e.g., trauma

▶ **Table 37.2** Most common causes of acquired sensorineural hearing loss

Cause	Examples
Degenerative	Presbycusis
Idiopathic	
Infection	Ramsay Hunt syndrome, syphilis, meningitis
Ischaemia	Cerebrovascular accident, sickle cell disease
Inflammation	Ménière's disease, autoimmune disease, e.g., rheumatoid arthritis, sarcoidosis
Neoplastic	Vestibular schwannoma
Trauma	Noise, temporal bone fracture
Iatrogenic	Surgical, ototoxicity
Neurological	Multiple sclerosis

- *Stenosing otitis externa* results in progressive inflammatory narrowing of the external auditory canal with eventual formation of a deep ear canal fibrous plug. The underlying tympanic membrane is usually normal. Once the otitis externa has burnt out, surgical correction may be considered in order to restore hearing although stenosis recurs in up to 60% of cases. The fibrous plug is removed down to the healthy tympanic membrane. A bony canalplasty is usually carried out and the deep ear canal can then be grafted using a split-skin graft. Alternatively, a number of different implantable bone conduction hearing aids (IBCHAs) can be used and these provide excellent hearing outcomes albeit with the inconvenience of having to wear an aid.

- *Exostoses* result from repeated prolonged exposure to cold water. This causes an hyperostotic reaction resulting in formation of several bony swellings in the deep ear canal. It is most commonly seen in surfers. When small, they do not cause any problems, but large ones can completely occlude the external auditory canal. Progression can be stopped through appropriate ear plugging during exposure to cold water. This may avoid the need for intervention. Large ones can be removed by carrying out a bony canalplasty.

- *Osteomas* are benign neoplasms of the bony external auditory canal. They are solitary, have a pedunculated base, and usually arise at the

bony margin of the tympanic ring. These features differentiate them from exostoses. In the same way as exostoses, they can occlude the external auditory canal when large. It is usually a straightforward matter to fracture the osteoma at its base and remove it although formal canalplasty may be required in some cases.

37.6 Tympanic Membrane

Perforations of the tympanic membrane do not cause conductive hearing loss when small but large ones often do. While the primary aim of tympanoplasty is to close the tympanic membrane, a secondary effect in those with an associated conductive hearing loss is often improvement in hearing.

37.7 Ossicular Chain

37.7.1 Ossicular Fixation

- *Tympanosclerosis and fibrous adhesions* resulting from inactive chronic otitis media may result in fixation of the ossicular chain. In many cases tympanosclerotic plaques can be removed although great care needs to be taken around the stapes superstructure as excessive manipulation can result in sensorineural hearing loss or even a dead ear. Fibrous adhesions can be carefully divided and the laser can be extremely helpful in this setting. Traditional hearing aids and IBCHAs may also be offered as an alternative to middle ear surgery.

- *Otosclerosis* results in the formation of new, abnormal bone at the fissula ante fenestram, a small connective tissue filled cleft between the oval window and cochleariform process. The new bone fixes the stapes and prevents the conduction of sound through the ossicular chain. Occasionally, the otosclerosis can also affect the cochlea resulting in sensorineural hearing loss. In most cases, it is an autosomal dominant condition with variable penetrance. As with other forms of conductive hearing loss, rehabilitation options include traditional hearing aids and IBCHAs. Stapedectomy is, however, a very successful surgical solution that, in experienced hands, can close the air-bone gap to less than 10 dB in 90% of cases. It involves removal of the arch of the stapes, formation of a small fenestrum in the footplate of the stapes, and placement of a piston through the fenestrum that is hooked around the long process of the incus proximally. There is a 1 to 2% risk of dead ear with stapedectomy.

37.7.2 Ossicular Erosion

- *Chronic otitis media* with or without cholesteatoma can result in erosion of the ossicular chain, particularly the long process of the incus. As a result, the ossicular chain becomes discontinuous and can no longer transfer sound to the inner ear. Again, traditional hearing aids and IBCHAs may be used to rehabilitate hearing but surgical reconstruction may also be considered. Localised erosion of the long process of incus can be repaired with bone cement. More extensive ossicular damage can be reconstructed using a partial or total ossicular replacement prosthesis (PORP or TORP) depending on whether the stapes superstructure is present or absent, respectively. Some surgeons may also remove, modify, and then transpose the incus. Success rates are variable with the most important factor being the status of the stapes arch. If present, the reconstruction is more stable and successful closure to within 15 dB air-bone gap closure can be achieved in 70% of cases compared to 50% if the arch is absent.

37.7.3 Ossicular Subluxation and Fracture

Trauma to the temporal bone can result in fracture through the middle and inner ear. Middle ear involvement most often results in subluxation of the incus but fracture of the stapes superstructure can also occur. Options for hearing rehabilitation in those with conductive hearing loss are the same as those for ossicular erosion.

Middle Ear Space

Otitis media with effusion is the commonest form of acquired hearing loss in children with up to 80% of children experiencing at least one episode during childhood. It is characterised by a non-purulent fluid collection filling the middle ear that interferes with the function of the tympanic membrane and ossicular chain. Most cases settle spontaneously, but persistent effusions

can be treated by drainage via a myringotomy followed by placement of a ventilation tube across the tympanic membrane. Alternatively, a hearing aid may be used but they do not address the underlying pathology and are associated with poor compliance.

37.8 Sensorineural Hearing Loss

Sensorineural hearing loss is not usually amenable to surgical correction until the loss is profound at which point cochlear implantation can be used to electrically stimulate the auditory pathway. When hearing loss is not profound, rehabilitation using traditional hearing aids is available. More recently, a number of active implantable hearing aids have been developed offering rehabilitation solutions in those that are outside the criteria for cochlear implantation but cannot use traditional hearing aids.

37.8.1 Presbycusis

With increasing age, there is loss of inner and outer hair cells within the cochlea as well as loss of cochlear nerve and central auditory neurons. This typically results in a high-frequency sensorineural hearing loss that progresses slowly over time. The age of onset and degree of hearing loss are variable between individuals.

37.8.2 Noise-Induced Hearing Loss

Short-term exposure to excess noise results in a reversible reduction in cochlear function termed temporary threshold shift. If such exposure is very prolonged (it takes 10 years of exposure for 8 hours a day at 90 dB or more to cause significant noise-induced hearing loss [NIHL] in an averagely sensitive individual), free radical formation results in loss of cochlear hair cells. The damage is most severe at the 4-kHz portion of the basilar membrane and this typically manifests as a notch at 4 kHz on pure-tone audiometry.

37.8.3 Vestibular Schwannomas

Vestibular schwannomas (often, inaccurately, called acoustic neuromas) are benign tumours originating from the Schwann cells lining the vestibular nerve as it passes from the brainstem, across the cerebellopontine angle (CPA) to the

H

internal auditory meatus. They are the commonest type of tumour to occur in the CPA. Ninety-five percent of tumours are associated with hearing loss. Eighty percent of tumours do not grow after diagnosis and do not require active treatment. They are usually monitored with serial imaging. Those that grow may be treated with stereotactic radiosurgery or with surgical resection. Any patient with a significant asymmetry in his or her sensorineural hearing thresholds should be screened for a vestibular schwannoma using MRI.

37.8.4 Iatrogenic Hearing Loss

Inadvertent injury to the inner ear can result from middle or inner ear surgery. There are also some types of surgery to the ear that, by the nature of the procedure, result in loss of sensorineural hearing, for example, removal of vestibular schwannomas. Sensorineural hearing may also be damaged by the use of certain drugs, for example, aminoglycosides and platinum-based chemotherapy drugs.

37.8.5 Idiopathic Sudden Sensorineural Hearing Loss

The incidence of idiopathic sudden sensorineural hearing loss is around 10 per 100,000 per year. It is usually unilateral. There are a number of theories as to how this type of hearing loss arises. This includes direct injury from a viral infection (mumps and herpes viruses are most often implicated), a vascular event, an autoimmune response and an abnormal cytokine-mediated response to certain stimuli such as a viral infection or physical or mental stress. Such hearing losses can spontaneously recover but recovery may be facilitated by the use of either oral or intra-tympanic steroids. A Cochrane review of steroid use in idiopathic sudden sensorineural hearing loss presently shows no statistical definite benefit in giving steroids as a treatment.

37.8.6 Labyrinthitis

Inflammation or infection of the inner ear structures is termed labyrinthitis. It results in acute failure of the vestibulocochlear system and presents with acute vertigo and profound sensorineural hearing loss. It should be differentiated from vestibular neuronitis in which only the vestibular system is affected. It may be of viral or bacterial aetiology. The most common viruses to be implicated are rubella, cytomegalovirus, mumps, measles and varicella (Ramsay Hunt syndrome). Bacterial labyrinthitis usually results from chronic otitis media or meningitis. There is no identifiable cause in some cases. Fibrosis of the cochlear duct can occur, especially with bacterial labyrinthitis, and this may make cochlear implantation in those that require rehabilitation of profound deafness very challenging. Cochlear implantation should be carried out urgently in patients with profound hearing loss due to meningitis in order to avoid this issue. It should be noted that meningitis can also damage the central auditory pathway limiting the outcomes of cochlear implantation.

37.8.7 Autoimmune Hearing Loss

Autoimmune hearing loss is characterised by rapidly progressive, fluctuating sensorineural hearing loss, most frequently in one ear but occasionally in both, that is often responsive to steroids. It is sometimes associated with vertigo. In many cases there is no obvious underlying medical condition but autoimmune-mediated diseases such as rheumatoid arthritis, polyangiitis with granulomatosis and sarcoidosis are all associated with sensorineural hearing loss. It can also be difficult to differentiate autoimmune hearing loss from endolymphatic hydrops and, in fact, the latter can be autoimmune mediated. The mechanism by which hearing loss develops is not fully understood, but it may be mediated by antibodies to a constitutively produced inner ear protein called heat shock protein 70. The mainstay of treatment for autoimmune hearing loss is steroids, delivered either orally or intratympanically. In a limited number of cases immunosuppressants such as methotrexate or azathioprine may be considered.

37.8.8 Endolymphatic Hydrops

The classic triad of episodic vertigo associated with fluctuating sensorineural hearing loss and tinnitus is the hallmark of Ménière's disease. The underlying pathology is an excess of endolymph resulting in expansion of the endolymphatic compartment and stretching of the neuroepithelial membranes of the inner ear. The pathophysiology is not fully understood but is likely to involve disordered endolymph metabolism that, in some, may be autoimmune mediated. There are many treatments available for Ménière's disease including intra-tympanic steroids or gentamicin, saccus surgery (drainage, duct clipping or duct avulsion), labyrinthectomy and vestibular nerve section. These treatments aim to improve the vertiginous element of symptoms and to not affect hearing or cause or increase tinnitus. Hearing loss is usually treated with appropriate aiding or, if profound, with cochlear implantation. Betahistine has recently been shown to be ineffective in Ménière's disease.

37.9 Audiological Rehabilitation of Hearing Loss

37.9.1 Implantable Bone Conduction Hearing Aids

Over the past 25 years, a number of different implantable bone conduction hearing aids have been developed. The earliest device, and still in widespread clinical use, is the bone-anchored hearing aid (BAHA [Cochlear]; Ponto [Oticon]). This consists of a titanium screw that is placed in, and osseointegrates with, the bone of the skull on the ipsilateral side. A percutaneous abutment is inserted into the screw and a vibrating sound processor is then clipped onto the abutment. The vibrations from the processor are carried by the abutment to the skull and the vibrations are then picked up by the cochlea, bypassing the poorly functioning conductive mechanism. More recently, a modified version without the abutment has been developed (BAHA Attract [Cochlear]). The Bonebridge device (MEDEL) is an alternative to the BAHA. It has two components, an external sound processor that attaches by magnetism to, and communicates with, an internal implanted component. The implanted component has a piezoelectric crystal within it. The signal from the sound processor stimulates vibration of the crystal and this passes through the skull to the cochlea. These are very effective ways of rehabilitating conductive hearing loss in those who do not wish to, or cannot, wear a traditional hearing aid and do not wish to have ossicular surgery.

37.9.2 Active Implantable Hearing Aids

There are currently three types of active implantable hearing aid in the market, the Vibrant Soundbridge (MEDEL), the Carina (Cochlear), and the Esteem (Envoy Medical). There are three main indications for implantation of these devices: (1) if traditional hearing aids cannot be used because of congenital atresia or recurrent otitis externa, (2) if the patient does not wish to wear traditional hearing aids, for example, if he or she likes the occlusion effect, and (3) if there is not enough gain from traditional aids but the hearing is too good for a cochlear implant. Each type of device is attached to the ossicular chain and actively drive the ossicular mechanism to maximise the signal entering the cochlea.

37.9.3 Cochlear Implantation

Cochlear implants are devices that electrically stimulate cochlear neurons to provide hearing in those with profound deafness. They have two components. The implantable part consists of an electrode array that is placed within the cochlea and a receiver stimulator package that is implanted under the skin behind the pinna. The external part looks like a large hearing aid and consists of a sound processor and its associated battery. The criteria for their use vary between countries. The 2009 NICE UK guidelines for cochlear implantation are out of date and are currently being updated. The 2009 criteria were a PTA hearing loss of greater than 90 dB in the better hearing ear between 2 and 4 kHz and sentence testing scores worse than 50% when delivered at 60 dB in quiet conditions. Most units now use a threshold of PTA loss of 70 dB. They have revolutionised hearing rehabilitation in the profoundly deaf allowing congenitally deaf children to learn normal speech and attend mainstream schools and allowing deaf adults to return to work and enjoy being able to communicate with family and friends again.

37.9.4 Auditory Brainstem Implantation

If an individual is profoundly deaf but cannot be implanted with a cochlear implant because of destruction of the cochlea or because of absence or loss of the cochlear nerve, then the only way to rehabilitate the hearing is to stimulate the auditory pathways upstream of the cochlear nerve. An auditory brainstem implant (ABI) offers the opportunity to stimulate the auditory pathways from the cochlear nucleus. It works in a very

H

similar way to a cochlear implant, but instead of having a linear array of electrodes, the electrodes are arranged in a paddle which is placed on the cochlear nucleus. Outcomes are significantly worse than those achieved with cochlear implants because of the non-tonotopic arrangement of the cochlear nucleus and the presence of other adjacent brainstem nuclei that can also be stimulated by the electrode. Patients with neurofibromatosis type 2 who have had bilateral vestibular schwannomas removed are the most common recipients of ABIs.

37.9.5 Rehabilitation of Unilateral Profound Hearing Loss

The only way to restore hearing to the deaf ear in an individual with unilateral profound sensorineural hearing loss is to use a cochlear implant. There is accumulating evidence that this provides some improvement in sound localisation and the ability to hear in a noisy environment. There are also a number of means by which sounds from the deafened side can be transferred to the hearing side. Contralateral routing of signal (CROS) aids consist of two hearing aid–like devices, one of which consists of a microphone placed in the deafened ear and the other consists of a speaker placed in the hearing ear. IBCHA can also be implanted on the deafened side with their vibrations being transferred transcranially to the hearing ear.

37.9.6 Hearing Therapy and Assistive Devices

There are means by which those suffering with hearing loss can be assisted other than with hearing aids or implantable hearing devices. Advice regarding listening tactics can be very helpful, for example, school children sitting at the front of class or, in those with unilateral hearing loss, sitting with the good ear adjacent to the person with whom they are conversing. There are also assistive devices available such as louder door bells and telephones. For those with a hearing aid loop system, FM systems and Bluetooth can all send sound signals directly into the hearing aid, enhancing the

listening experience. Hearing therapists have an important role in providing these forms of hearing rehabilitation. Prevention is also important; for example, for those exposed to excess noise, appropriate ear protection will avoid significant NIHL.

37.10 Conclusion

The differential diagnosis of hearing loss is very extensive, but the precise cause is often identifiable by taking a detailed history, undertaking a careful examination, and performing pure-tone audiometry. In some cases, cross-sectional imaging may also be helpful. Most types of hearing loss, with the exception of profound losses, can be rehabilitated using traditional hearing aids. In conductive hearing loss, ossicular reconstruction or implantable bone conduction hearing aids may also be considered. For sensorineural and mixed hearing losses, active implantable middle ear hearing aids are also available. For those with profound hearing loss, cochlear implantation offers the opportunity to restore functional hearing. The field of implantation otology is rapidly developing and now provides options for rehabilitation of almost any type of hearing loss.

Further Reading

Hearing loss in adults: assessment and management. NICE Guideline, No. 98. National Guideline Alliance (UK). London: Royal College of Physicians (UK); 2018 Jun. https://www.nice.org.uk/guidance/ng98/resources/hearing-loss-in-adults-assessment-and-management-pdf

Related Topics of Interest

Pure-tone audiometry
Impedance audiometry
Hearing aids
Cochlear implants
Ménière's syndrome
Noise-induced hearing loss
Age-associated hearing loss
Sudden hearing loss
Vestibular schwannoma
Otosclerosis
Labyrinthitis

38   HIV in Otolaryngology

This is an important subject, as about 80% of patients who are human immunodeficiency virus (HIV) positive will develop ear, nose and throat (ENT) manifestations. A patient with newly diagnosed HIV infection needs to be adequately counselled and staged and then managed according to the stage. Combination anti-retroviral therapy (ART) is offered to all individuals regardless of CD4+ count.

38.1 Aetiology

Acquired immunodeficiency syndrome (AIDS) is caused by two of four retroviruses that cause disease in humans, namely HIV-1 and HIV-2. The other two are human T-lymphotropic virus types I and II (HTLV-I and HTLV-II) and transmitted in the same way as HIV and associated with several types of lymphoma and leukaemia.

AIDS is defined as the development of a complication of immunosuppression, such as malignancy or opportunistic infection, in a HIV-positive individual *or* immunosuppression such that the CD4+ T-cell count is less than 200 cm^3. Immunisation and prophylaxis should be discussed and initiated but the detail of this is beyond the scope of this chapter.

38.2 Pathology

HIV-1 is prevalent worldwide, while the less virulent HIV-2 is found mainly in West Africa. HIV infects cells bearing the CD4+ antigen, which acts as a virus receptor. Such cells are monocytes, macrophages and T-helper cells. In HIV-1, the glycoprotein, gp120, binds to CD4+ and allows the virus to enter the cell. Viral replication may occur in cells in which HIV-1 DNA has been integrated (productive infection), although in some cells containing integrated HIV-1 DNA, the virus does not replicate except when the cell is activated by antigenic stimulation (latent infection), for example, Epstein–Barr virus or cytomegalovirus infection. Ultimately, a functional impairment and depletion of T-helper cells occurs. The ultimate consequence is a compromise of the host immune system. Immunosuppression places the victim at risk of developing opportunistic infections and unusual malignancies, particularly B-cell lymphoma and Kaposi's sarcoma.

Although the time from being infected with HIV-1 to development of AIDS is variable, most infected individuals in developed countries will develop AIDS about 8 to 11 years after infection with HIV, in the absence of treatment. It is estimated that a quarter of patients with HIV in the west are undiagnosed and some of these individuals will only be eventually diagnosed when they present with AIDS. This has significant implications regarding their prognosis because those patients with an early diagnosis of HIV have a near-normal life expectancy. Present World Health Organization (WHO) guidelines support the recommendation to initiate combination anti-retroviral therapy (ART) immediately in HIV-positive patients regardless of their CD4+ cell count. There are various methods of transmission, but all demand close contact with infected body fluids, particularly blood. High-risk groups include intravenous drug users, homosexual males, prostitutes, lorry drivers (a significant percentage use prostitutes), heterosexual contact with an infected partner and children of infected mothers. Although transfusion of blood products, particularly in haemophiliacs, resulted in a significant number of HIV cases in the 1980s and 1990s, all blood donated for transfusion in the United Kingdom and United States is screened for HIV-1 and HIV-2 by testing for both antibody to the viruses and for p24, a protein in the virus coat (this test is called the enzyme-linked immunosorbent assay [ELISA] combination test), and also a screen for the viral RNA which will be positive earlier than the combination test. The combination test may be positive as early as 10 days after exposure but may take as long as 3 months. The viral RNA test will usually be positive within 5 to 10 days of exposure. This has greatly reduced the risk of blood transfusion transmission but not eradicated it because of the short time it takes for seroconversion (the interval between infection and the appearance of antibody/measurable virus).

38.3 ENT Manifestations of HIV Disease

HIV patients are prone to a variety of conditions, their incidence increasing as the CD4+ count reduces. These include Kaposi's sarcoma, lymphoma, HIV-associated generalised lymphadenopathy, immune reconstitution inflammatory syndrome (IRIS, an increase in HIV symptoms that occurs within 3 months of commencing ART), recurrent aphthous ulceration and unusual infections may develop. These unusual infections include tuberculosis, atypical mycobacterial infection, herpes zoster and herpes simplex infection, human papilloma virus (HPV) infection, toxoplasmosis, histoplasmosis, cryptococcal infection and fungal infection, particularly candidiasis and aspergillosis.

1. Otological otitis media and externa (particularly fungal) are more common. Kaposi's sarcoma of the pinna or external auditory meatus, a sensorineural hearing loss and vertigo may occur.

2. Rhinological acute and chronic rhinosinusitis may occur with unusual organisms because of the debilitated state of the patient. Epistaxis may occur due to HIV-associated thrombocytopenia. Kaposi's sarcoma and lymphomas may be found in the nasopharynx.

3. Oropharyngeal The oral cavity is one of the most commonly affected sites. Kaposi's sarcoma is not uncommon. Severe candidiasis is frequent and may spread to involve the pharynx and larynx. Herpes simplex ulceration tends to be widespread and persistent for many weeks. Oral hairy leukoplakia, HPV infection, gingivitis and periodontal disease and squamous cell carcinoma may occur. Xerostomia is a frequent symptom.

4. Neck cervical lymphadenitis may be due to HIV-associated generalised lymphadenopathy, IRIS, lymphoma, leukaemia, lymphoproliferative disorders including multicentric Castleman's disease and metastatic squamous cell carcinoma. Unusual organisms such as atypical *Mycobacterium* may form a neck abscess.

38.4 Investigations

The diagnosis of HIV infection depends on detecting the virus or the host response to it in the blood. Usually, this is done by identifying a specific antibody, using first an ELISA as a screen. This is done in combination with testing for p24 antigen (the combination HIV p24 antigen and HIV antibody test) followed by Western blot confirmation. Plasma HIV RNA assays give useful information when measured sequentially about both disease progression and response to anti-viral treatment.

Monitoring of the CD4+ T-cell count is a measure of immune function and disease progression. Opportunistic infections are diagnosed by appropriate sampling and microbiological culturing. Neoplastic lesions are confirmed histologically on biopsy. Other investigations (e.g., radiology) are dictated by the clinical conditions.

38.5 Management

The management of HIV infection as it presents to the ENT surgeon and the management of the patient to avoid the risks of infection pose separate problems. The occurrence of unusual organisms requires a high index of suspicion to make the diagnosis, followed by appropriate therapy. Radiotherapy and chemotherapy may be used for Kaposi's sarcoma and lymphomas.

38.6 Risk of Infection

The risk of infection to a health care worker from a HIV-positive patient is extremely low and invariably relates to blood exposure. To reduce this risk, two sets of common sense recommendations have developed.

• Universal precautions should be adopted for all patients and involve the use of gowns and gloves to avoid blood contamination. All non-intact skin surfaces should be covered, and sharps should be handled with appropriate caution.

• Theatre precautions apply to any invasive procedure on a proven or suspected HIV-positive patient. A high level of discipline is required in these cases. The most senior or experienced surgeon/clinician should operate and theatre/ancillary staff should be kept to a minimum. All staff should be fully gowned and double gloved and boots and eye protection should be worn. Drapes should be disposable and double bagged at the end of the procedure. The patient need not be last on the list, but the theatre should be thoroughly cleaned with hypochlorite solution prior to the next case. There is no evidence of infection risk from the anaesthetic system, but sensible hygienic measures should be employed.

Should exposure occur when treating an HIV-positive patient, post-exposure prophylaxis (PEP) should be considered according to the exact nature of the exposure. PEP should be instituted within 48 hours of exposure, so immediate advice from occupational health and/or an HIV specialist is vital. Appropriate serological monitoring is required over a period of several months.

The government announced in 2014 that dentists or surgeons who are HIV positive and who are taking ART and have an undetectable viral load may perform surgery. Such doctors are not expected to disclose their HIV status to patients because of the negligible risk of transmission.

38.7 Follow-Up and Aftercare

Patients are best cared for by a hospital where there is a team with a special interest in managing HIV-infected patients.

Further Reading

Sanjar FA, Queiroz BEUP, Miziara ID. Otolaryngologic manifestations in HIV disease—clinical aspects and treatment. Braz J Otorhinolaryngol. 2011; 77(3):391–400

Tshifularo M, Govender L, Monama G. Otolaryngological, head and neck manifestations in HIV-infected patients seen at Steve Biko Academic Hospital in Pretoria, South Africa. S Afr Med J. 2013; 103(7):464–466

Related Topics of Interest

Rhinosinusitis—appropriate terminology
Salivary gland diseases

H

39 Hypopharyngeal Carcinoma

The hypopharynx extends from the lower limit of the oropharynx at the level of the hyoid bone down to the lower level of the cricoid cartilage at the opening of the oesophagus. For the purposes of tumour classification, the UICC recognises three anatomical sites:

1. *Post-cricoid* (The pharyngo-oesophageal junction). Extends from the level of the arytenoid cartilages and connecting folds to the inferior margin of the cricoid cartilage, thus forming the anterior wall of the hypopharynx.
2. *Piriform fossa* This extends from the pharyngoepiglottic fold to the opening of the oesophagus. It is bounded medially by the arytenoids and aryepiglottic folds and laterally by the inner surface of the thyroid cartilage.
3. *Posterior pharyngeal wall* Extends from the superior aspect of the hyoid bone (floor of the vallecula) to the level of the inferior border of the cricoid cartilage.

39.1 Pathology

More than 90% of tumours of the hypopharynx are squamous cell carcinomas. Other epithelial and mesodermal tumours of benign and malignant behaviour do occur, but they are rare.

Carcinoma of the hypopharynx is an uncommon disease with a prevalence of less than 1 per 100,000 population and constitutes 5 to 10% of upper aerodigestive tract malignancies. It is a disease of the elderly and the incidence is higher in men than in women. The post-cricoid site is unusual in that women have a higher incidence. Tobacco smoking and alcohol are the main aetiological agents. Approximately 2% of patients with the Paterson–Brown–Kelly syndrome (iron deficiency anaemia, glossitis, angular stomatitis, pharyngeal web, koilonychia and splenomegaly) will develop post-cricoid carcinoma. A few patients who had irradiation for thyrotoxicosis many years ago present with pharyngeal carcinoma after a latent period of over 30 years.

Hypopharyngeal tumours are sometimes so advanced when first seen that it is difficult to determine the site of origin, but the piriform fossa (60–70%) is the most common site, with posterior pharyngeal wall tumours (10–20%) and post-cricoid carcinoma (5–15%) occurring less often. Tumours

of the posterior pharyngeal wall and the upper iriform fossa tend to be exophytic, whereas an ulcerated lesion is typical of the other parts of the hypopharynx. Tumours of the lateral wall of the piriform fossa may invade the thyrohyoid membrane and present as a palpable neck mass which may represent direct extension of the tumour rather than an enlarged lymph node. Medial wall tumours invade the aryepiglottic fold and into the paraglottic space, causing fixation of the vocal cord and consequent hoarseness. Dissemination of hypopharyngeal tumours in the submucosal lymphatics leads to a high incidence of 'skip lesions'. Approximately 5 to 10% of patients have a second tumour in the oesophagus or lungs. Hypopharyngeal tumours also have a propensity to metastasise to cervical lymph nodes. The piriform fossa has the richest lymphatic drainage, around two-thirds of these patients will have lymph node metastases at presentation (level IV), with half of these being bilateral. Post-cricoid tumours tend to spread to paratracheal nodes (level VI). The incidence of distant metastases at presentation is higher than for any other head and neck cancer.

39.2 Clinical Features

Early symptoms include soreness, odynophagia, the sensation of a lump or discomfort in the throat. There may be referred otalgia via the auricular branch of the vagus nerve (Arnold's or Alderman's nerve). Later the patient will usually present with dysphagia, at first for solids then for fluids. Hoarseness may occur as a result of invasion of the larynx or vocal cord paralysis. The patient with advanced disease may have anorexia and weight loss. There may be a history of food sticking and repeated aspiration which will cause pneumonia. Determination of weight loss, comorbidity and performance status (Karnofsky or WHO) are essential as morbidity and mortality rates are higher in patients with poor parameters.

Fibre-optic laryngoscopy may reveal an obvious tumour or oedema of the arytenoids with pooling of saliva in the piriform fossa. A Valsalva manoeuvre can be useful to open the piriform fossae for a better view. There may be vocal cord fixation. The neck must be examined for lymph node metastases and occasionally a direct extension of the tumour through the thyrohyoid membrane is palpable as a neck mass. Laryngeal crepitus may be lost as the prevertebral fascia is invaded, particularly in post-cricoid tumours.

39.3 Investigations

1. **Laboratory tests:** A full blood count to exclude anaemia and biochemical tests (U&Es and liver function tests [LFTs]) are required as electrolyte disturbances and malnutrition are not infrequent.

2. **Radiography:**
   - For those patients who present with a neck mass, an ultrasound-guided fine-needle aspiration biopsy (USSgFNAB) will be the first investigation. This will help delineate the presence of nodal disease (enlarged nodes, round shape with loss of fatty hilum) and confirm squamous cell carcinoma (sensitivity and specificity over 90%).
   - Contrast-enhanced computed tomography (CT) or magnetic resonance imaging (MRI) should be used to assess the extent of the disease. Scans should be performed prior to biopsy as this will distort the images and may affect staging and treatment discussions. The key determinants for staging and treatment are the site and size of the tumour, the tumour's upper and lower limits, the presence of thyroid cartilage invasion, the possibility of prevertebral fascia invasion (likely to be considered inoperable and incurable) and the presence of cervical node metastases. MRI is preferable to CT scanning in delineating the soft tissue extent and spread of tumour but can overestimate thyroid cartilage invasion.
   - A CT scan of the chest is mandatory to exclude metastases and may demonstrate any consolidation due to aspiration.
   - A barium swallow can be used to help demonstrate the extent and limits of a hypopharyngeal tumour or oesophageal lesion.
   - Positron emission tomography CT (PET-CT) is recommended for advanced hypopharyngeal cancers for assessment of the inferior extent of disease and in assessment of post-treatment residual disease or recurrence.

3. **Endoscopy:** Panendoscopy performed under general anaesthetic allows assessment of the tumour and a representative biopsy to be taken.

Laryngoscopy and oesophagoscopy can evaluate the site, size and extent of the lesion, with the upper and lower limits (the distances will be measured on the endoscope from the upper incisors) particularly needing to be assessed. Bronchoscopy can be performed to look for spread to the trachea and oesophagoscopy may reveal skip lesions or a synchronous oesophageal primary, but the addition of bronchoscopy (to the so-called triple endoscopy of laryngoscopy and oesophagoscopy with bronchoscopy) is not mandatory, unless imaging is suspicious, as chest imaging is much improved. Digital examination of the tumour is appropriate if there is superior spread. Palpation of the patient's neck while he or she is under the general anaesthetic allows further confirmation of nodal disease and assessment of mobility of the nodes.

39.4 Staging of Hypopharyngeal Carcinoma

When the patient has had a clinical assessment, radiological analysis and histological confirmation of squamous carcinoma, the UICC/AJCC stage should be conferred. Nodal stage is identical to that of the other head and neck subsites. The 8th edition UICC/AJCC primary site T stage for hypopharyngeal carcinoma is as follows:

T1	Tumour limited to one subsite of hypopharynx and/or 2 cm or less in greatest dimension.
T2	Tumour invades more than one subsite of hypopharynx or an adjacent site, or measures more than 2 but less than 4 cm in greatest dimension.
T3	Tumour measures more than 4 cm in greatest dimension, or with fixation of the hemilarynx, or extension to the oesophagus.
T4a	Tumour invades any of the following: thyroid/cricoid cartilage, hyoid bone, thyroid gland, oesophagus or central compartment soft tissues (strap muscles or subcutaneous fat).
T4b	Tumour invades pre-vertebral fascia, encases carotid artery or involves mediastinal structures.

Stage grouping is based on the TNM status:

Stage I	T1	N0	M0
Stage II	T2	N0	M0
Stage III	T3	N0	M0
	T1,T2,T3	N1	M0

Stage IVA	T4a	N0 N1	M0
	T1,T2,T3,T4a	N2	M0
Stage IVB	T4b	Any N	M0
	Any T	N3	M0
Stage IVC	Any T	Any N	M1

39.5 Management

Management will depend on the age and general condition of the patient, the site and extent of the disease and the patient's/carer's wishes. Decisions will be made in partnership with the patient and with the expertise of the head and neck cancer multidisciplinary team.

Hypopharyngeal carcinoma generally has a poor prognosis even with extensive surgery, and 60% of patients suffer local recurrence within a year; most mortality occurs within a year or two of diagnosis. Because of the low survival and high recurrence rate, the choice of treatment is particularly important. The optimal treatment modality should provide the best chance of cure, the lowest mortality and morbidity, the shortest hospital stay and the highest chance of good upper aerodigestive tract function (speech and swallowing).

These patients are usually in poor general condition and malnourished. Performance status will affect treatment decisions regarding fitness for surgery or suitability to receive chemotherapy. Pre-treatment nutritional assessment and placement of a nasogastric (NG) or percutaneous gastrostomy (PEG) will be necessary and any deficit in nutritional status should be proactively managed.

All patients should have elective treatment to their neck. In patients with an N0 neck, the overall risk of occult nodal metastases may be as high as 40%. Bilateral nodal involvement is also common. Therefore, treatment of both sides of the neck and the retropharyngeal lymph nodes with either surgery or radiotherapy is essential. Metastases are most common in levels II, III, and IV. A lateral selective neck dissection is therefore appropriate if surgery is the preferred modality.

Treatment may consist of radiotherapy, surgical resection, combined therapy or palliative therapy. The choice of modality remains controversial as no treatment type has been shown to be superior in terms of disease control and survival.

1. **Radiotherapy and chemoradiation:** Early hypopharyngeal cancer (Stage I/II) may be treated with radiotherapy, with the option of salvage surgery if there is a recurrence. Radiotherapy should be intensity modulated (IMRT) and comprise of 70 Gy in 35 fractions to the primary and involved lymph nodes (or an elective 50 Gy in 25 fractions to the N0 neck). In selected cases, radiotherapy can be given to the primary tumour and a neck dissection carried out for nodal metastases. Late disease (Stage III/IV) can be treated with primary chemoradiation if cartilage is not extensively involved and the vocal cords are not paralysed. Concomitant chemotherapy confers a survival advantage over radiotherapy alone. Patients who are 70 or less should be offered this. Cisplatin is usually given (100 mg/m^2) every 3 weeks. Carboplatin is an alternative if there is reduced renal function. Side effects of radiotherapy treatment include lethargy, weakness, dry mouth, mucositis, altered taste, pharyngeal stenosis, neck musculature stiffness and pain and vascular complications. Chemotherapy potentiates these side effects.

2. **Surgery:** Early disease can be treated with transoral endoscopic laser, transoral robotic surgical excision or open partial pharyngolaryngectomy. Elective selective neck dissection (levels II–V) in all cases is mandatory. Surgical resection is preferred for large tumours or in the presence of bulky cervical metastases. It should be offered to 'fit' patients in the setting of a compromised larynx or significant dysphagia. In view of the propensity to submucosal extension of disease, generous surgical margins are recommended with 1.5 cm superiorly, 3 cm inferiorly, and 2 cm laterally. A lateral pharyngotomy can be performed for posterior wall tumours and the defect repaired with a radial forearm free flap. Extensive and circumferential lesions will require total pharyngolaryngectomy and then reconstruction of the residual defect. A variety of techniques to reconstruct have been used and each has its own advantages and limitations. The main complications are failure of the graft or flap, post-operative fistula and stenosis, which are all more likely if there has been previous radiotherapy. The choice of reconstruction often depends largely on the experience of the unit.

  • Radial forearm flap: This is easy to raise and ideal as a patch graft for partial pharyngeal excisions, but it is relatively small and associated with stricture when used in tubing for circumferential excisions.

- Anterolateral thigh flap: This is a perforator flap with a low donor site morbidity and is easily tubed. When inserted over a salivary bypass tube, it has a lower rate of stenosis compared to other flaps, and minimal donor site morbidity. It is claimed that voice outcomes are better than with jejunum.
- Jejunal flap: It is easily positioned into a circumferential defect and is a reliable free flap, but it is prone to stenosis and subjects the patient to potential abdominal surgery complications.
- Gastro-omental flap: Sometimes favoured in salvage pharyngolaryngectomy reconstruction (post-chemoradiotherapy). The omentum is highly vascular and thought to offer some protection to the carotids from rupture, improve vascularity of the overlying skin and possess anti-inflammatory properties. It can be bulky making neck closure difficult and is another flap which subjects the patient to an abdominal procedure.
- Gastric pull-up: A stomach pull may be necessary if the inferior extent of the tumour is too low for closure within the neck or if the inferior extent necessitates removal of the oesophagus to ensure clearance. It is an abdominal procedure and mediastinal, with a significant mortality rate of up to 15%.

On the 7th to 10th post-operative day, if there is no evidence of graft failure or leak, the patient can be tested with a methylene blue or contrast swallow. If there is no evidence of extravasation, the patient can be commenced on fluids and then soft diet. Most patients will require thyroid, calcium and calciferol replacement for life. Speech rehabilitation is difficult in these patients, and although there are some encouraging reports with low-pressure speech valves, many will require a mechanical voice (e.g., Servox) device.

3. **Combined therapy:** Hypopharyngeal cancer can be treated surgically with a total pharyngolaryngectomy and reconstruction with adjuvant radiotherapy. Post-operative radiotherapy is carried out within 6 weeks of surgical resection as a combined treatment, with the aims of destroying metastases and maximising the recurrence-free life interval. It is indicated if surgical resection margins are close to or involved in tumour, in most large tumours requiring surgery, when there is vascular or perineural invasion, more than two lymph nodes are involved, or if there is extracapsular rupture.

4. **Palliation:** This therapy is for those patients with advanced end-stage disease, severe intercurrent illness, poor general condition, distant metastases or those who refuse curative treatment. Palliative radiotherapy can be offered to produce tumour shrinkage and symptom relief from bleeding or pain. Tracheostomy for airway obstruction or protection of the airway from aspiration may be required. A PEG may be required for hydration and nutrition.

39.6 Follow-Up and Aftercare

Patients should be regularly reviewed in the clinic and their nutritional status and swallowing ability should be monitored along with a careful examination for primary and secondary recurrence. Most recurrence (60%) occurs within the first year of treatment. For early disease, the 5-year survival is reasonable (up to 60%), but in Stage III and IV disease, the 5-year survival is poor (15–20%), with an overall 5-year disease-specific survival rate of 30 to 35%.

Further Reading

Hall SF, Groome PA, Irish J, O'Sullivan B. Radiotherapy or surgery for head and neck squamous cell cancer: establishing the baseline for hypopharyngeal carcinoma? Cancer. 2009; 115(24):5711–5722

Jones AS, Roland NJ, Husband D, Hamilton JW, Gati I. Free revascularized jejunal loop repair following total pharyngolaryngectomy for carcinoma of the hypopharynx: report of 90 patients. Br J Surg. 1996; 83(9):1279–3

Lefebvre JL, Andry G, Chevalier D, et al; EORTC Head and Neck Cancer Group. Laryngeal preservation with induction chemotherapy for hypopharyngeal squamous cell carcinoma: 10-year results of EORTC trial 24891. Ann Oncol. 2012; 23(10):2708–2714

Patel RS, Goldstein DP, Brown D, Irish J, Gullane PJ, Gilbert RW. Circumferential pharyngeal reconstruction: history, critical analysis of techniques, and current therapeutic recommendations. Head Neck. 2010; 32(1):109–120

Pracy P, Loughran S, Good J, Parmar S, Goranova R. Hypopharyngeal cancer: United Kingdom National Multidisciplinary Guidelines. J Laryngol Otol. 2016; 130(Suppl 2):S104–S110

Related Topics of Interest

Globus pharyngeus
Laryngeal carcinoma
Oral cavity carcinoma
Oropharyngeal carcinoma
Ototoxicity

40 Imaging in ENT

40.1 Computed Tomography

CT is primarily used to delineate bony anatomy.

1. Unenhanced CT scans are indicated for:
   - Trauma.
   - Assessment of sinus anatomy (▶ Fig. 40.1) and benign sinus disease prior to functional endoscopic sinus surgery.
   - Assessing bone invasion in sinonasal or other head and neck tumours.
2. High-resolution CT (HRCT) of the temporal bone is used for assessment of bony anatomy in the middle and inner ear (▶ Fig. 40.2 and ▶ Fig. 40.3).
3. CT can also be useful for staging head and neck cancer in patients who have contraindications to MRI.

Modern multi-slice CT scanners acquire data volumetrically, allowing multi-planar reconstruction of CT images. This is particularly useful in oncology and in complex anatomical evaluation of the temporal bone.

It is important to remember that CT uses radiation. Although the doses received are now much lower on modern scanners, it is essential to limit its injudicious use, particularly in children.

CT is contraindicated in pregnancy. The use of intravenous (IV) iodinated contrast media is contraindicated in those with a history of allergy to IV iodine (not topical iodine) and in strongly atopic patients. IV contrast can be given cautiously in these patients as long as there is medical backup. Steroid use pre-injection is no longer thought to confer any benefit and is not used. Patients with renal impairment should not be given IV contrast unless absolutely necessary and in those circumstances, there should be involvement of the renal team pre-scan and for follow up with urinary function tests.

40.2 Magnetic Resonance Imaging

MRI provides markedly superior definition of soft tissues in any imaging plane and is preferable, for example, in delineating the extent of any head and neck lesion.

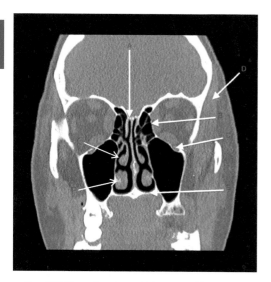

Fig. 40.1 Normal anatomy of sinuses on CT. A, cribriform plate; B, lamina papyracea; C, inferior orbital nerve; D, temporalis muscle; E, hard palate; F, inferior turbinate; G, middle turbinate

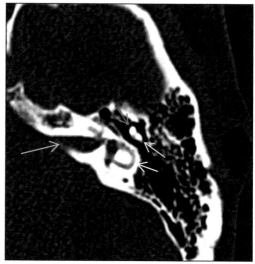

Fig. 40.2 Normal anatomy of the middle/inner ear on CT. *Red arrow*, head of malleus; *green arrow*, short process of incus; *blue arrow*, internal auditory canal; *yellow arrow*, lateral semi-circular canal

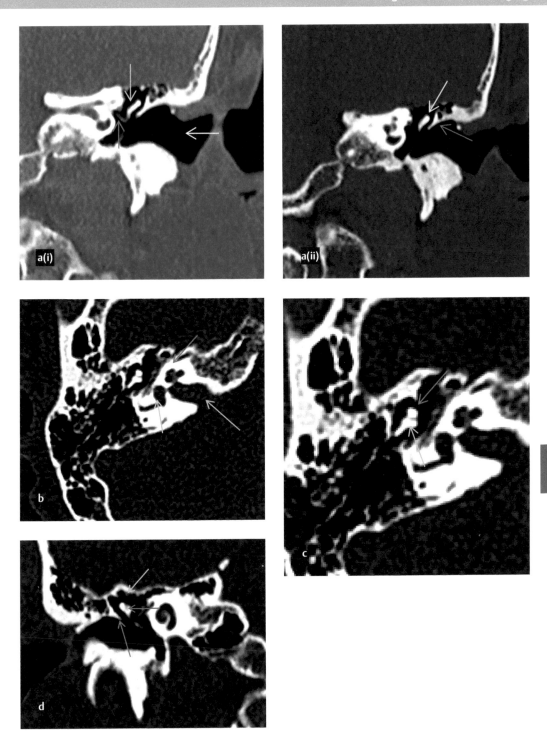

Fig. 40.3 (a–d) Normal anatomy of the middle/inner ear on CT. (a[i]) *Red arrow*, stapes inserting into oval window; *blue arrow*, long process of incus; *yellow arrow*, external auditory canal, (a[ii]) *red arrow*, scutum; *green arrow*, malleus; (b) *red arrow*, cochlear; *blue arrow*, internal auditory canal; *green arrow*, vestibule (c) *red arrow*, head of malleus; *green arrow*, long process of incus; (d) *red arrow*, scutum; *green arrow*, epitympanum or attic region; *blue arrow*, head of malleus

There are several MRI weightings and sequences, which can be used to answer specific diagnostic problems.

- *T1-weighted (T1W) images* In these images, the fluid signal in cerebrospinal fluid (CSF) or in the globes appears dark, whereas fat appears bright or white. T1W images are useful to look at the extent of tumours as they tend to grow through and obliterate the fat planes. The loss of the normal fat in bone marrow in the mandible and within skull base foramina on a T1W image is particularly useful in staging.

- *T2-weighted (T2W) images* In these images, fluid appears to be of high signal and fat is also bright or white. T2W images are useful for looking for high signal fluid necrosis in metastatic lymph nodes from a squamous cell carcinoma (SCC) and for distinguishing a sinus tumour from surrounding fluid secretions.

- *Diffusion-weighted imaging* uses the diffusion of water molecules to generate contrast. It is useful to differentiate cholesteatoma from fluid secretions. The water molecules in cholesteatoma are not free to diffuse (i.e. they are restricted) and so appear bright on a diffusion-weighted scan. Diffusion-weighted imaging has also been used to differentiate tumour recurrence from post-radiation changes and has a role in imaging the brain of patients who have suffered an acute stroke.

- *Gadolinium* is a paramagnetic contrast agent used in MRI. It behaves in exactly the same way as iodine-based contrast media described in the CT section. Fat-saturated T1W images post-gadolinium are used to demonstrate enhancement (an increase in signal) and are useful for showing enhancement in the wall of a necrotic lymph node or for enhancing tumours. Fat saturated means that the bright fat signal is suppressed or removed from the image, leaving the pathology more conspicuous.

- *Short-tau inversion recovery (STIR) sequence* is a T2W scan with fat signal suppression. This shows pathology and fluid as 'white' in the image and therefore more conspicuous than in an ordinary T2W image. This sequence is of great value in the delineation of head and neck cancers.

MRI cannot be used in patients with cardiac pacemakers, iron-containing brain clips, certain cardiac prosthetic valves and implants, and in the first trimester of pregnancy. Gadolinium should also be used with caution in patients with renal impairment. Patients can have an anaphylactic reaction to IV gadolinium; however, this is less common than with IV iodinated contrast.

▶ Table 40.1 shows patterns of tissue characterisation, where observation of signal on T1W and T2W images allows identification of tissue type, and it also relates the MR characterisation to CT appearance.

40.3 Ultrasound

Ultrasound is a very useful technique for the assessment of masses in the neck, thyroid goitres and for suspected salivary gland pathology. It does not involve any radiation exposure. It can be linked with ultrasound–guided-fine needle aspiration (FNA), performed as an out-patient procedure at the time of diagnostic scanning.

A high frequency (7.5–10 mHz) hand-held probe is placed directly on the neck and the fine needle can be visualised directly entering individual lesions as small as 1 cm in diameter. As a technique, however, it is very operator-dependent

▶ **Table 40.1** Patterns of tissue characterisation

Tissue	Signal T1 weighted	MR intensity Signal intensity	CT image appearance
Water (CSF, oedema)	Low (black)	High (white)	Dark grey
Fat	High (white)	High (white)	Very dark grey
Malignant/inflamed tissue	Intermediate (grey)	Intermediate (grey)	Grey
Cortical bone (Air) Fast-flowing blood)	Signal void (black)	Signal void (black)	White Black Grey

Abbreviation: CSF, cerebrospinal fluid.

requiring an ultrasonologist with specific technical skills who performs head and neck ultrasound regularly.

40.4 Positron Emission Tomography and Computed Tomography

Positron emission tomography–computed tomography (PET–CT) scan uses radioactive glucose in the form of fluorodeoxyglucose (FDG) as the tracer. The FDG is injected into the patient and it accumulates in areas of high metabolic activity. This will include normal structures such as the brain and heart. The tracer is excreted by the kidneys and therefore the urinary tract will also show increased activity. Increased activity is also a feature of tumours, referred to as PET positive lesions.

PET and CT images are acquired during the scan and the images are then fused by software to allow a map of functional activity onto structural landmarks. In head and neck, the two main indications are for investigation of a primary of unknown origin (▶ Fig. 40.4) and for patients with suspected recurrent head and neck cancer. FDG PET/CT is expensive and confers a high radiation dose to the patient; however, the advantage over structural imaging alone outweighs this.

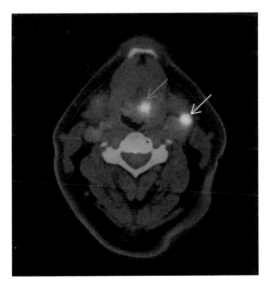

Fig. 40.4 FDG PETCT fused image at the level of the tongue base. *Red arrow*, T1 primary SCC left tongue base; *green arrow*, metastatic left level 2 lymph node

40.5 Sentinel Node Imaging

Sentinel node imaging for head and neck is indicated in patients with early (T1) oral cavity tumours and an N0 neck on conventional imaging.

The primary tumour is injected per orally with 40 Mbq of technetium 99m nano-colloid and then dynamic and static nuclear medicine images as well as delayed SPECT/CT images are taken for localisation.

The patient then undergoes surgery the day after the sentinel node imaging and the first order drainage node is identified with a gamma probe in theatre and removed. The whole of the node is sectioned and analysed for tumour involvement. If the node is positive for metastatic disease, the patient is offered a formal neck dissection at a later date. If negative, the patient undergoes 2 years of ultrasound neck surveillance, with three monthly ultrasound scans, to identify any nodal recurrence.

40.6 Plain Films

Following the increased use of complex diagnostic techniques such as CT and MR, plain films are rarely used for diagnostic purposes in ENT. The Royal College of Radiologists' guidelines recommend that 'plain films of the sinuses are not routinely indicated'. The radiation dose of a 4 projection sinus series is equivalent to 25 chest X-ray doses or 10 weeks of background radiation.

Lateral soft-tissue views of the neck are of limited value in isolation. They may demonstrate opaque foreign bodies, but many foreign bodies are likely to be non-opaque. Contrast swallows are more accurate in this situation.

40.7 Contrast Swallow

A contrast swallow is indicated in the investigation of dysphagia or symptoms suggestive of motility disorders.

Barium swallows are of superior sensitivity in demonstrating pharyngeal pouches, pharyngeal webs (the web is a linear line indenting the anterior aspect of the barium column at the level of C5/C6) and cricopharyngeus hypertrophy (indents the posterior column of barium at the C6/C7 level). Digital screening is preferred to reduce radiation dose. Image acquisition is preferably at the rate of 2 frames per second during a bolus swallow.

Motility disorders are best assessed using dynamic video swallow fluoroscopy.

Water soluble contrast swallows (using non-ionic relatively inert contrast media) are indicated when the history suggests that aspiration into the lungs is a real risk (if barium is used in these circumstances it may lead to resistant chest infection or permanent lung damage), when perforation of the oesophagus is suspected or a surgical anastomosis is being evaluated (barium used in these circumstances will remain in the soft tissues if a leak is present, obscuring the area for further follow-up studies and being a viscous thick suspension it is less likely to demonstrate small oesophageal leaks than water soluble contrast).

Imaging in Otology

40.8 Cholesteatoma

Congenital cholesteatoma presents as an avascular mass behind an intact tympanic membrane and usually occurs in children or young adults with a male predominance. HRCT of the temporal bones shows a well-defined mass in the middle ear cleft with or without ossicular erosion.

In acquired cholesteatoma imaging shows a mass in Prussak's space in the attic region of the middle ear cleft (pars flaccida). Ossicular erosion is seen in 70% of pars flaccida cholesteatoma. There may also be erosion of the scutum and lateral epitympanic wall. Pars tensa cholesteatoma is less common and is typically seen in the posterior mesotympanum. Differential diagnosis for all types of cholesteatoma would include cholesterol granuloma, glomus tympanicum or fluid opacification of the middle ear cleft.

HRCT is usually used as the first line of investigation to look for a middle ear mass with associated bone erosion. MRI with diffusion-weighted imaging is helpful to differentiate cholesteatoma from fluid or post-surgical change. Cholesteatoma is typically avascular and does not enhance post-gadolinium; however, it may show peripheral enhancement due to granulation or scar tissue.

40.9 Vestibular Schwannoma

The typical appearance of a vestibular schwannoma is of an enhancing mass at the cerebellopontine (CP) angle or within the internal auditory meatus.

MRI is usually the first line of investigation in patients presenting with sensorineural hearing loss and/or tinnitus. High-resolution T2W images of the CP angles give excellent detail of the vestibulocochlear nerves (▶Fig. 40.5 and ▶Fig. 40.6) and can be used as a screening tool for vestibular schwannoma. Larger tumours may show central areas of cystic degeneration (▶Fig. 40.7) shown on both T2W and post-gadolinium scans.

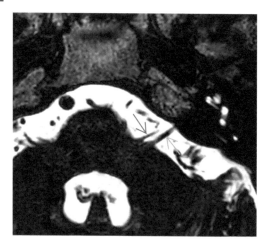

Fig. 40.5 Normal anatomy of the IAM on axial high-resolution T2W MRI. *Red arrow*, 7th or facial nerve; *blue arrow*, 8th or vestibulocochlear nerve

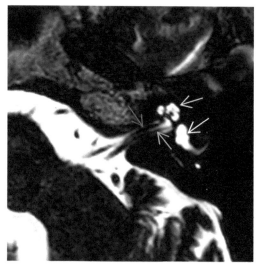

Fig. 40.6 Normal anatomy of the IAM on axial high-resolution T2W MRI. *Red arrow*, cochlear nerve; *green arrow*, cochlea; *blue arrow*, vestibular nerve; *yellow arrow*, vestibule

I

Schwannomas can significantly increase in size on serial scans due to interval cystic degeneration. Large areas of cystic change make these tumours less suitable for radiotherapy treatment compared to solid tumours. Bilateral vestibular schwannomas occur in neurofibromatosis type 2 (▶Fig. 40.8a, b).

The main differential diagnoses of a CP angle lesion are:

- Facial nerve schwannoma.
- Epidermoid cyst.
- CP angle meningioma.

CP angle meningiomas tend to have a broad flat base towards the temporal bone as well as a mushroom cap and typically enhance uniformly post-contrast, often with a dural tail.

40.10 Cochlear Otosclerosis

This condition involves lysis of the bone surrounding the cochlea and is of unknown aetiology. In the acute phase, the bone appears lytic, later becoming sclerotic in the healing phase. Typically, focal lytic areas are seen in the bone surrounding the cochlea giving a halo appearance. MRI post-contrast shows curvy linear enhancement around the cochlea. HRCT of the temporal bones is the best imaging modality, allowing better delineation of the bony anatomy. Differential diagnosis in adults includes otosyphilis in the lytic phase and Paget's disease and fibrous dysplasia in the sclerotic phase.

40.11 Cholesterol Granuloma

Cholesterol granulomas are also referred to as cholesterol cysts or 'chocolate ear'. Clinically, these appear as a bluish discoloration behind the tympanic membrane. The typical radiological appearances are that of a well-defined expansile mass in the middle ear cavity or mastoid region, which is bright on both T1W and T2W images. On both CT and MRI the mass fills the middle ear cleft causing erosion of the ossicles and expansion of the bony margins. The mass is bright on T1W and T2W images due to underlying haemorrhage. There is no enhancement post-contrast.

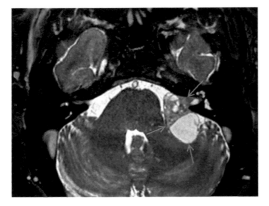

Fig. 40.7 Axial T2W high-resolution MRI of the IAMS. *Red arrows* outlining a left solid/cystic vestibular schwannoma

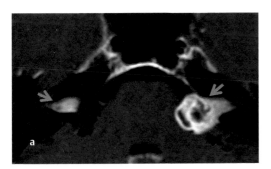
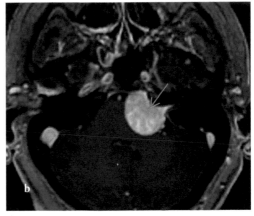

Fig. 40.8 (a, b) Axial T1W image of the IAMS post-gadolinium. *Red arrow heads*, bilateral acoustic neuromas in a patient with neurofibromastosis type 2; *red arrow*, left CP angle meningioma with a broad base and extension into the left IAM.

40.12 Glomus Tympanicum Paraganglioma

These are benign tumours that arise from the glomus bodies on the cochlear promontory. Clinically, they present with a vascular mass behind the tympanic membrane and pulsatile tinnitus. On HRCT of the temporal bones, they are seen as a mass in the middle ear cleft with a flat base overlying the cochlear promontory. On MRI, these typically show enhancement post-gadolinium. Differential diagnosis would include cholesteatoma.

40.13 Acute Otitis Media and Mastoiditis

This results from infection within the middle ear cleft and mastoid air cells. On HRCT of the temporal bones there may be fluid opacification within the middle mastoid air cells and occasionally destructive changes within the bony septations in the mastoid region. Post-contrast CT and MRI may show diffuse enhancement of inflammatory tissue. It is important to look for associated intracranial spread of inflammation with meningeal enhancement or cerebral abscess in the adjacent temporal lobe. Complications include subperiosteal abscess, meningitis/cerebral abscess, dural venous sinus thrombosis and extension to the petrous apex, causing petrous apicitis.

40.14 Squamous Cell Carcinoma of the External Auditory Canal

Typical imaging appearances are that of a mass with underlying bone destruction, which is best shown on a HRCT of the temporal bones. Typically, the middle ear structures are spared. MRI shows an enhancing mass and allows extent of the soft tissue involvement, including the adjacent temporal mandibular joint, and to assess for intracranial extension. The adjacent parotid gland should be scrutinised for metastatic nodes.

40.15 Bell's Palsy

MRI is reserved for atypical presentations. The typical finding is of marked asymmetrical enhancement post-gadolinium at the fundus and within the labyrinthine segment of the facial nerve. Abnormal facial nerve enhancement may persist on imaging after full clinical improvement.

Imaging in Rhinology

40.16 Sinonasal Polyposis

The first line of imaging is usually in the form of CT sinuses that show anything from solitary to multiple bilateral sinonasal polyps. The surrounding bone may become thinned due to pressure and disease in the ethmoid region may lead to lateral bulging of the lamina papyracea into the orbits. The maxillary ostium is often expanded and blocked. Fluid or a bubbly appearance of mucous in the sinuses indicates that there may be an acute sinusitis element. Sometimes, the degree of bone thinning can be difficult to differentiate from a malignant process. On MRI, fluid/mucous shows high signal on a T2W images. Polyps usually have a characteristic high signal appearance and show peripheral enhancement and low signal central change on the T1W images post-contrast. MRI, particularly T2W coronal images, can be helpful to identify underlying low signal tumour from high signal polyps.

40.17 Antrochoanal Polyp

This often has a dumb bell appearance and will expand the maxillary ostium. The maxillary sinus and middle meatus are usually completely opacified. These polyps appear of low attenuation on CT, high signal on T2W MRI and do not enhance post-contrast.

40.18 Mucocele

Mucoceles result from mucous retention within an obstructed sinus leading to expansion of the sinus and impingement on adjacent structures. There is usually dehiscence of the wall of the sinus. Frontal and ethmoid mucoceles can cause extrinsic compression of the globe resulting in proptosis. The best imaging clue is an expanded opacified sinus with thinning or dehiscence of the bony wall. Mucoceles appear of varying signal intensity on MRI. Proteinaceous contents may show a very high T1W signal. Chronic inspissated mucous can also appear low signal or black mimicking air. Mucoceles do not enhance and this helps to differentiate them from a sinus tumour.

40.19 Non-Invasive Fungal Sinusitis

This condition is usually seen in immunocompromised patients. The presence of fine linear calcifications within an opacified sinus is strongly suggestive of underlying fungal infection. There are usually signs of accompanying chronic sinusitis with thickening and sclerosis of the walls of the affected sinus. On MRI, the T1W images may show low signal change within an obstructed sinus due to the underlying solid mycetoma. Occasionally, if the extent of fungal involvement in a sinus is marked, the sinus may appear 'black', which can mimic an aerated sinus. CT is therefore better than MRI for initial diagnosis.

40.20 Wegener's Granulomatosis

CT is initially used for delineation of sinonasal involvement. These patients may develop a soft-tissue opacification in the paranasal sinuses and nose, typically associated with septal and bone destruction particularly along the medial walls of the maxillary sinuses and of the turbinates. With advanced disease orbital involvement can occur. Other complications include meningeal enhancement and neurological complications from vasculitis.

40.21 Juvenile Angiofibroma

The typical presentation is that of a vascular mass in the nasal passage found in young male patients. The mass is centred at the sphenopalatine foramen and often results in expansion of the pterygopalatine fossa with potential for bone remodelling and destruction. These tumours extend from the region of the sphenopalatine foramen into the nasal passages. If the tumours are large there is potential for central skull base foramina involvement and extension into the middle cranial fossa. CT is the best imaging tool to show the extent of bone involvement. On MRI these tumours are intensely vascular and show flow voids within them, which, together with the expansion of the pterygopalatine fissure and sphenopalatine foramen, is the best diagnostic clue.

40.22 Inverted Papilloma

The typical imaging appearances are that of a mass centred on the middle meatus obstructing the maxillary ostium and causing opacification of this sinus. There may be associated bone remodelling. These tumours enhance and can appear lobulated post-contrast. In 10% of cases calcification is seen on CT within the tumours. On MRI these tumours have a lobulated cerebriform pattern. Radiological follow-up is usually indicated as these tumours have a high recurrence rate and an association with SCC.

40.23 Paranasal Sinus Squamous Cell Carcinoma

Paranasal sinus SCC usually presents on imaging as an enhancing mass with bone destruction. The most common site is within the maxillary sinuses. Staging of these tumours depends on the extent of local tumour spread and key areas of involvement include orbital extension, intracranial extension, perineural spread along the inferior orbital nerve, pterygopalatine foramen or cavernous sinus, invasion of the skin of the cheek and the infratemporal fossa. Imaging should also include an assessment of the neck for nodal disease. T2W images are useful for delineating intermediate signal tumour from high signal secretions. Fat saturation images post-gadolinium to cover the skull base are essential to look for perineural spread.

40.24 Anatomical Variants of the Paranasal Sinuses

- The cribriform plates can be defined as types I, II or III according to the Keros classification (see ▶ Table 40.2). Low lying type III cribriform plates have the highest risk of iatrogenic injury and CSF leak.
- Agger nasi cells result from pneumatisation of the agger mound and can extend into the frontal recess causing mechanical obstruction.

▶ **Table 40.2** Keros classification

Keros classification	
Type I	1–3 mm (26.3% population)
Type II	4–7 mm (73.3% population)
Type III	8–16 mm (0.5% population)

161

- Concha bullosa refers to a pneumatised middle turbinate. When enlarged, these can narrow the middle meatus and osteomeatal complex resulting in obstruction. Inflammation and fluid opacification can also occur within the concha bullosa, resulting in a bullitis.
- Haller air cells are ethmoid air cells that have projected inferiorly along the medial aspect of the orbital floor and can obstruct the maxillary ostium if enlarged.
- The uncinate process may be elongated and deviated medially abutting the middle turbinate and obstructing the middle meatus. Careful inspection of the bone within the cribriform plates and lamina papyracea is required on CT to exclude any areas of dehiscence prior to surgery.

Head and Neck Imaging

40.25 Benign Cervical Lymph Nodes

Ultrasound is the best modality to image cervical lymph nodes as it allows an assessment of their size, shape and morphology. Ultrasound is quick, relatively inexpensive, avoids ionising radiation, but is operator dependant. Benign or reactive lymph nodes typically have an oval shape, have a long to short axis of more than 2, show a fatty or white hilum and show hilar blood flow on colour Doppler imaging (▶Fig. 40.9). Pathological lymph nodes tend to be rounded or lobulated, have a long to short axis of less than 2, lose their fatty hilum and show disorganised flow on colour Doppler imaging (▶Fig. 40.10).

The size of benign lymph nodes is variable and in teenagers and young adults, benign reactive nodes can be several centimetres in length. The width of the node rather than the length is usually measured to predict whether the node is benign or pathological. The jugulodigastric node tends to be the largest and normally has a width of less than 15 mm. Retropharyngeal nodes below the skull

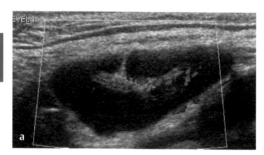

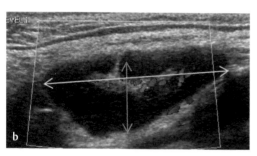

Fig. 40.9 (a, b) Normal lymph node anatomy on ultrasound showing an oval shape, long (*yellow arrow*) > short (*red arrow*) axis ratio > 2; white fatty hilar stripe; Hilar blood flow

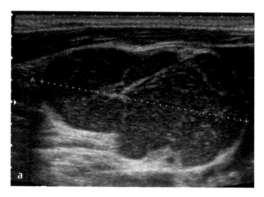

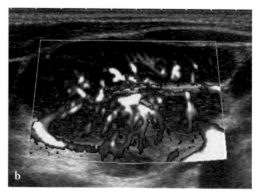

Fig. 40.10 (a, b) Ultrasound image of a pathological lymph node. Typical appearance of a pathological node with a round/lobulated shape; hypoechoic echotexture; loss of white fatty hilar stripe; disorganised blood flow on colour doppler

base tend to be the smallest and have a width of less than 5 mm. The width of the remaining neck nodes is generally taken to be less than 10 mm; although, this does vary in the literature.

A comparison of the ultrasound appearance of benign and malignant nodes is given in ▸Table 40.3.

▸ **Table 40.3** Comparison of the ultrasound appearance of benign and malignant nodes

Benign lymph nodes	Malignant lymph nodes
Oval shape	Round or lobulated
Solid	Necrosis typical of metastatic nodes from SCC or papillary thyroid cancer
Fatty hilum	Loss of fatty hilum
Hilar blood flow	Disorganised peripheral blood flow
Uniform echogenicity	Hypoechoic or 'darker'
Size variable however tend to be longer than wider, i.e. the long to short axis ratio > 2	Size variable however tend to be rounded, i.e. the long to short axis ratio < 2
Single node	Clustering of nodes is suspicious

Abbreviation: SCC, squamous cell carcinoma.

40.26 Metastatic Nodes from Squamous Cell Carcinoma

Metastatic nodes from SCC show areas of necrosis or cystic change within the node that can be seen on ultrasound, CT and MRI. Post-IV contrast, the nodes may show peripheral ring enhancement with central fluid change. Ultrasound combined with FNA has the highest sensitivity and specificity for detecting lymph node metastases compared to other imaging modalities. Extracapsular spread is difficult to detect early on imaging and is usually a histological finding. When present on imaging the margins of the nodes appear indistinct and there is usually oedema around the nodes, which may encase the carotid sheath indicating a poor prognosis. ▸Fig. 40.11 shows a metastatic right level 2 node from a right tonsillar primary.

40.27 Metastatic Node from an Unknown Primary Origin

PET–CT is currently indicated to assess patients with a metastatic node proven to be from an SCC on FNA but without any obvious primary tumour either clinically or on cross-sectional imaging. The usual sites detected by PET–CT are in the tonsils, tongue base or nasopharynx.

I

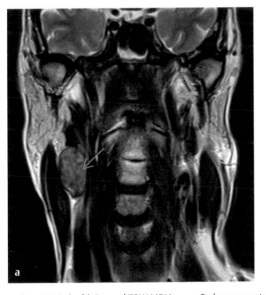
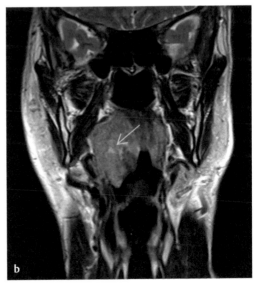

Fig. 40.11 (a, b) Coronal T2W MRI image. *Red arrow,* metastatic right level 2 lymph node from SCC of the right tonsil; *green arrow,* primary SCC right tonsil

40.28 Lymphoma

Lymphomatous nodes tend to be solid not cystic, involve multiple nodal stations and appear high signal on fat-saturated images (STIR) and dark/hypoechoic on ultrasound. The nodes tend to enhance uniformly post-IV contrast.

40.29 Metastatic Nodes from Papillary Thyroid Cancer

Metastatic nodes from papillary cancer of the thyroid tend to be cystic and show micro-calcifications similar to the primary tumour. The nodes are more usually seen in levels 4 and 6 on imaging.

40.30 Thyroid Nodules

Thyroid nodules are common and present a diagnostic dilemma as most are found incidentally on imaging for other reasons, that is CT and PET–CT. The majority of thyroid nodules will be benign; however, differentiating which nodules are benign from malignant can be challenging on imaging.

Ultrasound is the best imaging technique to evaluate thyroid nodules. The American Thyroid Association has developed an imaging strategy to guide the need for FNA and prevent over-investigation. Suspicious thyroid nodules that require FNA are those which have the following appearances on ultrasound:

- Solid and hypoechoic/darker than surrounding thyroid/strap muscles.
- Irregular margins (infiltrative, lobulated).
- Micro-calcifications.
- Taller-than-wide shape.
- Rim calcifications with small extrusive soft tissue component.
- Extension outside of thyroid.

Papillary cancers and associated nodal metastases typically show micro-calcification and may be cystic on ultrasound. Follicular lesions tend to be more solid and uniform in echotexture. Anaplastic cancers are more frequently seen in older patients and appear as a diffusely hypoechoic/dark infiltrating mass with invasion of adjacent structures such as the trachea and carotid sheath. These are usually staged with CT or MRI rather than ultrasound. Lymphoma also appears as a diffusely hypoechoic/dark echotexture and differentiation

from a thyroiditis can also be difficult—the diagnosis is usually established clinically and on biopsy.

Benign nodules tend to be of similar echogenicity or brighter than normal thyroid tissue. Purely cystic nodules do not need an FNA unless required for cosmetic reasons. Colour Doppler is no longer felt useful in differentiating benign from malignant nodules.

The use of PET–CT is resulting in the increased detection of FDG positive thyroid nodules and these should always undergo FNA, as there is a 30% risk of these being a well differentiated thyroid cancer.

40.31 Salivary Glands

- *Benign tumours* Pleomorphic adenoma appears as well-defined, solid and darker than normal parotid tissue on ultrasound. Ultrasound-guided FNA can be used to give a cytological diagnosis. MRI pre-surgery can be helpful to define the relationship of the tumour to the expected course of the facial nerve (▶ Fig. 40.12). Surgical tumour 'spillage' can result in multi-focal nodular areas of recurrence on post-operative imaging. Deep lobe pleomorphic adenoma presents as a parapharyngeal space mass and either arises in ectopic salivary gland tissue or from the deep lobe of parotid. Differential diagnosis includes a schwannoma. These lesions can be difficult to biopsy percutaneously and may require per oral biopsy. Twenty percent of Warthin's tumours are multiple or bilateral and they are typically partly cystic on imaging.

- *Nodes* The normal parotid gland has between 3 and 32 benign intra-parotid lymph nodes and is a first-order nodal site for tumours of the skin of the upper face, external ear and scalp. Parotid metastases should therefore be considered in patients presenting with a cystic parotid mass and with a history of SCC of the skin in the scalp/facial region.

- *Malignant tumours* Malignant parotid tumours are typically poorly defined on imaging with infiltration of the overlying skin and deeper structures in the masseteric space. Patients usually present with a rapidly growing mass and there may be clinical evidence of facial nerve palsy. Adenoid cystic carcinoma of the parotid gland can range in appearance on imaging from low-grade and well-defined to high-grade and poorly defined masses. This type of carcinoma

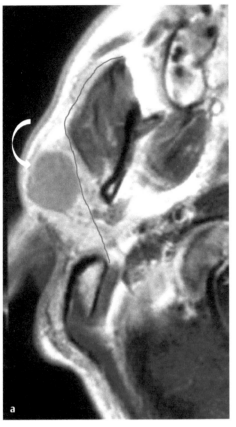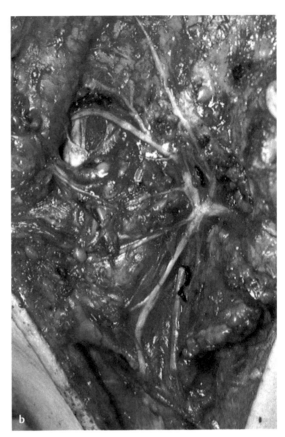

Fig. 40.12 (a, b) Axial T1W image of the right parotid gland. The approximate path of the facial nerve is shown by the *red line* indicating the route from the stylomastoid foramen and through the parotid gland lateral to retromandibular vein. This divides the parotid into deep and superficial lobes. The well defined pleomorphic adenoma is seen in the superficial lobe (*curved arrow*).

can spread perineurally and therefore it is important that pre-operative imaging with MRI post-gadolinium enhancement covers the whole of the facial nerve pathway to identify tumour spread along the nerve.

40.32 Cystic Neck Masses

- *Thyroglossal duct cyst* On imaging the cysts are well defined; however, the wall of the cyst may become thick and enhance post-contrast, if infected. Less than 1% are associated with a thyroid carcinoma, most commonly papillary carcinoma and, therefore, it is treated with complete surgical resection of the entire cyst and tract.

- *Laryngocele* On imaging these appear as thin-walled air or fluid-filled cystic lesions that communicate with the laryngeal ventricle. The wall of the laryngocele may become thick and enhance, if infected. Secondary laryngoceles result from an underlying glottic SCC obstructing the laryngeal ventricle and therefore careful attention to this area on imaging is required.

- *Branchial cleft cyst* There are four types of branchial cleft anomalies/cysts. Type 1 usually occur at the level of the parotid gland or preauricular region, type 2 in the region of level 2 within the neck (▶Fig. 40.13), type 3 in the upper to mid-neck and type 4 anywhere from the left pyriform sinus apex to the thyroid lobe. The diagnosis of a branchial cleft cyst should be made with caution in adults presenting with a cystic neck mass. In these patients a cystic metastatic node from a squamous primary origin should be

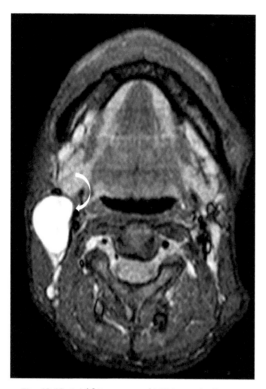

Fig. 40.13 Axial fat suppressed MRI image in the region of the tongue base. Fat suppressed image showing a right level 2 branchial cyst (*curved arrow*).

excluded before the diagnosis of a branchial cyst is assumed. The patient should be worked up as per protocol, which usually involves exclusion of an underlying occult primary tumour with MRI and PET–CT.

- *Ranula* Also known as a sublingual gland mucocele or mucous retention cyst and can be simple (above the mylohyoid muscle) or plunging/diving when it has extended outside of the sublingual space into the submandibular space. On imaging they typically appear as simple cystic lesions that communicate with the sublingual space/gland and may show an enhancing wall, if infected.

- *Dermoid cyst* It appears as well-defined oral cavity masses that typically have fatty, fluid or mixed contents. Fat is seen as bright on both DT1W and DT2W images and loses signal or becomes dark on the fat-suppressed (STIR) images. These are typically midline and the presence of fat helps to differentiate these from other cystic neck lesions.

- *Lymphangioma* On imaging they appear as uni- or multi-loculated non-enhancing cystic neck masses, which can occur in any head and neck space and may reach several centimetres in size. CT or MRI is best to delineate the extent of the lesion and typically there is no enhancement post-contrast.

Further Reading

The Preoperative Sinus CT. Avoiding a "CLOSE" call with surgical complications. William T. O'Brien, Stefan Hamelin, Erik K. Weitzel Radiology. 2016(October)

Trotta BM, Pease CS, Rasamny JJ, Raghavan P, Mukherjee S. Oral cavity and oropharyngeal squamous cell cancer: key imaging findings for staging and treatment planning. Radiographics. 2011; 31(2):339–354

Christe A, Waldherr C, Hallett R, Zbaeren P, Thoeny H. MR imaging of parotid tumors: typical lesion characteristics in MR imaging improve discrimination between benign and malignant disease. AJNR Am J Neuroradiol. 2011; 32(7):1202–1207

van der Jagt MA, Brink WM, Versluis MJ, et al. Visualization of human inner ear anatomy with high-resolution MR imaging at 7T: initial clinical assessment. AJNR Am J Neuroradiol. 2015; 36(2):378–383

Head and Neck Cancer | Guidance and Guidelines | NICE. Available at: https://www.nice.org.uk/guidance/qs146/chapter/quality-statement-2-clinical-staging

Learned KO, Lev-Toaff AS, Brake BJ, Wu RI, Langer JE, Loevner LA. US-guided biopsy of neck lesions: the head and neck neuroradiologist's perspective. Radiographics. 2016; 36(1):226–243

Schwartz KM, Lane JI, Bolster BD Jr, Neff BA. The utility of diffusion-weighted imaging for cholesteatoma evaluation. AJNR Am J Neuroradiol. 2011; 32(3):430–436

Ultrasound "U" classification of thyroid nodules: radiology reference article. Availabe at: https://radiopaedia.org/articles/ultrasound-u-classification-of-thyroid-nodules-1

Wong KT, Lee YY, King AD, Ahuja AT. Imaging of cystic or cyst-like neck masses. Clin Radiol. 2008; 63(6):613–622

Hoang JK, Eastwood JD, Tebbit CL, Glastonbury CM. Multiplanar sinus CT: a systematic approach to imaging before functional endoscopic sinus surgery. AJR Am J Roentgenol. 2010; 194(6):W527–36

41 Impedance Audiometry

41.1 Physics and Physiology

The middle ear and mastoid air cells communicate with the nasopharynx via the eustachian tube. As a closed system, air is being continually absorbed by the lining mucosa to create negative middle ear pressure. Swallowing allows the eustachian tube to open by the pulling action of tensor levi palatini and salpingopharyngeus. The levator levi palatini and tensor tympani complete the list of four muscles that open and close the eustachian tube. Air in the nasopharynx is at atmostpheric pressure and therefore on swallowing air flows up the eustachian tube from the nasopharynx to the middle ear and will equalise middle ear pressure. Sound transmission from the external to the inner ear is optimal when the compliance of the middle ear system is maximal, that is, when the pressure in the middle ear is equal to the pressure in the external auditory meatus.

Compliance (or admittance) is the measure of this system to allow the passage of sound energy through it, and is inversely related to impedance. *Impedance* is the resistance to the passage of sound energy. The mass, stiffness and frictional resistance of the medium through which the sound wave travels contribute to the impedance, which at low frequency is stiffness dominated. Strictly speaking, compliance is the reciprocal of stiffness, so impedance measurements at low frequency are usually referred to as the compliance.

41.2 Basic Principles

Impedance audiometry consists of three tests:

1. Tympanometry.
2. Acoustic reflex testing.
3. Static compliance (rarely used).

All three tests work on the same basic principle. The test probe consists of a sound producer, a sound receiver and a device for altering the air pressure within the external auditory meatus (EAM). The probe has a soft plastic or rubber tip to allow an airtight seal in the EAM. A test tone is emitted (226 Hz, 70 dB) into the EAM, of which some will be absorbed (admitted) by the middle ear system (drum and ossicles) and some reflected. The reflected sound energy is measured by the probe microphone. The compliance (the amount of sound absorbed by the middle ear system) can be determined either by measuring the reflected sound level in the ear canal or more commonly by measuring the amount of energy required to keep the sound level constant at varying ear canal pressures. The compliance will be maximal when the ear canal pressure is equal to middle ear pressure, when there is no pressure differential across the tympanic membrane. A tracing of the compliance as ear canal pressure alters allows this and other parameters to be determined. The tone frequency of 226 Hz is used as at this sound frequency the middle ear system is stiffness dominated, and compliance (measured in mmho) is directly proportional to the closed air volume and so can predict ear canal volume (1 mmho = ~ 1 mL). In very small infants (usually < 6 months old), the system is hypercompliant and so a 1-kHz tone is often used instead.

41.3 Tympanometry

This test is the most commonly used aspect of impedance audiometry and is particularly useful in evaluating children with otitis media with effusion. Here compliance is measured continuously while the pressure in the EAM is automatically varied from +200 to –400 daPa. This gives a graphical result which can be classified into one of three groups (▶ Fig. 41.1).

- **Type A:** Maximal compliance occurs when the pressure in the EAM is between +50 and –100 daPa. A normal maximal middle ear admittance or compliance value is between 0.3 and 1.6 mL. A low value for maximal compliance (type As) indicates stiffness of the middle ear system as in tympanosclerosis or otosclerosis. A high (type Ad) or unrecordable peak of compliance indicates excess mobility of the middle ear system as in ossicular discontinuity or atelectasis.

- **Type B:** A low-value flat or horizontal compliance trace occurs, implying persistently low compliance. This is usually taken to indicate fluid in the middle ear cavity, and in young children (< 7 years) with glue ear can be correlated with audiometric hearing loss. A type B tympanogram will also occur in the presence of a perforation

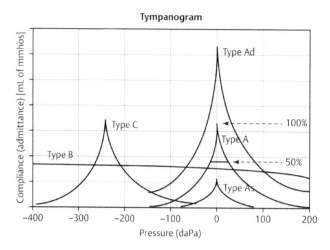

Tympanogram

Fig. 41.1 Diagram of the three curves.

in the tympanic membrane, but the ear canal volume will be large (> 6 mL) because it is measuring that of the middle ear cleft too. It can occasionally be useful in confirming this diagnosis or to test the patency of a ventilation tube.

- **Type C:** This group gives a peak compliance when the pressure in the EAM is less than –100 mmH$_2$O. This indicates a significant low pressure in the middle ear system and is a sign of eustachian tube dysfunction. The C curve can be subdivided into C1, when the peak is between –100 and –199 daPa, and C2, when the peak occurs at less than –200 daPa.

41.4 Acoustic Reflex Measurement

Acoustic reflexes are measured at the ear canal pressure producing maximum compliance, which corresponds to middle ear pressure. Ipsilateral reflexes are recorded using the tympanometry probe; contralateral reflexes use a monaural headset to deliver sound to the non-probe ear. It is usual to test at 0.5, 1, 2, and 4 kHz. A sound intensity of 70 to 90 dB above the pure-tone threshold at that frequency is required to elicit a reflex in a normal-hearing subject, although in one who has a recruiting sensorineural hearing loss a reflex may be present only 10 dB above threshold.

The compliance, which is constant for the ear canal pressure selected, is recorded as a horizontal line and shows a dip on contraction of stapedius muscle, representing a reduction in compliance. The stapedial reflex is a complex crossed reflex and demands an intact afferent arm, brainstem and seventh cranial nerve. As such, the acoustic reflex can provide diagnostic information with regards to the site of a neurological lesion based on the pattern of response to ipsi- and contralateral testing.

It is important to remember that a conductive hearing loss of only 5 dB may result in an absent ipsilateral and contralateral reflex (for reasons that have not been satisfactorily explained), although it is not until there is a 15-dB air–bone gap that the reflex is absent in 50% of cases. Adaption (stapedial reflex decay) is determined by producing a persistent tone in the test ear and measuring the reflex in the contralateral ear. Normal adaption occurs only after 10 seconds, decay being no more than 50%.

Summary of the value of measuring the acoustic reflex is as follows:

a. Assesses the integrity of the facial nerve up to the branch to stapedius tendon.
b. Assesses recruitment and stapedial reflex decay, the latter in particular being an accurate pointer in distinguishing a cochlear (recruiting) from a retrocochlear (abnormal decay) lesion.
c. Can indicate the presence of a conductive hearing loss.
d. Can assess brainstem function.

41.5 Static Compliance

The compliance is measured with an air pressure of +200 daPa in the EAM, and this figure is subtracted from the maximal compliance, regardless of the pressure in the EAM at which this occurs. The normal range for this is from 0.3 to 1.6 mL. A figure greater than 2.0 mL implies the presence of a tympanic membrane perforation.

41.6 Calibration

Daily checks of the equipment must be carried out by the tester using a test probe cavity and known normal middle ear. Detailed objective calibration should not exceed 12 months.

41.7 Subject Preparation

History and otoscopy must be performed prior to tympanometry. The subjects should have the procedure explained to them and they should be informed to sit still and avoid swallowing and talking during the procedure.

41.8 Conclusion

Impedance audiometry is rapid and easy to use. It provides an objective measure of middle ear function, can help to distinguish cochlear from retrocochlear hearing loss, as well as localising brainstem and facial nerve lesions. It is, however, essential that the results are interpreted in the context of the other clinical findings.

Further Reading

Katx J. Handbook of Clinical Audiology. 7th ed. Philadelphia, Baltimore, New York: Wolters Kluwer; 2015

British Society of Audiology—Recommended Procedure—Tympanometry. Date: August 2013, Correction: June 2014, Due for review: August 2018

Related Topics of Interest

Clinical assessment of hearing
Facial nerve palsy
Otitis media with effusion

I

42 Labyrinthitis

Labyrinthitis is an inflammation of the labyrinth and may be classified into perilabyrinthitis, paralabyrinthitis, serous labyrinthitis and suppurative labyrinthitis. Bacterial labyrinthitis is rare in our post-antibiotic era and is usually secondary to meningitis or acute otitis media. Cooksey–Cawthorne exercises will accelerate recovery and central compensation from reduced labyrinthine function caused by an episode of labyrinthitis but should only be commenced once the initial acute phase of symptoms has settled.

42.1 Labyrinthine Fistula

A labyrinthine fistula is a bony erosion of the labyrinthine capsule to expose and sometimes rupture the endosteum of the labyrinth. The endosteum is the thin layer of periosteum separating the membranous labyrinth from the dense cortical bone covering the semicircular canals. A breach results in a perilymph fistula and may cause vertigo and a dead ear. A fistula most commonly occurs in the dome of the lateral semicircular canal.

42.2 Tullio's Phenomenon

The Tullio phenomenon is defined as vertigo in the presence of loud sounds. The phenomenon occurs when sound energy is transmitted from a mobile stapes footplate to the labyrinth which is distensible only when there is a fistula. Historically, the phenomenon occurred after a fenestration procedure was performed in the presence of a mobile footplate, this scenario arising in the 1950s in patients with so-called adhesive otitis. Adhesive otitis was a term applied to patients with a history of chronic middle ear disease without cholesteatoma, who had developed a conductive hearing loss in the presence of a mobile stapes and an intact ossicular chain but no obvious tympanosclerosis. Probably such patients had an undiagnosed ossicular erosion or otosclerosis. The Tullio phenomenon may also arise in those with endolymphatic hydrops when it is thought to be secondary to sound energy transmission from the footplate to the distended saccule which may be touching the undersurface of the footplate. It may also arise in patients who have had mastoid surgery when either the disease or the surgery has created a labyrinthine fistula, usually of the lateral semicircular canal.

42.3 Fistula Sign

In the presence of a labyrinthine fistula, raising the ipsilateral ear canal pressure may cause conjugate deviation of the eyes away from the affected ear. The mechanism is pressure transmission to the labyrinth causing endolymph movement and stimulation of the labyrinthine sense organs. This occurs either directly if there is labyrinth endosteum exposed to the ear canal after mastoid surgery or indirectly if endosteum is covered by disease (e.g., cholesteatoma) that can transmit the pressure wave. On occasion, it may occur by a similar mechanism to the Tullio phenomenon. Releasing the pressure allows the deviated eyes to return to the midline.

42.4 Perilabyrinthitis

Perilabyrinthitis is a syndrome caused by a labyrinthine fistula *after mastoid surgery* in the presence of retained labyrinthine function. The fistula may have been present, but silent, before surgery. For example, when secondary to cholesteatoma, the mass of the cholesteatoma sac prevents distension of the labyrinthine endosteum. Alternatively, the fistula may be iatrogenic. The hallmarks of perilabyrinthitis are the Tullio phenomenon and a positive fistula sign. Vertigo may also arise in perilabyrinthitis on windy days when the wind, which is cooler than air in the external ear canal, produces a thermal gradient across the labyrinth and a difference in the specific gravity of endolymph at each end of the semicircular canal to cause circulation of the endolymph within the canal (i.e., causes eddy currents).

Conservative treatment consists of occluding the meatus with cotton wool when outdoors. Surgical treatment involves covering the fistula with bone pâté or temporalis fascia and a temporalis muscle flap reinforced with fibrin glue, or a combination of these.

42.5 Paralabyrinthitis

This is vertigo occurring in the presence of chronic suppurative otitis media (CSOM) when inflammation close to the endosteum of the labyrinth causes an irritative nystagmus (nystagmus towards the affected ear because the irritation pushes the eyes away from the affected ear with a rapid correction—the nystagmus—towards the affected ear).

42.6 Serous and Suppurative Labyrinthitis

Acute vestibular failure causing sudden-onset vertigo is most commonly due to an injury to the vestibular receptors from a neurotrophic virus. The percentage of receptor injury defines the severity of symptoms, the length of time to obtain full compensation and the likelihood of repeated episodes of decompensation. Serous labyrinthitis is a retrospective diagnosis and depends on there being some recovery of cochlea and vestibular function after an attack of acute labyrinthitis. The symptoms and signs are identical to suppurative labyrinthitis except in the latter the loss of inner ear function is irreversible and there is an identifiable cause of the suppuration (meningitis or both acute and chronic otitis media).

42.7 Aetiology

Bacterial or serous labyrinthitis is a potential consequence of meningitis or otitis media and may occur by either direct bacterial invasion (suppurative labyrinthitis) or through the passage of bacterial toxins and other inflammatory mediators into the inner ear (serous labyrinthitis). Labyrinthitis is the most common complication of otitis media, accounting for a third of intracranial and extracranial complications. Bacterial labyrinthitis from otitis media is rare in the post-antibiotic era, but bacterial meningitis remains a significant cause of hearing loss. Bacteria can spread from cerebrospinal fluid (CSF) via the cochlear aqueduct or internal auditory canal directly to the labyrinth. Inflammation of the labyrinth from bacterial toxins or neurotrophic viruses (serous labyrinthitis) may also occur. Hearing loss, tinnitus and vertigo occur in about 20% of children with meningitis. Meningitis often affects both ears, whereas otogenic infection typically causes unilateral symptoms.

Bacterial infections of the middle ear or mastoid most commonly spread to the labyrinth through a dehiscent horizontal semicircular canal. Usually, the dehiscence is the result of erosion by a cholesteatoma. When suppurative labyrinthitis occurs, it is almost always associated with cholesteatoma. Profound hearing loss, severe vertigo, ataxia and nausea and vomiting are common symptoms of bacterial labyrinthitis.

42.8 Clinical Features

The labyrinthitis is usually secondary to CSOM but may also be a complication of acute suppurative otitis media (ASOM) via the round window, or meningitis or rarely it may be blood borne. In addition to the presence of the clinical features of the precipitating cause, there is an acute onset of violent, overwhelming vertigo that is so severe that it inhibits the perception of tinnitus and hearing loss. There may be a short period of irritative jerk nystagmus towards the affected ear, but soon a paralytic jerk nystagmus to the healthy ear ensues. Tiny movements of the head exacerbate the vertigo so that the patient prefers to lie completely still on their side and in the presence of a paralytic nystagmus the affected ear will be uppermost. In this position, the patient will tend to voluntarily look in the direction of the affected side (especially when he or she has visitors), reducing the drive from the unaffected ear so that the corrective nystagmus and therefore the vertigo will be less severe. This can be understood when we explain the normal labyrinth causes conjugate deviation of the eyes to the opposite side so that if one labyrinth is paralysed, the opposite labyrinth will become dominant and deviate the eyes to the side of the affected ear, the nystagmus occurring as a corrective measure. Initially, there is third-degree nystagmus on optic fixation (nystagmus in any direction of lateral gaze). As compensation occurs, second-degree nystagmus develops (nystagmus when gazing straight ahead or looking in the direction of the nystagmus) and then first-degree nystagmus (nystagmus only when looking in the direction of the nystagmus). Finally, there is absence of nystagmus on optic fixation.

42.9 Investigations

The diagnosis is made on the clinical features occurring in the presence of a precipitating factor. If possible, the ears should be examined under the microscope after removal of all external ear canal debris. If there is an open mastoid cavity, there may be a visible labyrinthine fistula. If there are no features to suggest meningitis, the important diagnosis not to miss is a cerebellar abscess. Here the symptoms and signs are different but may be difficult to recognise in a patient continuously

L

vomiting. An enhanced computed tomography (CT) or preferably an enhanced magnetic resonance imaging (MRI) scan will be necessary in these circumstances. Sequential pure-tone audiometry and electronystagmography (ENG) will allow the monitoring of recovery although hearing loss and vestibular failure are permanent with purulent labyrinthitis.

42.10 Management of Labyrinthitis

Treatment of both the precipitating factor and symptomatic relief of the labyrinthitis is necessary.

- An ear culture swab and appropriate antibiotics, broad spectrum until results of the swab are available.
- Bed rest, avoiding head movements.
- Vestibular sedatives.
- Intravenous fluids if vomiting.
- If the precipitating factor was CSOM, exploration of the mastoid after recovery from the acute symptoms should be considered. A labyrinthine fistula may have arisen from chronic osteitis or cholesteatoma. The chronic disease should be eradicated and if a fistula is identified, the treatment is described above.

42.11 Follow-Up and Aftercare

After recovery from the acute infection, Cooksey–Cawthorne exercises may accelerate central compensation. They should be started once the acute spinning sensation has settled, which is often not for several weeks and occasionally several months.

Even with complete central compensation, patients with unilateral labyrinthine failure will still be unsteady in certain circumstances. The loss of vestibulocochlear input means that vestibulo-occular input becomes more important as does the proprioreceptor input from joint receptors to the higher vestibular centres. If one of these inputs is reduced or lost too, then profound vertigo may occur even with full vestibulocochlear compensation. Vertigo may therefore occur:

- In the dark.
- During a severe illness(allows inhibition of central compensation).
- With a peripheral neuropathy as it may affect the function of the peripheral proprioceptors.

- As an age affect, with reducing sight and proprioreceptor input occuring with age.

42.12 Labyrinthitis Ossificans

Labyrinthitis ossificans is the pathological ossification of the fluid-filled spaces of the inner ear, following an injury to the bony labyrinth and cochlea. It may therefore follow an episode of serous or suppurative labyrinthitis. The basal turn of the scala tympani is the commonest site for labyrinthitis ossificans and the corollary of this is that decisions regarding cochlear implantation must be made as soon as possible in such patients.

42.13 Future Advances

Growth factors and antioxidant cocktails may provide protection to the labyrinth from progressive damage and may allow regeneration of vestibular receptors. Antioxidants reduce sensory hair cell loss due to cisplatin and the protective function of antioxidants to gentamicin ototoxicity and to acoustic trauma has also been demonstrated. Neurotrophic factors and antioxidants may therefore have a significant future role to play in the protection and recovery of inner ear receptors from injury, but presently there is no evidence that any specific medication or vitamin supplement will enhance recovery of vestibular or cochlear receptors from injury.

Further Reading

B, ovo R, Ciorba A, Martini A. The diagnosis of autoimmune inner ear disease: evidence and critical pitfalls. Eur Arch Otorhinolaryngol. 2009; 266(1):37–40

Staecker H, Dazert S, Malgrange B, Lefebvre PP, Ryan AF, Van de Water TR. Transforming growth factor alpha treatment alters intracellular calcium levels in hair cells and protects them from ototoxic damage in vitro. Int J Dev Neurosci. 1997; 15(4–5):553–562

Wu JF, Jin Z, Yang JM, Liu YH, Duan ML. Extracranial and intracranial complications of otitis media: 22-year clinical experience and analysis. Acta Otolaryngol. 2012; 132(3):261–265

Related Topics of Interest

Suppurative otitis media—complications
Suppurative otitis media—acute
Vestibular function tests
Vertigo

43 Laryngeal Carcinoma

43.1 Pathology

Squamous cell carcinoma of the larynx represents approximately 1% of all malignancies in men. It is about five times commoner in males than in females. The incidence increases with age, with three-quarters of all diagnoses in patients over 60, but the peak age of presentation is not until the eighth decade. Tobacco and alcohol, individually and synergistically, are the main causes. In contrast to oropharyngeal cancer, it appears that human papilloma virus infection is not a major cause. There are other histological tumours of the larynx in addition to squamous cell carcinoma. Verrucous carcinoma is a distinct variant of well-differentiated squamous cell carcinoma. Adenocarcinoma, adenoid cystic carcinoma, fibrosarcoma, chondrosarcoma and lymphomas are all rare.

For classification purposes, the larynx is divided into three regions of which each includes a number of subsites:

1. **Supraglottis:** This comprises the larynx superior to the apex of the ventricle. It includes the ventricle, vestibular folds, arytenoids, aryepiglottic folds and the epiglottis (laryngeal surface, tip and lingual surface).
2. **Glottis:** This comprises the vocal cords and the anterior and posterior commissures. It extends from the apex of the laryngeal ventricle to 1 cm below. Some authorities hold that the superior and inferior borders of the glottis correspond to the superior and inferior arcuate lines, respectively.
3. **Subglottis:** This extends from the inferior border of the glottis to the lower border of the cricoid cartilage.

43.2 Clinical Features

The clinical features of malignant disease are dictated by the primary tumour, secondary deposits and the general effects of cancer. The symptoms and signs of a laryngeal tumour depend on the subsite involved and the way in which it is related to the upper aerodigestive tract. Hoarseness is the commonest, and often the only, presenting symptom. Dyspnoea and stridor are late symptoms and usually indicate an advanced tumour. Pain is an uncommon symptom but may occur with supraglottic tumours. Patients with a cancer in this site may complain of a unilateral sore throat and there may be referred otalgia. Dysphagia indicates invasion of the pharynx. Swelling of the neck may be due to direct penetration of the tumour outside the larynx or to lymph node metastases. Cough and throat irritation are occasional symptoms. Anorexia, cachexia and foetor imply advanced disease.

There should be a general examination to identify distant metastases and an assessment of the overall physical status of the patient. Fibre-optic laryngoscopy should allow an inspection of the primary tumour site and size. Vocal cord mobility should also be assessed. The two areas which are difficult to examine by this technique are the subglottis and the laryngeal ventricle and should be carefully examined at microlaryngoscopy under general anaesthesia. The neck should be carefully palpated for the presence of enlarged lymph nodes. Examination must include an assessment of the number, mobility and level of the nodes. Laryngeal tumours usually metastasise to the upper deep cervical lymph nodes, but supraglottic tumours may cause bilateral nodes, and some subglottic tumours may spread to the upper mediastinal nodes.

43.3 Investigations

1. Blood tests A full blood count and serum analysis are baseline investigations. The serum analysis may show deranged liver function raising suspicion of liver metastases, or hypoproteinemia, which may indicate malnourishment and a possibility of poor wound healing.

2. Magnetic resonance imaging (MRI) or computed tomography (CT) scans of the larynx and neck provide further information about the primary tumour. Both modalities are acceptable, and choice often depends on local protocols. MRI with contrast is preferable to show soft tissue disease, but high-resolution CT is useful in evaluation of the integrity of thyroid cartilage. Imaging may also detect the presence of impalpable or occult nodes. A CT scan of the chest and upper abdomen is required to exclude metastases and to assess intercurrent

L

lung disease. Distant metastases are unusual in laryngeal carcinoma (1–5%).

3. At microlaryngoscopy, the patient should have all the larynx subsites inspected systematically. It should routinely involve the use of straight (0-degree), and angled (30- or 70-degree) endoscopes. Photographs should be taken and the tumour's position and extension should be recorded by means of diagrams in the case notes. An adequate and representative biopsy is essential for accurate histology. While the patient's neck muscles are relaxed under general anaesthetic, the neck should be palpated for nodes which may not have been noted previously. Cord mobility should be assessed as the patient wakes, if not recorded previously.

The information obtained will allow tumour staging according to the current UICC/AJCC TNM classification and appropriate management.

43.4 Staging

Laryngeal tumours are diverse in their behaviour and prognosis and thus there have been many endeavours to classify them. Clinical staging attempts to group together features which may share prognosis or certain treatments. In cancer of the larynx, clinical staging is the only generally reliable criterion of any prognostic significance, but some parts of the T staging are subjective. Therefore, even with this standard, there may be considerable variability between surgeons in T-stage assignment for a given tumour, particularly in T3 tumours. An accurate anatomical description of tumour extent (with a case file diagram and photograph) is therefore essential in treatment selection. The 8th edition of the UICC/AJCC staging system defines T stage as listed below.

43.4.1 Supraglottis

T1   Tumour limited to one subsite of the supraglottis.
T2   Invasion of more than one subsite of the supraglottis or glottis or adjacent region outside the supraglottis (e.g., mucosa of tongue base).
T3   Confined to larynx with a fixed vocal cord or invades the post-cricoid area, pre-epiglottic or paraglottic space, base of tongue, inner cortex of thyroid cartilage.

T4a   Extends beyond the larynx. Invading through thyroid cartilage and/or trachea, soft tissues of the neck including extrinsic tongue muscles, strap muscles, thyroid gland and oesophagus.
T4b   Tumour invades prevertebral space, encases carotid artery or mediastinal structures.

43.4.2 Glottis

T1(a)   Tumour limited to one vocal cord.
T1(b)   Involves both vocal cords.
T2   Tumour extends to supraglottis and/or subglottis or impaired cord mobility.
T3   Confined to the larynx with a fixed vocal cord and/or invades paraglottic space and/or inner cortex of thyroid cartilage.
T4a   Extends beyond the larynx. Invading through thyroid cartilage and/or trachea, soft tissues of the neck including extrinsic tongue muscles, strap muscles, thyroid gland and oesophagus.
T4b   Tumour invades prevertebral space, encases carotid artery or mediastinal structures.

43.4.3 Subglottis

T1   Tumour limited to subglottis.
T2   Extends to vocal cords with normal or impaired mobility.
T3   Limited to larynx with vocal cord fixation.
T4a   Extends beyond the larynx. Invading through thyroid cartilage and/or trachea, soft tissues of the neck including extrinsic tongue muscles, strap muscles, thyroid gland and oesophagus.
T4b   Tumour invades prevertebral space, encases carotid artery or mediastinal structures.

N stage is identical to that of other head and neck sites and covered in Chapter 9, Cervical Lymphadenopathy.

Stage grouping is based on the TNM status:

Stage I	T1	N0	M0
Stage II	T2	N0	M0
Stage III	T3	N0	M0
	T1,T2,T3	N1	M0
Stage IVA	T4a	N0N1	M0
	T1,T2,T3,T4a	N2	M0
Stage IVB	T4b	Any N	M0
	Any T	N3	M0
Stage IVC	Any T	Any N	M1

The presence of palpable lymph nodes is the most important factor in determining prognosis, but assessment of lymphadenopathy is subjective. About one-third of patients with no palpable lymph nodes have histologically involved nodes, and a similar number of palpable nodes are not invaded by tumour. The supraglottis has a rich lymphatic drainage, and a high proportion of these tumours spread to cervical lymph nodes. The subglottis drains to paratracheal and mediastinal nodes in addition to cervical lymph nodes. The glottis has virtually no lymphatic drainage, so metastases usually only occur when the tumour has spread to involve the supraglottis and subglottis, the so-called transglottic tumour. The lymphatics and patterns of spread are important and have a significant effect on overall management, particularly in the management of the neck.

43.5 Management

Following assessment, the patient will be discussed at a head and neck MDT meeting. Each patient will fall into one of the following categories depending on his or her age, general condition and tumour stage: curative or palliative treatment.

Curative treatment will involve either radiotherapy (RT), chemoradiotherapy (CRT), surgery or a combination of these modalities.

Palliative care may include pain relief, tracheostomy, insertion of a percutaneous gastrostomy, palliative radiotherapy, chemotherapy and occasionally surgery (e.g., laser debulking).

43.6 Surgery

- Preservation laryngeal surgery is an option with early disease (Stage I/II) and can be used in highly selected advanced tumours. Transoral endoscopic laser microresection (TLM) and transoral robotic surgery (TORS) are both options. Open partial laryngeal surgery (laryngofissure cordectomy, vertical partial laryngectomy, supracricoid laryngectomy) is an option, but less used now because of the easier option of TLM. (For more details please refer to Chapter 44, Laryngectomy).

- More advanced tumours (Stage III/IV disease) treated by surgery are likely to need a total laryngectomy, usually with postoperative radiotherapy.

Patients who present with stridor should have endoscopic debulking (ideally with a laser to reduce bleeding) when possible. Tracheostomy, although not desirable, may be necessary.

- Management of the neck will depend on nodal status. Elective treatment of the neck is not necessary for glottic tumours, but supraglottic tumours have a high incidence of overt and occult nodal metastases and the N0 neck usually needs elective treatment in these cases. Elective bilateral dissection of levels II to IV, with inclusion of level I if tongue base involvement and level VI if subglottic spread, is recommended. Node-positive disease in cancers from all sites of the larynx can be treated by modified radical neck dissection.

43.7 Radiotherapy

- In early disease, radiotherapy schedules typically use 50 to 52 Gy in 16 fractions and 53 to 55 Gy in 20 fractions over 3 to 4 weeks. Elective treatment of the neck is not required for glottic tumours, but supraglottic tumours should have elective irradiation to levels II to IV. Acute toxicity from RT includes skin reactions, mucositis, odynophagia, thick and sticky secretions and hoarse voice, but most of these resolve after 6 weeks of completion of treatment and late complications are unusual. Conventional RT alone may be suboptimal for the treatment of advanced laryngeal cancer. Altered fractionation regimens (including acceleration and hyperfractionation) improve locoregional control and overall survival compared with standard fractionated RT for head and neck cancer patients who elect or are selected to receive RT alone (albeit at the cost of higher mucosal toxicity).

- In advanced disease, the standard treatment for many years was total laryngectomy and postoperative RT. Disease control and survival figures were reasonable, but it was recognised that the loss of the larynx in total laryngectomy has a major impact on the quality of life of the patient. Treatment has therefore been directed towards larynx-preservation strategies.

There have been several trials that establish the use of RT and chemotherapy as an alternative to total laryngectomy. The Veterans Affairs Laryngeal Cancer Study Group (VALCSG) established that induction chemotherapy and RT (IC + RT) yielded

L

similar overall survival (68% at 2 years) compared to total laryngectomy followed by adjuvant RT for Stage III to IV laryngeal cancer with high rates of larynx preservation (64% at 2 years). Patients who had recurrent or residual disease following chemotherapy and RT underwent a salvage laryngectomy. Rates of salvage laryngectomy were significantly lower for T3 versus T4 disease (29 vs. 56%, p = 0.001). Subsequently, the Radiation Therapy Oncology Group (RTOG) 91-11 trial demonstrated that concurrent CRT was superior to IC + RT and RT alone in terms of laryngeal preservation (88 vs. 75 vs. 70%, respectively, at 3 years), although overall survival in each treatment arm was similar. The use of concurrent CRT for locally advanced head and neck cancers, including laryngeal cancers, is now considered the standard of care. Standard concurrent chemotherapy regimens include cisplatin (100 mg/m$_2$) on days 1, 22, and 43 of RT and carboplatin/5-FU on weeks 1 and 5 of RT.

Concurrent CRT is associated with a significant increase in acute and late toxicity compared with RT alone. Over 40% of patients develop severe late toxicity, including a reduction in speech and swallowing function which can lead to lifelong dependence on a feeding tube (13% of patients 2 years after treatment) and have a profound effect on quality of life. This has led to the assertion that 'laryngeal preservation' does not always equate to reasonable 'laryngeal function' and a small percentage of patients will require a total laryngectomy for functional reasons. Older age, advanced T stage, larynx/hypopharynx primary site and neck dissection after chemoradiotherapy all increase the risk of severe late toxicity after CRT. The benefit of chemotherapy is not significant above 70 years of age, so it is not used in these patients.

An alternative to concurrent CRT for patients with laryngeal cancer who cannot receive it is cetuximab. This is a monoclonal antibody which competitively inhibits the cell surface epidermal growth factor receptor. Cetuximab has been shown to improve locoregional control and overall survival over RT alone in a study of patients with locally advanced (Stage III/IV) head and neck cancer (27% of whom had laryngeal cancer). Toxicities of cetuximab include rash and hypersensitivity reactions, but it does not increase the risk of radiation-related mucositis.

43.8 Glottic Tumours

T1 glottic tumours: RT and TLM are the two most commonly used treatment modalities. Open partial laryngeal surgery is an option, but less used now because of the often preferred option of TLM. Survival outcomes and local control rates are similar for T1a(90–95%), but they have not been compared in randomised trials. In the case of T1b disease, the control rate is slightly lower (85–90%). Single-modality treatment should be the aim.

T2 glottic tumours: They can be similarly managed by radiotherapy or by TLM. Long-term voice outcome for T2 glottic cancers is generally accepted to be better after RT than TLM. Voice outcome for TLM is dependent on the extent of the resection and if the resection involves the anterior commissure.

T3 glottic tumours: Most T3 glottic tumours are amenable to treatment by larynx-preserving CRT. TLM or open partial laryngeal surgery +/- postoperative RT is sometimes an alternative. Open partial laryngeal procedures which might be considered include vertical partial laryngectomy (VPL), frontolateral VPL, supraglottic laryngectomy, supracricoid partial laryngectomy and extended supraglottic laryngectomy. Elective treatment of the N0 neck is recommended to at least lymph node levels II to IV bilaterally, because of the risk of occult nodal metastases. If there is node-positive disease, it is recommended that levels II to V be treated on the involved side.

T4 glottic tumours: CRT is an option if there is no significant cartilage invasion. Otherwise these tumours should be treated with total laryngectomy and post-operative radiotherapy. The VALCSG study showed reduced tumour response to CRT and higher rates of salvage laryngectomy for T4 tumours (56% for T4 vs. 29% for T3 tumours). Treatment of the neck should be by elective selective neck dissection irrespective of the nodal status (N0 or N+) with a comprehensive inclusion of levels II to VI. Patients with nodal disease treated by CRT who experience a complete response on post-treatment positron emission tomography CT(PET-CT) do not require any further intervention.

43.9 Supraglottic Tumours

T1–T2 supraglottic cancer: These can be treated by radiotherapy, TLM, TORS or less frequently open partial conservation surgery (supraglottic laryngectomy). Survival outcomes are similar with RT and surgery (75–95%), but swallowing function outcomes with surgery are not as good. Patient selection is therefore imperative, and single modality should be the aim to reduce morbidity from combined treatment. In view of the rich lymphatic supply of the supraglottis, all patients should have elective treatment of bilateral lymph node levels II to IV—either with RT or selective neck dissection. In patients who present with nodes, concurrent CRT or surgery followed by post-operative RT is recommended.

T3–T4 supraglottic cancer: Most cases of T3 supraglottic cancer are suitable for nonsurgical larynx preservation strategies with concurrent chemoradiation. TLM or open supraglottic laryngectomy with post-operative RT is an option in elected cases. In the N0 neck, elective treatment (SND or RT) is recommended to lymph node levels II to IV bilaterally. In node-positive disease, lymph node levels II to V should be treated on the involved side. As per the PET-NECK clinical trial, patients with N2 or N3 neck disease, who undergo treatment with CRT to their laryngeal primary and experience a complete response with a subsequent negative post-treatment PET-CT scan, do not require an elective neck dissection. In contrast, patients who have a partial response to treatment or have increased uptake on a post-treatment PET-CT scan should have a neck dissection.

43.10 Subglottic Tumours

Pure subglottic cancer is very unusual. The subglottis becomes involved in extensive glottic and transglottic carcinoma. Small tumours may be treated by radiotherapy, but these tumours often present late and the patient often needs a total laryngectomy. It is important that the upper mediastinum is included in the radical treatment regimen.

43.11 Follow-Up and Aftercare

Patients who have had potentially curative treatment should be carefully examined for signs of primary recurrence, neck node spread and distant metastases, and have their weight recorded in the outpatient clinic on a regular basis. This should be monthly for the first 6 months, then every 2 months for 6 months, every 3 months for 12 months, then 6 monthly for the next 3 years. Some units continue to monitor patients as the incidence of second primary tumours is in the region of 10 to 20%. A baseline MRI scan, or for those treated by CRT a PET-CT scan, 12 weeks post-treatment should be undertaken. All patients should have the option of voice restoration following laryngectomy and will require speech therapy. They will also require monitoring of their thyroid function and calcium levels.

Further Reading

Ambrosch P. The role of laser microsurgery in the treatment of laryngeal cancer. Curr Opin Otolaryngol Head Neck Surg. 2007; 15(2):82–88

Forastiere AA, Zhang Q, Weber RS, et al. Long-term results of RTOG 91–11: a comparison of three nonsurgical treatment strategies to preserve the larynx in patients with locally advanced larynx cancer. J Clin Oncol. 2013; 31(7):845–852

Jones TM, De M, Foran B, Harrington K, Mortimore S. Laryngeal cancer: United Kingdom National Multidisciplinary guidelines. J Laryngol Otol. 2016; 130(S2):S75–S82

Thomas L, Drinnan M, Natesh B, Mehanna H, Jones T, Paleri V. Open conservation partial laryngectomy for laryngeal cancer: a systematic review of English language literature. Cancer Treat Rev. 2012; 38(3):203–211

Wolf GT, Fisher SG, Hong WK, et al; Department of Veterans Affairs Laryngeal Cancer Study Group. Induction chemotherapy plus radiation compared with surgery plus radiation in patients with advanced laryngeal cancer. N Engl J Med. 1991; 324(24):1685–1690

Related Topics of Interest

Cervical lymphadenopathy
Laryngectomy
Neck dissection
Radiotherapy and chemotherapy for head and neck cancer
Tracheostomy

L

44 Laryngectomy

The choice between surgery and radiotherapy as the primary treatment for carcinoma of the larynx should be made according to the likely effective control of the cancer, the general health of the patient, the relative consequences of the treatment and the informed decision of the patient. With either laryngectomy or radiotherapy, there is invariably some or total loss of normal voice and compromise of airway protection, and general function. Although patients may undergo speech rehabilitation and may swallow well after total laryngectomy, the main handicap associated with this procedure, according to quality-of-life studies, appears to be the need for a permanent stoma. Transoral laser microsurgery (TLM) is now a standard of care and transoral robotic surgery (TORS) is increasingly utilised. There is considerable geographic variation in the use of open conservational approaches which attempt to preserve as much of the larynx and its function as possible (used sparingly in the United Kingdom, but popular in Italy, Spain and South America). The goals of all partial laryngeal surgery are to control cancer and obtain a functional outcome of speech and swallowing without the need for a permanent tracheostomy. Laryngectomy techniques also have an importance in less common malignant neoplasms of the larynx (adenocarcinoma, verrucous carcinoma, fibrosarcoma, chondrosarcoma, etc.), which are invariably treated by surgery. It is apparent that the modern surgeon should not manage laryngeal cancer based on one surgical option (total laryngectomy). The repertoire must include conservative techniques and surgical voice restoration.

44.1 Types of Laryngectomy

1. Endoscopic transoral resections
   a. Transoral laser microsurgery.
   b. Transoral robotic surgery.
2. Vertical partial resection
   a. Cordectomy.
   b. Hemilaryngectomy (frontal, lateral and frontolateral).
3. Horizontal partial resection
   a. Epiglottectomy.
   b. Supraglottic laryngectomy.
4. Near-total laryngectomy
   a. Supracricoid partial laryngectomy.
   b. Vertical subtotal laryngectomy.
5. Total laryngectomy

44.2 Pre-Operative Management

In clinic, fibre-optic laryngoscopy should allow an inspection of the primary tumour's site and size. Vocal cord mobility should also be assessed. The two areas which are difficult to examine by this technique are the subglottis and the laryngeal ventricle, both of which should be carefully examined at microlaryngoscopy under anaesthetic. The neck should be carefully palpated for the presence of enlarged lymph nodes.

A computed tomography (CT) or magnetic resonance imaging (MRI) scan of the larynx should be obtained prior to endoscopy and biopsy before there is distortion of the anatomy. A microlaryngoscopy should always be performed by the surgeon who is going to perform any subsequent procedure. This will allow a representative biopsy to be obtained, the tumour to be staged and the appropriate operation planned. Straight (0-degree) and angled (30- and 70-degree) rigid endoscopes should be used to carefully and systematically assess the extent of the tumour. Photographs should be taken and tumour diagrams carefully documented.

With the accumulated information, the patient's case should be discussed in the Head & Neck MDT meeting. Close attention to the extent of the disease and the anatomical landmarks of the larynx should form the basis of dialogue regarding the patients' suitability for a particular type of laryngectomy. This will be in conjunction with a thorough knowledge of their general condition, intercurrent disease, performance status and social (home and caregiver) circumstances. It is imperative that written confirmation of the histological diagnosis must be in the case notes before undertaking any laryngeal resection.

The patient should have a clear explanation of the diagnosis and what it means. The surgical and non-surgical options of treatment, if applicable, should be discussed and recorded in the case file. The operation chosen should be described in some detail. It should be remembered that this situation will be distressing for the patient, who should have a relative or close friend present. The patient should be warned before any treatment that there is no guarantee of cure. Specifically, for a total laryngectomy the patient must be warned that the voice box will be lost and a new technique to speak will need to be learned, a permanent end tracheostomy will be necessary and thyroid and parathyroid supplements may be needed for life following the operation. The possibility that a partial procedure may culminate in an eventual total laryngectomy (residual disease requiring further excision or a poorly functioning larynx after partial surgery) should be discussed and the patient's written consent obtained on this understanding.

Assessment and counselling by a speech therapist prior to any procedure is essential. It is often reassuring for patients (particularly those who may need a total laryngectomy) to meet someone who has previously undergone the procedure. The patient should undergo nutritional assessment and any deficit be addressed. On occasion when prolonged aspiration is predicted, or patients are malnourished from dysphagia, percutaneous endoscopic gastrostomy (PEG) tube insertion may be necessary. The patients' performance status and fitness should be well known before the MDT discussions and particularly if partial surgery is contemplated, any doubt about their respiratory system should be checked with respiratory function tests.

44.3 Transoral Laser Microsurgery

The CO_2 laser has a high coefficient of extinction in water which limits its penetration and collateral effects. It provides an ideal and precise cutting instrument for laryngeal lesions. Endoscopic TLM is commonly used for T1–T2 glottic and supraglottic cancers, selected T3 cancers and debulking of tumours that present with airway obstruction. It has limitations when there is involvement of the anterior commissure or arytenoid cartilages as swallowing outcomes may not be as good as radiotherapy (RT) for these patients. There are also practical limitations imposed by the need

for a clear line of sight, so patients with restricted neck extension, limited mouth opening, unfavourable laryngeal and dental configuration (large and capped teeth or crowns) may have limited access to their tumour. This is important to document at the time of assessment so that the appropriate decisions are made at the Head & Neck MDT meeting. TORS solves some of these problems and so is finding increasing application.

The European Laryngology Society proposed the following classification of endoscopic cordectomies:

Type I   Subepithelial (severe dysplasia and carcinoma in situ), a resection of the epithelium.

Type II   Sublingamental (T1 vocal cord carcinoma with mobile cord), a resection of the epithelium, Reinke's space and vocal ligament.

Type III   Transmuscular (T1 tumours that reach the vocalis muscle without deeply infiltrating), a resection of those structures resected in type II and, in addition, vocalis muscle.

Type IV   Total cordectomy (T1 tumour infiltrating the vocal fold).

Type V   Extended cordectomy (T2 tumours infiltrating the arytenoid or ventricular fold) subdivided into Va, extended cordectomy encompassing the contralateral vocal cord and anterior commissure; Vb, extended cordectomy including the arytenoid; Vc, extended cordectomy including the subglottis; Vd, extended cordectomy to include the ventricle.

Type VI   Anterior commissurotomy with bilateral anterior cordectomy (T1b anterior lesions).

44.4 Hemilaryngectomy

This technique can be used to remove tumours confined to the vocal cord, with an adequate margin of healthy tissue. It involves removal of half of the thyroid cartilage, with the false and true vocal cords, part of the supraglottis and the upper half of the cricoid cartilage. The resulting gap can be left open to granulate or is closed by the strap muscles, fashioned to form a new fixed vocal cord. This procedure therefore has the advantage of allowing some protection of the airway and a reasonable voice for the patient. However, the procedure leaves the patient with a fixed hemilarynx and intensive speech and swallowing therapy is required as these patients can be difficult to rehabilitate. If, on histological examination, there has been incomplete resection of the lesion, either postoperative radiotherapy or total laryngectomy should be performed.

44.5 Supraglottic Laryngectomy

This is indicated for cancer of the supraglottis (epiglottis and laryngeal vestibule). The technique involves removing the entire supraglottis from the vallecula to the ventricle and joining the lower half of the larynx to the base of the tongue. A cricopharyngeal myotomy is considered an essential manoeuvre to make swallowing easier. Voice outcomes from this procedure are excellent. The operation is not suitable if the tumour extends to the base of tongue or vocal cords. It is not advisable if the patient is elderly and infirm, or if there is intercurrent lung disease. If the operation is to be carried out for post-radiotherapy recurrence, it is important that the extent of the original lesion is known.

44.6 Supracricoid Partial Laryngectomy

In the spectrum of procedures available for the surgical management of laryngeal carcinoma, the supracricoid partial laryngectomy (SCPL) falls between the vertical partial laryngectomy and the supraglottic laryngectomy, at one extreme and total laryngectomy at the other. There are two groups of SCPLs. The first is used for selected glottic carcinomas in which both true and false cords, the whole thyroid cartilage and a maximum of one arytenoid cartilage are resected. Closure is between the cricoid, the hyoid and the remaining epiglottis and tongue base, hence the name cricohyoidepiglottopexy.

The procedure used for selected supraglottic and transglottic carcinomas results in a more extensive resection, with removal of the entire epiglottis and pre-epiglottic space. In this case, closure is performed by a pexy between the cricoid and the hyoid and tongue base; therefore, the procedure is called cricohyoidopexy.

The aim of these two procedures is excision of tumour and to allow speech and swallowing without a permanent tracheostomy. Patients will often have a protracted period of aspiration, but eventually speak and swallow relatively well.

44.7 Total Laryngectomy

Total laryngectomy is indicated for the curative treatment of laryngeal carcinoma when the tumour is unsuitable for either chemoradiotherapy (e.g., T4 tumours invading through cartilage) or a partial resection. It is also indicated as salvage surgery in failed radiotherapy and as a palliative measure in some advanced cases of carcinoma. It may also be considered, as a last resort, in those who have no voice and have chronic aspiration due to palsy of the ninth, tenth and eleventh cranial nerves. The technique involves removing the hyoid bone, thyroid and cricoid cartilages and several rings of the proximal trachea and an ipsilateral thyroid lobectomy or total thyroidectomy (with preservation of the parathyroid glands). The main disadvantages of this procedure are the loss of normal voice and the need for a permanent end tracheostomy. Ideally, patients having a total laryngectomy should have a speech valve inserted at the time of primary surgery.

Pharyngocutaneous fistula following total laryngectomy is a problem that all surgeons are keen to avoid. It is more common in patients who are malnourished, those who have had previous radiotherapy or chemoradiation and those with chronic disease, all of which may affect healing (e.g., diabetes). If the patient has had previous RT or chemoradiotherapy (CRT), then many surgeons will place a pectoralis major flap over the repair line (a so-called defensive flap repair) to reduce the risk of fistula formation.

44.8 Emergency Laryngectomy

An emergency laryngectomy is one performed on a patient with airway compromise due to carcinoma, within 24 hours of presentation, without a prior tracheostomy. This is a rare occurrence and should be avoided by proper planning and if possible by establishing an airway when such patients present. The laser can be used to debulk the tumour and improve the airway, after laryngoscopy and biopsy. This has the advantage of

L

avoiding any surgical disturbance of the regional anatomy yet secures the airway while the biopsy results are awaited, the patient counselled and further treatment planned.

The rationale for emergency laryngectomy is based on the dismal prognosis for any patient who develops a tumour recurrence in his or her tracheostome, so-called stomal recurrence. Performing a tracheostomy for the relief of airway obstruction due to carcinoma prior to any definitive treatment is associated with a high rate of stomal recurrence. This could be due to tumour seeding at the time of tracheostomy, to inadequate resection at laryngectomy or to a second primary tumour.

44.9 Voice Restoration

Pre-operative input from the SALT team will help with early rehabilitation. Speech exercises should aim to strengthen normal structures, compensate and increase range of movement, while swallowing assessments should identify aspiration and initiate helpful swallow manoeuvres. For total laryngectomy patients, there should be discussion regarding the options available for them: oesophageal voice, prosthetic speech valve or electrolarynx. Primary oesophageal speech depends on the patient's ability to swallow and regurgitate air, and good vibration of the pharyngo-oesophageal segment. It doesn't work well in patients who have salvage laryngectomy following chemoradiation. A prosthetic speech valve can be placed in a primary (at the time of laryngectomy) or secondary tracheo-oesophageal puncture. These valves generally work well, but there can be problems with extrusion, and central and peripheral leakage. The electrolarynx produces vibrations that resonate in the pharynx allowing speech. They are an option for temporary voice while patients are waiting for speech valves or have encountered complications with valves.

Further Reading

Ambrosch P. The role of laser microsurgery in the treatment of laryngeal cancer. Curr Opin Otolaryngol Head Neck Surg. 2007; 15(2):82–88

Forastiere AA, Zhang Q, Weber RS, et al. Long-term results of RTOG 91–11: a comparison of three nonsurgical treatment strategies to preserve the larynx in patients with locally advanced larynx cancer. J Clin Oncol. 2013; 31(7):845–852

Jones TM, De M, Foran B, Harrington K, Mortimore S. Laryngeal cancer: United Kingdom National Multidisciplinary guidelines. J Laryngol Otol. 2016; 130(S2):S75–S82

Thomas L, Drinnan M, Natesh B, Mehanna H, Jones T, Paleri V. Open conservation partial laryngectomy for laryngeal cancer: a systematic review of English language literature. Cancer Treat Rev. 2012; 38(3):203–211

Related Topics of Interest

Laryngeal carcinoma
Lasers in ENT
Stertor and stridor
Tracheostomy

L

45 Lasers in ENT

45.1 Introduction

LASER is an acronym for Light Amplification by the Stimulated Emission of Radiation. The possibility of laser light, which is monochromatic (same colour), coherent (intense and in phase) and collimated (parallel and unidirectional), and is therefore an extremely powerful and high-energy light beam, was first postulated by Einstein in 1917. It wasn't until 1960 that Dr T Maiman produced the first laser light using synthetic ruby crystals.

Laser light is produced traditionally by having a laser medium within a resonating chamber which has a fully reflective mirror at one end and a partially reflective and partially transmitting mirror at the other. When this medium is heated to its excited state by an electrical current (rather like throwing copper granules into a flame), the medium rises to its excited state, then drops back down to its ground (stable) state, emitting a photon of light, the wavelength of which is characteristic to its own atomic structure. This is called fluorescence. Copper emits green light of a specific wavelength (510.6 nm). Einstein postulated that if a population inversion occurred, that is, if more than 50% of the atoms were excited instead of being in the usual ground state, then those photons emitted through fluorescence would interact with other excited atoms, and cause the emission of an identical clone of itself, as the excited atom descended to its ground state (stimulated emission). If a single clone could be encouraged, then this would create a beam of laser light. This occurs because the emitted photons bounce around within the inside of the resonating chamber and only those parallel to the long axis of the chamber are able to escape through the partially transmitting mirror.

Over the years, solid-state lasers such as the Neodymium doped Ytrrium Aluminium Garnet (Nd–YAG) have been developed, and more recently diode lasers using gallium aluminium arsenide chips rather like a silicon chip microprocessor. These are smaller, cheaper and more reliable than the original resonating chamber lasers. Excimer lasers use a combination of resonating chamber and excimer recombination.

There are an almost infinite number of compounds that can be used as a laser medium. ▶ Table 45.1 is a short, but not comprehensive, list.

Lasers are useful in medicine because of the effect laser light has on tissue. In essence, lasers are a heat beam which can be very accurately focused when using high-quality lenses. Very small spots with very high-energy densities are therefore possible. Because this heat beam is solely of one wavelength, the different penetration of light through tissue can be used to advantage. Picture yourself holding a bright white light on your finger tip. Look at the other side and you will just see red. Of the visible spectrum, only red light gets through, the rest is absorbed. See ▶ Fig. 45.1a, b for a description of the characteristics of light transmission through tissue.

If a highly penetrating laser is required, for example, to slowly heat and coagulate large vascular tumours in a difficult area such as the trachea or main bronchi, choose a highly penetrating laser which won't suddenly vaporise a big hole in a blood vessel, for example, the Nd–YAG laser. If you want to delicately nibble off a vocal cord polyp with a no-touch technique, choose a delicate non-penetrating system such as the carbon dioxide (CO_2) laser.

45.2 Selective Photothermolysis and Thermal Relaxation

These two theories, developed in the 1980s, led to a great leap forward in the use of lasers clinically, particularly in ENT and dermatology.

Selective photothermolysis uses the fact that laser light can be selective. A laser light highly absorbed by oxidised haemoglobin, but poorly absorbed in other chromophores such as water and melanin should be chosen, and you have a wavelength that will vaporise blood vessels, but leave surrounding tissue such as skin, undamaged. Skin haemangiomas, where a tuneable dye laser, tuned to yellow light at 588 nm has been very effective in shrinking haemangiomas in children, is an example.

Thermal relaxation uses the fact that delivered energy can be confined to its target area without spreading and damaging surrounding tissue (thermal confinement). This happens if the laser light is delivered within a very short period of time, called the thermal relaxation time. Think of

▶ **Table 45.1** Compounds used as a laser medium

Name	Wavelength (nm)	Type	Clinical use
Ruby	694.3	Solid state—rod	Hair and tattoo removal
Copper	510.6	Resonating cavity	Vascular anomalies
Argon	454.6	Resonating cavity	Retinal lesions
Helium–neon (He-Ne)	632.8	Resonating cavity	Guide for CO_2 laser
Carbon dioxide	10,600	Resonating cavity	Wide ranging in surgery espcially skin and ENT
Nd–YAG	1,064	Solid-state crystal	Airway malignancy— debulking
KTP (potassium titanyl phosphate)	532	Solid-state crystal, or diode	Ear, some vocal cord
Erbium–YAG	2,940	Solid-state crystal	Skin, middle ear
Holmium–YAG	2,100	Solid-state crystal	ENT, especially cancer and turbinoplasty
			Renal tract stones
Thulium–YAG	2,000	Solid-state crystal	ENT—tongue base
Gallium Aluminium	530–900	Diode	Varicose veins, poss
Gallium-Arsenide		Diode	Turbinoplasty, hair removal
Tuneable dye	410–830	Resonating cavity	Skin, esp. haemangioma
Argon fluoride	193	Excimer	Cornea
Photodynamic therapy	500–800	Diode, tuneable dye, LED[a]	Cancer, retina, dental, prostate
QS[b] Nd–YAG	1064 QS	Solid-state crystal	Tattoo removal

[a]Light-emitting diode.
[b]QS, quality switching, delivers extremely high peaks of energy over extremely short time periods—causes plasma formation and a shattering effect on tattoo ink.

doing the ironing and touching the hot part of the iron. If you touch for the shortest time, your finger doesn't burn. If you touch for a second, you will get a superficial burn, with some deeper dermal damage and scarring.

Shuttering (like a camera shutter) allows a short on–off time of laser beam delivery. The energy levels need to be sufficient to have its effect, so that a shuttered pulse will just heat the target tissue and won't give an undesired effect of injuring surrounding tissue. For thermal confinement to be accurate and specific, a non-penetrating beam is most suitable. The CO_2 laser was developed for this application and a new technique of superpulsing the photon energy was used. Here separate laser pulses are stacked one on top of the other, to double the available energy but still deliver it within the thermal relaxation time of the target tissue (usually around 900–1,000 µs). This works well for vocal cord lesions or the skin. This same technique is used for cornea surgery, although here the risk of scarring is high and therefore an extremely non-penetrating laser is used, such as the argon fluoride excimer laser. This would be too delicate for the vocal cord; a nodule would take hours to remove.

Thermal confinement without superpulsing is still used in higher-powered laser systems for ENT use, the most modern of which is the Carl Zeiss computerised pattern generator (CPG).

45.3 Other Considerations

In some lasers, in particular, the CO_2 laser, the light beam will not travel down a fibre, such as a quartz fibre, as it is absorbed by the quartz. This means it cannot be inserted into parts of the body that are relatively inaccessible. Light channels for the CO_2 laser are not particularly effective. This confines its use mainly to skin and ENT surgery. Safety is always a concern, particularly with highly absorbed lasers such as the CO_2, which can cause corneal scarring, or the more penetrating lasers of 500- to 1,200-nm wavelength, which can cause

L

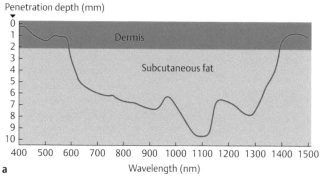

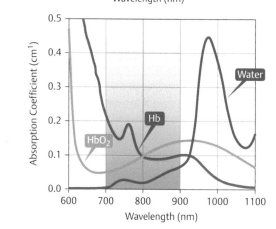

Fig. 45.1 (a, b) The three main light-absorbing compounds (chromophores) in tissue are water and hemoglobin oxidised and reduced. Low absorption for all three is around 900- to 1,100-nm wavelength of light. Skin is a good example, although melanin is another chromophore that may need to be taken into account here, depending on skin type. It has a similar absorption spec.

retinal damage. Also a laser beam has a great ability to set things on fire (an igniter), particularly in areas of high partial pressure of oxygen, such as the airway in general anaesthetic.

45.4 Specific Applications of Lasers in ENT

- *Head and neck cancer* Excision of cancer requires a good view of the margins—as removal must always be beyond but close to the margin unless reconstruction is being used. Therefore, this type of treatment is only for smaller lesions, usually T1 and T2. Using a combination of the CO_2 laser, operating microscope, micromanipulator, CPG scanning, and superpulsing, accurate and delicate removal of upper aerodigestive tract cancers can be achieved bloodlessly with excellent observation of the cancer margin—particularly in laryngeal and soft palate cancers. In more vascular areas such as the oropharynx,

the Holmium–YAG laser can be used under microscope control for close margin excision of tonsil and posterior pharyngeal wall cancer. Photodynamic therapy shows great promise for early head and neck cancer, and as a non-ablative treatment, it seems to give better functional results than other laser excision, and traditional surgery. This is particularly the case in oral cavity and early-stage oropharyngeal cancers (T1 and < 5 mm in depth).

- *Nose* Although much promise was initially shown when using lasers in the nose, only three areas have survived the test of time—inferior turbinate reduction, division of adhesions and vascular lesions such as hereditary haemorrhagic telangiectasia (HHT). Inferior turbinate reduction can be in the form of partial turbinectomy under local anaesthetic, or turbinoplasty under general anaesthetic. The former can be performed using special hand-pieces and the CPG or flash-scanned carbon dioxide laser using medium-diameter spot of

L

around 2 to 3 mm, the aim being to remove a moderate thickness of inferior turbinate mucosa at around the level of the nasal valve. Division of nasal adhesions uses the same laser parameters as partial turbinectomy. Turbinoplasty, where the inferior turbinate bone is partially removed, uses a different laser—one that cuts very hard tissue. This is the Holmium–YAG laser, used also for destruction of very hard renal tract stones, through its photoacoustic effect. Another advantage of this laser is that it is fibre delivered, so no special handpieces are required—the fibre is inserted through the nasal mucosa until it touches the turbinate bone, which is then partially destroyed using the laser. Vascular lesions such as HHT are very problematic as the lesions are very thin walled. The slightest trauma makes them bleed, and this includes laser light hitting the lesion. The Holmium–YAG laser has been shown to be more effective than others, since its high-energy pulse effectively blasts through blood, and hits the lesion underneath—something other commonly used lasers such as the KTP and Nd–YAG cannot do.

- *Throat (oropharynx)* Lasers can be used successfully in two main areas in the oropharynx: tonsil and soft palate. In the tonsil, the CPG-scanned CO_2 laser can be used with a 6.3-mm diameter spot, and relatively high-energy density, to vaporise the palatine tonsils. Using an operating microscope and micromanipulator, accurate removal of the tonsil under high magnification means that the tonsil edge, capsule/superior constrictor, is surgically defined. Vaporisation can be stopped just short of this point, meaning subtotal intra-capsular removal is achieved, with claimed reduction of bleeding risk and pain. This can also be performed under local anaesthesia with Xylocaine spray, then it is called tonsillotomy (not all patients are suitable for this due to mouth opening, gag reflex, hidden tonsils, etc.). Only a partial removal is possible with this procedure. The same technique can be used for posterior pharyngeal wall lymphoid aggregates. The soft palate/uvula complex can also be debulked using the CO_2 laser, a procedure known as laser-assisted uvulopalatoplasty (LAUP).

- *Ear* As excellent, delicate bone-cutting lasers, often used in dentistry it is a surprise that the CO_2 and Erbium–YAG laser are not more widely used in the United Kingdom for middle ear surgery, although in Germany and the United States they are quite widely employed in this area. This is because photons have no real mass, and can cut through structures such as the stapedius tendon, stapes crurae, etc. with ease. Currently in the United Kingdom, the KTP laser is used to denature/soften the stapes footplate in stapedotomy, and in expert hands for cholesteatoma surgery will reduce rates of recurrence.

- *Throat (larynx)* The CO_2 laser is the main system used in this area. The main advantage of using this system in the larynx is that there is no touching of mucosa so that scarring and trauma to normal mucosa is minimised—no grabbing, pulling, etc. Lesions for histology can be cut off at the neck, with a low-pressure suction holding the lesion as it is released and sent for histology. Other lesions such as nodules can be vaporised flush with vocal cord mucosa under high magnification. With thermal confinement technology, the overall effect means benign lesions are removed without the shearing effect of scissors, and the inevitable damage caused by handling with microforceps, yet with minimal lateral heat spread and scarring. Other conditions advantageously treated in this way include laryngeal papilloma, cordotomy, webbing. Arytenoidectomy requires a more coagulating laser, such as the KTP.

- *Skin* The CO_2 laser in thermal confinement mode is an excellent system for use in facial skin. Indications range from the ageing face (laser skin resurfacing), vaporisation of benign skin lesions such as epithelial nevi, hamartomas and sebaceous hyperplasia, such as rhinophyma. Using a variable-diameter CPG-scanned beam, facial skin can be sculpted using the CO_2 laser without scarring, if laser parameters are set appropriately. The Erbium–YAG laser can also be used for similar applications, as a more delicate (but less effective) alternative, for example, in fractional resurfacing. Haemangiomas and other vascular lesions such as veins, spider nevi, small arteriovenous malformations can be treated using selective photothermolyis principles, with the tuneable dye laser and long-pulsed KTP laser.

- *Others* Some experts have used diode lasers and fine, sculpted tips as a 'hot knife' to treat delicate parts of the body, such as the free edge of the vocal cord. Others use the Ho–YAG laser to break through the lateral nasal wall in dacryocystorhinostomy. Some ENT surgeons are involved in lower airway treatments, sometimes for obstructing malignancy using the Nd–YAG laser with tip cooling so that high powers can be used without tip carbonisation. In facial plastics, the long-pulsed diode laser is effective at treating the Fitzpatrick types 1 to 4 skin for permanent hair reduction, and the q-switched Nd–YAG laser for vaporising pigment in the facial tattoo. In transoral robotic surgery (TORS), the thulium–YAG laser is used preferentially for excision of tongue base lesions, as it offers a good combination of delicacy and hemostasis.

45.5 Safety

Lasers are dangerous tools. However, with the principles outlined, they are very much part of the ENT surgeon's armamentarium. The following rules regarding safety for a class 4 laser apply:

1. Designated laser environment with appropriate signage. This entails signs on all theatre access doors when the laser is in use with theatre doors ideally locked or/and signage instructing theatre personnel outside of the laser theatre not to enter.
2. Laser safety officer and laser supervisor appointed and appropriately trained.
3. All laser users should attend regular update courses.
4. Anaesthetic consideration—use a non-inflammable anaesthetic agent and mix oxygen with air, nitrogen and helium but not nitrous oxide because of the risk of an airway fire. Use a laser ET tube that is reflective and ensure the endotracheal cuff is inflated with saline and not air.
5. Patient consideration—saline-soaked drapes over exposed face and taped eyes (or patient wears safety goggles) when under general anaesthetic.
6. Surgeon and theatre staff considerations—all theatre personnel to wear safety goggles. The microscope eyepieces provide the surgeon with adequate protection.
7. Laser considerations—these high-powered systems can overheat. Regular maintenance and checking of the aiming beam and laser output is required.
8. Instruments—use non-reflective scopes with airway/laryngeal/pharyngeal work.
9. Adequate suction—this is required for both smoke extraction when the laser is vaporising tissue and as a joint suction/traction tool when dissecting tissue (e.g., when performing an arytenoidectomy).

Further Reading

Oswal V, Remacle M, Jovanvic S, Zeitels SM, Krespi JP, Hopper C. Principles and Practice of Lasers in Otorhinolaryngolgy– Head and Neck Surgery. The Netherlands, Kugler Publications; 2014

Related Topics of Interest

Laryngectomy
Papilloma of the larynx
Oropharyngeal carcinoma
Robots in ENT/head and neck surgery

L

46 Literature Review and Statistics

The medical literature industry has exponentially grown in the internet era. It is common for inboxes to be flooded by emails purporting ground-breaking data from the latest study accompanied by an expert commentary or two. Authors, even early on in their career, are regularly invited to contribute to 'open access' journals with promises of wide exposure for their work on a global platform, contributing to the increasing volume of litera-ture. Thus, there is a clear need for clinicians and researchers, irrespective of their stage in the career pathway, to acquire the necessary skills to be able to assess the relevance, impact and application of a paper to their practice. The journal the article is published in, its origin and provenance should not be an indication of its trustworthiness and relevance; instead, readers should approach the paper as they would any other using critical appraisal skills and tools, arriving at their own judgements. Unless a systematic approach is used to evaluate a research paper, the reader can be lulled into a false sense of security by the head-line results. This chapter will not only provide such a framework, but also offer a pragmatic view as many questions in the surgical literature, espe-cially in a small surgical specialty such as ours, will be unable to accrue the highest quality of evidence to guide practice in all areas.

46.1 Peer Review

Almost all journals nowadays use an online plat-form for article submission and peer review. Once an article has been submitted to a journal, it is sub-jected to a quality check to ensure that it meets the journal style. Based on the editorial board and journal policies, a quick assessment of the content is made to ensure that the topic will be of interest to the readership and is appropriate to the journal, usually by a senior editor, after which the paper is sent out for peer review. The peer review pro-cess requires reviewers to critically evaluate an article that is submitted to a journal and make recommendations to the editor on the scientific merit and suitability of the paper for publication. A critical review takes significant time and effort, especially when starting out, but is a very useful skill to acquire. Unfortunately, many reviewers, often chosen for their prominence in a specialty, are unable nor have the time to do this properly.

Journals with higher-impact factors usually tend to have a more robust peer review process.

▶ Table 46.1 is a list of journals ranked by impact factors, one of the metrics used for journal citation, as per the Web of Science Core Collection maintained by Clarivate Analytics (formerly the intellectual property of Thomson Reuters), which ranks 12,090 publications across 256 disciplines in science, social science, arts and humanities. The list enumerates the top five journals in the list to give the reader a perspective of the specialties residing at the top, followed by some prominent otolaryngology journals. Different biomedical specialties have different citation patterns and what is high-impact factor in one field is not necessarily high in another. To help place this list in context, here are some facts: Otorhinolaryngology is ranked 170 among 234 journal categories, rang-ing from Acoustics through Linguistics to Zoology. The aggregate impact factor of Otolaryngology journals is 1.768; the categories at the top of this have broader scope, and include entities like nanosciences, cell sciences and chemistry with aggregate impact factor of greater than 5.5. Within the medical specialties, critical care medicine tops the categories with an aggregate impact factor of 4.483.

46.2 Literature Review

An important component of literature evalua-tion is the skill to carry out a literature review. To enable a good evaluation, the study should be assessed alongside existing research work to determine its importance. Searching for relevant literature is a skill that is best learnt by attend-ing dedicated courses and requires a period of study that will teach the technical terms, guide-lines and methodology needed to perform a comprehensive search.

46.3 Critical Appraisal

Critical appraisal (CA) of a study can be boiled down to one question 'Are the methodology and results robust enough to persuade me to adopt the study recommendations to my patient population?' The primary focus of a CA should be on the adequacy of study methods. An inadequate description of the methodology will not allow a

L

▶ **Table 46.1** Impact factor for selected journals in 2016 based on the Web of Science, maintained by Clarivate Analytics

Rank	Journal	Impact factor
1	CA A cancer journal for clinicians	187.04
2	NEJM	72.046
3	Nature reviews drug discovery	57
4	Chemical reviews	47.928
5	Lancet	47.831
19	Lancet oncology	33.9
22	Cell	30.41
23	Nature medicine	29.886
48	BMJ	20.785
167	PLOS medicine	11.862
252	Cancer Research	9.122
856	Oral Oncology	4.794
1829	Head and Neck	3.376
2277	Trends in hearing	3.024
2378	JAMA otolaryngology head and neck surgery	2.951
2454	Hearing research	2.906
2564	Ear and hearing	2.842
3129	Clinical otolaryngology	2.523
3236	Laryngoscope	2.471
3509	Rhinology	2.35
3709	Otolaryngology—head and neck surgery	2.276
4189	Dysphagia	2.077
4326	Otology and neurorotology	2.024
5408	European archives of otorhinolaryngology	1.66
8805	Journal of laryngology and otology	0.844
9368	Laryngo-rhino-otologie	0.732
9422	HNO	0.723
10145	B-ENT	0.578

Note: In any given year, the impact factor of a journal is the number of citations, received in that year, of articles published in that journal during the two preceding years, divided by the total number of articles published in that journal during the two preceding years.

comprehensive appraisal of the study's relevance, reliability and applicability.

Critical appraisal of the literature has come a long way since inception, thanks to the pioneering work of Sir Muir Gray, who set up the Critical Appraisal Skills Programme (CASP) in 1993. Research methodologists realised early on that using checklists for systematic literature evaluation permits a rapid and comprehensive assimilation of critical appraisal skills. Since then, many organisations set up task groups to generate checklists, scoring systems and visual aids for the purpose (▶ Table 46.2). These include University of Alberta, University of Adelaide, University of Bristol, Cardiff University, McMaster University, National Institute for Health and Care Excellence, University of Oxford, University of Sheffield, Scottish Intercollegiate Guidelines Network, University of South Australia and independent ventures such as the GRACE initiative. The rest of this chapter describes the steps and pitfalls that will allow the reader to meet this aim, largely set along the principles of the

▶ **Table 46.2** Common checklists used for the various study types

Study type	Checklist
Randomised controlled trials	CASP Cochrane RoB tool EPOC RoB tool GATE CAT SURE
Nonrandomised controlled trials	EPOC RoB tool GATE CAT SURE
Systematic reviews and meta-analyses	CASP AMSTAR 2 SURE GATE CAT
Case-controlled studies	GATE CAT CASP
Cohort and cross-sectional study	GATE CAT Cochrane RoB tool EPOC RoB tool Newcastle–Ottawa scale EPHPP GRACE CASP
Economic evaluations	CHEERS CASP NICE
Qualitative studies	SURE CASP
Diagnostic accuracy studies	CASP QUADAS-2

Abbreviations: AMSTAR, a measurement tool to assess systematic reviews (http://www.amstar.ca/index.php); CASP, Critical Appraisal Skills Programme (http://www.casp-uk.net/casp-tools-checklists); EPHPP, Effective Public Health Practice Project (http://www.ephpp.ca/tools.html); EPOC, Effective Practice and Organisation of Care (http://epoc.cochrane.org/); GATE CAT, Graphic Appraisal Tool for Epidemiology Critically Appraised Topics (https://www.fmhs.auckland.ac.nz/en/soph/about/our-departments/epidemiology-and-biostatistics/research/epiq/evidence-based-practice-and-cats.html); GRACE, Good ReseArch for Comparative Effectiveness initiative (https://www.graceprinciples.org/about-grace.html); NICE Guidelines, The Manual Appendix H. pp7–20; QUADAS, Quality of primary diagnostic accuracy studies; SURE, Specialist Unit for Review Evidence (http://www.cardiff.ac.uk/specialist-unit-for-review-evidence/resources/critical-appraisal-checklists); RoB, Risk of Bias; Newcastle–Ottawa scale (http://www.ohri.ca/programs/clinical_epidemiology/oxford.asp).

CASP. Some of these organisations have recorded videos of their critical appraisal teaching programme, available for free online.

46.4 Reporting Guidelines

Akin to critical appraisal checklists, reporting guidelines (RG) have evolved, the purpose of which is to ensure accurate and transparent information is provided about study methods and findings. The framework of RG helps researchers to report all relevant aspects of a study, and permits peer reviewers to assess adequacy of reporting. The best known of all RGs is the CONSORT statement, first published in 1996 (revised in 2001 and 2010). The profusion of RGs led to the creation of the EQUATOR (Enhancing the QUAlity and Transparency Of health Research; http://www.equator-network.org/) network, an 'umbrella' organisation that brings together research methodologists, guideline development groups, journal editors, peer reviewers and funders. The EQUATOR site is a one-stop shop which lists RGs for 384 study types, thus ensuring that one is available for almost any study being written up. ▶ Table 46.3 identifies RGs for the main study types. It is common practice for funders and high-impact journals to demand a RG checklist at the time of submission of the report. In addition to this, specialty specific guidelines also exist; for instance, the STROCSS statement (STrengthening the Reporting Of Cohort Studies in Surgery) and PROCESS guidelines (Preferred Reporting Of CasE Series in Surgery) are specifically meant for surgical cohort and case series in the surgical specialties. Despite the profusion of RGs, they are not fully enforced by journals, primarily owing to resource constraints.

46.5 Critical Appraisal Checklists versus Reporting Guidelines

It should be noted that RG and CA checklists are distinct and have different purposes. It has been said that use of RGs is like 'turning the light on before you clean up a room: It doesn't clean it for you, but does tell you where the problems are*. To extend this

---
*LaCombe MA, Davidoff F. On Being a Doctor 2. Ann Intern Med. ;132:671–672.

▶ **Table 46.3** Reporting guidelines for main study types. For more information on these reporting guidelines please visit the EQUATOR website (http://www.equator-network.org/).

Study type	Reporting guideline
Randomised controlled trials	CONSORT
Systematic reviews and meta-analyses	PRISMA; MOOSE
Observational studies	STROBE
Economic evaluations	CHEERS
Qualitative studies	SRQR, COREQ
Diagnostic accuracy studies	STARD, TRIPOD
Study protocols	SPIRIT, PRISMA-P
Clinical practice guidelines	AGREE, RIGHT
Search strategies	PRESS

analogy further, a critical appraisal helps the visitor to the room to sift through the 'dirt' and understand the problems better. It is the author's practice to carefully study the RG checklist if published with the paper. This will help focus the CA on the areas where the RG has identified deficiencies.

46.6 Risk of Bias Assessment

It is crucial for the critical appraiser to have the skills to identify the risk of bias across a variety of studies. Bias is a systematic error in the results or inferences of study; bias should not to be confused with imprecision. In the presence of bias, replication of the same study would reach the same wrong conclusion, but imprecision refers to random error and replications of the same study will provide different answers. It must be recognised that bias is not a dichotomous variable, qualified by its presence or absence. On the other hand, the critical appraiser should consider the degree to which bias was prevented by the study design and implementation; given that bias is nearly always present to some degree, the appraiser must consider how bias might influence the results and their applicability. For instance, bias in a systematic review, despite uniform and consistent results about the effect size of an intervention's effect will reduce the strength of recommendation.

The Cochrane collaboration has defined an excellent risk of bias (RoB) tool, as have other organisations. The Cochrane collaboration also offers Webinars on RoB which is highly recommended. Bias is regularly discussed and taught across the curriculum and this section will not go into detail on the various types of bias.

46.7 Steps to a Critical Appraisal

1. Identity the category of the article.
   The questions being asked to determine the quality of a study should be tailored to the type of publication. Common article types that are usually critically evaluated and form the focus of journal clubs include systematic reviews, randomised controlled trials (RCTs) and diagnostic studies; in rarer diseases and the epidemiological literature, cohort studies will be the focus. Less common designs include case-control studies, economic evaluations, qualitative studies and clinical prediction rules. ▶ Fig. 46.1 depicts an algorithm for identifying quantitative (experimental and observational) study designs.

2. Peruse the abstract.
   The first question to ask is if the study addresses a clearly focused question. Asking a focused question is a skill, and most researchers early in their career often struggle with this step for a proposed piece of research. There are important lessons in framing the research question that a novice trainee can learn from the publication of a well-planned and executed study. The focused question should include the following elements within it, best summarised as PICO: The Patient population being studied should be succinctly and clearly described; the Intervention being studied should be mentioned with appropriate amount of detail, as should the Comparator; the Outcomes used to measure the study results should be clearly set out as part of this

L

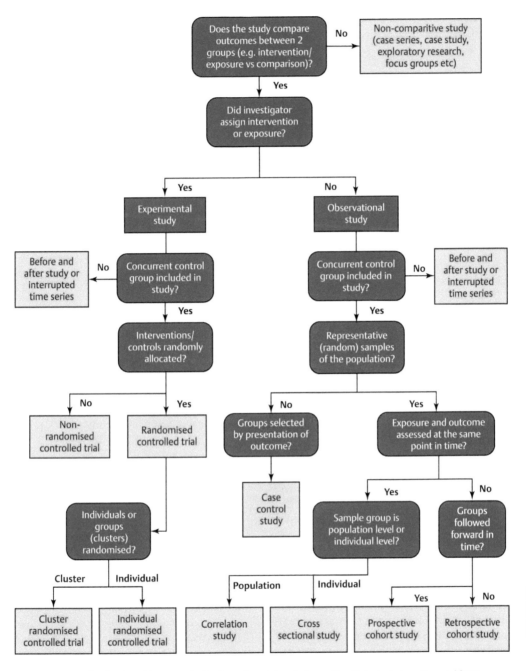

Fig. 46.1 Algorithm for classifying quantitative (experimental and observational) study designs. Sourced from National Institute for Health and Care Excellence Developing NICE guidelines: the manual appendix H. July 2015:3.

framework. The PICO should be available in the abstract itself, and where journals opt for a structured abstract, this information is readily identified. If, on perusing the abstract, any of the elements of PICO is not clear and if it does not apply to the reader's practice, the abstract

▶ **Table 46.4** CASP methodology: systematic review and meta-analysis

Are the results valid?	Is the question focused?	• Are the elements of PICO well described?
	Has the right type of papers been searched for?	• Did the included papers address the question posed by the review? • Were inclusion criteria for papers appropriate? • Were appropriate study designs looked for and included?
	Were important and relevant studies included?	• Did the methodology include the following elements critical to a systematic review? Search strategy for appropriate electronic databases, follow up on references from identified papers, identify and contact subject experts, identify unpublished work, search for non-English language literature.
	Was the quality of studies assessed?	• Was a validated checklist used to assess quality?
	Was it reasonable to pool the results?	• Were the results similar from study to study (i.e., homogeneous) and thus suitable for pooling? • If pooling was done despite variable results, were these justified?
	Is the question focused?	• Are the elements of PICO well described?
What are the results?	Overall results?	• Are the presented headline results numerically appropriate? • Have they been appropriately expressed (NNT, odds ratio, etc.)
	How precise are they?	• Are confidence intervals set out?
Will they help locally?	Applicability to local population	• Does the population being studied sufficiently differ from the local population? • Is the setting different?
	Were all outcomes considered	• Would the reader like to have seen any other information?
	Do benefits outweigh harm and costs	• Is there a cost-effectiveness analysis?

may well be the only component of the paper that is read. The PICO format, evidently, will not apply to all study types.

3. Systematic approach to performing CA of the study.
A systematic approach to CA can be ingrained by using existing checklists and tools designed for the purpose. In the early stages of CA, and especially when appraising topics that are outside the expertise of the reviewer, the author would certainly recommend that a CA checklist appropriate to the study be used as an aide-memoire; with time and practice, there is a lesser need for these checklists to be referred to as frequently. While several checklists and graphic models exist for CA (▶ Table 46.2), the author's preference is for the CASP framework, a programme with a long pedigree that is internationally recognised and used. The CASP framework aims to appraise the paper using questions grouped under three domains. ▶ Table 46.4, ▶ Table 46.5 and ▶ Table 46.6 set out the CASP framework for systematic reviews/meta-analyses, randomised controlled trials and cohort studies. Checklists for other study types can be found at the CASP website (http://www.casp-uk.net/). The following is a high-level description of the tool.

4. Is the study valid?
Based on the category of the article, ethical approval may be needed, and this should form part of the CA. Any study's worth should hinge on its methodological quality, and thus, this section should be the first port of call when looking at the full text. The methodology of

L

▶ **Table 46.5** CASP methodology for randomised trials

Domain	Question	Items to look for
Are the results valid?	Is the question focused?	• Are the elements of PICO well described?
	Was the assignment of patients to treatments randomised?	• What was the randomisation procedure? • Was the allocation sequence concealed from researchers and patients?
	Were all the patients who entered the trial properly accounted for at its conclusion?	• Was the trial stopped early? • Were patients analysed in the groups to which they were randomised?
	Were patients, researchers, and health care personnel blind to treatment?	
	Were the groups similar at the start of the trial?	• Age, sex, social class
	Aside from the experimental intervention, were the groups treated equally?	• Investigations • Follow-up protocol • Management of side effects
What are the results?	How large was the treatment effect?	• What outcomes were measured? • Is the primary outcome clearly specified? • What results were found for each outcome?
	How precise was the estimate of the treatment effect?	• Confidence intervals
Will they help locally?	Can the results be applied in your context?	• Do you think that the patients covered by the trial are similar enough to the patients to whom you will apply this? If not, how do they differ?
	Were all clinically important outcomes considered?	• Is there other information you would like to have seen? • If not, does this affect the decision?
	Are the benefits worth the harms and costs?	• Even if this is not addressed by the trial, what do you think?

a study is also the key element that influences the strength of recommendation when commissioners and guideline developers assess the applicability of a study (http://www.gradeworkinggroup.org/), and thus its impact. The CASP framework to assess validity uses screening questions followed by a detailed assessment of the validity. These questions will vary depending on the study type.

• *Case-controlled study* These designs are especially common in the surgical literature, given the complexity of setting up and running surgical trials. The reader should first identify if a case-controlled study is the most appropriate way to answer the issue under scrutiny and if the literature has other robust datasets that have answered the question using other designs. There should be clarity on why the authors did not go for a superior

design as opposed to case-controlled study. Detailed screening questions will include if the cases were recruited in an acceptable way, precisely defined within the population and if the time frame was relevant to the disease and exposure. Bias will be inevitable in such a design and it should be clear if the controls were reasonably well matched to the cases. The study methodology should be precise about the exposure or the intervention in the groups and if appropriate, subjective/objective measurements were used for the purpose. Was a uniform set of measurements used both in the cases and the controls? Once again, the reader should specifically look for confounding factors as these may have a bigger role to play than with other study designs.

• *Cohort study* Screening questions to assess the validity in this study type would include

L

► **Table 46.6** CASP methodology for cohort study

Domain	Question	Items to look for
Are the results valid?	Is the question focused?	• Elements of PICO
	Was the cohort recruited in an acceptable way?	• Cohort representative of a defined population • Inclusion of the appropriate population at risk
	Was the exposure accurately measured to minimise bias?	• Use of subjective or objective measurements • Measurements are validated instruments • Subjects classified into exposure groups using same definition
	Was the outcome accurately measured to minimise bias?	• Use of subjective or objective measurements • Measurements are validated instruments • A reliable system was established for detecting all cases • Measurement methods were similar in the different groups • Subjects and/or the outcome assessor blinded to exposure, if appropriate
	Have the authors identified all important confounding factors?	
	Have they taken account of the confounding factors in the design and/or analysis?	• Look for restriction in design, and techniques, e.g., modelling, stratified, regression, or sensitivity analysis to correct, control, or adjust for confounding factors
	Was the follow-up of subjects complete enough?	
	Was the follow-up of subjects long enough?	• The good or bad effects should have had long enough to reveal themselves • The persons that are lost to follow up may have different outcomes than those available for assessment • In an open or dynamic cohort, was there anything special about the outcome of the people leaving, or the exposure of the people entering the cohort?
What are the results?	What are the results of this study?	• What are the bottom line results? Have they reported the rate or the proportion between the exposed/unexposed, the ratio/the rate difference? • How strong is the association between exposure and outcome (RR)? • What is the absolute risk reduction (ARR)?
	How precise was the estimate of the treatment effect?	• Confidence intervals, if given
	Do you believe the results? ☐ Yes ☐ Can't tell ☐ No HINT:	Consider ☐ Big effect is hard to ignore! ☐ Can it be due to bias, chance, or confounding? ☐ Are the design and methods of this study sufficiently flawed to make the results unreliable? ☐ Bradford Hill's criteria (e.g., time sequence, dose–response gradient, biological plausibility, consistency)

L

▶ **Table 46.6** (*Continued*) CASP methodology for cohort study

Domain	Question	Items to look for
Will they help locally?	Can the results be applied in your context?	☐ A cohort study was the appropriate method to answer this question ☐ The subjects covered in this study could be sufficiently different from your population to cause concern ☐ Your local setting is likely to differ much from that of the study ☐ You can quantify the local benefits and harms
	Do the results of this study fit with other available evidence?	
	What are the implications of this study for practice?	Consider: ☐ One observational study rarely provides sufficiently robust evidence to recommend changes to clinical practice or within health policy decision making for certain questions observational studies provide the only evidence ☐ Recommendations from observational studies are always stronger when supported by other evidence

a good description of PICO and if the cohort was recruited in an acceptable way within a well-defined population or if heterogeneity existed in the cohort. Following this, further detailed questions regarding validity would be on how the exposure was measured and how bias was minimised within the study, appreciating that there will be inevitable bias given the design of the study. Additionally, within a cohort study it is important to ensure that a robust system was established to detect all instances of disease occurrence and if confounding factors were identified and addressed as appropriate. Finally, the reader should ensure that the follow-up period in a cohort study was long enough to capture the outcomes of interest.

- *Randomised controlled trial* The assessment of validity in an RCT would include how patients were assigned to the comparative arms at the time of randomisation, if allocation sequence was concealed from researchers and patients, if the trial stopped early, and if the intention to treat paradigm followed. It is also important to ask if the patients and the personnel running the study were blinded to the intervention and if the groups were similar at the start of the trial, and if apart from the experimental intervention, patients were managed similarly throughout the trial. Was the sample size and power calculation generated using robust pilot data?

- *Systematic review and meta-analysis* An important consideration in a meta-analysis is whether it was reasonable to statistically pool the results of the review, as heterogeneity across trials in meta-analyses is inevitable and if this was clinically acceptable.

5. What are the results?
Once the reader judges the methodology to be valid, the results can be studied. Again, based on the study type the questions being asked will vary.

- *Case-controlled study* Consider the strength of the association between exposure/intervention and outcome as expressed by the odds ratio (OR) and if the results have been adjusted for confounding, as this can sometimes explain the association. It is especially important to assess if the adjustment made a big difference to the OR. The reader should identify if p values and confidence intervals have been used as estimates of the risk.

- *Cohort study* CA of the results should assess if the rate difference between the exposed and unexposed groups are reported, the strength of association between exposure and outcome (risk ratio) and the absolute risk reduction (ARR). Does the reported association meet Bradford Hill's criteria for causation (▶ Table 46.7)?

L

▶ **Table 46.7** Bradford Hill's criteria for investigating causality in epidemiological studies

Strength of the association.

Consistency across other studies.

Specificity of the causative link to the population.

Temporal association between cause and effect.

Biological gradient, indicating a link between strength of exposure and effect.

Plausibility, with evidence of a plausible mechanism.

Coherence between epidemiological and laboratory findings.

Experimental evidence.

Analogy with similar factors.

- *Randomised controlled trial* In an RCT, the reader should scan the results with a view to ensuring the following questions have been answered: how large was the treatment effect and how precise was the estimate of the treatment effect (expressed as *p* values and confidence intervals)? If these data are sufficiently robust, the next logical question is whether the results of the study can be translated to the context of the reader's practice, paying special attention to the demographic and clinical characteristics of the trial population. Most trials will report the harms and costs and these will need to be considered if the trial recommendations are to be adopted to the local practice.

- *Systematic review and meta-analysis* In the setting of a meta-analysis, the pooled results, the confidence intervals, the number needed to treat are assessed to see if these are significant and applicable to the local population. Usually, harms and cost will not be part of a systematic review and thus, more information from the local network to define the cost of the recommended intervention prior to implementing a practice change.

46.8 Tips on Writing an Effective Paper

The following section identifies what peer reviewers expect from authors and defines the contents of the different sections of a paper being written up.

Introduction The introduction of the research report will have two major objectives. It provides the context for the study and includes the background information and specifies the aims of the study that form the paper. This is the section reviewers are least likely to read, but often referred to by the reader naïve to the subject. The introduction should aim to be concise, yet providing reasonable depth to engage the reader. In a prospective study, time may have elapsed between the initial write-up when the grant was applied for, and this section may need significant revision and updating.

Methodology This section should have sufficient detail that enables a subsequent researcher to repeat the study and extend the study as appropriate. The methodology should be explicit and provide enough information that will help the reader decide the robustness of the study. Statistical analysis should be very clearly mentioned including cutoff points where the statistical outcomes are thought to be significant. As discussed above, this is the section that makes or breaks a paper in the reviewers' eyes, and significant attention should be paid when drafting this up. Often, for prospective studies, the methods section will have been fully written up in the protocol and may have been peer reviewed by funders. In these instances, submission to a journal will need significant rewriting to bring it under the journal's word limit. Care should be taken to ensure that important information is not lost in the process of pruning the methodology. It is often useful to get a reader who is not familiar with the study to re-read this section.

Results This is the section that should be written up first. The results should identify if the objectives of the study have been fulfilled and set out clearly the findings based on the proposed outcome measures. Results should be presented without interpretation, allowing the readers to make their own judgment on the results in the light of current knowledge and practice. The results section should also include figures and tables that add to the data being presented in the results section without duplicating unnecessary information.

Discussion: This section should place the results obtained in perspective without repeating the results of the earlier section. Several journals will ask for a structured discussion section, thus enabling a focused write-up. Most experienced readers will skip to the section that provides information on the weakness and the strengths of the study and the proposed next steps that will move the science forward.

Further Reading

Critical Appraisal Skills Programme. CASP Checklist. http://www.casp-uk.net/. Accessed December 30 2017

L

47 Mastoid Surgery

Mastoid surgery (mastoidectomy) is a procedure performed to remove the mastoid air cells. It is used to treat mastoiditis and chronic suppurative otitis media, both with and without cholesteatoma. It is also used for access when inserting cochlear implants or as part of lateral skull base surgery for vestibular schwannomas and to access temporal bone tumours such as paragangliomas (glomus tumours) and epidermoid cysts.

There are six different types of mastoidectomy:

1. Cortical mastoidectomy also called simple mastoidectomy or Schwartze's procedure.
2. Radical mastoidectomy—Removal of posterior and superior canal wall, meatoplasty and exteriorisation of the middle ear.
3. Canal wall up mastoidectomy also called closed-cavity mastoidectomy or combined-approach tympanoplasty in which the posterior and superior ear canal walls are kept intact.
4. Canal wall down mastoidectomy or modified radical mastoidectomy in which the ear canal wall is removed and one cavity created and the middle ear repaired with tissue grafts.
5. Canal wall reconstruction mastoidectomy where either a modified radical mastoidectomy is done and the cavity is reduced in size by repairing the ear canal wall as well as the middle ear or the medial portion of the posterior canal wall and superior canal wall are removed by a combined permeatal inside out and cortical mastoidectomy approach. The removed canal wall is then reconstructed with conchal cartilage.
6. Subtotal or total petrosectomy. Every mastoid cell is removed plus or minus the bone down to soft tissue.

There are also the lateral and total temporal bone resections used for cancers.

47.1 Procedure Principles

Mastoidectomy procedures are typically performed under non-paralysing general anaesthesia to allow the use of a nerve integrity monitor. High-speed drills, a microscope, microinstruments and increasingly otoendoscopes are used. The surface landmarks of the bony external ear canal, zygomatic root, spine of Henle and mastoid tip, allow the surgeon to initiate bone removal in the correct location. The first steps are always identifying the tegmen and saucerising the edges of the mastoid cavity using the largest burr possible.

Safe mastoid surgery requires routine identification of key anatomical structures after identifying the tegmen (middle fossa floor), then sigmoid sinus and diagastric ridge, then external auditory canal, lateral semicircular canal, short process of the incus and facial nerve. Microscopic surgery is now being augmented with endoscopes to examine and remove disease from areas challenging to visualise such as sinus tympani, supratubal recess, epitympanum, facial recess, perilabyrinthine air cells and retrofacial air cells.

1. Cortical mastoidectomy—Consists of opening the mastoid cortex and identifying Koerner's septum and the aditus ad antrum. Removal of mastoid air cells is undertaken without affecting the middle ear. This is typically done for mastoiditis.
2. Radical mastoidectomy—Removal of posterior and superior canal wall, meatoplasty and exteriorisation of the middle ear. A radical mastoidectomy is a canal wall down mastoidectomy in which the tympanic membrane and ossicles are not reconstructed, thus exteriorising the disease. The eustachian tube is often obliterated with soft tissue to reduce the risk of a chronic otorrhoea.
3. Canal wall up mastoidectomy—A complete or canal wall up mastoidectomy necessitates removal of all of the mastoid air cells along the tegmen, sigmoid sinus and presigmoid dural plate. The posterior and superior canal walls are kept intact. A posterior tympanotomy via a facial recess approach is usually included.
4. Canal wall down mastoidectomy—It includes a complete mastoidectomy in addition to removal of posterior and superior canal wall and a meatoplasty. The tympanic membrane is left in place or reconstructed. A meatoplasty is always performed to decrease the risk of developing moisture in the cavity and to facilitate future debridement. It entails removal of a varying amount of the conchal cartilage, post-auricular periosteum and cartilaginous ear canal while preserving as much external ear canal skin as possible.

5. Canal wall reconstruction mastoidectomy—The removal of bone is the same as an open-cavity mastoidectomy. The canal wall is reconstructed to avoid a cavity. This is done with some or all of cartilage, soft tissue free grafts, pedicled flaps, bone or occasionally artificial tissue. This is covered with vascularised flaps and leaves a normal-looking ear canal. The middle ear is reconstructed in the same way as a modified radical mastoidectomy. This avoids the long-term drawbacks of canal wall down mastoidectomy while offering surgeons excellent exposure of the middle ear and mastoid. In the world literature, this is the most common type of mastoid surgery and has the highest chance of curing cholesteatoma.

A modification of this is to just remove the medial portion of the posterior canal wall and also the medial superior wall in a combined inside out/cortical mastoidectomy approach to expose the cholesteatoma from both sides of the posterior canal wall but with much wider access than a total canal wall-up technique with posterior tympanotomy.

6. Subtotal and total petrosectomy—It consist of a complete removal of the mastoid bone all to way down to the dura of the middle and posterior fossa and the removal of the mastoid tip and the middle ear. It usually involves sacrificing and blind sacking the ear canal and obliterating the eustachian tube.

47.2 Incisions

Either an endaural or post-aural incision is used. Both are equally popular in the United Kingdom. A properly performed endaural incision will allow good access to the attic, tegmen and sigmoid sinus even in well-aerated mastoids. It provides better access to the sinus tympani and is ideally suited for a small-cavity mastoidectomy. It will not allow sufficient posterior access for a subtotal petrosectomy unless extended. Some surgeons routinely perform a subtotal petrosectomy removing bone behind the venous sinus to allow the post-auricular soft tissues to fall into the smooth defect, obviating the need for an obliteration procedure. A post-aural incision is usually used to perform a posterior tympanotomy for combined-approach tympanoplasty and to access the round window in cochlear implants where it also provides access for the implant bed.

47.3 Complications

Facial nerve injury Permanent facial nerve paralysis (~ 0.1%). A transient facial weakness can be seen in the immediate post-operative period from local anaesthetic. Controversy exists as to whether facial nerve monitoring is helpful in reducing the risk of post-operative facial nerve injury, but from a medicolegal point of view, it is mandatory.

Hearing loss A temporary or permanent conductive hearing loss is very common. A significant sensorineural hearing loss is rare (~ 1%).

Tinnitis Temporary tinnitus is common after surgery. Occasionally, the tinnitus is permanent and troublesome (~ 2%).

Vertigo Temporary vertigo and/or dizziness are frequently seen in patients undergoing otological surgery. Permanent vestibular symptoms are quite rare after mastoidectomy (~ 0.1%). Sometimes a labyrinthine fistula is found at the lateral or anterior parts of the lateral semicircular canal and cholesteatoma matrix can be left over the fistula so as not to expose it and risk a dead ear if a canal wall down procedure is being performed. Otherwise temporalis muscle and fascia or bone pate should be immediately placed over the fistula if the surgeon decides to remove matrix.

Change in taste The chorda tympani nerve may be stretched or traumatised causing an altered sensation of taste, typically described as a metallic or sour taste on the affected side. This sensation may be persistent but often resolves over a period of months. The chorda tympani nerve is often divided in mastoid surgery for cholesteatoma and patients may fleeting complain of reduced taste which usually quickly settles unless the patient is a supertaster.

Dural injury Dural exposure without breach needs no treatment. A cerebrospinal fluid leak should be repaired when noticed but often necessitates admission, elevation of the head of the bed and, in refractory cases, placement of a lumbar drain.

Vascular injury The sigmoid sinus is one of the initial landmarks used in mastoid surgery. Injury typically results in copious venous bleeding. Since the sigmoid sinus is a low-flow system, gentle pressure, Surgicel or crushed muscle stops the bleeding. An arterial injury to the petrous carotid artery should be taken to interventional neuroradiology immediately after tamponading the vessel with crushed muscle.

M

47.4 Long-Term Monitoring

Patients with cholesteatoma need to be followed up long term. Recurrence occurs in about 25% of patients in whom the canal wall was preserved when performed by experienced and competent otologists although some surgeons have a much lower rate of recurrence (Hamilton quotes < 5% recurrence) and up to 20% of patients in whom a canal wall down procedure was performed. In patients undergoing canal wall up procedures, a second-look procedure 6 to 12 months after the initial surgery allows for assessment and removal of residual disease. Non-echoplanar diffusion-weighted magnetic resonance imaging (DW-MRI) may in some cases detect pearl-like recurrences down to 2 mm in size and avoid the need for a second look.

There has been a debate for years on the canal wall up versus canal wall down techniques. There is now a consensus that the patient and the disease should dictate the procedure used. It is, however, more commonly the surgeon who does this. There is also consensus that if a canal wall up procedure is used, endoscopes are useful and that if a canal wall down mastoidectomy is done, then canal wall reconstruction with the patients tissue such as vascularised flaps should be done at the same time. There is no consensus that lasers improve outcome or reduce complications. However, some surgeons have accepted very small recurrence rate of less than 10% in children with cholesteatoma when using the canal wall up technique and a laser with even better results for adults who typically have less aggressive disease. The incidence of recurrence is therefore undoubtably related to the technique and the experience/expertise of the surgeon.

The most common procedure done worldwide is the small-cavity mastoidectomy with repair. It has had a recent resurgence, as it is suited to endoscopic ear surgery.

The surgery is performed by following the disease from the front backward starting by removing bone medially through the ear canal. The epitympanum is progressively enlarged, and the posterior canal wall is removed from the inside out. Bone removal is limited to that necessary to remove all of the cholesteatoma and the defect is repaired using cartilage and fascial grafts.

Such a subcortical, or inside-out, mastoidectomy combines the advantages of canal wall up and canal wall down techniques but may commit the surgeon to a canal wall down operation if the cholesteatoma is in a well-aerated mastoid. Some surgeons, with large cholesteatomas, will start the procedure with an inside-out approach and then proceed with excision of the residual disease with a cortical mastoidectomy approach. This, therefore, approaches the disease from both the external ear canal and mastoid and is by definition a type of combined approach tympanoplasty. It does not, however, involve a posterior tympanotomy because this portion of bone has already been excised in the initial inside-out approach. The medial canal wall and attic defect is reconstructed with conchal cartilage with attached perichondrium. If a canal wall down procedure is necessary, then a vascularised canal wall reconstruction is often needed.

47.5 Advantages and Disadvantages of the Canal Wall-Up Procedure

- Normal appearance.
- Hearing aids easy to fit.
- No routine cleaning required because the canal is usually self-cleaning.
- High tolerance for water exposure.
- A second-stage procedure is necessary to check for recurrent cholesteatoma and if found, a third or fourth procedure may then be necessary.
- Needs complex scanning (if radiological expertise to interpret the scan is available) and follow-up.
- High rate of recurrent or persistent cholesteatoma for most surgeons.

47.6 Advantages and Disadvantages of the Canal Wall-Down Procedure

- Enlarged meatus.
- Hearing aids difficult to fit.
- Annual or biannual canal cleaning needed forever and should the cavity become infected, then the cleaning may need to be more frequent.
- Some cavities persistently discharge.
- Dizziness may develop after exposure to water or cold air.
- Usually a single procedure.
- Low rate of recurrent cholesteatomas.

M

47.7 Advantages and Disadvantages of Mastoidectomy with Canal Wall Reconstruction Procedures

- Small meatoplasty meatus.
- Hearing aids fit.
- Usually no canal cleaning needed.
- High tolerance for water exposure.
- Might be a single procedure if the cholesteatoma is small and the surgeon confident of complete removal without the need for a cortical approach in a small-cavity mastoidectomy.
- Lowest rate of recurrent cholesteatomas.

The decision about how to manage the canal wall sometimes can only be made when the operation has begun and a better understanding of the extent of disease has emerged. If a canal wall up procedure has been planned, some intra-operative findings favour a canal wall down technique such as involvement of the sinus tympani, or the medial end of the canal wall, cholesteatoma wedged laterally between the heads of the ossicles in the epitympanum and medial canal wall, ostitis or friable cholesteatoma in the area around the opening to the eustachian tube or in the most inferior parts of the middle ear space, and defects in the canal wall. A small-cavity approach, removing the most medial portion of the bony ear canal may overcome some of the access difficulties mentioned in the above scenarios.

For a canal wall up procedure to be done, favourable features are a functioning eustachian tube with a well-maintained middle ear space and adequate communication between the mastoid and the middle ear space through the aditus ad antrum or a facial recess posterior tympanotomy. It is important to eliminate the bony epitympanic defect with a cartilage or bone graft, that is, repair the scutum and attic.

When a canal wall down procedure is done, there is removal of the lateral and posterior walls of the epitympanum so that the tegmen mastoideum and tegmen tympani become a smooth, featureless plane; sometimes amputation of the mastoid tip; extensive saucerisation of the lateral margins of the cavity; lowering of the posterior bony external auditory wall to the level of the facial nerve; lowering of the medial end of the external auditory canal towards the floor of the hypotympanum and enlargement of the meatus by removing or transposing the anterior end of the helix and superior part of the choncal cartilage.

Further Reading

Sanna M, Sunose H, Mancini F, Russo A, Taibah A. Microsurgical Management of Middle Ear and Petrous Bone Cholesteatoma. New York, NY: Thieme. In press

Belal A, Reda M, Mehana A, Belal Y. A new staging system for tympano-mastoid cholesteatoma. J Int Adv Otol 2012;8:63-68

Harris AT, Mettias B, Lesser TH. Pooled analysis of the evidence for open cavity, combined approach and reconstruction of the mastoid cavity in primary cholesteatoma surgery. J Laryngol Otol. 2016 Mar;130(3):235-241

Related Topics of Interest

Cholesteatoma
Suppurative otitis media—chronic

M

48 Medicolegal Aspects of ENT

Medical negligence is a civil tort that may occur when a patient suffers harm due to the action, or inaction, of a doctor entrusted with his or her care. For a claim in negligence to succeed, the claimant must prove three things:

1. That the doctor owed them a duty of care.
2. That the doctor's practice fell below an acceptable standard of care.
3. That the patient suffered harm as a *direct result* of that substandard care.

The claim process must commence within the required statutory time frame.

If negligence is proven, it results in liability for compensation to the injured patient for the harm suffered as a result of the negligence. This is in contrast to the tort of battery where the defendant is liable for *all* the harm and consequences of the tort, whether or not these could have been predicted. The size of any quantum awarded is usually directly related to the severity of the harm suffered and is often relatively modest. The majority of extremely large awards are related to loss of earnings, or the requirement for ongoing and future care provision.

Let us consider each of these points in turn.

48.1 Duty of Care

It is usually easy to prove a duty of care. If a patient consults with a doctor and the doctor offers advice or treatment, he or she has undertaken a duty of care towards that patient. This means he or she should make the care of that patient 'his or her first concern'.

48.2 Standard of Care

For many years, the courts used the Bolam principle alone to judge the standard of medical care delivered. This principle states:

'he is not guilty of negligence if he has acted in accordance with a practice accepted as proper by a responsible body of medical men skilled in that particular art'.

However, in 1998, the common interpretation of Bolam was modified by the case of *Bolitho*, which concerned the management of a child

suffering from respiratory failure. In this ruling, the judges agreed that it was not enough merely to demonstrate that the doctor's management was in line with that, '*accepted as proper*' by other medical experts if, '*the professional opinion is not capable of withstanding logical analysis*'.

Until *Bolitho*, it was customary for the courts to accept the opinion of doctors without question. However, with this ruling the courts took back control and made it clear that if the judge felt that medical opinion did not withstand scrutiny then he was, '*entitled to hold that the body of opinion is not reasonable or responsible*'.

48.3 Harm

In order to prove negligence, the claimant must prove that *on the balance of probability* (i.e., with a likelihood of > 50%) the contested harm occurred as a *direct result* of the doctor's action or inaction, *but for* his actions, the harm would have been avoided. This is often the hardest point of the three to prove and the reason that many claims fail. For example, a patient bringing a claim against a surgeon who did not diagnose cancer promptly would have to prove that this delay *directly* harmed his or her clinical outcome.

48.4 Negligence in the Context of Invalid Consent

A patient may successfully sue his or her doctor in negligence if he or she proves that the information he or she was given, and on which he or she based his or her consent to treatment, was deficient in some way. If he or she can demonstrate this and convince the court the following.

- He or she would not have agreed to treatment if he or she had been in possession of the correct information.
- The harm he or she suffered was as a direct result of this treatment.

Then, the claim may be successful. Since the Montgomery judgement, the standards required of the consent process have become much more demanding (see Chapter 14, Consent and Capacity).

M

48.5 Claims

Medical negligence claims fall into three broad groups:

1. Delay in, or failure to make, a diagnosis.
2. A recognised complication occurs after a procedure (usually surgical).
3. An adverse outcome of treatment (both medical and surgical).

In the first group, the delay in diagnosis is normally easily proven although there may be legitimate reasons for the delay. Typical scenarios include a patient with vague otological symptoms who is later found to have an acoustic neuroma; patients with globus-like symptoms who are subsequently found to have oesophageal cancer; or otalgia with tongue base or tonsillar carcinoma. A harder task for the claimant is to demonstrate that they have suffered definite harm as a result of the delay.

In the second group the case may be argued on the point that the surgeon's skills were inadequate, but is more normally fought around the quality and content of the consent process. Typical cases revolve around nerve damage and include facial nerve damage in ear and parotid surgery, accessory nerve damage in neck surgery, particularly lymph node biopsy, and recurrent laryngeal nerve damage in thyroid surgery. The use of nerve monitoring can be helpful but certainly does not guarantee avoidance of risk and interestingly, in the majority of such cases seen by the author, nerve monitoring was used! Other cases that often fall into this category are orbital complications and cerebrospinal fluid (CSF) leaks following endoscopic sinus surgery.

The criticism of a surgeon's skill is normally easily defended, particularly if it is an operation that the surgeon performs regularly and for which he or she has audit data to support his or her (usually good) outcomes, and lack of complications, with or without monitoring devices. However, it is an argument for avoiding 'occasional surgery' in modern practice. With regards to consent, the claimant will argue that they were not made aware that a certain complication might occur, or if they were, that the exact ramifications of said complication were not fully explained, and had this been done, they would not have proceeded with said procedure.

Further, it is extremely important to explain to the patient the option of no treatment at all, and the potential consequences of that. This can be more easily defended with supportive and thorough documentation.

Finally, the third group represents a more difficult area and in fact on closer examination, these cases often progress because of a failure of communication between clinician and patient. Often there are unrealistic expectations of outcome, and a subsequent failure to acknowledge this in an angry patient. Typical cases include dissatisfaction with appearance after cosmetic surgery, failure to address symptoms with nasal surgery or poor hearing after ear surgery (despite addressing any infective issue). If these cases prove unsuccessful in litigation, they may often result in a complaint to the regulator (GMC) by an unhappy patient or his or her family. Patients who feel they have been pressured into having surgery are often found in this group.

48.6 Medical Records

The primary purpose of medical records is to support ongoing patient care. They provide a crucial source of information in a health care system where shift work and frequent handovers are increasingly the norm. However, as alluded to above, good-quality, contemporaneous notes with a clear demonstration of the clinician's available information and management thought processes will represent the best defence against any complaint, medicolegal or otherwise. Complaints can often take several years to surface and the notes should be comprehensive enough to provide an accurate record of the events in question.

In its guidance on record keeping the GMC states, 'Record your concerns, including any minor concerns, and the details of any action you have taken, information you have shared, and decisions you have made relating to those concerns'.

Therefore, records must:

- Be clear, accurate and legible, including date and time, and signed to allow identification of the author.
- Be made contemporaneously or as soon as possible after each episode of patient care.
- Record every consultation relevant to that patient whether that occurs in the clinic, at the bedside, by telephone or even discussions with relatives.
- Allow health care professionals accepting handover of care to follow the sequence of

M

treatment decisions, the reasons for them and future management plans.

- Not be altered, amended or added to after the original episode of care. If corrections are necessary, the original entry should be scored through with one line, leaving it legible, and the replacement entry signed and dated.
- Avoid abbreviations.
- Record abnormal test results and the subsequent actions taken.

48.6.1 Electronic Patient Records

Electronic patient records are becoming more widespread and overcome the problem of illegibility. Care must still be taken to make a full entry into these records and hospitals must have systems in place to make regular backups, to avoid their loss during any technical 'glitch'. Any entry into computer-generated notes, including alterations, will be logged and date and time stamped to provide an audit trail of activity.

48.6.2 Storing Records

Records must be stored securely and protected against loss, damage and breaches of confidentiality. In the private sector, the patient's consultant is responsible for arranging appropriate storage of the records and the notes are the doctor's property. The patient has the right to access his or her records under the Data Protection Act 1998. Independent practitioners must be registered with the Information Commissioner under the Data Protection Act 1998.

48.6.3 Retaining Records

The Private and Voluntary Health Care (England) Regulations 2001 dictate for how long various medical records in the independent sector must be retained before destruction. For uncomplicated adults the norm is 8 years.

48.6.4 Sharing Records and Patient Information

Confidentiality must be preserved when sharing patient information in whatever format. E-mails

containing patient information sent outside of a trust should therefore be encrypted, and paper records moved between sites must be kept secure at all times.

48.7 Conclusion

There is no way to guarantee avoidance of complaints in medicine or surgery in particular, but sage advice to minimise the risk can probably be summarised as follows:

1. Take time to establish a good relationship with your patients.
2. Take time to explain the diagnosis and any treatment plans, and make sure your patient understands. This may mean multiple clinic visits. Remember that consent is an ongoing process and not a single event.
3. Don't pressure patients to have surgery, even if you think it is the right thing to do; they may not agree!
4. Finally, document fully and clearly everything you do, and the reasons for your actions or inactions.

Further Reading

General Medical Council. Good Medical Practice: consent guidance expressions of consent. http://www.gmc-uk.org/guidance/ethical_guidance/consent_guidance_expressions_of_consent.asp. Accessed October 30, 2016

Bolam v Friern Hospital Management Committee (1957) 2 All ER 118

Bolitho v City Hackney Health Authority (1998) AC 232

Montgomery v Lanarkshire Health Board [2015] UKSC 11, [2015] All ER(D) 113 (Mar)

General Medical Council. Good. Medical Practice 2013

The Private and Voluntary Health Care (England) Regulations. 2001 No 3968, Schedule 3, Part 1. Found at www.legislation.gov.uk

Related Topic of Interest

Consent and capacity

M

49 Ménière's Disease

In 1861, Prosper Ménière gave a presentation to the French Academy of Medicine describing a series of patients who experienced episodic vertigo and hearing loss. Contrary to the dogma of the time, he suggested that vertigo could have an otological rather than neurological cause. Subsequently, his name was used to define the condition characterised by episodic vertigo, sensorineural hearing loss and tinnitus. A sensation of aural fullness commonly accompanies this classical triad of symptoms.

The pathophysiology of Ménière's disease remains obscure though high-resolution magnetic resonance imaging (MRI) scans have confirmed the association with endolymphatic hydrops. Diagnosis is based on a clinical history of episodic vertigo, hearing loss and tinnitus and observing a fluctuating sensorineural hearing loss on audiometry. There is currently no cure for Ménière's disease, but there are many options for controlling the symptoms. Intra-tympanic injections of steroids or gentamicin have usurped many previous treatments.

49.1 Pathophysiology

The exact cause of Ménière's disease remains unknown. There is an association with endolymphatic hydrops, an expansion of the scala media and membranous labyrinth, the endolymphatic compartment of the inner ear. Modern high-resolution MRI studies suggest that when strict criteria for Ménière's disease are applied, all Ménière's disease patients have hydrops. However, endolymphatic hydrops may be seen in other conditions and has been identified in postmortem studies of people with no history of dizziness. There have been various suggestions as to how endolymphatic hydrops could cause the clinical symptoms of Ménière's disease. These include simple mechanical distortion of inner ear structures or rupture of Reissner's membrane, causing mixing of high potassium endolymph and low potassium perilymph with consequent disruption of normal hair cell function. Repeated attacks are thought to result in hair cell loss. Several triggers for endolymphatic hydrops have been suggested including autoimmune disease, allergy and viral infections. A genetic predisposition is seen in some cases of Ménière's disease and in a small percentage of these, individual gene mutations have been identified.

49.2 Clinical Features

The classical presentation of Ménière's disease is of a short prodromal period of increasing unilateral tinnitus and aural fullness followed by vertigo and low-frequency sensorineural hearing loss. The vertigo typically lasts between 20 minutes and several hours and is frequently accompanied by nausea and vomiting. However, atypical presentations are frequently encountered, hindering the diagnostic process. Because of the diagnostic difficulties, several attempts have been made to produce defining criteria for the condition. The most commonly cited criteria are those of the American Academy of Otolaryngology—Head and Neck Surgery, Committee on Hearing and Equilibrium (▶Table 49.1). A more recent set of criteria has been published by an international working group (▶Table 49.2).

Ménière's disease is said to start most commonly in the fifth, sixth or seventh decades of life though there are reports of onset in both the elderly and childhood. The course of Ménière's disease is unpredictable with some people experiencing long periods of remission whereas for others the attacks are frequent. The condition tends to lessen or 'burn out' with time and vertigo ceases in 71% of cases by 8.3 years. In the early stages of the disease, the hearing often returns to normal between attacks but with progressive attacks, a degree of permanent hearing loss usually develops. Although Ménière's disease typically presents unilaterally, there is a long-term risk of clinical symptoms in both ears.

Epidemiological studies have given wildly varying estimates of prevalence from 4 to 513 per 100,000. Part of this variation may be explained by different racial susceptibilities to Ménière's disease—Caucasians are thought to be at greater risk than other races. However, some of the discrepancy is almost certainly due to different trials using different diagnostic criteria and methodological weaknesses in the studies. Older studies are likely to have included patients who would now receive a diagnosis of vestibular migraine which

M

▶ **Table 49.1** Criteria for Ménière's disease by the American Academy of Otolaryngology—Head and Neck Surgery

Certain Ménière's disease	Definite Ménière's disease, plus histopathological confirmation (made on autopsy).
Definite Ménière's disease	Two or more definitive spontaneous episodes of vertigo 20 minutes or longer, audiometrically documented hearing loss on at least one occasion, tinnitus or aural fullness in the treated ear. Other causes excluded.
Probable Ménière's disease	One definitive episode of vertigo, audiometrically documented hearing loss on at least one occasion, tinnitus or aural fullness in the treated ear. Other causes excluded.
Possible Ménière's disease	Episodic vertigo without documented hearing loss, or sensorineural hearing loss, fluctuating or fixed with dysequilibrium but without definitive episodes. Other causes excluded.

Source: Produced by the American Academy of Otolaryngology—Head and Neck Surgery, Committee on Hearing and Equilibrium, 1995.

▶ **Table 49.2** Criteria for Ménière's disease, 2015

Definite Ménière's disease	Two or more spontaneous episodes of vertigo, each lasting 20 minutes to 12 hours. Audiometrically documented low- to medium-frequency sensorineural hearing loss in one ear, defining the affected ear on at least one occasion before, during, or after one of the episodes of vertigo. Fluctuating aural symptoms (hearing, tinnitus, or fullness) in the affected ear. Not better accounted for by another vestibular diagnosis.

Source: Produced by an international working group, comprising the Classification Committee of the Bárány Society, the Japan Society for Equilibrium Research, the European Academy of Otology and Neurotology (EAONO), the Equilibrium Committee of the American Academy of Otolaryngology—Head and Neck Surgery (AAO-HNS), and the Korean Balance Society, 2015.

is a common differential diagnosis of the condition. Women and overweight patients seem more prone to Ménière's disease. Ménière's disease has several comorbidities: conditions associated with immune or autonomic dysfunction may coexist as can allergic conditions. This list of comorbidities includes arthritis, chronic fatigue syndrome, rhinitis, eczema, irritable bowel syndrome, gastro-oesophageal reflux, migraine and psoriasis.

When patients are assessed in the ENT clinic, they are generally in the period between attacks and consequently physical examination is often normal. Benign paroxysmal positional vertigo can coexist with Ménière's disease, so patients should undergo Dix–Hallpike testing.

49.3 Investigations

The diagnosis is still predominantly reached by taking a clear medical history, performing serial audiometry, and by excluding other causes. Classically the audiometric loss is described as a fluctuating low-frequency sensorineural loss, but other patterns may be seen. This is particularly so in the later stages of the condition when mid- and high-tone losses are common. Tympanometry is helpful as many patients with Ménière's disease

are told by primary care physicians that the aural fullness they experience is due to eustachian tube dysfunction. Acoustic reflex testing is often normal.

Electrocochleography (ECoG) may show an enhanced negative summating potential indicative of altered cochlear function. Caloric tests may demonstrate impaired vestibular function on the affected side though testing is almost always carried out in the period between attacks and it is therefore not unusual for the caloric tests to be normal. Glycerol dehydration testing works on the principle that dehydrating the cochlea and thus reducing the endolymphatic hydrops will produce an improvement in the audiogram and the ECoG; it can be used as a pre-operative assessment of the potential response to conservative surgery but is unpleasant for the patient as it causes nausea and headache.

Both cervical and ocular vestibular-evoked myogenic potential (VEMP) tests have been investigated as potential diagnostic tools for Ménière's disease. Most studies of this modality show low specificity and sensitivity so the role of VEMPs seems limited. Clearly, vertigo, tinnitus and hearing loss are not unique symptoms to Ménière's disease.

Other causes of intermittent vertigo should also be excluded and, as with any asymmetrical

M

audiovestibular symptoms, it is essential to exclude a cerebellopontine angle tumour such as a vestibular schwannoma. A diagnostic MRI scan of the internal auditory meatuses should be performed. MRI is also now being used to directly visualise endolymphatic hydrops; gadolinium is administered either as an intra-tympanic injection or as an intra-venous bolus. After an interval of several hours, a high-resolution MRI in a 3T scanner is performed. The gadolinium contrast accumulates in the perilymph but not the endolymph allowing demarcation to be made between the two compartments. Presently, this is generally a research tool, but it seems likely that it will at some stage enter routine clinical practice. Interestingly, initial studies using this technique suggest that bilateral hydrops is common in patients with Ménière's disease, even if their Ménière's symptoms are unilateral.

49.4 Management

Many treatment modalities have been tried in the management of Ménière's disease. It is one of the truisms of medicine that when there are many treatment options it is because none of them are perfect and this aphorism certainly seems to apply in the case of Ménière's disease. Much of the research that has been undertaken in the field has been, and continues to be, of poor quality and all too often when a systematic review and meta-analysis of a treatment is attempted, the conclusion is that the evidence is inadequate.

Treatment can be either medical or surgical and can be regarded as a therapeutic ladder, climbing from the simple to the complicated, from the non-invasive to the invasive. Some of the treatments that have been used are listed in ▶ Table 49.3.

49.4.1 Medical, Conservative

Medical treatment usually starts with advice on diet, particularly advice to reduce salt, fluid and caffeine intake. There is no robust scientific evidence to support any of this advice. Betahistine, a histamine analogue, given at a dosage of 16 mg three times daily, is widely prescribed, but there is no good-quality evidence to support this practice. Vestibular sedatives, such as prochlorperazine and cinnarizine, are without doubt useful in short-term symptom control and are best prescribed to be taken at the onset of any attack. Mycostatin (nystatin) has been suggested as a possible Ménière's disease treatment, but this was based on

▶ **Table 49.3** Some of the treatment options that have been used in the management of patients with Ménière's disease

Medical treatments, conservative	Low-salt diet
	Low-caffeine diet
	Restriction of fluid intake
	Betahistine
	Diuretics
	Vestibular sedatives
	Allergy therapy
	Mycostatin (nystatin)
	Calcium channel blockers
	Intra-tympanic steroid injection
	Intra-tympanic depot steroid injection
	Intra-tympanic antiviral (ganciclovir) injection
	Intra-tympanic prostaglandin analogue (latanoprost) injection
Medical treatments, destructive	Intra-tympanic gentamicin injection
Surgical treatments, conservative	Endolymphatic sac and duct surgery
	Grommet
	Grommet and pressure device
	Sacculotomy
	Division of intra-tympanic muscles
Surgical treatments, destructive	Vestibular nerve section
	Vestibulocochlear nerve section
	Labyrinthectomy

Note: Modalities present in this table but not discussed in the main text have insufficient evidence to ascertain efficacy.

M

a small, retrospective, uncontrolled study and it is difficult to envisage a pharmacological mechanism by which it could work. Diuretics, particularly thiazides, are sometimes prescribed but there is no good study to demonstrate any greater efficacy than placebo in this condition. One conservative treatment option that has been demonstrated to show benefit is the use of intra-tympanic steroid injections, particularly with regards to vertigo control. Benefit is, however, often short lived. By injecting steroids within a thermosensitive gel that remains in the middle ear for up to 3 months, it is hoped that prolonged inner ear exposure to steroids can be achieved. A pilot trial has shown modest benefit and further work is underway. Intra-tympanic injection of other drugs, namely, antiherpetic antiviral drugs and prostaglandin analogues, has not shown benefit.

Medical treatment is generally said to provide adequate symptom control in about 70 to 80% of patients though with most treatment regimens it remains unclear whether this is due to the treatment or psychological reassurance and the placebo effect. Tinnitus management strategies, hearing rehabilitation and vestibular rehabilitation exercises may be needed for some patients.

49.4.2 Medical, Destructive

Chemical labyrinthectomy using gentamicin is increasingly popular, relying on gentamicin's property of being selectively toxic to vestibular hair cells but not auditory hair cells. When injected intra-tympanically, gentamicin achieves good vertigo control though there is an associated risk of causing hearing loss. As with all ablative procedures, this treatment carries a risk of long-term imbalance.

49.4.3 Surgical, Conservative

The simplest surgical procedure is the insertion of a grommet in the affected ear. This procedure is without any logical or scientific support and any effect is probably attributable to the placebo effect. It is possible to insert a grommet and then use a positive pressure device to transmit low-pressure pulses through the lumen of the grommet into the middle ear and thence to the inner ear. Systematic review of this technique found no evidence of its benefit.

Surgical decompression of the endolymphatic sac has been used with the aim of treating the underlying pathophysiological abnormality without destroying the function of the ear and thereby offering control of the vertigo at the same time as hearing preservation. This is accomplished via a cortical mastoidectomy approach to the sac as it lies in the posterior cranial fossa. Decompression is achieved by exposing the sac with or without opening the sac and inserting a shunt to provide prolonged drainage. Systematic review of this technique has found no evidence of its benefit. Furthermore, a Danish sham study was performed in 1981, in which sac surgery was prospectively and randomly compared with simple cortical mastoidectomy. The participants in the study were blinded to the treatment that they received, and no significant difference was seen between the two surgical options.

49.4.4 Surgical, Destructive

Vestibular nerve section, which abolishes input from the troublesome labyrinth to the brain while preserving hearing achieves a high rate of vertigo control, but as a stand-alone procedure it has the disadvantage of requiring a neurosurgical approach. Surgical labyrinthectomy achieves similar rates of vertigo control and remains a useful option for patients who have lost all hearing in the affected ear. Some surgeons have combined a transmastoid labyrinthectomy with a translabyrinthine vestibular nerve section, arguing that this is the most certain way to fully ablate vestibular function.

49.5 Follow-Up and Aftercare

Although Ménière's disease is uncommon, because it is a chronic condition, affected patients account for a significant proportion of the patients seen in neuro-otology clinics. Various studies have suggested that this figure is 10 to 20% of the clinical workload in such units. In addition to specific Ménière's treatments, hearing, tinnitus and balance rehabilitation may be required.

M

Further Reading

American Academy of Otolaryngology-Head and Neck Foundation, Inc.. Committee on Hearing and Equilibrium guidelines for the diagnosis and evaluation of therapy in Ménière's disease. Otolaryngol Head Neck Surg. 1995; 113(3):181–185

James AL, Burton MJ. Betahistine for Ménière's disease or syndrome. Cochrane Database Syst Rev. 2001(1):CD001873

Lopez-Escamez JA, Carey J, Chung WH, et al; Classification Committee of the Barany Society. Japan Society for Equilibrium Research. European Academy of Otology and Neurotology (EAONO). Equilibrium Committee of the American Academy of Otolaryngology-Head and Neck Surgery (AAO-HNS). Korean Balance Society. Diagnostic criteria for Ménière's disease. J Vestib Res. 2015; 25(1):1–7

Tyrrell JS, Whinney DJ, Ukoumunne OC, Fleming LE, Osborne NJ. Prevalence, associated factors, and comorbid conditions for Ménière's disease. Ear Hear. 2014; 35(4):e162–e169

Wright T. Ménière's disease. BMJ Clin Evid. 2015; 2015:2015

Related Topics of Interest

Vertigo
Vestibular function tests
Labyrinthitis
Perilymph and labyrinthine fistula

M

50 Nasal Reconstruction

50.1 Introduction

The causes of tissue loss requiring nasal reconstructive surgery are many and varied, although the majority of patients will have undergone nasal skin cancer excision. Other nasal reconstruction cases follow trauma, complications of surgery, recreational drug use, vasculitis or congenital conditions.

With an ageing population, the incidence of nasal skin cancer is rising, and basal cell carcinoma is the most common tumour in patients undergoing surgery. Reconstructive nasal surgery for squamous cell carcinoma is rare, and there are very few cases of malignant melanoma.

When managing malignancy of the external nose, it is of paramount importance to completely excise the tumour before reconstructing the defect. Nasal skin basal cell carcinomas, particularly those on the nasal tip, often extend for some distance beyond the limit of the visible tumour making the excision margin difficult to judge. Mohs' micrographic surgery is therefore recommended for nasal skin tumours because this technique gives the combination of a high cure rate with tissue resection kept to a minimum.

50.2 Principles of Nasal Reconstruction

In addition to skin, the defects requiring reconstruction may involve nasal mucosa, cartilage and bone. Defects of nasal bone requiring reconstruction are fortunately rare.

An informed discussion with the patient is vital before a nasal reconstruction is undertaken. In most cases, there are different options for the reconstruction, and the patient's concerns regarding the aesthetic outcome must be understood regardless of their age. Although a more straightforward technique may be possible, this may result in a less favourable aesthetic outcome than if a more complex procedure is used. Sufficient discussion of these issues takes time, and for this reason it is recommended that the patient is seen on two occasions. Photographs of previous cases are useful to help explain the surgical options, and patient involvement in the decision making is essential.

Defects may be defined as partial or full thickness. In a full-thickness defect, all three layers (inner lining of vestibular skin or mucosa, cartilage and skin) need to be reconstructed. The fundamental principle of nasal reconstruction is to replace each of these three layers using 'like with like' tissue where possible.

50.3 Reconstructive Techniques

A detailed description of the techniques used in nasal reconstruction is beyond the scope of this chapter, and an overview is given. For a comprehensive description, the reader is directed towards the recommended texts in Further Reading.

50.3.1 Inner Lining

Reconstruction of the inner lining of vestibular skin or mucosa is of paramount importance and often the most challenging part of a nasal reconstruction. Without a well-vascularised inner lining to support overlying cartilage grafts, healing is compromised, and contraction and alar retraction often results.

Small, non-marginal mucosal defects of a few millimetres can be closed primarily after mobilising the surrounding mucosa. Inner lining defects at the alar margin of up to 1 cm can be reconstructed by extensive mucosal mobilisation and advancing a bipedicled flap of mucosa. A cephalic releasing incision is often required, and tension must be avoided.

Larger defects require a rotation flap from the septum. A favoured technique is to use a septal hinge flap. This involves mobilisation of a sizable, ipsilateral, anteriorly based flap, which is dissected free posteriorly and folded anteriorly. The posterior free edge of the flap is sutured at the reconstructed alar margin, temporarily closing the nasal cavity. This mucosal flap is divided within the nasal cavity 4 weeks later at the same time as division of the skin flap pedicle.

In certain cases, generally non-cancer reconstructions, it is possible to turn down nasal tip or sidewall skin towards the alar margin to form the inner lining. The size of the skin defect to be reconstructed is therefore increased. This can actually improve the aesthetic outcome allowing more aesthetic scar placement in keeping with the nasal subunit principle of nasal reconstruction as described further.

50.4 Cartilage in Nasal Reconstruction

Cartilage support of the overlying skin is vital if the result of a nasal reconstruction is to be both functionally and aesthetically favourable. Conchal cartilage has a natural curvature ideal for alar reconstruction. This can be harvested with low morbidity and is preferred to septal cartilage.

Conchal cartilage grafts used in alar reconstruction do not directly replace a deficient lower lateral cartilage, rather they are positioned along the alar margin in a non-anatomical position. The inner lining is sutured to the skin around the marginal cartilage graft. This is important to prevent alar retraction.

Even in cases where the lower lateral cartilages remain intact, cartilage support is required in the reconstruction of small alar margin and soft triangle defects to prevent notching and retraction. A notch at the alar margin of only a few millimetres will catch the eye, and achieving a smooth, symmetrical alar margin is a key outcome in the aesthetic aspect of nasal reconstruction.

50.5 Reconstruction of the Nasal Skin

The external nose can be divided into nine nasal subunits: the tip, dorsum, columella and paired alar, soft triangle and sidewall. These subunits are based on the natural shadowing and contouring of the nose.

The aesthetic subunit principle proposes that if a defect occupies more than 50% of a subunit, the remainder of the subunit should be excised. Scars are then located at the border of a subunit, making them less visible. There are, however, times when the subunit principle should be adapted for aesthetic benefit. For instance, a hemi-tip defect may be reconstructed with a central tip scar preserving skin over the contralateral hemi-tip. The skin over the rhinion on the dorsum of the nose is very thin and is only removed if involved in tumour resection. In alar defects, it is advisable to preserve a few millimetres of the lateral alar skin adjacent to the nasofacial sulcus and avoid placing scars in the sulcus where they are actually more visible.

It is also important to reconstruct the nose separately from the cheek, and where a defect extends onto the cheek, the cheek skin should be advanced to the nasal sidewall margin.

50.6 Options for Skin Reconstruction

When considering the reconstruction of nasal skin defects, several factors are considered. These include the size, location and depth of the defect, and associated comorbidity such as diabetes, smoking and previous radiotherapy. If structural cartilage grafting is required, a vascularised flap is generally required rather than a skin graft.

50.6.1 Skin Grafts

Full-thickness skin grafts may be used to reconstruct certain smaller defects. They give the best results in areas where the nasal skin is thin such as the bony dorsum or sidewall. Where the skin is thicker, particularly over the nasal tip, full-thickness skin grafts generally do not give a good cosmetic result because of a poor contour match.

More favourable results on the tip of the nose may be achieved using a composite skin and fat graft from the forehead. These grafts give a much improved contour, although they are limited to defects no larger than about 1 cm, and are not as reliable as a vascularised forehead flap.

50.6.2 Local Flaps

Local flaps are useful to reconstruct smaller defects of the nasal tip, dorsum and sidewall. Caution is advised for defects within 0.5 cm of the alar margin because alar retraction can occur post-operatively. Distortion of the nasal tip, prominence of the main lobe and telangiectasia can be seen with bilobed flaps, particularly for larger defects. For this reason, some authorities prefer a composite skin and fat graft.

50.6.3 Pedicled Flaps

Large defects and those which are full thickness require a pedicled flap. These flaps generally provide a favourable skin match and contour. Two varieties are commonly used for nasal reconstruction.

1. Melolabial flap
   For the melolabial, also known as the nasolabial flap, skin from the cheek is rotated and used to reconstruct the nasal defect. The flap is interpolated, indicating that it bridges normal skin and the alar base. This is important, because

N

it preserves the nasofacial sulcus. This flap is particularly suited to smaller defects limited to the nasal alar. Where the defect extends to the alar margin, a cartilage graft is required to prevent retraction or notching of the nasal alar. The scar for this flap is placed in the melolabial crease and gives a favourable result in older patients with lax skin and a well-formed crease.

This flap is a relatively minor procedure compared to the forehead flap described later, and easier to live with between the first stage and flap division 4 weeks later. In younger patients without a formed melolabial crease the visible facial scar and cheek asymmetry make this flap far less suitable. The vascularity of this random pattern flap is also less reliable than the paramedian forehead flap, and caution is required before this flap is used in smokers.

2. Paramedian forehead flap
   Larger skin defects affecting the nasal tip, sidewall and dorsum are usually reconstructed using a paramedian forehead flap. This is the so-called 'workhorse' flap of nasal reconstruction and the whole of the nasal skin can be replaced with this flap if required. It is based on the supratrochlear artery. The flap is also interpolated, has a reliable vascularity, and the forehead skin has a good colour and texture match to the adjacent nasal skin. The resulting

donor site scar is also favourable if the forehead is closed with meticulous surgical technique. Although the forehead flap can be divided as early as 2 weeks, it is recommended to be patient and divide the flap at 4 weeks to give the optimum result.

50.7 Refinement Procedures

A number of patients require subsequent refinement procedures which are best delayed for several months to allow swelling to settle, wound contraction and scar maturation. Following reconstruction of the nasal alar and sidewall, creation of an alar crease may be required as a secondary procedure. This relatively minor procedure may be performed under local anaesthetic and the improved symmetry imparts a major aesthetic enhancement to the reconstruction result.

Further Reading

Baker SR, Nafficy S. Principles of Nasal Reconstruction. St Louis, MO: Mosby; 2002

Burget GC, Menick FJ. Aesthetic Reconstruction of the Nose. St Louis, MO: Mosby Year Book; 1994

Related Topics of Interest

Reconstructive surgery
Rhinoplasty

N

51 Nasal Trauma

The commonest causes of nasal trauma are assault, road traffic accident and sports injuries. Injury to the nose may result in a combination of soft tissue injury, fracture of the nasal bones, fracture or dislocation of the septum, septal haematoma, cerebrospinal fluid (CSF) leak and facial bone fracture. Evidence shows nasal bone fractures may be mobile up to about 3 weeks' post-injury and manipulation under anaesthesia (MUA) may be successful up to 27 days post-injury.

51.1 Classification of Fracture of the Nasal Bones

An isolated nasal fracture is usually caused by low-velocity trauma. If the nose is fractured by high-velocity trauma, then facial fractures are often an accompaniment. Nasal fractures are classified on a 1 to 3 scale depending on their severity and extent.

- Class 1 fracture: Usually due to a frontal or fronto-lateral blow and results in a vertical fracture of the septum (Chevallet's septal fracture) with a unilateral depressed or displaced distal portion of the nasal bone.

- Class 2 fracture: Nearly always due to lateral trauma and results in a horizontal (Jarjavay's septal fracture) or C-shaped fracture of the septum involving the perpendicular plate of the ethmoid and the septal cartilage in combination with a fracture of the frontal process of the maxillae. The fracture therefore involves displacement of both nasal bones to the side opposite the blow.

- Class 3 fracture: Indicates that the velocity of the trauma has been even greater and results in a nasal fracture which extends to include the ethmoid labyrinth. The perpendicular plate of the ethmoid rotates backward and the septum concertinas into the face, raising the tip of the nose and revealing the nostrils. There is a marked depression of the nasal bones, which are pushed under the frontal bones, and there is an apparent widening of the space between the eyes (telecanthus).

51.2 Clinical Features

Trauma to the nose may be part of a more extensive injury to the facial skeleton and base of skull.

It should be remembered that the most important consideration in maxillofacial injuries is the maintenance of an airway. A history of trauma to the midface accompanied by epistaxis, a noticeable nasal deformity and nasal airway obstruction are the usual complaints. Nasofrontoethmoid fractures may produce symptoms of diplopia and epiphora. It is important to carefully record the time and nature of the trauma, previous episodes of nasal or facial trauma, and whether the nasal deformity is new or old. Trauma to the head and neck should be noted as should any other injuries. Tenderness, periorbital and/or facial haematoma and soft tissue swelling of the nose, face and periorbital areas may make the initial assessment difficult. It is appropriate in uncomplicated cases to reassess the patient 5 to 10 days after the injury. The nasal swelling is often accompanied by periorbital and sub-conjunctival ecchymosis.

The most difficult injury to assess and therefore the easiest to misdiagnose is the class 1 injury. Here, there is a depressed fracture of the injured side but not of the opposite nasal bone. If there is minimal nasal/facial soft tissue swelling, this may give the false impression of the whole nasal skeleton being deviated to the side opposite the injury. This may result in the surgeon at an MUA, trying to push a fixed uninjured contralateral bone towards the midline rather than elevating the depressed fracture on the injured side. A class 1 fracture may be missed if there is more significant facial oedema because the position of the depressed segment may be masked by the oedema, giving the impression of just a soft tissue injury. One can therefore appreciate the importance of not just observing the nasal shape, but palpating the nasal bones when standing behind a seated patient and asking oneself is this a class 1 or a class 2 fracture.

A class 2 fracture results in the whole nasal skeleton (i.e., both nasal bones) being displaced. This is sometimes a fracture where the left and right nasal bones move as a single fragment and in this case an MUA might just involve pushing this fragment back into position. Commonly, however, there is also a depressed fracture of the side subject to the blow and in these cases the MUA must also involve elevating and stabilising this depressed segment. If the depressed fracture is missed, the patient will have a residual and noticeable nasal bone deformity. This is one of the reasons why class

N

2 fractures can be associated with an unsatisfactory position after an MUA. Some class 2 fractures, however, are unstable and may redisplace because of an overlapping septal fracture. The nasal septum should be carefully examined to determine if there is any deformity or septal haematoma. The septum may be difficult to assess because of oedema; gentle probing of the septum with a Jobson Horne speculum will allow a more accurate assessment of whether a septal haematoma is present. Ocular movements should be tested and fifth nerve function (infra-orbital sensation) and dental occlusion should be checked. All injuries should be carefully documented contemporaneously in the case notes, supplemented with drawings and occasionally photographs. The documentation is not only good medical practice, but may be important for medicolegal purposes.

51.3 Investigations

In most simple uncomplicated fractures, no investigations are required, but in more serious injuries, radiographs are the most important investigation. They should include views of the skull, face and nasal bones depending on the extent and severity of the injury. They may be important for medicolegal purposes. A computed tomography (CT) scan on bone setting may delineate maxillo-facial fractures when there is uncertainty.

51.4 Management

51.4.1 Soft Tissue Injury

Wounds are thoroughly cleaned and any foreign bodies removed. Appropriate antibiotic and antitetanus cover should be given. Abrasions are best left open. Small lacerations can be closed with Steri-Strips, but larger lacerations should be closed with fine monofilament sutures. Lacerations through the upper and lower nasal cartilages should be treated by closing the wound in layers, the cartilage being opposed with fine absorbable monofilament sutures such as Monocryl or PDS.

51.4.2 Nasal Fracture

- Treatment is not required in some patients because there is no fracture or bony deformity. These patients should be reassured and reviewed again when the swelling has subsided.

It is also inappropriate to try and manipulate a long-standing deformity as this will result in a failure to reduce.

- It is possible to reduce a simple class 1 fracture under local anaesthetic before any swelling appears if it is seen early enough. Disimpaction and realignment can usually be achieved with laterally applied digital pressure and Walsham's forceps, one blade in the nasal cavity and the other outside (with skin protection). If the fracture is seen later and there is much swelling, manipulation should be delayed for 5 to 7 days. Manipulation should ideally be performed at 10 to 14 days post-injury because the nasal bones may fix after this. Recent evidence suggests, however, that many nasal fractures are still reducible up to 27 days after injury, so the cut-off for attempting an MUA can be raised to nearly 4 weeks from the date of injury.

- Class 2 fractures have a propensity to redisplace owing to overlapping of the fractured ends of the septal cartilage and the perpendicular plate of the ethmoid. Some authorities therefore suggest manipulation of the nasal bone should be accompanied by an excision of the septal fracture and overlapping segments. The problem with this is that the septum is often very difficult to assess in the first few weeks after injury due to septal oedema taking 3 to 4 weeks to settle. Also, if an attempt is made to perform a septoplasty at this stage, the mucoperichondrial flaps are friable and tear easily. Moreover, the septal cartilage will be subject to further trauma and another month of healing. Some authorities argue that this increases the risk of cartilage resorption and a residual dorsal nasal saddle. Most experienced ENT surgeons would therefore just perform an MUA of the nasal bones and assess the residual septal deformity 3 months post-injury.

- A class 3 fracture will require an open reduction. The depressed nasal bones need to be disimpacted and elevated into position. The bones are then supported with wires via an incision over the nasofrontal angle. The septum is approached through a Cottle incision with the aim of pulling the rotated septal cartilage forward and downward. Malunion following nasal trauma will require treatment by a formal septorhinoplasty.

N

51.4.3 Septal Haematoma

Blood may collect beneath the mucoperichondrium of the nasal septum. It may follow nasal trauma, but it can also occur as a complication of septoplasty surgery and, rarely, blood dyscrasias. There is a unilateral boggy nasal swelling that may completely occlude one nostril. Bilateral nasal obstruction may also occur, caused by a soft swelling on one side of the septum displacing the opposite side or if there is cartilage necrosis. If this is missed or not treated correctly, a septal abscess, further cartilage necrosis, and a saddle deformity may ensue. Aspiration may suffice if the haematoma is small, but incision and drainage with quilt suturing (to obliterate the dead space) is required for most haematomas or if a small collection re-accumulates. The patient should be given a course of antibiotics to reduce the risk of a secondary septal abscess.

51.4.4 Cerebrospinal Fluid Leak

The presence of clear rhinorrhoea at any stage following nasal trauma should raise the suspicion of a CSF leak. The cribriform plate is extremely thin and is the commonest area of fracture. Confirmation of the diagnosis is obtained by testing a sample of the fluid for the presence of β_2-transferrin (this is a protein present in perilymph and CSF). Fluorescein injected into the CSF via a lumbar puncture can be collected from the leak in the nose. A high-resolution (0.5 mm) coronal CT scan of the anterior skull base may delineate the fracture. Until the leak ceases, the patient is at a small risk of meningitis and pneumococcal and meningococcal vaccination is advised. Some leaks will close spontaneously with a week or two of bed rest in the 30-degree head up position, but some will require surgical repair (see Chapter 32, Functional Endoscopic Sinus Surgery).

Further Reading

Perkins V, Vijendren A, Egan M, McRae D. Optimal timing for nasal fracture manipulation—Is a 2-week target really necessary? A single-centre retrospective analysis of 50 patients. Clin Otolaryngol. 2017; 42(6):1377–1381

Rohrich RJ, Adams WP Jr. Nasal fracture management: minimizing secondary nasal deformities. Plast Reconstr Surg. 2000; 106(2):266–273

Related Topics of Interest

Examination of the nose
Septal perforation
Functional endoscopic sinus surgery

N

52   Nasopharyngeal Tumours

The nasopharynx (also known as the post-nasal space) is situated behind the nasal cavities. It is the upper one-third of the pharynx and separated from the oropharynx below by the superior surface of the soft palate. The undersurface of the body of the sphenoid bone forms the roof of the nasopharynx as it slants inferiorly to form the posterior wall in front of the atlas and axis vertebrae. The lateral wall of the nasopharynx is formed by the opening of the eustachian tubes superiorly and the superior constrictor muscle inferiorly. The space formed by the eustachian tube opening and posterior wall of the nasopharynx is the fossa of Rosenmüller.

Nasopharyngeal tumours can be described under four specific groups:

1. Nasopharyngeal carcinoma (NPC).
2. Other nasopharyngeal tumours (e.g., lymphoma, salivary gland tumours).
3. Angiofibroma.
4. Adenoids (see Chapter 1, Adenoids).

52.1 Nasopharyngeal Carcinoma

52.1.1 Pathology

NPC is rare in Western populations (1 per 100,000 population) but has a predilection for those of Southern Chinese (Cantonese) or Hong Kong extraction (20–30 per 100,000 population) forming 20% of all malignancies in these people and 80% of their head and neck cancers. Migrating members of these communities maintain their increased risk. It is more common in men, and although it can occur in young patients (< 30 years of age), it has an average presentation of 50 years of age. NPC can be divided into three subtypes based on the World Health Organization (WHO) classification, which divides the cancer based on its light microscopic appearance.

- Type 1: Keratinising squamous cell carcinoma (SCC).
- Type 2: (a) Non-keratinising SCC (b) undifferentiated carcinoma.
- Type 3: Basaloid SCC.

Non-keratinising SCC is the commonest in both high- and low-incidence areas.

52.2 Aetiology

The consensus view is that in the genetically predisposed, a carcinogen is triggered by an environmental cofactor to transform nasopharyngeal epithelial cells. This appears to be an interaction between the environmental, immunological and genetic factors.

Environmental: The environmental factor most widely implicated is salted preserved fish (containing dimethylnitrosamine), a staple diet of the Hong Kong boat people, the male population of which comprises the world's highest at-risk population group.

Immunological: Latent Epstein–Barr virus (EBV) infection is endemic in this group and the evidence for EBV being the carcinogen is compelling. Southern blot and polymerase chain reaction consistently detect DNA sequences of EBV in NPC cells. NPC cells consistently express two species of EBV proteins; EB nuclear antigen 1 and latent membrane protein 1 detectable by immunofluorescence. Plasma antibodies to *viral capsid antigen* and to *early antigens* (one of which is an EBV DNAse) are seen, titres of the latter have been cited as a potential predictor of tumour relapse after radiotherapy. EBV is associated with all types of NPC but is more commonly present in the non-keratinising types. EBV is an interesting virus and is associated with other tumours and diseases including the following:

- Burkitt's lymphoma (a monoclonal B-cell non-Hodgkin's lymphoma).
- T-cell lymphoma.
- Hodgkin's lymphoma.
- Infectious mononucleosis.

Genetic factors: The human leucocyte antigen allele A2 without BW46 or B17 is associated with long-term survival. The A2 BW46 allele combination is associated with intermediate-term survival while the occurrence of B17 is associated with short-term survival.

52.3 Clinical Features

NPC usually arises from the fossa of Rosenmüller and patients typically present with a mixture of

N

nasal and ear symptoms, often combined with a neck mass and occasionally cranial neuropathies:

- Nasal symptoms: Nasal obstruction, discharge, epistaxis.
- Lymphadenopathy: Seventy percent of patients will have metastatic lymph node involvement at presentation and in a large Hong Kong series this was the mode of presentation in 40% of patients.
- Ear symptoms: Hearing loss due to otitis media with effusion. Referred otalgia.
- Cranial nerve neuropathies: Cranial spread can cause cranial nerve palsies to II, III, IV, V, and VI and laterally spread to the parapharyngeal space damaging V, IX, X, XI, and XII. When a tumour has become so advanced, patients will typically have mandibular nerve paralysis with partial loss of facial, palatal and pharyngeal sensation and involvement of the pterygoid musculature causing trismus. Involvement of the cervical sympathetic trunk and the ninth to twelfth cranial nerves causes Horner's syndrome, vocal cord, pharyngeal, palatal, shoulder and tongue paralysis and pain. Paralysis of III and IV and upper two divisions of the fifth cranial nerves will cause diplopia, facial hypoaesthesia and headaches.

NPC may present as a cancer of unknown primary. It often spreads submucosally from the fossa of Rosenmüller so that no nasopharyngeal abnormality is visible, although there may be metastatic lymph node disease. Adult patients who present with a unilateral middle ear effusion and/or a neck mass should be treated with suspicion and caution. Endoscopic examination of the nasopharynx with attention to the fossa of Rosenmüller is mandatory.

52.4 Investigations

Ultrasound-guided fine-needle aspiration biopsy (USSgFNAB) should be undertaken on all patients who present with a neck node. The polymerase chain reaction to EB virus genome has been used to diagnose NPC in patients with a malignant neck node with an occult primary.

Computed tomography (CT) and magnetic resonance imaging (MRI) scans are complementary. CT is the investigation of choice to assess skull base and paranasal sinus involvement. MRI imaging including a short tau inversion recovery (STIR) sequence to suppress fat clearly defines the tumour margins in soft tissue and will best define

meningeal/cranial involvement and the presence and extent of metastatic neck disease.

In the assessment of distant metastases, CT of chest and upper abdomen has now been surpassed using positron emission tomography CT (PET-CT), which is now recommended by NICE guidelines for NPC.

A biopsy of the fossa of Rosenmüller is obtained under either a local or general anaesthetic. In cases presenting with a cancer of unknown primary, it may be necessary to perform targeted biopsies of the area. Biopsies should be done after staging scans to avoid false artefacts.

52.5 Staging

Several staging systems have been developed for NPC which has made it difficult to compare treatment results using differing modalities and results between centres. In contrast to other sites of the head and neck, N staging is different for NPC reflecting the different pathology of these tumours. The eighth edition of the UICC/AJCC staging system is as follows:

52.5.1 T Stage

T1   Tumour confined to nasopharynx or extends to oropharynx and/or nasal cavity without parapharyngeal involvement.

T2   Tumour with extension to parapharyngeal space and/or infiltration of the medial pterygoid, lateral pterygoid and/or prevertebral muscles.

T3   Tumour invades bony structures of skull base cervical vertebra, pterygoid structures and/or paranasal sinuses.

T4   Tumour with intra-cranial extension and/or involvement of cranial nerves, hypopharynx, orbit, parotid gland and/or infiltration beyond the lateral surface of the lateral pterygoid muscle.

52.5.2 N Stage

NX   Regional lymph nodes cannot be assessed.

N0   No regional lymph node metastasis.

N1   Unilateral metastasis, in cervical lymph node(s), and/or unilateral or bilateral metastasis in retropharyngeal lymph nodes, 6 cm or less in greatest dimension, above the caudal border of cricoid cartilage.

N

N2 Bilateral metastasis in cervical lymph node(s), 6 cm or less in greatest dimension, above the caudal border of cricoid cartilage.

N3 Metastasis in cervical lymph node(s) greater than 6 cm in dimension and/or extension below the caudal border of cricoid cartilage.

Stage grouping is based on the TNM status:

Stage I	T1	N0	M0
Stage II	T1	N1	M0
	T2	N0, N1	M0
Stage III	T1, T2	N2	M0
	T3	N0, N1, N2	M0
Stage IVA	T4	N0, N1, N2	M0
Stage IVA	Any T	N3	M0
Stage IVB	Any T	Any N	M1

52.6 Management

Radiotherapy (RT) is the mainstay for the treatment of nasopharyngeal carcinoma. Intensity-modulated radiotherapy (IMRT) facilitates dosimetric coverage of the tumour volume and sparing of normal organs, including the parotid gland, reducing the risk of xerostomia, thereby improving quality of life. There is evidence confirming improvement in overall survival in patients treated concurrently with chemoradiation (CRT) compared with RT alone. Cisplatin is usually used concurrently with radiation and a combination of cisplatin and fluorouracil may be used in the neoadjuvant setting. The most commonly used chemotherapy schedule is cisplatin 100 mg/m^2 on days 1, 22 and 43 of RT.

Surgery plays a limited role in the treatment of NPC. It is used to obtain tissue from the nasopharynx for diagnosis, for biopsy of neck node (USSgFNAB or core biopsy), and possibly to deal with otitis media with effusion. The rate of otorrhoea is higher if grommets are inserted after RT, so repeated paracentesis, aspiration and a hearing aid are recommended instead. Radical neck dissection may control radio-resistant nodes and post-radiation cervical node recurrence. In selected patients, salvage surgery may be indicated for nasopharyngeal recurrence.

Stages I and II Patients with early disease can be treated with RT alone (IMRT should be used) with disease-free survival rates of 85 to 90%. The dose to the primary tumour should be 70 Gy in 35 fraction and at least 50 Gy in 25 fraction to the bilateral neck. Patients with Stage II disease who are N1 (T1/T2 N1) can be treated with RT alone but will often have CRT. It has been shown that IMRT alone has as good results as CRT in Stage II disease and with less toxicity.

Stages III and IV Concurrent CRT is the standard for care of advanced nasopharyngeal carcinoma. Five-year survival rates are 50 to 60%. A dose of 70 Gy with concurrent cisplatin is used. The field will include the target volume of gross tumour, the nasopharynx and pterygopalatine fossa, the skull base and clivus, the sphenoid and posterior ethmoid sinuses and posterior nasal cavity, retropharyngeal lymph nodes and the parapharyngeal space. Prophylactic irradiation must include elective treatment of uninvolved levels I to V.

Residual and recurrent disease Surgery for recurrence is associated with less morbidity than re-irradiation. Nasopharyngectomy and neck dissection are the first options for locoregional residual disease or recurrence. A variety of approaches to the nasopharynx have been used. Transcranial approaches have a high morbidity, transnasal and transantral approaches give poor access, but endoscopic resection of smaller recurrences is possible. The anterolateral approach with maxillary swing is probably the most used and gives the best access. Recurrent and residual neck disease is likely to require a radical neck dissection as there will be a high likelihood of extracapsular spread of disease. Free flap and pedicled flaps may be required to replace skin and brachytherapy wires may be used. Re-irradiation can be used for local recurrences but should be considered as a second-line treatment.

52.7 Follow-Up and Aftercare

Assessment of treatment response should be by endoscopic examination and neck palpation and a baseline MRI and PET-CT scan at 3 months. It can take up to 3 months for NPC to disappear histologically, which can make interpretation of post-treatment biopsies difficult and there needs to be caution in diagnosis of residual/recurrent disease.

52.8 Other Nasopharyngeal Tumours

- Non-Hodgkin's lymphoma.
- Extra-medullary plasmacytoma (predilection for the nasopharynx and paranasal sinuses).
- Paediatric nasopharyngeal tumours: ectodermal (dermoids, teratomas); neuroectodermal (encephalocele, meningocele); dysontogenetic (craniopharyngioma, chordoma).

N

52.9 Angiofibroma

Angiofibroma occurs almost exclusively in young adult males, and although benign, it is locally aggressive. It is histologically benign and comprises fibrous tissue with a variable proportion of vascular tissue, often with large endothelial spaces. Tumour blood vessels typically lack smooth muscle and elastin fibres, which contribute to its propensity for bleeding. It arises from the postero-lateral wall of the nasal cavity and the superolateral nasopharyngeal wall. The sphenopalatine foramen, pterygopalatine fossa and choanae are the usual sites of tumour origin.

52.9.1 Clinical Features

The tumour expands to erode or compress surrounding fissures, foramina and tissues. The commonest symptoms are epistaxis and nasal obstruction. It may expand laterally into the pterygo-palatine fossa, through the pterygo-maxillary fissure and into the infra-temporal fossa, expanding superiorly to erode the pterygoid plates, the greater wing of the sphenoid and the skull base foramen. Anterosuperior expansion into the nasal cavity, paranasal sinuses, parasellar region, cavernous sinus and orbit may also occur. Presenting signs are similar to NPC except there is a smooth mass filling the nasopharynx on endo-scopic or mirror examination. A high index of suspicion for any nasopharyngeal mass is essential because angiofibroma should not, as a rule, be biopsied as it may cause significant haemorrhage that may be difficult to control. In particular, it must not be confused with a large adenoid pad.

52.9.2 Investigations and Treatment

An MRI scan is the investigation of choice to define the extent and vascularity of the tumour. Typically, a lobulated non-encapsulated soft tissue mass is demonstrated centreed on the sphenopalatine foramen. A T1 image will show an intermediate signal, T2 a heterogeneous signal, where flow voids appear dark and gadolinium contrast shows prominent enhancement. The presence of prominent flow voids leads to a 'salt and pepper appearance' on most sequences and are characteristic. CT is particularly useful at delineating bony changes. Digital subtraction angiography shows the branches of the external carotid system to be the primary feeders (94%). The main supply comes from the internal maxillary artery, but ascending pharyngeal or vidian arteries may contribute to the blood supply. Surgery is the treatment of choice for all but the smallest tumours as they may continue to expand and are typically poorly radio-sensitive. The feeding vessels should be embolised 1 to 2 days pre-operatively.

Endoscopic surgery is the approach of choice in early stages (Fisch I and II), whereas, in advanced disease (Fisch III and IV) open and/or endo-scopic approaches are feasible. Tumours limited to the nasal cavity, nasopharynx, ethmoid and sphenoid sinus endoscopic methods compare favourably with external approaches with significantly reduced morbidity. In tumours of greater extent, a midfacial degloving or, if the cribriform plate is involved, a craniofacial approach are most widely advocated and these may need to be combined with an infra-temporal approach. Post-operative radiotherapy or stereotactic radiosurgery is an option in long-term control of juvenile angiofibroma, particularly those that extend to anatomically critical areas unsuitable for complete resection, but chemotherapy and hormone therapy are ineffective.

Further Reading

Baujat B, Audry H, Bourhis J, et al; MAC-NPC Collaborative Group. Chemotherapy in locally advanced nasopharyngeal carcinoma: an individual patient data meta-analysis of eight randomized trials and 1753 patients. Int J Radiat Oncol Biol Phys. 2006; 64(1):47–56

Lee AW, Ngan RK, Tung SY, et al. Preliminary results of trial NPC-0501 evaluating the therapeutic gain by changing from concurrent-adjuvant to induction-concurrent chemoradio-therapy, changing from fluorouracil to capecitabine, and changing from conventional to accelerated radiotherapy fractionation in patients with locoregionally advanced naso-pharyngeal carcinoma. Cancer. 2015; 121(8):1328–1338

López F, Triantafyllou A, Snyderman CH, et al. Nasal juvenile an-giofibroma: current perspectives with emphasis on manage-ment. Head Neck. 2017; 39(5):1033–1045

Simo R, Robinson M, Lei M, Sibtain A, Hickey S. Nasopharyn-geal carcinoma: United Kingdom National Multidisciplinary Guidelines. J Laryngol Otol. 2016; 130(S2):S97–S103

Xu C, Zhang LH, Chen YP, et al. Chemoradiotherapy versus ra-diotherapy alone in stage ii nasopharyngeal carcinoma: a systemic review and meta-analysis of 2138 patients. J Cancer. 2017; 8(2):287–297

Related Topics of Interest

Adenoids
Cervical lymphadenopathy

N

53 Neck Dissection

A primary carcinoma arising from the upper aerodigestive tract may ultimately drain into the lymph nodes of the neck, which forms an efficient barrier to the further spread of the disease. The prognosis for the patient regardless of the site of the primary tumour is worse if there are cervical lymph nodes involved at presentation. Only 50% of such patients will survive longer than 5 years.

Treatment of cervical lymph nodes is either elective (in the clinically negative neck) or therapeutic (in the clinically positive neck). The modality chosen is usually the same as that used for the primary tumour. The surgical treatment of malignant neck nodes is by some form of neck dissection (ND). Broadly speaking, radiotherapy alone (RT) will only be effective in the curative treatment of cervical lymph node metastases if they are less than 2 cm in diameter. Concomitant chemotherapy (CR) is now advocated in advanced nodal disease, with the advantage that it precludes the need and morbidity of surgery, which can be kept in reserve for the treatment of any recurrence.

The choice of treatment modality and when it should be used can be controversial. It is a subject of debate in many multidisciplinary team (MDT) meetings. The discussion regarding elective (prophylactic) therapy in the N0 neck is now supplemented, in oral cavity cancer, by the increasing role of sentinel node biopsy. Furthermore, in cases treated by neck dissection as primary modality, there may be a requirement for adjuvant treatment. The rupture of the lymph node capsule by tumour (extracapsular spread [ECS]) is a bad prognostic sign. Fifty percent of nodes with a diameter greater than 3 cm exhibit this. Post-operative RT or CR to the neck following neck dissection is indicated in the presence of ECS and positive surgical margins.

53.1 Classification

The classification suggested by the American Academy's Committee for Head and Neck Surgery and Oncology is still used, but there is an increasing trend to divide neck dissections into two broad types with subdivisions: comprehensive (removal of levels I–V) and selective (less than five levels). The need for less extensive surgery in the chemoradiation era has led to calls for revision of the system. Radical neck dissection is the standard basic procedure, and all others represent one or more alterations to this procedure. Modified radical neck dissection involves the preservation of one or more non-lymphatic structures routinely removed in radical neck dissection. Selective neck dissection (SND) involves the preservation of one or more lymph node groups routinely removed in radical neck dissection. Extended radical neck dissection involves removal of additional lymph node groups or non-lymphatic structures relative to the radical neck dissection (i.e., a superior mediastinal dissection in patients with subglottic or cervical oesophageal tumours).

1. Radical neck dissection.
2. Modified radical neck dissection.
3. Selective neck dissection.

(a) Supraomohyoid neck dissection. (b) Posterolateral neck dissection. (c) Lateral neck dissection. (d) Anterior compartment neck dissection.

4. Extended radical neck dissection.

53.1.1 Radical Neck Dissection

This operation refers to the removal of lymph nodes in the anterior and posterior triangles extending from the inferior border of the mandible superiorly to the clavicle inferiorly, the midline anteriorly and the anterior border of the trapezius muscle posteriorly. The cervical lymph node groups routinely removed are as follows: submental and submandibular; upper, middle and lower jugular (deep cervical); and the posterior triangle group. The submandibular gland, spinal accessory nerve, internal jugular vein and sternocleidomastoid muscle are also removed. Extended radical neck dissection consists of removal of all the structures in a radical neck dissection along with one or more additional lymph node groups (e.g., retropharyngeal nodes, parotid nodes, levels VI/VII) or non-lymphatic structures (e.g., parotid gland, hypoglossal nerve, digastric muscle, external carotid artery or skin) or both.

53.1.2 Modified Radical Neck Dissection

Modified radical neck dissection (MRND) consists of a monobloc removal of the cervical lymph nodes from levels I through V as with an RND. The procedure is modified by preservation of just the accessory nerve (Type I) or the accessory nerve and internal jugular vein (Type II), or the accessory nerve, internal jugular vein and sternocleidomastoid muscle (Type III), see ▶ Table 53.1.

The jugular vein preservation is of great importance when bilateral neck dissections need to be performed, but the main advantage from this procedure is that the risk of frozen shoulder (due to accessory nerve resection) is avoided. MRND is considered to result in regional control rates similar to those achieved by RND if patients are carefully selected. It is known in patients with a positive node that the risk of occult metastases in apparently uninvolved levels of the neck is high. Level V is the least likely to be involved (3–7% involvement in RND specimens).

53.1.3 Selective Neck Dissection

SNDs are based on the knowledge of predictability and distribution of nodal metastases from the different primary sites. SND is effective as MRND for controlling regional disease in N0 neck for all primary sites. Prophylactic SND neck is now advocated in the patient who has a primary tumour

▶ **Table 53.1** Modified radical neck dissection classification

Type I	Spinal accessory nerve preservation
Type II	Spinal accessory nerve and internal jugular vein preservation
Type III	Spinal accessory nerve, internal jugular vein and sternomastoid preservation

▶ **Table 53.2** Procedures, levels, and indications for patients with N0 disease

Type	Levels	Indication
Supraomohyoid dissection	I, II, and III	Oral cavity tumours
Lateral neck dissection	II, III, and IV	Larynx and hypopharynx
Posterolateral neck dissection	II, III, IV, and V	Skin tumours (SCC, melanoma)
Anterior compartment	VI	Thyroid cancer

Abbreviation: SCC, squamous cell carcinoma.

with a high incidence (> 15–20%) of occult nodes (oral cavity, oropharynx, supraglottic larynx and hypopharynx). This in fact includes almost all primary sites except for T1 and T2 glottic cancers and T1 oral cavity. Thus, for patients with N0 disease, ▶ Table 53.2 describes procedures that are an option, which levels are dissected and what the common indications are.

The levels or sublevels removed during SND should be precisely stated in the operation notes, and the pathology specimen clearly marked. There is good evidence for reduced long-term morbidity with SND compared to the comprehensive types (MRND and RND). There is often debate as to when to dissect level 2b lymph nodes as there is additional morbidity incurred by skeletonising the spinal accessory nerve.

53.2 Complications of Neck Dissection

1. Immediate.
   - Haemorrhage (from either end of the internal jugular vein or other ligated vessel).
   - Chyle leak may occur if the thoracic duct has been inadvertently damaged. If noticed intra-operatively, this should be repaired immediately. If noted in post-operative period, the patient should have a non-fat diet and a non-suction drain inserted. Parenteral nutrition and return to theatre may be required.
   - Nerve palsies (phrenic, vagus, marginal mandibular branch of the facial, lingual, hypoglossal, sympathetic trunk, brachial plexus). The risk of marginal mandibular nerve damage can be reduced by ensuring the plane of dissection over the submandibular gland is deep to the investing layer of capsular fascia. Ligating the facial vein and raising the flap deep to the vein will also help avoid injury to the nerve. The accessory nerve is best identified at the upper end of the internal jugular vein and followed through the sternomastoid muscle. It can be identified as it enters the posterior triangle at Erb's point, which is 1 cm superior to where the greater auricular nerve curves over the posterior border of the sternomastoid muscle. The phrenic nerve can be protected if dissection of the posterior triangle is performed superficial to the prevertebral fascia which covers the nerve.

N

2. Intermediate.
   - Facial oedema.
   - Cerebral oedema (usually after a synchronous or staged bilateral neck dissection).
   - Wound infection.
   - Wound breakdown (poor surgical technique, previous radiotherapy, diabetes, poor nutritional status).
   - Rupture of the carotid artery (may be a sequel to wound breakdown).

3. Late.
   - Frozen shoulder due to accessory nerve damage. It is less likely to occur if the cervical nerve branches of C3 and C4 are preserved as they pass under the fascia of the floor of the posterior triangle and communicate with the accessory nerve or supply trapezius directly.
   - Lymphoedema will usually settle over time with massage.
   - Recurrence in the glands or skin.

53.3 Consent for Neck Dissection

Patients should be consented for the anaesthetic and general risks of operation (wounds, drains, haematoma, infection and numbness) and procedure-specific risks to cranial nerves (marginal mandibular, lingual, hypoglossal, accessory and vagus), wound breakdown, chyle leak, brachial plexus risk, phrenic nerve risk and carotid artery damage (stroke and death). They should be consented for the possibility of further treatments including RT/chemoradiotherapy (CRT).

53.4 Bilateral Neck Dissection

The possibility of bilateral nodal disease should be considered especially when the primary site involves the tongue base, nasopharynx or supraglottic larynx, or when the primary site crosses the midline. The presence of bilateral neck nodes is not an independent poor prognostic sign, but there is a reduced 5-year survival. The use of RT and CRT has reduced the need for bilateral surgery, but it is still necessary when surgery is chosen for treatment of the primary site and when there is recurrence/residual disease after CRT.

Most cases of bilateral dissection will have a MRND or SND. Bilateral synchronous RND would be a rare undertaking now and carries a significant morbidity and a mortality of about 3%. Many of the complications can be reduced by either staging the procedure with an interval of 6 weeks or longer or performing a modified procedure on the opposite side to preserve the internal jugular vein. The most serious complication is that of raised intra-cranial pressure. Ligation of one internal jugular vein results in a threefold increase in the intra-cranial pressure, but when the second side is tied, there is a tenfold increase in pressure. In this instance, the patient should have a temporary tracheostomy, be nursed, propped up in the bed and may require an infusion of mannitol (500 mL of 10% mannitol over 4 hours). The most critical period is the first 12 hours post-operatively. Over the following 8 to 10 days after the operation, the intra-cranial pressure tends to fall, though it never returns to its normal level.

53.5 Salvage Neck Dissection

Many patients with N2/N3 disease will be treated with CRT as per positron emission tomography (PET) neck protocols. The current standard of care is a PET–computed tomography (PET-CT) performed 12 weeks following CRT and neck dissection being offered to those who have an equivocal or incomplete response. The extent of salvage neck dissection is a matter of debate, with an increasing trend to a limited neck clearance with the involved node level alone or an adjacent level. Management of advanced recurrence in the neck is contentious. Prognosis is poor and surgery complicated. RND may be used, but there is often increased morbidity in previously treated necks with a high risk of wound breakdown and need for free flap or pedicled pectoralis flap reconstruction. However, patients can live a considerable time with regional recurrence and intervention to prevent neck fungation as a palliative procedure to improve quality of life may be considered in specific cases.

Further Reading

D'Cruz AK, Vaish R, Kapre N, et al; Head and Neck Disease Management Group. Elective versus therapeutic neck dissection in node-negative oral cancer. N Engl J Med. 2015; 373(6):521–529

Ferlito A, Robbins KT, Shah JP, et al. Proposal for a rational classification of neck dissections. Head Neck. 2011; 33(3):445–450

Mehanna H, Wong WL, McConkey CC, et al; PET-NECK Trial Management Group. PET-CT surveillance versus neck dissection in advanced head and neck cancer. N Engl J Med. 2016; 374(15):1444–1454

N

Paleri V, Urbano TG, Mehanna H, et al. Management of neck metastases in head and neck cancer: United Kingdom National Multidisciplinary Guidelines. J Laryngol Otol. 2016; 130(S2):S161–S169

Robbins KT, Clayman G, Levine PA, et al; American Head and Neck Society. American Academy of Otolaryngology—Head and Neck Surgery. Neck dissection classification update: revisions proposed by the American Head and Neck Society and the American Academy of Otolaryngology-Head and Neck Surgery. Arch Otolaryngol Head Neck Surg. 2002; 128(7):751–758

Related Topics of Interest

Cervical lymphadenopathy
Hypopharyngeal carcinoma
Laryngeal carcinoma
Oral cavity carcinoma
Oropharyngeal carcinoma

N

54 Neck Swellings

Neck swellings are common findings that present in all age groups and represent a variety of diverse pathologies. The old surgical aphorism, 'consider the anatomical structures and then the pathology that can arise from these', is never more appropriate than when one contemplates the causes of a lump in the neck.

54.1 Anatomy

Several structures are palpable in the normal neck. In females, the cricoid cartilage is often the most palpable laryngeal structure; whereas in men, it is the thyroid cartilage. The mastoid tip is readily palpable behind the ear. Between the mastoid tip and the angle of the mandible, the transverse process of the C1 vertebra is sometimes palpable, especially in thin females. This is more likely in elderly patients when osteoarthritis can cause a slight rotation of the cervical spine. This leaves one side of the C1 transverse process prominent (neck slightly rotated to the left leaves a slightly prominent right side of C1 transverse process) and the other side a little retracted. This can be mistaken for a retromandibular parotid mass or hard upper cervical node. The carotid bulb or bifurcation can also be felt pulsating at about the level of the hyoid bone just underneath the sternocleidomastoid muscle (SCM) and can be mistaken as a mass.

Remember the normal glandular structures which are consistent in their location. The thyroid gland is a bilobed structure located along the midline of the neck, either side of the trachea, above the sternal notch and below the cricoid cartilage. The parotid gland is a pyramidal structure found in front of the ear or pinna, and extends from the cheek bone (zygomatic process of maxilla and zygomatic arch) above, down and behind to the mastoid tip, below into the upper neck near the hyoid bone and forward onto the cheek for about 2 to 3 cm. The submandibular gland is located below the posterior half of the mandible and above the hyoid bone. It does not extending beyond the angle of the mandible. It can readily be bimanually palpated intraorally between the fingers of both hands.

The SCM muscle joins the mastoid tip to the sternoclavicular joint and the medial one-third aspect of the clavicle. It is an important landmark dividing the neck into anterior and posterior triangles (▶ Fig. 54.1).

Within each side of the neck there are located more than 100 lymph nodes, usually impalpable, and distributed mainly along the jugular chain. They are located within each of the five clinically and anatomically described levels of the anterior neck and in the single but divided level in the posterior neck. The posterior border of the SCM separates the anterior neck from the posterior neck. There are other major structures within the neck, such as nerves, blood vessels, muscles, cartilages and bones. Knowledge of their anatomical outline should allow the examiner to consider any abnormal enlargement or swellings in each anatomical location to be included within a differential diagnosis.

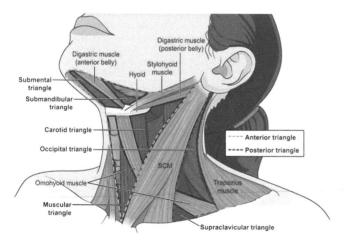

Fig. 54.1 Triangles of the neck. SCM, sternocleidomastoid. (Reproduced from Dyleski R, Linstrom C, Pitman M, et al. Anatomy of the neck. Total Otolaryngology. Head and Neck Surgery. 1st ed. New York, NY: Thieme; 2014.)

54.2 Differential Diagnosis

Reaching a diagnosis requires some knowledge of the potential pathology. It is difficult to present an exhaustive list of the potential causes of a neck swelling, but a simple classification is as follows:

- Congenital: lymphangiomas, dermoids, thyroglossal cysts.
- Developmental: branchial cysts, laryngoceles, pharyngeal pouches.
- Skin and subcutaneous tissue: sebaceous cyst, lipoma.
- Thyroid swellings: multi-nodular goitre, solitary thyroid nodule, firm/hard/woody thyroid swelling (possibly anaplastic carcinoma or thyroiditis).
- Salivary gland tumours: benign (e.g., pleomorphic adenoma, Warthin's tumour) or malignant tumour (e.g., mucoepidermoid, adenoid cystic).
- Tumours of the parapharyngeal space: deep lobe parotid tumour, chemodectoma.
- Reactive neck lymphadenopathy: tonsillitis, glandular fever, HIV.
- Malignant neck node: carcinoma metastases, carcinoma of unknown primary, lymphoma. In practical terms, the diagnosis is reached from the patient's age, the history, physical examination of the neck, the lump's location, a thorough examination of the upper aerodigestive tract and the results of appropriate tests and investigations.

54.3 Clinical Assessment

54.3.1 History

The first consideration should be the patient's age group. In general, neck masses in children and young adults are more commonly inflammatory than congenital and only occasionally neoplastic. However, the first consideration in the older adult should be that the mass is neoplastic. The duration of symptoms is one of the most important historical points. Inflammatory disorders are usually acute in onset and resolve within 2 to 6 weeks. Cervical lymphadenitis is often associated with a recent upper respiratory tract infection. In contrast, congenital masses are often present since birth as a small, asymptomatic mass which enlarges rapidly after a mild upper respiratory tract infection. Metastatic carcinoma tends to have a short history of progressive enlargement.

Transient post-prandial swelling in the submandibular or parotid area is suggestive of salivary gland duct obstruction. Bilateral diffuse tender parotid enlargement is suggestive of parotitis, most commonly mumps.

One must also be mindful that associated symptoms both specifically from the mass and from symptoms suggestive of a systemic process such as fever, night sweats, fatigue or weight loss (consider lymphoma) must be sought and documented. Symptoms of a sore throat or upper respiratory tract infection may suggest an inflammatory cervical lymphadenopathy. Persistent hoarseness of voice, sore throat, pain on swallowing, cough and sensation of a lump in the throat are risk symptoms of an upper aerodigestive tract malignancy. The symptoms are particularly relevant in patients who are over the age of 40 years and who smoke cigarettes.

54.3.2 Examination

A full head and neck examination including fibre-optic examination of mucosal surfaces of the pharynx and larynx is important, especially when suspecting a malignancy. The overlying skin colour and texture, and the location, mobility and consistency of a neck mass can often place it within a general aetiological group—congenital, nodal/inflammatory, vascular, salivary, thyroid or possibly neoplastic. Congenital masses may be tender when infected or inflamed, but are generally soft, smooth and mobile. A tender, mobile mass or a high suspicion of inflammatory adenopathy with an otherwise negative examination may warrant a clinical trial of a broad-spectrum antibiotic and a review after 2 weeks. Chronic inflammatory masses and lymphomas are often non-tender and rubbery and may be mobile or feel like a 'matted mass' of nodules. In older age groups, the submandibular and parotid glands may become ptotic (droopy) and mimic a neck mass, and can cause concern to patients.

54.4 Investigations

Ultrasound scan can delineate the position, size and sometimes the nature of a neck lump. It may delineate impalpable nodes and thyroid nodules. It can help diagnose a thyroglossal cyst and confirm the presence of a normal-looking thyroid gland prior to excision. The shape of a lymph node

N

(normally oval with a fatty hilum) can be altered by malignant disease (round shape with irregular margins and infiltrated hilum). Although ultrasound (US) is performed with a view to guiding an ultrasound-guided fine-needle aspiration biopsy (USSgFNAB) it should be noted that a biopsy may not be indicated if the size and nature of the lump is obviously benign. An inadequate biopsy may require a repeat USSgFNAB, a US-guided core biopsy or even an open biopsy, depending on the clinical picture.

A computed tomography (CT) scan can distinguish cystic from solid lesions, define the origin and full extent of deep, ill-defined masses, and when used with contrast can delineate vascularity or blood flow. Magnetic resonance imaging (MRI) is useful for parapharyngeal and skull base masses and for assessment for unknown primary carcinomas. With contrast, it is good for vascular delineation and MRI angiography may substitute for arteriography in the pulsatile mass or mass with a bruit or thrill. A positron emission tomography CT (PET-CT) scan is the investigation of choice in a patient with an unknown primary cancer.

Blood tests may help in specific circumstances. This will usually include a full blood count (FBC) and erythrocyte sedimentation rate (ESR). Viral serology (Epstein–Barr virus, cytomegalovirus, and toxoplasmosis) may be useful and patients with a thyroid nodule should have thyroid function tests.

Cervical lymphadenopathy, thyroid nodules and salivary gland tumours are topics covered in other chapters.

54.5 Haemangiomas

These are common congenital lesions usually presenting within the first year of life and often resolve spontaneously within the first decade. They are thought to be the result of hyperplasia of endothelial cells. Haemangiomas often appear bluish on the overlying skin and are compressible. Diagnosis is usually clinical, but MRI may help define the extent of the lesion, especially when involving the airway. Treatment is generally non-surgical and to await spontaneous resolution. The aggressive proliferative type has been treated using propranolol orally, but this must be given under specialist hospital care because of its side effects. The duration of treatment remains controversial but should be given until the expected proliferative phase has elapsed.

Steroids are an option and surgery is only reserved for haemangiomas potentially obstructing or damaging adjacent structures (the eye or airway).

54.6 Lymphangiomas

These are formed from abnormalities of lymphatic channels. There are three types of lymphangioma: simple (thin-walled channels), cavernous (dilated lymphatic spaces) and cystic hygroma (cysts of varying sizes). Simple and cavernous lesions arise principally in the lips, cheek and floor of the mouth. Cystic hygromas usually arise in the lower neck. Lymphangiomas usually remain unchanged into adulthood. A lymphangioma mass is usually an asymptomatic soft, doughy, ill-defined and rarely present with pressure effects. Ultrasound and/or MRI scan may be useful to confirm the diagnosis. Not all lesions need intervention and can be observed, but treatment with surgical excision or injection of sclerosants can be used. Surgical removal is generally considered to be the treatment of choice. Picibanil (OK-432) is a lyophilised mixture of group A *Streptococcus pyogenes* with a capacity to produce a selective fibrosis of lymphangiomas.

54.7 Sebaceous Cysts

These are common masses presenting in all age groups. They are slow growing but may become fluctuant and painful when infected. Diagnosis is made clinically; the overlying skin is adherent to the underlying mass and a punctum is often seen. Excisional biopsy confirms the diagnosis and is curative.

54.8 Lipoma

Lipomas or fatty lumps are the most common benign soft tissue tumour in the neck. They present as a poorly defined, soft mass usually presenting after the fourth decade. They are usually discreet, asymptomatic, soft to palpate and deep to the skin. Occasionally they can grow very large and be deeply seated between muscles and nerves. An US or MRI scan will confirm the diagnosis and extent of the lesion. Fine-needle aspiration cytology (FNAC) can be helpful to confirm a clinical diagnosis but smears are often described as inadequate or showing only fat. Surgery is generally for cosmetic reasons but may be indicated when there appears to be an increase in size (risk of liposarcoma) or doubt about the diagnosis.

54.9 Branchial Cleft Cyst

Four theories regarding aetiology have been proposed: (1) They arise from elements of squamous epithelium within a lymph node. This is the current consensus view. (2) They arise from remnants of the first pharyngeal pouch. (3) They are remnants of the cervical sinus. (4) They are remnants of the duct connecting the thymus to the third pharyngeal pouch. Branchial cysts are lined by stratified squamous epithelium and contain lymphoid tissue in their wall. They usually present in young adults, 60% on the left and 60% in males.

They most often present during or after an upper respiratory tract infection, as a sudden onset of a tender oval mass. The mass is located in the upper neck at the junction of the upper and middle third of the anterior border of the SCM. If presentation is as an acute infected process, then the lesion should be treated with antibiotics followed by elective interval surgery. The differential diagnosis is between a solid mass—most likely to be a lymphoma at this age group. In patients elder than 40 years, such a presentation could represent a cystic metastasis from a papillary thyroid carcinoma or a cystic metastasis from a primary oropharyngeal squamous cell carcinoma. It is imperative that a primary of unknown origin is excluded in these patients prior to a planned excision (thorough examination of the upper aerodigestive tract and a PET-CT scan). Treatment is surgical excision of the mass with histological confirmation of the true nature of the cystic process.

54.10 Thyroglossal Duct Cyst

These are cysts along the tract of the obliterated thyroglossal duct. The thyroid gland arises from the second and third branchial arches. It migrates inferiorly from the base of tongue (foramen cecum) to the lower neck anterior to the trachea during the third to seventh week of gestation. Failure of the tract to involute may lead to cyst formation. They may contain elements of thyroid tissue and may even be the sole source of functioning thyroid tissue. Therefore, an ultrasound scan is performed to help with diagnosis and confirmation of whether there is a normal gland present. Ninety percent of thyroglossal cysts are midline and 9% left-sided, occurring between the body of the hyoid bone and the cricoid cartilage. Most occur in childhood (mean age 4 years). They move with swallowing and tongue protrusion as they are ultimately attached on their deep aspect to the larynx. Infection causes the rapid onset of diffuse swelling, pain, and tenderness. Thyroglossal cysts should not be incised and drained as this may cause an ugly sinus which is difficult to excise in toto and in continuity with the deflated cyst. A long course of antibiotics and repeat aspiration of the cyst, if the child allows, are recommended. The tract may climb anterior or posterior to the body of the hyoid to the tongue base. The body of the hyoid and preferably a wedge of tongue base should therefore be included in the excision of the cyst (Sistrunk's procedure). Following this procedure, the recurrence rate varies from 2 to 8%. If the hyoid body is not removed, the recurrence rate rises to 85%.

54.11 Laryngocele

Only about 30 occur each year in the United Kingdom, 80% in men with a mean age of 55. They arise from the laryngeal saccule (sinus of Morgagni), expanding internally to present in the vallecula or externally through the thyrohyoid membrane. In most subjects raising the intra-laryngeal pressure causes no expansion of the saccule. In those in whom the saccule expands, perhaps because of a wider than usual true cord to false cord distance (wide neck) or because the false cord is compressed against the saccule to create a one-way valve, coughing, sneezing or trumpet playing may fully develop the laryngocele. They are occasionally associated with a ventricular carcinoma, so microlaryngoscopy with angled rigid endoscopes is recommended prior to definitive treatment.

An intermittent neck swelling is the usual presentation, perhaps with hoarseness, cough or pain. It is usually impalpable but may become both visible and palpable on performing the Valsalva manoeuvre. Fibre-optic laryngoscopy may reveal fullness of the ipsilateral false cord. Plain antero-posterior and lateral neck radiographs or a neck CT may show an air-filled sac. Laryngoceles may obstruct the larynx, so the safest treatment is excision, which includes the upper half of thyroid

N

cartilage on the side of the laryngocele so that its neck can be ligated. Transoral laser surgery can also be used in selected cases.

54.12 Tumours of the Parapharyngeal Space

This space is described in neck space infection. Parapharyngeal tumours expand either medially, when the tonsil will be displaced towards the midline, or laterally to present in the upper deep cervical region. It is therefore important to exclude a metastatic node as a cause of the swelling. However, the common tumours are as follows:

- Lipomas.
- Parotid deep lobe tumours.
- Neurogenic tumours.
- Carotid aneurysm.

Parotid tumours are the commonest and are discussed elsewhere (see Related Topics of Interest).

Neurogenic tumours develop from neural crest cells which have differentiated into Schwann cells or sympathicoblasts. Schwann cells give rise to neurofibromas and schwannomas, the sympathicoblasts to ganglioneuromas and chemodectomas (carotid body tumours, glomus vagale and glomus jugulare tumours).

a. Neurofibromas arise from endoneural fibrous connective tissue and are composed of a mass of spindle cells which can entwine nerve fibres, sometimes causing weakness or paralysis of the involved nerve.

b. Schwannomas are benign tumours of the neurolemma or sheath of Schwann and so tend to be encapsulated. Their expansion may compress the involved nerve, giving rise to reduced function, but paralysis is unusual. In the parapharyngeal space a painless neck mass is usually the only sign.

c. Chemodectomas arise from paraganglionic tissue at three common sites in the neck. On the medial side of the carotid bulb are found highly vascular tumours arising from the carotid body cells; these carotid body tumours are rare except in high-altitude population centres such as Mexico City. Vagal paragangliomas arise from paraganglionic tissue within the perineurium of the vagus, the glomus vagale tumour, which, if it involves the ganglion nodosum just below the jugular foramen, is referred to as a glomus jugulare. The cells are not functionally active. Patients present with a slow-growing painless lump in the neck or a mass pushing the tonsil medially. Vagal nerve paragangliomas present with pulsating tinnitus and syncope. Glossopharyngeal (IX), vagal (X), accessory (XI) and hypoglossal nerve (XII) palsies may arise if the tumour expands at the skull base. Carotid body tumours present with a pulsatile mass which is only mobile in the horizontal plane (Fontaine's sign) and occasionally with an audible bruit. Malignant change rarely, if ever, occurs in chemodectomas of these three sites. Occasional reports of metastases in the literature may be confusing a chemodectoma with a large-cell neuroendocrine carcinoma. Chemodectomas may occur rarely at other sites, particularly the larynx.

A carotid aneurysm may be caused by atheroma, trauma or infection. If expanding or causing transient ischaemic attacks, it can be resected and replaced with a reversed saphenous vein graft or an endovascular (stent-graft) repair.

54.12.1 Investigations

An MRI scan will delineate the position, the size and the vascularity of the mass. If a carotid body tumour (CBT) is suspected, an MR angiogram will define the tumour circulation and its principal feeding vessels and will define a cranial cross-circulation, all of which must be known prior to surgery. Shamblin's staging classification is listed below.

Class I CBT	Localized CBT with minimal vascular attachment
Class II CBT	Partially surrounds carotids
Class III CBT	Encases carotids so surgical resection will be difficult and may require temporary interruption of cerebral circulation.

Interventional radiology to embolise larger feeding vessels prior to surgical resection is helpful.

54.12.2 Treatment

The management of these patients requires a multidisciplinary team. There may be a genetic predisposition and some patients may have a

228

pheochromocytoma. The mass will, as a rule continue to expand so that symptoms may progress. A tissue diagnosis may not be possible. For these reasons, surgery is the treatment of choice for parapharyngeal tumours. The parapharyngeal space can be approached by either a transcervical, transparotid or transmandibular route. The vagus and the hypoglossal nerves are at risk of injury. There is also a small, but definite, risk of stroke from surgery particularly in Shamblin class III lesions. A significant proportion of young patients will refuse surgery if presented with all the facts. Recent publications have suggested that carotid body tumours may be radiosensitive and radiotherapy may be indicated either as adjuvant treatment or in those unfit or unwilling to have surgery.

54.13 Follow-Up and Aftercare

Follow-up of all parapharyngeal mass patients post-operatively for 5 years, except those who had a lipoma, is indicated. Glossopharyngeal and vagal nerve injury may give rise to aspiration and a hoarse voice, although symptoms gradually settle, especially if an experienced speech therapist is involved in rehabilitation. A vocal fold palsy is treated as discussed elsewhere (see Chapter 122, Vocal Fold Paralysis).

Further Reading

Addams-Williams J, Watkins D, Owen S, Williams N, Fielder C. Non-thyroid neck lumps: appraisal of the role of fine needle aspiration cytology. Eur Arch Otorhinolaryngol. 2009; 266(3):411–415

Cozens NJ. A systematic review that evaluates one-stop neck lump clinics. Clin Otolaryngol. 2009; 34(1):6–11

MacGregor FB, McAllister KA. Neck lumps and head and neck tumours in children. Br J Hosp Med (Lond). 2008; 69(4):205–210

Roland N, Bradley PJ. Neck swellings. BMJ. 2014; 348:g1078

Suárez C, Rodrigo JP, Mendenhall WM, et al. Carotid body paragangliomas: a systematic study on management with surgery and radiotherapy. Eur Arch Otorhinolaryngol. 2014; 271(1):23–34

Related Topics of Interest

Cervical lymphadenopathy
Neck space infection
Vocal fold paralysis
Salivary gland neoplasms
Salivary gland diseases
Thyroid disease—benign
Thyroid disease—malignant
Examination of the head and neck

N

55 Neck Space Infection

55.1 Introduction

To understand deep neck space infection, it is important to have a clear understanding of the anatomy of the numerous fascial spaces within the neck. The spaces are interconnected, and so infection can spread from one space to another. Nerves and blood vessels pass through the spaces and the bones of the skull base, vertebrae and mandible are in close proximity. A delay in diagnosis or treatment can result in significant complications including osteomyelitis, vascular erosion or thrombosis. The management principles common to all neck space infections include the early identification and immediate management of any airway compromise, early use of empirical parenteral broad-spectrum antibiotics (while waiting for culture and sensitivity), drainage of any abscess (surgical or by aspiration) and management of any complications.

55.2 Anatomy

The superficial fascia of the neck is deep to the dermis and encloses the platysma muscle. The space deep to this contains superficial blood vessels and lymph nodes as well as the cutaneous nerves. The deep cervical fascia forms three distinct fibrous layers, the investing layer, the pretracheal layer and the prevertebral layer, in addition to the carotid sheath. The deep cervical fascia supports the viscera, muscles and vessels of the neck (▶Fig. 55.1, ▶Fig. 55.2).

55.2.1 Investing Layer

Attached posteriorly to the ligamentum nuchae, the superior nuchal line, occipital protuberance and the mastoid process, the investing layer encloses the anterior and posterior triangles of the neck. It splits to enclose trapezius and sternomastoid. Anteriorly, it is attached to the hyoid bone and splits to enclose the submandibular glands. Superiorly, it is attached to the mandible; it splits to enclose the parotid glands in a dense fascia and attaches to the zygomatic arch and skull base superiorly to the parotid gland. The stylomandibular ligament is formed by a condensation of the fascia between the styloid process and the angle of the mandible. Inferiorly, the fascia is attached to the clavicle and the manubrium.

55.2.2 Pretracheal Layer

Superiorly attached to the thyroid and cricoid cartilages, the fascia ensheaths the thyroid and parathyroid glands and invests the infra-hyoid muscles. Inferiorly, the fascia extends into the mediastinum and blends with the fibrous pericardium. Laterally, the fascia blends with both the investing layer deep to sternomastoid and the carotid sheath.

Fig. 55.1 Transverse section of infra-hyoid neck.

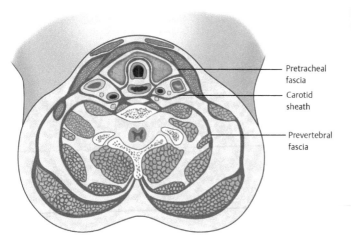

Pretracheal fascia

Carotid sheath

Prevertebral fascia

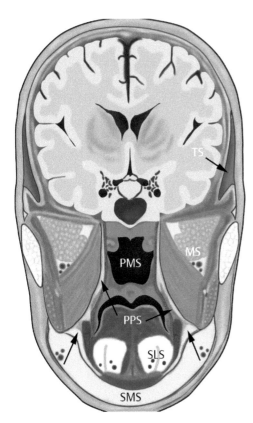

Fig. 55.2 Coronal view of fascial spaces.
TS, temporal space; MS, masticator space;
PMS, pharyngeal mucosal space; PS, parotid space;
PPS, parapharyngeal space; SM, submandibular space.

55.2.3 Prevertebral Layer

Attached to the ligamentum nuchae, the pre-vertebral fascia invests the prevertebral muscles and forms the floor of the posterior triangle. Superiorly, it is attached to the base of the skull, in front of the atlas. Inferiorly, the fascia extends into the thorax and attaches to the anterior longitudinal ligament of the vertebral column, at the level of T3. An abscess behind this fascia cannot extend below T3 unless the fascia is breached.

55.3 Retropharyngeal Space

Immediately anterior to the prevertebral fascia is a potential space extending from the skull base to the diaphragm. That portion behind the pharynx is the retropharyngeal space. There is no anatomical barrier preventing an abscess tracking inferiorly into the superior and posterior mediastinum, although the inflammatory reaction usually localises the abscess to the retropharyngeal space. The retropharyngeal space communicates laterally with the parapharyngeal space.

55.4 Parapharyngeal Space

The parapharyngeal space is a potential space immediately lateral to the oropharynx and naso-pharynx, the styloid process dividing it into an anterior or pre-styloid and a posterior or post-styloid compartment. The latter contains the carotid sheath, which is firmly attached on its lateral aspect to the investing layer of deep fascia on the deep aspect of sternomastoid but has only loose areolar tissue lying medially and posteriorly. Infection may therefore spread from the pre-styloid to the post-styloid compartment by passing medial to the carotid sheath or from the retropharyngeal space to the post-styloid compartment (and vice versa) by passing posterior to the carotid sheath. An abscess in the post-styloid compartment may track further laterally to point just behind the posterior aspect of sternomastoid. In the pre-styloid compartment, a collection may extend as far forwards as the fascia surrounding the submandibular gland, just anterior to the sternomastoid but above the hyoid bone.

55.5 Infra-Temporal Fossa

The infra-temporal fossa lies beneath the base of skull between the sidewall of the pharynx and the ascending ramus of the mandible. It is bounded posteriorly by the styloid process and the anterior wall of the carotid sheath, anteriorly by the posterior wall of the maxilla and superiorly by the infra-temporal surface of the greater wing of the sphenoid. The infra-temporal fossa therefore is equivalent to the pre-styloid compartment of the parapharyngeal space.

55.6 Submandibular Space

The submandibular space is bound by the mucosa of the floor of the mouth superiorly and by the mylohyoid muscle and deep fascia investing the submandibular gland inferiorly.

N

55.7 Clinical Presentation

The clinical features of deep neck space infections are variable; while some patients will present in extremis with severe pain, dysphagia, stertor, stridor and obvious neck swelling, others may have little or no temperature, no neck swelling but a sore throat and some neck stiffness. It is important to have a high index of suspicion and take a thorough history.

55.8 Common Symptoms and Signs

Pyrexia.
Malaise.
Dehydration.
Respiratory distress.
Stridor.
Stertor.
Trismus.
Drooling.
Dysphagia/odynophagia.
Hoarseness.
Referred otalgia.
Neck swelling.
Reduced/painful neck movement.

55.9 Investigations

Patients should have routine blood tests looking specifically for raised inflammatory markers, septic patients should have blood sent for culture. Pus should be sent for aerobic and anaerobic culture. In immunocompromised patients fungal and tuberculosis (TB) culture should also be requested.

In the past, lateral plain X-rays of the neck were the standard initial investigation. While ultrasound can be effective in differentiating an abscess from cellulitis, CT with contrast is now regarded as the imaging investigation of choice. CT is helpful both in determining the presence and location of neck infections in children; it is less helpful in differentiating abscess from lymphadenitis and cellulitis. Magnetic resonance imaging (MRI) gives improved soft tissue definition without the use of radiation, but its use is limited due to time constraints especially in children, for whom general anaesthesia is often required. MR angiography may be needed if there is suspicion of the involvement of major neck vessels. Both CT and ultrasound can be used to assist in the aspiration of abscesses and so may prevent the need for open incision and drainage.

Any pus from aspiration or drainage should be sent for culture and the determination of antibiotic sensitivities. The organisms which may be responsible are numerous, including both aerobic and anaerobic organisms. Both gram-positive and gram-negative organisms can be cultured.

55.10 Management

Patients with a small collection (< 2.2 cm on computed tomography [CT]), without airway compromise who are otherwise fit and well, may respond to a period of medical management with appropriate broad-spectrum antibiotics. However, septic patients, those with airway compromise or complications, need surgical intervention. Surgery is also indicated for those who have failed to respond to antibiotics after 48 hours or with progressive symptoms in spite of antibiotics. Ultrasound-guided drainage can be effective for patients with well-defined unilocular abscesses in the absence of airway compromise. Whilst parapharyngeal and retropharyngeal abscesses, which are pointing in the pharynx, may be drained intra-orally, an external approach is required for most cases.

55.11 Specific Neck Space Infections

Citelli's abscess and *Bezold's abscess*, both complications of acute suppurative otitis media and *peritonsillar abscess* have been described earlier (see Related Topics of Interest).

55.12 Prevertebral Abscess

This is seen in adults, usually associated with cervical spinal tuberculosis. A prevertebral abscess may also be a consequence of iatrogenic trauma. The attachment of the fascia limits the inferior extent to the vertebral body of T3. The usual presentation is with a progressively painful and tender neck with limitation of movement. Occasionally, collapse will cause acute spinal cord compression, requiring urgent drainage of the abscess and cord decompression.

A contrast-enhanced CT scan of the neck is the investigation of choice (▶Fig. 55.3). Aspirating the abscess allows a sample to be subjected to a Z–N stain. A positive result does not distinguish between tuberculosis and atypical mycobacterial infection, but it may allow empirical

N

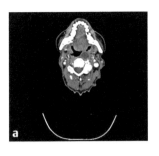

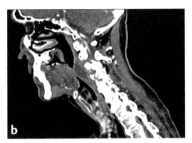

Fig. 55.3 (a, b) Prevertebral abscess.

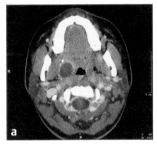

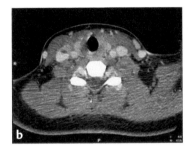

Fig. 55.4 (a, b) Parapharyngeal abscess complicated by Lemierre's syndrome.

anti-tuberculosis treatment to be instigated while the culture and sensitivity result is awaited.

55.13 Retropharyngeal Abscess

This is predominantly seen in children less than 4 years old. Older children have fewer retropharyngeal nodes and adults have only the node of Rouviere. The condition is seen in adults when a prevertebral TB abscess ruptures *through* the prevertebral fascia. Suppuration of retropharyngeal nodes may follow an upper respiratory tract infection (URTI) from lymphatics draining infected tonsils, teeth, pharynx or paranasal sinuses, although occasionally the source is an unsuspected foreign body. The child becomes increasingly toxic, may dribble, and have stertor or dysphagia. The neck is held rigidly and may become hyperextended. Symptoms mimic laryngotracheobronchitis and acute epiglottitis, although in the latter case the history is longer. It is safer not to examine the throat because of the risk of rupture of the abscess leading to inhalation or tracking of the abscess into the mediastinum.

55.13.1 Investigations

An inspiratory lateral soft tissue neck radiograph, the neck extended to prevent the retropharyngeal soft tissues causing a pseudomass, will show the widened retropharyngeal space and narrow oropharyngeal airway. An increase in the retropharyngeal soft tissue density of more than 7 or 14 mm in the retrotracheal area is highly suspicious of a retropharyngeal or retrotracheal abscess. An expiratory radiograph in a normal child can also cause widening of the retropharyngeal soft tissues, so the X-ray must be interpreted as part of the overall clinical picture before treatment decisions are made.

CT with intravenous contrast will show an abscess as a hypodense mass in the retropharyngeal space with peripheral ring enhancement. A CT scan gives more information than the lateral neck X-ray as the extent of the abscess and its relationship with the surrounding soft tissues and the adjacent major blood vessels can be assessed (▶ Fig. 55.4).

55.13.2 Treatment

In the absence of airway distress, intravenous antibiotics and close observation may obviate the need for incision and drainage of the abscess in the tonsillectomy position. The child may need to remain in intensive care unit (ICU) for 24 to 48 hours until the retropharyngeal soft tissue swelling settles.

55.14 Parapharyngeal Abscess

Sixty percent arise from tonsillitis or peritonsillitis and 30% from an abscess of the root of the

N

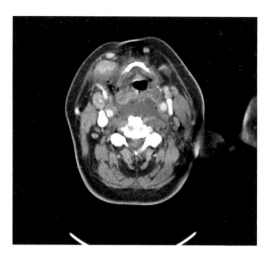

Fig. 55.5 Retropharyngeal abscess with spread to the parapharyngeal space and widening of the prevertebral soft tissue.

lower third molar, which lies below the mylohyoid line. Mastoiditis or a pharyngeal foreign body are unusual causes. There are potentially life-threatening complications including internal carotid artery rupture, internal jugular vein thrombosis and mediastinitis (▶ Fig. 55.5).

55.14.1 Clinical Features

These are similar to a peritonsillar abscess; trismus, soft palate oedema, often torticollis and the tonsil may be pushed medially. There is a hot, red, tender swelling which may be firm, fluctuant or diffuse. It lies most commonly behind the posterior aspect of the upper or middle third of the sternomastoid because infection most commonly drains from the pre-styloid to the post-styloid compartment and thereafter laterally. Diagnosis is confirmed following contrast-enhanced CT imaging.

55.14.2 Treatment

The commonest organism causing a parapharyngeal abscess is *Streptococcus milleri*. Repeat fine-needle aspiration of the abscess and intravenous antibiotics, either co-amoxiclav and/or ceftriaxone and metronidazole are the combination of choice. In patients with a penicillin sensitivity, meropenem may be substituted for co-amoxiclav and in patients with a definite allergy to penicillin and therefore possible cross-reactivity with a

cephalosporin, vancomycin and metronidazole should be used. If the patient is immunocompromised, Tazocin may be recommended, but it is important to discuss this with a consultant microbiologist. These may obviate the need for formal incision and drainage. *S. milleri* infection is associated with the formation of multiple abscesses and often significant tissue destruction so that repeated CT or MRI scanning may be required in a patient who is not improving as expected.

55.15 Submandibular Abscess (Ludwig's Angina)

In over 80% of patients' infection arises from a root abscess of the lower premolars or the first and second molars. There may be no history of dental pain if the root is close to the inner table of mandible, which gives way early. The remaining cases are secondary to tonsillitis. A mixed population of aerobic and anaerobic organisms is usually present with *S. milleri* being the main pathogen. The choice of antibiotics is similar to retropharyngeal and parapharyngeal abscess.

55.15.1 Clinical Features

Floor of mouth oedema secondary to cellulitis can progress rapidly to endanger the airway. The tongue is pushed posterosuperiorly and there is trismus and dribbling. The submandibular region is red, hot, swollen and tender.

Imaging with contrast-enhanced CT gives a good indication of the extent of the abscess and the likelihood that incision and drainage will be needed (▶ Fig. 55.6).

55.15.2 Treatment

If the airway is not in immediate danger, fine-needle aspiration of the abscess and intravenous antibiotics are usually adequate. If there is no rapid response to intravenous antibiotics or if the airway is becoming precarious, incision and drainage are necessary. The insertion of a nasopharyngeal tube will secure the airway prior to intubation.

55.16 Lemierre's Syndrome

It is a complication of a bacterial throat infection in otherwise healthy adults and refers specifically to

N

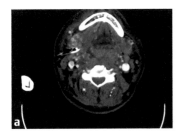 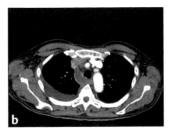

Fig. 55.6 (a, b) Parapharyngeal abscess complicated by Lemierre's syndrome.

thrombophlebitis of the internal jugular vein (IJV). The spread of anaerobic infection from a peritonsillar or parapharyngeal abscess to the nearby IJV provides access for bacteria to spread throughout the bloodstream. Clot formation in the IJV can result in septic pulmonary or other emboli at distant sites. Patients present with a persistent fever followed by a sore throat and then neck tenderness with or without swelling. The diagnosis is usually confirmed following CT scanning which demonstrates the IJV thrombosis and associated local soft tissue swelling.

55.16.1 Treatment

The syndrome is potentially fatal and so early diagnosis and treatment is of paramount importance. With high-dose anti-anaerobic antibiotics (clindamycin, metronidazole or imipenem), the treatment should be prolonged because of the endovascular infection. The neck or other distant abscesses may need to be drained, and the IJV may need to be ligated to prevent further septic embolisation.

Further Reading

Johannesen KM, Bodtger U. Lemierre's syndrome: current perspectives on diagnosis and management. Infect Drug Resist. 2016; 14:221–227

Kang SK, Lee S, Oh HK, et al. Clinical features of deep neck infections and predisposing factors for mediastinal extension. Korean J Thorac Cardiovasc Surg. 2012; 45(3):171–176

Lawrence R, Bateman N. Controversies in the management of deep neck space infection in children: an evidence based review. Clin Otolaryngol. 2017; 42:156–163

Sinnatamby CS. Last's Anatomy: Regional and Applied. 12th ed. London: Churchill Livingstone; 2011

Related Topics of Interest

Tonsil disease
Otitis media with effusion

56 Neck Trauma

Neck trauma can be rapidly fatal due to bleeding, airway obstruction, pulmonary complications and spinal injury. Because initial assessment and management of a trauma victim may be the keys to a favourable outcome, it is important to exclude conditions that can cause death within minutes by correctly assessing and managing the patient at the trauma scene, during transportation, and on arrival at the emergency unit.

56.1 Initial Management

56.1.1 Resuscitation

Initial resuscitation is based on the *advanced trauma life support (ATLS)* principles with specific attention to the airway, major cervical vessels, C spine and pulmonary complications.

56.1.2 Spinal Protection

Protect the spine with a hard cervical collar and employ spinal precautions until spinal injury has been excluded.

56.1.3 Secure the Airway

- Assess and secure the airway if there is airway obstruction, a rapidly expanding haematoma, massive external bleeding, and in an unconscious patient with a Glasgow coma score of less than or equal to 8.
- Most patients can be safely intubated by rapid-sequence induction and direct laryngoscopy.
- Blind, awake intubation is not advised with penetrating neck wounds when patients are drunk and unruly as deaths have been attributed to blind intubation in such circumstances.
- When endotracheal intubation is not possible, perform a cricothyroidotomy rather than a tracheostomy due to its speed and simplicity, and convert it to a formal tracheostomy to avoid subglottic stenosis only once the patient has been stabilised.
- The trachea may be intubated directly through an open penetrating tracheal wound.
- Take care not to overinflate the cuff of the endotracheal tube above 30 cm H_2O to prevent mucosal ischaemia and subsequent tracheal

stenosis. Digital palpation to determine balloon pressure is unreliable; therefore, use either a pressure gauge or employ the 'leak test'. If a patient is to be transported by air, fill the cuff with saline to avoid expansion of the cuff at altitude.

56.1.4 Control Bleeding

- Lay a patient with a penetrating neck wound flat and cover the wound with an occlusive dressing to prevent air embolism.
- Control bleeding with external digital pressure or by inserting a 20-FG Foley urinary catheter into the wound and inflating the balloon with water.
- Should a patient remain hypotensive despite fluid resuscitation, exclude neurogenic shock caused by spinal cord injury.

56.1.5 Radiology

- Exclude spinal injury with anteroposterior, lateral and open-mouth cervical spine X-rays.
- Prevertebral air and surgical emphysema should raise the possibility of a pharyngeal or oesophageal penetrating injury or a pneumothorax.
- Chest X-ray (anteroposterior [AP] and lateral) is necessary to exclude mediastinal air, a pneumothorax or haemothorax or a widened mediastinum that occurs with intra-thoracic great vessel or oesophageal injury.
- Females of childbearing age must have a pregnancy test done prior to undergoing further radiological examinations.

56.1.6 Define Cervical Injuries

- Avoid probing a wound as this may precipitate major bleeding from a vascular injury.
- Identify entrance and exit gunshot wounds to estimate the likely course of the tract and to predict anatomical structures that might be injured.
- In the absence of an exit wound, locate the bullet with cervical and chest X-rays to determine the course of a tract.
- Note whether saliva, chyle or cerebrospinal fluid is draining from a wound.
- Palpate the neck for surgical emphysema.

- Look for 'hard signs' of vascular injury such as ·bleeding, an expanding haematoma, a pulse deficit (check superficial temporal artery pulses) and auscultate the neck for a bruit.
- Do a neurological examination looking for Horner's syndrome, and cranial nerve, spinal cord and brachial plexus injuries.

56.1.7 History

With the patient stabilised, proceed to take a detailed history including questions that might indicate oesophageal, vagal or recurrent laryngeal nerve injury.

56.2 Penetrating Neck Trauma

56.2.1 Zones of Neck

Unlike the cervical levels used with head and neck cancers, trauma surgeons divide the neck into three zones that indicate structures most at risk of injury. Most important vessels and viscera are situated anterior or deep to the sternocleidomastoid muscle.

- Zone I encompasses the base of the neck and extends from the thoracic inlet inferiorly to the cricoid cartilage superiorly. It contains large vessels (subclavian artery and vein, brachiocephalic vein, common carotid artery, aortic arch, internal and external jugular veins), trachea, oesophagus, thyroid, the thoracic duct on the left side and the apex of the lung.
- Zone II encompasses the midsection of the neck and extends from the cricoid cartilage to the angle of the mandible; structures at risk of injury include the carotid and vertebral arteries, internal and external jugular veins, larynx, pharynx, oesophagus, cranial nerves X to XII and sympathetic trunk.
- Zone III extends above the angle of the mandible to the base of the skull and contains the parotid gland, pharynx, internal and external carotid arteries and its branches, internal jugular vein, cranial nerves V, VII, IX to XII and the sympathetic trunk.

56.3 To Explore or to Observe

Massive bleeding, an expanding haematoma, or a large tracheal wound requires immediate surgery. Debate revolves around how to manage the stable patient, and would depend in part on the available diagnostic resources.

- Modern imaging, flexible endoscopy and endovascular studies and interventions have improved our ability to evaluate cervical injuries and have permitted a switch from mandatory surgical exploration towards more selective, conservative management.
- Mandatory exploration for all penetrating trauma that breached the platysma used to be the standard of care, but was associated with high negative explorations rates.
- Proponents of selective exploration point to high rates of negative explorations and excellent specificity of angiography, oesophagography, oesophagoscopy and flexible laryngotracheo-bronchoscopy to exclude significant injury; many injuries such as thyroid, pharyngeal and selected venous trauma can be managed conservatively.
- The safety of a selective conservative approach has been confirmed in prospective clinical studies while other studies have shown that clinical examination and special investigations can exclude significant injury.

56.4 Special Investigations

The question today is no longer whether penetrating cervical trauma can be managed non-surgically, but what the indications are for special investigations, and what investigations should be done. ▶Table 56.1 lists investigations required for a selective conservative approach to be followed in a haemodynamically stable patient.

56.5 Selective Conservative Management

- Investigations related to symptoms and signs (▶Table 56.1) should have been completed.
- Patients must be haemodynamically stable without active bleeding or an expanding haematoma.
- They are admitted to a high care unit and undergo 4-hourly examinations, have haemoglobin checked regularly and are kept nil by mouth should they need to be taken to the operating room.
- Temperature spikes must be investigated.
- Patients are fed after 24 hours if they remain afebrile and stable, and may be discharged from hospital after 48 hours of observation.

N

▶ **Table 56.1** Investigations required relating to symptoms and signs, only in haemodynamically stable patients

Symptom	Sign	Investigation
Dysphagia Odynophagia Haemoptysis Haematemesis	Saliva leaking from wound Blood in nasogastric tube Prevertebral air on lateral X-ray Widened mediastinum Transmediastinal injury Pneumomediastinum	Contrast swallow or endoscopy
Hoarseness	Aspiration	Flexible laryngoscopy
Bleeding	Haemorrhage from neck wound controlled with a Foley catheter cervical haematoma Pulsatile haematoma Pulse deficit (arm or temporal) Bruit Transmediastinal injury Unexplained neurology Retained knife blade Widened mediastinum	Angiography (CTA)
	Severe subcutaneous emphysema Large air leak Pneumothorax, not expanding	Bronchoscopy

56.6 Retained Objects

- Not all metal foreign bodies, for example, bird-shot pellets need to be removed, as they become walled off by scar tissue and are generally quite innocuous.
- Should retained foreign bodies, for example, knives have to be removed, it should be done in the operating room under general anaesthesia.
- Anteroposterior and lateral X-rays are first done to identify vital structures that may have been injured. Computed tomography (CT) scans may provide additional information about the anatomical relationships.

56.7 Vascular Trauma

- All high-velocity gunshot wounds undergo surgical exploration.
- Angiography is reserved for stable patients with large haematomas, bruits, pulse deficits, a widened mediastinum or when bleeding requires tamponade with a Foley catheter.
- CT angiography (CTA) has a 90 to 100% sensitivity and specificity to detect arterial injury.
- A blunt carotid cerebrovascular injury needs to be excluded with a CTA in the following scenarios:
  - Unexplained neurological abnormality.

- Major facial fractures particularly Le Fort 2 and 3.
  - Fractures of C1 to C3.
  - Fracture through the foramen transversarium.
  - Cervical spine fracture with subluxation.

- In penetrating trauma, vascular continuity of the common or internal carotid arteries should be restored if possible in the absence of focal neurological deficits and profound coma. In a comatose patient and/or central neurological deficit, the surgeon has to decide whether to repair or ligate the common or internal carotid artery.
- Vertebral artery injury may present with acute bleeding or with late complications such as bleeding, thrombosis, false aneurysm, arteriovenous (AV) fistula and stroke. An AV fistula may present with a haematoma, thrill, bruit, neurological deficits or cardiac failure. Most vertebral artery injuries can be managed by angiographic embolisation. Should it be discovered at surgery, the vessel is ligated.
- Endovascular management of arterial trauma is being used more frequently with graft-covered stents inserted to seal post-traumatic false aneurysms and AV fistulae of key arteries. Traumatic AV fistulae of non-essential vessels in stable patients including the vertebral artery

N

with adequate contralateral flow are best managed with selective embolisation.

56.8 Hypopharyngeal Injury

- Hypopharyngeal injury is suspected with injuries of zones I and II, and with symptoms of odynophagia, dysphagia, dysphonia, haemoptysis, haematemesis and surgical emphysema.
- Flexible nasopharyngoscopy may reveal oedema, blood in the pharynx or a perforation.
- Although contrast swallow is unreliable, direct pharyngoscopy is accurate.
- Perforations with minimal leakage may be managed conservatively. The neck wound is not sutured, but left open to drain into a bag. The patient is fed via a nasogastric tube and is kept nil by mouth. Broad-spectrum antibiotics are administered for 5 days. A contrast study is repeated on day 7 to determine whether the leak has sealed. If sealed, the nasogastric tube is removed and the patient is fed orally.

56.9 Oesophageal Injury

- Penetrating oesophageal injury is uncommon.
- It is critical to minimise diagnostic and treatment delays as infective complications are related to the time delay between the trauma and definitive management.
- Clinical evaluation has a sensitivity of 80%, specificity of 64% and accuracy of 72%.
- Haemodynamically stable patients with symptoms and signs as listed in ▶ Table 56.1 should undergo water-soluble contrast oesophagography, the sensitivity of which is over 90%. If an obvious leak is suspected but not apparent, then barium may be administered.
- CT oesophagograms have acceptable diagnostic accuracy.
- Flexible oesophagoscopy is done when a strong clinical suspicion of a perforation persists in the presence of a negative oesophagogram.
- In an unconscious, intubated patient, endoscopy is preferred.
- The oesophagus is repaired in a single layer with good drainage.
- With concomitant tracheal injury, sternocleidomastoid or strap muscle is interposed to reduce the risk of a tracheo-oesophageal fistula.

56.10 Tracheal Injury

- Tracheal injuries may present with a 'blowing neck wound', surgical emphysema, haemoptysis, hoarseness, pneumomediastinum or tension pneumothorax.
- The priority is to secure the airway. Nasotracheal or orotracheal intubation should be avoided, as it may cause a false passage, is being overly cautious. Tracheobronchial disruptions can be bypassed using a rigid bronchoscope, or by intubating over a flexible bronchoscope. Tracheotomy may be indicated with massive surgical emphysema.
- Minor tracheal injuries are managed expectantly.
- Communication with the pleural space and a large air leak following placement of an intercostal drain indicate a need for surgical intervention.
- Tracheal repair is done with interrupted sutures. When there is an adjacent oesophageal injury, the repair is bolstered by a local muscle flap. A tracheotomy or an endotracheal tube may be used to initially protect the tracheal repair.

56.11 Laryngeal Injury

- Patients present with odynophagia, dysphonia, stertor, stridor, haemoptysis and airway obstruction.
- Like tracheal injuries, laryngeal injury is often associated with oesophageal, vascular and spinal injury.
- The priority is to secure an airway.
- The larynx is assessed by the voice quality, the airway and fibre-optic examination.
- If concerns exist about a displaced fracture of the thyroid or cricoid cartilage requiring surgical reduction and fixation, a CT scan is appropriate.

56.12 Summary

- Initial resuscitation is based on the *ATLS* principles.
- Clinical examination and special investigations can exclude significant cervical visceral and vascular injury.
- The safety of a selective conservative approach in stable patients has been established.

N

239

- All high-velocity gunshot wounds should undergo surgical exploration.
- Avoiding treatment delays is critical to favourable outcomes in oesophageal trauma.

Further Reading

Advanced Trauma Life Support® (ATLS®) program, American College of Surgeons (ACS) Committee on Trauma. https://www.facs.org/quality-programs/trauma/atls. Accessed June 21, 2018

Weigelt JA, Thal ER, Snyder WH III, Fry RE, Meier DE, Kilman WJ. Diagnosis of penetrating cervical esophageal injuries. Am J Surg. 1987; 154(6):619–622

Related Topics of Interest

Examination of the head and neck
Neck space infection
Nasal trauma
Temporal bone fractures

N

57 Noise-Induced Hearing Loss

57.1 Aetiology and Background

The ear is a sound-sensitive organ but can be damaged by excessive noise levels. Excessive noise can arise from a variety of sources: occupational, such as factory machinery, building sites, and high-impact tools and military firearms; recreational, such as shooting, home power tools, standing too close to speakers at concerts or nightclubs and personal stereos. Motorcycling and car air bags are also recognised causes of noise damage.

Changes in manufacturing industries, machinery designs and regulations have led to a change in the pattern of noise exposure and consequent complaints, with more frequent presentation, in a medicolegal setting, of tinnitus and hyperacusis. New industries, such as call centres, have brought novel forms of noise exposure with damaging consequences, such as 'acoustic shock'.

Worldwide though, noise-induced hearing loss (NIHL) is still one of the leading causes of sensory disability. Occupational deafness is a compensable disease and legislation exists to protect the employee (Health and Safety at Work Act). European legislation stipulates a first action level at 80 dB(A) for an 8-hour working day, at which point an employer is obliged to monitor the hearing levels of his or her workforce and to monitor noise levels at the workplace. At the second action level of 85 dB(A), he or she is statutorily obliged to provide a hearing protection programme to include hearing protection, monitoring and efforts to reduce sound levels at source.

57.2 Pathology

Biological variability (inherited or genetic susceptibility) means that individuals are not affected equally by the same noise exposure. However, with increasing noise levels above 90 dB(A), a greater proportion of the exposed population will exhibit pathological changes. The susceptibility of individuals to NIHL seems to be the same as the susceptibility to presbycusis indicating the inherited susceptibility to both conditions is linked.

Initially, noise exposure may lead to temporary threshold shift (TTS), which is a recoverable phenomenon. There are no obvious pathological changes in TTS and the condition may be due to metabolic 'exhaustion' of the hair cells of the cochlea. It is thought that repeated episodes of TTS may predispose patients to presbycusis at an earlier age compared to those who have not had such episodes.

There is substantial experimental evidence from animal studies that shows a change in cochlear blood flow associated with acoustic stimulation. With increasing and repeated noise exposure, there is permanent mechanical and metabolic damage, initially to the outer hair cells (OHCs) of row 1, and subsequently to the OHCs in rows 2 and 3 and the inner hair cells. Damage also occurs to the supporting pillar cells and the stria vascularis. The audiometric hearing loss tends to parallel the loss of hair cells.

57.3 Clinical Features

TTS may be perceived as tinnitus and pressure in the ears following excessive noise exposure. Permanent threshold shift (PTS) is frequently asymptomatic initially and is often found on routine screening audiometry carried out in the workplace. Such screening is a requirement of any hearing protection programme. When PTS becomes symptomatic, the first complaint is usually reduced understanding for speech, especially when there is background noise. As hearing loss becomes more profound, the patient complains more of being hard of hearing. Unfortunately, tinnitus is a frequent accompanying symptom in NIHL occurring in 40% of such patients. Examination will usually be normal (unless the patient has had previous middle ear disease).

57.4 Acoustic Shock

Acoustic shock is found, typically, in call centre workers who are under some pressure to process high volumes of calls in a defined time period. The sound comes through their headsets and may be the result of a technical malfunction, or a malicious act by the individual on the other end of the phone line. The sound is unexpected and is perceived as both loud and unpleasant by the affected individual, although when measured it may be less than classically damaging sound levels

N

of 85 dB(A) or above. Objective hearing loss is rarely a feature, but multiple symptoms and high levels of psychological distress are often described. Common otological symptoms include hyperacusis (84%), otalgia (81%), tinnitus (50%), imbalance (48%) and hearing loss (18%), while anxiety, sleep disturbance and headaches are also frequent. Theories exist that the problem represents a combination of an excessive 'startle' response, and/or a form of post-traumatic stress disorder. There is a view that myoclonic activity of the tensor tympani muscle may be involved.

57.5 Assessment and Investigations

A good history is the key to diagnosis and is essential in personal injury medicolegal cases to provide apportionment of disability if more than one type, or episode, of noise exposure has occurred. It is important to be sure that there has been sufficient noise to cause damage, and the efforts required to communicate with colleagues at work can be a useful guide. An unprompted description of post-exposure tinnitus can also be suggestive.

It is also essential when assessing any patient/claimant with NIHL to consider alternative explanations for the hearing loss; non-syndromic hereditary and degenerative causes are not uncommon. Cerebellopontine angle tumours may produce a unilateral asymmetrical, high-tone sensorineural hearing loss or intermittent tinnitus, occasionally necessitating a magnetic resonance imaging (MRI) scan.

The cornerstone of investigation though is a pure-tone audiogram, with both air and bone conduction to identify any conductive hearing loss. The usual clinical frequencies should be tested as well as 3 and 6 kHz. The classical audiometric pattern is of a high-tone hearing loss with a notched appearance centred on 4 or 6 kHz, with some recovery at 8 kHz. However, the classic notch is often absent or less obvious, particularly in the presence of significant age-associated hearing loss or other causes of hearing loss. Furthermore, the presence of a significant notch at 4 kHz on its own is not pathognomonic of NIHL. There are numerous reports of 4-kHz notches in individuals with no history of noise exposure. Significant audiometric loss at frequencies below 2 kHz is extremely uncommon in NIHL. If present, it should raise suspicion of some other process.

An uncooperative or unreliable claimant may require evoked-response audiometry.

57.6 Management—Clinical

Damage to the cochlea caused by noise is cumulative and irreversible. Once diagnosed, further deterioration should be prevented by adequate protective measures or, better still, avoidance of further exposure. Awareness of the potential hazards of noise can encourage prophylactic measures to be taken both at work and recreationally, for example, the use of earplugs and muffs. Counselling from a hearing therapist, regarding the hearing loss and frequent tinnitus, is helpful to minimise disability. Hearing aids may be required. There are increasing research reports of the use of pharmacological agents to protect the cochlea metabolically from the effects of noise. This involves taking antioxidants to mop up free radicals within the cochlea and particularly vitamins A, C, and E. There is also evidence that magnesium and zinc also have a protective effect.

57.7 Management—Medicolegal

Occupational NIHL became a compensable disorder in 1975, and as such a scheme exists to calculate the disability and hence the amount of compensation. If the individual has worked for 10 years or more in one of the prescribed occupations, he or she may be entitled to statutory DSS compensation. The hearing loss is calculated based on the average hearing levels at 1, 2, and 3 kHz ([4 × better ear + 1 × worst ear], divided by 5). The entry point is 50 dB HL, which equates to a 20% disability. The disability payments are relatively modest with a 20% disability attracting a payment of £33.60 per week and complete deafness (100% disability) £168 (2016 figures).

The second and more common option is to pursue a civil claim where the burden of proof is on the claimant. To succeed, he or she must demonstrate on the balance of probabilities that are as follows:

- There has been exposure to excessive noise.
- The hearing damage has been a consequence of that exposure.
- There was a foreseeable risk of injury from that exposure.

The case must be brought in time (3 years from the time of awareness). A specialist solicitor should

N

coordinate the case and can be found through the employee's union or work federation, or through the citizen's advice bureau. Frequently these claimants do not present until they start to suffer the additional effects of age-associated hearing loss. Medical report writing then becomes an exercise in separating the contribution of age and noise from the total hearing loss. Coles, Lutman and Buffin (CLB) have suggested an analytical approach to the shape of the audiogram as an aid to predicting the likelihood of NIHL. Since 2007, and the judgement in a group action by textile workers in Nottinghamshire, there has been a much greater reliance on the CLB guidelines; in fact, many solicitors will not proceed with a claimant's case if their audiogram does not meet the relevant criteria. This does provide a degree of certainty and clarity, but a lack of conformity does not exclude the diagnosis. Nor does it help in cases where non-hearing loss symptoms dominate. Lutman et al have produced a follow-up paper to their guidelines which attempts to provide quantification of the noise-induced component of any high-tone hearing loss.

Tinnitus, if present, should be graded for severity and, again, the various contributions to its aetiology should be apportioned. Guidance for severity grading has been published. By and large, the courts tend to accept that the cause of any tinnitus (and hyperacusis) is the same as the cause of any coexisting hearing loss, and in the same relative proportions if there are multiple contributions, such as age and noise, among others. Tinnitus following noise exposure without apparent hearing loss is a little more controversial. This does not apply if the onset of tinnitus followed closely from a specific incident, such as an episode of acute acoustic trauma.

The report should also include a section on prognosis in respect to both hearing loss and tinnitus. In particular, comment should be made regarding the need (either current or predicted) for any hearing aids or rehabilitative treatment, and, if possible, some indication of their costs.

57.8 Follow-Up and Aftercare

Continuing advice and review by a hearing therapist is recommended to minimise disability. Subsequent monitoring audiometry may be required.

Further Reading

Alvarado JC, Fuentes-Santamaría V, Melgar-Rojas P, et al. Synergistic effects of free radical scavengers and cochlear vasodilators: a new otoprotective strategy for age-related hearing loss. Front Aging Neurosci. 2015; 7:86

Baguley DM, McCombe AW. Noise induced hearing loss. In: Gleeson M, ed. Scott-Brown's Otolaryngology, Head and Neck Surgery. 7th ed. London: Hodder Arnold;2008:3548–3557

Coles RRA, Lutman ME, Buffin JT. Guidelines on the diagnosis of noise-induced hearing loss for medicolegal purposes. Clin Otolaryngol Allied Sci. 2000; 25(4):264–273

Le Prell CG, Henderson D, Fay RR, Popper AN, Eds. Noise-Induced Hearing Loss, Scientific Advances. New York, NY: Springer; 2012

Lutman ME, Coles RRA, Buffin JT. Guidelines for quantification of noise-induced hearing loss in a medicolegal context. Clin Otolaryngol. 2016; 41(4):347–357

McCombe A, Baguley D, Coles R, McKenna L, McKinney C, Windle-Taylor P; British Association of Otolaryngologists, Head and Neck Surgeons. Guidelines for the grading of tinnitus severity: the results of a working group commissioned by the British Association of Otolaryngologists, Head and Neck Surgeons, 1999. Clin Otolaryngol Allied Sci. 2001; 26(5):388–393

McFerran DJ, Baguley DM. Acoustic shock. J Laryngol Otol. 2007; 121(4):301–305

Nottinghamshire and Derbyshire Deafness Litigation (NDDL), Neutral Citation Number: [2009] EWCA, Civil division 499

Related Topics of Interest

Non-organic hearing loss
Pure-tone audiometry

N

58   Non-Healing Nasal Granulomata

A granulomatous reaction is a specific type of chronic inflammation characterised by the local accumulation of macrophages and their morphologically and functionally diverse derivatives. These comprise the epithelioid cell and the multinucleate giant cell. Usually surrounding and interacting with these cells is a zone of lymphocytes. Most nasal granulomata are formed because of specific chronic infections. The most important of these are tuberculosis, atypical mycobacterial infection, syphilis, leprosy and fungal infections. Non-specific granulomata occurs when no infectious agent can be defined and comprises sarcoidosis and granulomatosis with polyangiitis (GPA), which, until the nomenclature changed in 2011, was previously known as Wegener's granulomatosis.

58.1 Granulomatosis with Polyangiitis

Wegener in 1939 described a granulomatous disease of unknown aetiology comprising destructive lesions of the upper and lower respiratory tracts and glomerulonephritis. Histological examination showed granulomata formation and necrotising vasculitis. With GPA, there is usually multisystem involvement, affecting not only the three classical systems but also virtually every organ in the body including the ear. Occasionally, only a single system is affected by the disease.

58.1.1 Pathogenesis

Current knowledge suggests that an infection, perhaps of viral aetiology or due to *Staphylococcus aureus*, in susceptible individuals triggers an immunological response to produce the features of GPA.

58.1.2 Clinical Features

- In the nose, active GPA classically causes a sanguineous discharge, crust formation, friable, ulcerated mucosa and nasal obstruction. Septal cartilage may erode to cause a septal perforation. Loss of dorsal nasal support may occur resulting in a saddle deformity in advanced or untreated disease.

- Chest features comprise a cough, haemoptysis and dyspnoea. Oliguria and micro- or macroscopic haematuria suggest renal involvement.

- GPA may affect the external and middle and inner ear. External ear symptoms comprise inflammation of the pinna or external auditory canal with otalgia, canal oedema, canal ulceration with granulations and serosanguinous discharge. Middle ear involvement may cause myringitis, tympanic membrane perforation, a mucosanguinous discharge, ossicular erosion, fallopian canal inflammation and erosion, a facial nerve palsy, middle ear mucosal oedema, granulomata formation and a conductive hearing loss. Vertigo, tinnitus and a sensorineural hearing loss suggest vestibulocochlear involvement.

- There may also be laryngeal, pharyngeal and oral cavity ulceration with mucositis and friable lesions. The appearances of active areas of involvement are similar to a carcinoma and the diagnosis can only be made by a representative biopsy.

- Secondary infection may occur with malaise, lethargy, loss of appetite and weight loss. Untreated, there is a 93% 2-year mortality.

58.1.3 Investigations

- A chest radiograph may show single or multiple opacities up to 5 cm in diameter compatible with areas of infarction with or without cavitation. Alveolar infiltrates, pleural opacities or atelectasis may be present.

- Urinalysis may show red cells, protein and casts. Creatinine clearance declines. Renal biopsy, if indicated, shows focal necrotising glomerulonephritis and vasculitis.

- Cytoplasmic antineutrophil cytoplasmic antibody (c-ANCA) is usually positive in GPA. Recent meta-analysis looking at patients with active GPA, for c-ANCA, calculated a sensitivity of 91% and a specificity of 78 to 100% for patients with disseminated disease but just 60 to 70% for those with upper aerodigestive tract disease without lung, renal or other system involvement. Between 20 and 40% patients have raised titres against perinuclear ANCA (p-ANCA). Both antibodies are detected by indirect immunoflu-orescence. Both antibodies are directed against proteinase 3 and therefore low-titre samples can be checked by an antigen-specific enzyme-linked immunosorbent assay. Titres parallel changes in disease activity.

- A representative biopsy of an active area of inflammation with symptoms and signs of either isolated or systemic GPA is necessary and sufficient to make the diagnosis. Random biopsies of normal-looking upper respiratory mucosa in subjects suspected of having GPA will never show features of GPA and therefore the biopsy of an active area is stressed.

58.1.4 Treatment

The disease is usually managed by a physi-cian with a special interest in GPA. Long-term, low-dose antibiotic therapy aimed at preventing an infectious trigger and/or immunosuppressive therapy aimed at dampening the immunological response is the current strategy. Low-dose cotri-moxazole shows promise in reducing relapse in many patients. It has been shown to increase host cytotoxicity and enhance intra-cellular killing. Cell-mediated immunity against viruses involves the intra-cellular killing of free virus particles and the killing of virus-infected cells by macrophages. Cotrimoxazole's mechanism of action may be to enhance virus killing suffi-ciently to prevent immune complex formation which causes inflammation and granuloma formation when deposited in the microcircula-tion (see Further Reading). Cyclophosphamide and prednisolone are the current immunosup-pressive drugs of choice, the dose of which is adjusted to reduce side effects to a minimum while maintaining remission. Methotrexate and azathioprine have similar efficacy in maintaining remission and are alternative immunosuppressive agents in patients who do not tolerate cyclophosphamide. In patients with resistant or fulminant disease, plasma exchange, high-dose intravenous steroids or extracorporeal immunoadsorption with protein are treatment options. Rituximab, a monoclonal antibody that targets B cells, has shown great promise as an alternative treatment to cyclophospha-mide. Disease activity can be monitored by the erythrocyte sedimentation rate (ESR) and serum C-reactive protein levels.

58.2 Sarcoidosis

Sarcoidosis is a multisystem inflammatory dis-ease of unknown aetiology and is characterised histologically by the formation of non-caseating granulomata. The disease may be insidious, presenting as general malaise and lethargy. The lungs and intra-thoracic lymph nodes are the most commonly affected sites on imaging (90% of patients), but only 50% of patients have lung symptoms at diagnosis. Indeed, 5% of patients with sarcoidosis are systemically asymptomatic and are diagnosed incidentally by having a chest X-ray. In the head and neck, sarcoidosis may present with sinonasal, salivary gland and pharyngolaryngeal symptoms as well as having dermatological manifestations.

58.2.1 Clinical Features

- Sinonasal disease may present with symptoms of chronic rhinosinusitis, particularly nasal obstruction and rhinorrhoea. Rhinorrhoea may be mucoid, mucosanguineous, or, if there is a secondary sinusitis, mucopurulent in nature. Nasal crusting from necrosis of the septum may occur. A watery eye may occur from inflam-mation of the lacrimal apparatus. Examination shows a generalised nodular appearance of nasal mucosa with rhinitis. There may be sep-tal and turbinate ulceration and necrosis with crusting and a septal perforation.
- Supraglottic and subglottic nodules and muco-sitis may occur, and subglottic stenosis has been described.
- Heerfordt's syndrome is a rare manifestation of sarcoidosis and comprises uveitis, parotitis, chronic fever and facial nerve palsy (from granu-lomatous parotitis).
- Lofgren's syndrome (chronic fever, bilateral hilar lymphadenopathy and polyarthralgia) is com-mon in Scandinavian patients but uncommon in African American patients.
- Lupus pernio is the most specific cutaneous lesion but erythema nodosum may also occur.

58.2.2 Investigations

Diagnosis relies on a biopsy of representative tissue showing the features of sarcoidosis in patients with symptoms and signs compatible with sarcoid. About 60% of patients have a raised

N

angiotensin-converting enzyme (ACE) level at diagnosis (non-caseating granulomata secrete ACE) and the ACE level is thought to correlate with total body load of granulomata. It may therefore be used in those patients with a diagnosis of sarcoid to monitor disease activity, but it cannot be used to make a diagnosis of sarcoid as the sensitivity is only 60% and specificity 70%.

58.2.3 Treatment

The disease is overseen by a clinician (usually a chest physician) with an interest in sarcoidosis. Otolaryngology treatment comprises nasal saline rinses and intra-nasal steroids for sinonasal disease. Crusting and sinusitis are treated with topical antibiotic applications and oral antibiotics as appropriate. More active disease, particularly disease affecting the airway or associated with a facial palsy, may require systemic steroids, monoclonal antibody treatment or immunosuppressive medication.

58.3 Other Autoimmune Granulomatous Disease

58.3.1 Relapsing Polychondritis

Relapsing polychondritis is a rare autoimmune disease to cartilage and tissue containing glycosaminoglycan. A perichondrial infiltrate of polymorphs, macrophages and plasma cells occurs at the chondro-dermal junction which may progress to granuloma formation with granulations. The nasal septum, pinna, tracheal rings and laryngeal cartilage (particularly the epiglottis and cricoid) may be involved and half the patients have polyarthritis. Antibodies to collagen type II should be requested and the diagnosis is made from the clinical features and histology from involved cartilage.

58.3.2 Lupus Erythematosus

Lupus erythematosus (LE) is an autoimmune disease most commonly occurring in young women. Overall the F:M ratio is about 7:1, but the ratio is variable depending on the subtype of LE. There are three main types:

1. Discoid.
2. Subacute cutaneous lupus erythematosus (SCLE).
3. Systemic lupus erythematosus (SLE).

Discoid is the mildest form and is a subtype of chronic cutaneous lupus erythematosus, affecting only the superficial tissues. It presents as raised erythematous plaques with hypopigmented edges and a negative antinuclear antibody and lupus erythematosus cell test. SCLE is a subtype of acute cutaneous lupus erythematosus and is a non-scarring photosensitive dermatosis which presents with papulosquamous (psoriasiform) or annular lesions in sun-exposed skin, particularly the neck, chest, shoulders and arms but usually not the face. Half the patients with SCLE have SLE (but only 10% of patients with SLE have SCLE) which means those patients with SCLE should have investigations for SLE to see if there is evidence of pleuritic, pericarditis, renal or neurological involvement.

SLE is a multisystem chronic autoimmune disorder. The F:M ratio is about 10:1. The classic presentation is a triad of fever, joint pain and a rash, commonly a malar rash, in a young adult woman. The presentation and activity of SLE, however, is protean. It can affect any organ system and the activity ranges from indolent to fulminant. There may be other subtypes of LE present, including SCLE and discoid, in patients with SLE. If it is suspected, the patient should be urgently referred to a rheumatologist.

Treatment of LE depends on its activity but usually comprises intralesional and systemic corticosteroids, antimalarials such as hydroxychloroquine and immunosuppressive drugs such as methotrexate, azathioprine, cyclophosphamide, and monoclonal antibody therapy (rituximab and belimumab).

58.3.3 Syphilis

Tertiary syphilis produces a granulomatous reaction, the pathological lesion being the gumma. This can invade mucous membrane, cartilage, or bone, the bony septum being the site most commonly involved. The usual presentation is nasal swelling, putrid discharge, bleeding, and crusting. A red nodular swelling which can be diffuse or localised may be visible. The treponema pallidum haemagglutination assay (TPHA) and fluorescent treponemal antibody (FTA) serological tests for syphilis are positive and a biopsy of the lesion shows perivascular cuffing of arterioles by chronic inflammatory cells and endarteritis. Treponemal enzyme immunoassay (EIA) for treponemal immunoglobulin G (IgG) and IgM may be performed for primary

N

and secondary syphilis or to confirm TPHA or FTA results. There may be a septal perforation, erosion of the nasal bridge with a saddle deformity, stenosis of the nares, or atrophic rhinitis.

58.3.4 Tuberculosis

Tuberculosis affects mainly the cartilaginous septum. In tuberculosis, there may be apple jelly nodules around the vestibular skin and signs of pulmonary involvement. Biopsy shows caseating granulomata and acid-fast bacilli may show on a Ziehl–Neelsen stain or following culture.

58.3.5 Leprosy

Leprosy is a chronic granulomatous infection caused by the acid-fast bacillus *Mycobacterium leprae*. It causes an initial cutaneous or mucosal reaction, which in the nose, mouth, or throat may be a single papule or multiple papules. Inflammation in the nose can lead to septal ulceration, septal perforation, and nasal hypoaesthesia. The immunological response to the disease then causes a peripheral neuropathy with its well-known disabling complications.

58.3.6 Scleroma

Scleroma is a disease affecting any area of the upper and lower respiratory tract and caused by a gram-negative diplobacillus, *Klebsiella* rhinoscleromatis. It is endemic in parts of South America, Southeast Asia, central and eastern Europe, and parts of Africa, but unusual in Western countries when it usually arises within the immigrant population. It usually has three stages of activity namely catarrhal, granulomatous, and cicatricial/sclerotic. Nasal symptoms are the most common and usually comprise nasal obstruction and foul-smelling mucopurulent rhinorrhoea. Epistaxis and nasal deformity occur as the disease progresses. Signs of a severe bacterial rhinosinusitis with mucosal injection and oedema, and mucopurulent discharge may be present on endoscopic examination. In the granulomatous phase, there may be submucosal swelling or rubbery nasal masses which arise from the mucocutaneous vestibular junction and occlude the nasal airway. Atrophic rhinitis such as crusting and septal perforation may occur in the cicatricial phase.

The diagnosis is made by culture of the diplobacillus. Mikulicz's cells (large macrophage with clear cytoplasm containing the encapsulated organism) and the Russell bodies (bright red homogeneous eosinophilic inclusion bodies in plasma cells and caused by the accumulation of immunoglobulins secreted by the plasma cell) are classically seen histologically when nasal masses in the granulomatous phase are biopsied. Ciprofloxacin, clindamycin, or a third-generation cephalosporins are the antibiotics of choice. They need to be continued for at least a month as the organism is difficult to kill because of its mucopolysaccharide coat.

58.3.7 Rhinosporidiosis

Rhinosporidiosis is a chronic disease which can affect any mucosal surface of the body and occasionally the viscera. Soft, sessile, or pedunculated polyps which are vascular and friable and often of strawberry appearance, develop on the mucosal or abraded skin surface. It is caused by *Rhinosporidium seeberi*. Recent ribosomal RNA (rRNA) gene analysis has placed the organism as an aquatic parasite of the class Mesomycetozoea, which causes similar disease in amphibians and fish. The organism has not been cultivated in vitro or transmitted to animals in the laboratory. It is transmitted by swimming in infected water. It is most commonly found in India and Sri Lanka.

The nose is the most commonly infected site and the disease is typically insidious in onset and runs a slow course. In the early stages a thick, sticky nasal discharge may be seen and there is usually a history of recurrent epistaxis. Thereafter, the soft polyps form typically around the nasal vestibule.

Treatment is surgical excision of the lesions. There have also been reports of successfully treating multisite involvement with a long course of dapsone.

58.4 High-Grade T-Cell Lymphoma

This was often confused with GPA, but with the advent of modern immunocytochemical techniques, a representative biopsy will allow an accurate diagnosis.

58.4.1 Clinical Features

The nasal features are similar to GPA, but there is little systemic disturbance and in particular no

N

bronchial or renal disease. There is progressive destruction of the midfacial structures. Untreated, the patient succumbs from secondary infection or cachexia.

58.4.2 Investigations

A representative biopsy will show huge numbers of small cells with a high incidence of mitoses. There may be zones of acute inflammatory cells if a secondary infection supervenes. Necrotising vasculitis and granuloma formation are absent. As the small cells may represent a poorly differentiated squamous cell carcinoma, malignant melanoma, neuroblastoma, or rhabdomyosarcoma, immunocytochemical analysis is necessary to confirm the diagnosis. Staging should be undertaken by a medical oncologist to determine optimum treatment.

58.4.3 Treatment

1. Antibiotics to control secondary infection.
2. Surgical debridement of necrotic tissue.
3. A curative dose of radiotherapy usually 60 to 66 Gy in 30 fractions if stage I disease followed by further debridement if indicated.
4. Reconstructive surgery to the nose and regions as required.

Further Reading

Falk RJ, Gross WL, Guillevin L, et al. Granulomatosis with polyangiitis (Wegener's): an alternative name for Wegener's granulomatosis. Ann Rheum Dis. 2011; 70(4):704

Specks U, Merkel PA, Seo P, et al; RAVE-ITN Research Group. Efficacy of remission-induction regimens for ANCA-associated vasculitis. N Engl J Med. 2013; 369(5):417–427

Related Topics of Interest

Sinonasal tumours
Rhinosinusitis—appropriate terminology

N

59 Non-Organic Hearing Loss

Non-organic hearing loss (NOHL) is a condition in which a patient consistently displays an apparent auditory deficit, when no true hearing loss exists, or exaggerates a real hearing loss.

This condition is usually encountered either in an adult, in whom there is an ongoing claim for compensation because of ototrauma (hearing loss from noise exposure, ototoxic drugs or trauma), or in a child with psychological disturbance. In the former group, the patient exaggerates an existing hearing loss to improve any compensatory payment. In the latter group, this psychosomatic symptom represents a cry for help in response to some current stressful event, although it may not always be possible to identify the stressor. The underlying hearing is usually normal.

59.1 Clinical Assessment

The diagnosis of NOHL depends primarily on a high index of clinical suspicion, particularly in those who may achieve a financial gain and in children without obvious pathology. The preliminary clinical investigation may reveal some inconsistencies which suggest the diagnosis:

- The patient appears to hear much better than the subsequent audiogram would suggest (but beware of lip readers).
- The pure-tone audiogram itself may be performed in an erratic and hesitant fashion.
- Patients complaining of a unilateral hearing loss may deny any hearing of a tuning fork placed on the mastoid process of the affected side. A patient with a genuine unilateral hearing loss would perceive the bone-conducted stimulus in the normal cochlea and report the perception of sound in one or both ears.
- Those patients who have some degree of psychological upset often appear completely unconcerned about the hearing loss but are often accompanied by an extremely concerned carer.

Unfortunately, in all patients who are pursuing a financial claim, a non-organic component must be excluded; it has been estimated to occur in up to 25% of cases.

59.2 Investigations

A plethora of tests exist to try and distinguish non-organic from organic hearing loss.

1. Tuning forks. These can be used as part of the clinical assessment in cases of apparent unilateral hearing loss, for example, the Stenger test (see Chapter 11, Clinical Assessment of Hearing), which can also be performed using an audiometer.

2. Pure-tone audiometry. In the truly deaf patient, pure-tone audiometry reveals consistent results. One should suspect a NOHL when pure-tone responses are inconsistent or when the patient denies hearing a sound over 70 dB above the threshold in the good ear, when applied to the bad ear. Such a sound should be audible in the good ear.

3. Impedance audiometry. The stapedius reflex threshold normally varies from 70 to 95 dB above the pure-tone threshold. There may be recruitment, so this is not invariably the case. Even then there is usually at least 20 dB between the reflex threshold and the pure-tone threshold. If the thresholds are within 20 dB or less, then a NOHL is likely.

4. Speech audiometry. This is often useful in making the diagnosis. Patients often find it more difficult to exaggerate their impairment to the same extent in speech as in pure-tone audiometry.

5. Otoacoustic emissions. Distortion product otoacoustic emissions (OAEs) can give useful information, particularly about the peripheral auditory system. Frequency-specific threshold measures can be provided.

6. Delayed speech feedback. The patient is asked to read aloud from a book. The voice is recorded and played back into the bad ear via headphones, the recording being delayed by milliseconds. If there is a genuine deafness, the patient will be able to read without pausing. If the patient is feigning deafness, then the

delayed speech feedback will alter the reading pattern causing the patient to stammer, slow down or shout.

7. Evoked-response audiometry. If knowledge of the auditory thresholds is required with some precision, as in medicolegal cases, electric response audiometry will be required. Cortical responses are preferred to brainstem-evoked responses as they provide more precise threshold levels and establish integrity of the entire auditory pathway.

59.3 Management

The aims in management are first to recognise that there is a NOHL and thereafter to ascertain the true auditory thresholds. Once it is indicated to the patient, without being confrontational, that the test has not shown the true thresholds, and an honourable escape route is provided, the NOHL will often disappear on repetition of testing. This may involve bringing the patient back for a repeat test while telling the patient their responses will improve on a repeat test because of the patient's better understanding what to do and what the test involves. Any true hearing loss can then be treated on its merits, including the provision of a hearing aid if required. Fortunately, in the younger, disturbed group the condition is usually short lived, rarely lasting more than a few weeks or months, as the stressing event disappears, or the patient develops appropriate coping strategies. Confrontation is rarely, if ever, successful. Strong reassurance that there is nothing serious present and that the hearing will improve in time is usually all that is required. A hearing aid may be provided for its placebo effect when there is great distress on the part of the patient or carers.

59.4 Follow-Up and Aftercare

In severe or prolonged cases (up to 20%) appropriate psychiatric referral may be required. Follow-up is only required to document the return of normal hearing.

Further Reading

Brooks DN, Geoghegan PM. Non-organic hearing loss in young persons: transient episode or indicator of deep-seated difficulty. Br J Audiol. 1992; 26(6):347–350

Katx J. Handbook of Clinical Audiology. 7th ed. Philadelphia, Baltimore, New York: Wolters Kluwer; 2015

Lynch C, Austen S. Non-organic hearing loss. In: Graham J, Baguley D, eds. Ballantyne's Deafness. 7th ed. West Sussex, UK:Wiley Blackwell; 2009:162–174

Related Topics of Interest

Clinical assessment of hearing
Evoked response audiometry
Impedance audiometry
Noise-induced hearing loss
Pure-tone audiometry
Speech audiometry

N

60 Nutrition in Head and Neck Cancer

Nutrition is a key modality in the treatment and effective management of patients diagnosed with head and neck cancer. Patients can be malnourished at presentation, and many patients undergoing treatment for head and neck cancer will need nutritional support. Early identification of high risk patients and intervention with nutrition support should be included as part of the planning for every patient when treatment options are being considered. This should include quality-of-life (QoL) issues to address psychosocial, rehabilitation and survivorship needs of patients and carers. The dietitian is a core member of the multiprofessional team and the team specialist for leading multidisciplinary discussion and decision making for all nutrition related issues.

60.1 Nutritional Screening and Monitoring

Nutritional screening of patients in an outpatient setting and on admission to hospital, identifies those at risk, allowing early nutritional intervention to correct deficiencies and optimise nutritional status prior to treatment.

Basic nutritional parameters to consider are:
- Nutritional intake (change in texture or volume).
- Impaired swallow.
- Weight change and body mass index (BMI).

Nutritional screening should be undertaken using a validated screening tool and continued regularly throughout treatment to monitor impact of treatment on nutritional status.

Validated screening tools available:
- Subjective global assessment (SGA).
- Patient-generated SGA.
- Malnutrition screening tool (MST).
- Malnutrition universal screening tool (MUST).

Screening should be undertaken weekly for inpatients to monitor the effects of nutritional intervention. Outpatients should have their weight recorded at each visit and unintentional weight loss of 2 kg within a 2-week period should be referred onto the dietitian.

60.2 Impact of Malnutrition

Patients with head and neck cancer are at risk of malnutrition due to the site of the disease, the disease process itself, the treatment and lifestyle factors such as excessive alcohol intake. *Unintentional* weight loss of 10% or greater in the preceding 6 months is a sign of malnutrition regardless of presenting BMI.

Morbidities associated with malnutrition include:
- Delayed wound healing.
- Increased risk of infection and post-operative infection.
- Reduced response to non-surgical treatments.
- Muscle wasting.

Early nutritional intervention can minimise nutritional losses and improve clinical outcomes.

60.3 Nutritional Assessment

A full nutritional assessment should be undertaken once patients are identified as being malnourished or at risk of malnutrition. This should consider a variety of parameters including ability to chew and swallow, changes in texture, changes in appetite, anthropometry (including percentage weight change), nutritional intake, biochemistry and social information. This should be reassessed throughout the patient's treatment.

60.4 Cancer Cachexia

Cachexia syndrome is a multifactorial problem that cannot be fully reversed by conventional nutritional support and leads to progressive functional impairment. Cytokine-induced metabolic alterations can prevent cachectic patients from regaining body cell mass during nutritional support and are not relieved by conventional nutritional intervention. As a minimal goal, body weight should be maintained and further loss prevented. The management approach should include assessment and ongoing monitoring with intensive nutritional support, anti-inflammatory treatment, symptom control as well as oncological treatment options to reduce the catabolic effect of the cancer.

N

60.5 Estimating Nutritional Requirements

Cancer itself does not have a consistent effect on resting energy expenditure (REE) but energy requirements will be affected by solid tumours, surgery in the last 7 days, oncological treatments, metabolic state, activity levels, nutritional status, phase of illness, age and sex.

Basic calculations for energy and protein requirements are highlighted below but may be less accurate for severely malnourished patients, multiple comorbidities or morbidly obese patients. Patients at risk of refeeding syndrome will require a different calculation for energy requirements.

Energy	25 to 35 kcal/kg/day dependant on activity level. It can increase further, if major complications occur.
Protein	0.8 to 2.0 g/kg/day for depleted or treatment complications.
Fluid	30 to 35 mL/kg/day, increases in infection and excessive fluid losses.
Vitamins and minerals	As per recommended daily amounts unless considered deficient.

60.6 Refeeding Syndrome

This potentially lethal condition can be defined as severe fluid and electrolyte shifts associated with metabolic abnormalities in patients who have had little or no food for more than 5 days, on the reintroduction of nutrition via the enteral (including nutritional supplements taken via the oral route) or parenteral feeding route.

Criteria for determining people at moderate or high risk of developing refeeding syndrome:

1. Patient has one or more of the following:
   - BMI less than 16 kg/m^2.
   - Unintentional weight loss greater than 15% within last 3 to 6 months.
   - Little of no nutritional intake for more than 10 days.
   - Low levels of potassium, phosphate or magnesium prior to feeding.
2. Or patient has two or more of the following:
   - BMI less than 18.5 kg/m^2.
   - Unintentional weight loss greater than 10% within last 3 to 6 months.

- Little or no nutritional intake for more than 5 days.
- A history of alcohol abuse or drugs including insulin, chemotherapy, antacids or diuretics.

60.7 Refeeding Syndrome Flow Chart

All patients requiring nutrition support whether via enteral (including oral) or parenteral route should be referred to the dietitian.

60.8 Nutrition Support

The aims of nutrition support are to:

- Maintain or improve food intake and mitigate metabolic derangements.
- Maintain skeletal muscle mass and physical performance.
- Reduce the risk of reductions or interruptions of scheduled anticancer treatments.
- Improve QoL.

Nutritional support should be considered in the following scenarios:

- BMI < 18.5kg/m^2.
- Unintentional weight loss > 10% over 3 to 6 months
- A BMI < 20 kg/m^2 and unintentional weight loss over 3 to 6 months.
- Minimal intake for more than 5 days.
- Increased nutritional requirements due to catabolism.

60.8.1 Types of Nutrition Support

Nutritional counselling should be tailored to meet the needs of the patient and be realistic for the patient to achieve. There are three main methods of nutrition support: oral, enteral and parenteral. Parenteral nutrition support is rarely used in the head and neck cancer setting. It should, however, be considered if required.

60.8.2 Oral Nutrition Support

Nutritional interventions include review of therapeutic diets, for example lipid lowering, and introduction of food fortification as first-line advice

N

to prevent nutritional decline. Patients may require more intensive nutritional support methods from the beginning of treatment over and above traditional food fortification methods with the early use of oral nutritional supplements, for example nutritionally complete liquid supplements. There are a variety of oral nutritional support products available. The choice will depend on patient preference, current macro and micro nutrient intake and local availability of nutritional products.

60.8.3 Enteral Nutrition Support

Tube feeding is indicated when patients are unable to take adequate nutrition orally (oral intake < 50% for more than 7 days) or early post-operative oral nutrition (within 24 hours) cannot be initiated. The choice of feeding route will depend on local arrangements and the optimal timing for decision making is at diagnosis. NICE 2016 guidance recommends clinical and non-clinical factors for risk stratification when selecting which people would benefit from short- or long-term enteral nutrition.

Short-term feeding routes (less than 30 days):

- Nasogastric, orogastric, nasojejunal, tracheo-oesophageal fistulae tubes.

Long-term feeding routes (more than 30 days):

- Endoscopically inserted gastrostomy, radiologically inserted gastrostomy, surgically inserted gastrostomy, gastro-jejunostomy and jejunostomy.

NICE guidelines on enteral feeding suggest that if enteral feeding is expected to be required for longer than 4 weeks then gastrostomy insertion is recommended. Despite these recommendations there remains considerable debate between the use of nasogastric and gastrostomy feeding tubes due to concerns about long-term tube dependency with gastrostomy tubes and reduced swallow function. Although the optimal method of tube feeding remains unclear, prophylactic tube feeding compared to reactive tube feeding or oral intake alone improves nutritional outcomes with reduced weight loss, and can therefore contribute towards clinical, financial and QoL outcomes.

Variation exists in the preferred method of insertion of gastrostomy tubes (whether endoscopic, radiological or open surgical) and is dependent on local policy. There are no nationally agreed selection criteria for gastrostomy placement in head and neck patients.

60.9 Enteral Nutrition

The type and volume of enteral nutrition will depend upon the patients' symptoms and current intake and is likely to change throughout and following treatment. There is no data to suggest a role for cancer specific enteral formulae and standard polymeric feeds should be used in this population group. There are a range of nutritionally complete feeds available. Local policies and feed contract arrangements determine the type and make.

60.10 Immune Enhanced Nutrition

Immunonutrition are feeds containing amino acids, nucleotides and lipids. There are no additional benefits to immunonutrition pre-operatively over standard nutrition support in patient with head and neck cancer.

60.11 Parenteral Nutrition

Parenteral nutrition is rarely used in head and neck cancer patients as there is usually adequate access to the gut and enteral nutrition can be delivered either orally or via an enteral feeding tube. Parenteral nutrition should be considered if enteral nutrition is not sufficient to meet nutritional requirements or is not feasible. This may be due to inability to access the gastrointestinal tract or the need for bowel rest.

60.12 Monitoring Nutritional Support

Ongoing monitoring of nutritional interventions is vital and should involve the whole multidisciplinary team as delivery can be challenging due to compliance.

60.13 Nutrition Considerations during Surgical Treatment

Surgery will induce catabolic stress to a greater or lesser extent which may result in a compromise in nutritional status. The disease process in head and neck cancer has significant impact on nutritional status and can have a negative influence on clinical outcomes.

N

▶ **Table 60.1** Potential side effects of surgery and nutritional implications

Side effect	Nutritional implications
Loss of taste	Surgery to the tongue, salivary glands or olfactory nerve can affect taste acuity, leading to reduced appetite.
Loss of smell	Loss of nasal airflow via the olfactory receptors in the nasal cavity can affect oral intake.
Difficulty in chewing	Partial or total inability to chew due to resection of mandible, dental extraction or trismus requiring texture modification.
Reduced lip seal, drooling and pocketing of food and fluid	Reduced pressure to move the bolus into the pharynx occurs due to surgery or nerve damage can reduce intake.
Oral regurgitation	Requires small frequent meals, remaining upright for 1 hour post meal.
Nasal regurgitation	Functional impairment of the soft palate or motor activity of the graft.
Poor wound healing	Flap failure, dehiscence at anastomosis, necrosis, higher risk with pre-existing malnutrition and infection.
Fistulae	In the oral cavity, pharynx or larynx caused by previous radiotherapy effecting tissue healing and swallowing requiring alternative feeding.
Risk of wound infection	At wound site or chest with extensive surgery increasing nutritional requirements.
Nerve injury	Damage of trigeminal, facial, glossopharyngeal, vagus, accessory, hypoglossal and recurrent laryngeal nerve affecting swallowing co-ordination, chewing and taste increasing risk of aspiration and fatigue during meals.
Aspiration	Requires enteral tube feeding.
Strictures and stenosis	May need dilatation/dietary texture modification.

Source: Adapted from Talwar BP. Head & Neck Cancer. In C. Shaw (ed) Nutrition and Cancer. Oxford: Wiley Blackwell Science Ltd. 2010. pp188–220

Studies have shown that the loss of lean body mass and poor nutritional status can lead to increased post-operative complications, toxicity, increased mortality and reduced QoL.

All head and neck cancer patients, whether undergoing curative or palliative surgery, should be enrolled on an enhanced recovery after surgery (ERAS) program. Nutrition interventions can occur at any stage of the pathway. Key components of pre-operative ERAS entails: pre-operative fluid and carbohydrate loading, avoiding prolonged fasting periods pre-operatively and mobilisation in the pre-operative phase. The potential side effects of surgery and nutritional implications are outlined in ▶ Table 60.1.

60.14 Pre-Operative Nutritional Support

Some patients may require nutrition intervention before surgery to correct nutritional deficits. Patients that should be considered for pre-operative intervention include those who are defined as malnourished.

ESPEN criteria for malnutrition are defined as:

- BMI < 18.5kg/m^2.
- Combined weight loss > 10% or > 5% over 3 months and reduced BMI or a low fat free mass index (FFMI).
- A reduced BMI is < 20 or < 22 kg/m^2 in patients younger and older than 70 years, respectively.
- A low FFMI is < 15 in females and < 17 kg/m^2 in males.

Mildly malnourished patients should receive nutritional support for 7 to 10 days and severely malnourished patients for 7 to 14 days even if this means the operation is delayed to optimise nutritional status.

60.15 Post-Operative Nutrition

Post-operative nutritional intervention will vary depending on the type and extent of surgery. All patients should follow ERAS guidelines and early post-operative tube feeding (within 24 hours is indicated in patients in whom early oral nutrition cannot be initiated or oral intake is < 50% required).

Regular dietetic review during the hospital stay is essential to optimise the patient's nutritional status with safe discharge.

60.16 Nutritional Management of Chyle Leaks

The management of chyle leaks may be conservative including dietary manipulation or further surgery. Confirmation of a chylous leak should be sought by biochemical analysis of the drainage fluid prior to commencing dietary restriction.

The principle aims of nutritional management are to reduce the flow of chyle whilst maintaining nutritional status, ensuring adequate fluid balance and replacing electrolyte losses.

The nutritional management is to use a fat free or high medium chain triglyceride (MCT) product. MCT is recommended because it is directly absorbed into the portal system resulting in less chyle production. In clinical practice fat free products are more accessible and practical than MCT feeds. If dietary manipulation is unsuccessful parenteral nutrition may be required. This should not be used as first line management except in extreme cases, for example very high-volume leaks (> 1,000 mls).

60.17 Nutritional Consideration During Radiotherapy with Chemotherapy

Intensive support to prevent treatment associated weight loss is recommended for patients before, during and after the course of radiotherapy with or without chemotherapy.

Oral intake can be impaired due to previous surgery and as a direct consequence of the radiotherapy and chemotherapy as outlined below. The potential side effects of radiotherapy and chemotherapy and nutritional implications are highlighted in ▶ Table 60.2 and ▶ Table 60.3.

▶ **Table 60.2** Potential side effects of radiotherapy and nutritional implications

Side effect	Nutritional implications
Taste changes	Can be diminished, distorted food aversion and reduced intake
Mucositis	Reduced oral intake due to pain and infection
Xerostomia	Requires artificial saliva, and food texture modification
Dysphagia	Pre-existing or post-treatment with tissue damage impairing wound healing can lead to NG/PEG placement
Swallowing impairment of oral phase	Reduced range of lingual motion and strength causing difficulty chewing, taste changes and fatigue during meals
Swallowing impairment of pharyngeal phase	Impaired tongue base movement, delayed trigger of the swallow, reduced pharyngeal contraction, reduced laryngeal function, reduced opening of the oesophageal sphincter resulting in impaired bolus clearance and aspiration
Aspiration	Silent or reactive coughing on food and fluid associated with fear of eating, can be due to lethargy, weakness and reduced alertness secondary to malnutrition
Trismus	Reduction in oral intake and dysphagia
Osteoradionecrosis	Can lead to pathological fractures, orocutaneous fistula which limit intake and can require NG/PEG placement
Impaired wound healing	Permanent tissue damage increasing risk of poor wound healing
Fatigue	Limiting physical function, as well as motivation with swallowing increasing time and effort at meals with an overall reduction intake
Dental caries	Due to poor oral hygiene, or exacerbated in the presence of xerostomia
Dehydration	Decreased salivary, reduced daily fluid intake, increased requirements from losses during treatment due to side effects

Abbreviation: NG/PEG, nasograstric/percutaneous endoscopic gastronomy.
Source: Adapted from Talwar BP. Head & Neck Cancer. In C. Shaw (ed) Nutrition and Cancer. Oxford: Wiley Blackwell Science Ltd. 2010. pp188–220

N

▶ **Table 60.3** Side effects of chemotherapy and nutritional implications

Sides effect	Nutritional implications
Severe mucositis	Can be exacerbated by the systemic effects of the drug that can impair wound healing
Nausea and vomiting	Systemic or anticipatory triggered by taste, smell and anxiety
Anorexia	Reduced appetite accompanied by reduced intake
Taste and Smell alterations	Diminished or distorted can result in food aversion and reduced intake
Diarrhoea	Risk of dehydration and intolerance to ONS/feed
Stomatitis	Can reduce oral intake
Nephrotoxicity/ototoxicity	Renal impairment can lead to nausea and loss of appetite, nutritional restrictions
Metabolic abnormalities	Can lead to increased energy expenditure and micronutrient deficiency

Source: Adapted from Talwar BP. Head & Neck Cancer. In C. Shaw (ed) Nutrition and Cancer. Oxford: Wiley Blackwell Science Ltd. 2010. pp188–220

Dietetic counselling with or without the use of oral nutritional supplements may not be sufficient to prevent nutritional decline in patients having treatment. This will result in patients experiencing weight loss and lean body mass reduction and can lead to malnutrition related morbidity, treatment interruption or discontinuation and hospital admissions.

Dysphagia alone is reported in 30 to 50% of patients undergoing chemoradiation. Clinical studies with randomised controlled trials have demonstrated the importance of initiating nutritional management as a prophylactic (before treatment) rather than interventional (during treatment) or reactive (when required due to nutrition decline) approach.

60.18 Nutritional Considerations during Palliative Chemotherapy and Radiotherapy

When head and neck cancer cannot be cured, chemotherapy and/or radiotherapy may be used to relieve symptoms and can cause side effects that affect oral intake. The goal of the treatment is to improve QoL and intervention may be required to support the patient's nutritional needs during this time. Intervention may include: dietary counselling, oral nutritional support (e.g. nutrition supplements) and in some circumstances enteral tube feeding. When considering enteral tube feeding in the palliative setting, life expectancy and risk of tube insertion complications must be considered.

60.19 Rehabilitation/ Survivorship

Rehabilitation should start at the point of diagnosis with referral as early as possible. Rehabilitation should be part of a co-ordinated approach to care across the whole patient pathway. At the end of rehabilitation patients should be equipped with the knowledge of important symptoms which would ensure that they reaccess care quickly. This may be achieved by delivering education in survivorship workshops and self-help support groups.

60.20 Quality of Life

Head and neck-specific validated tools exist to evaluate QoL. These tools may include factors relating to eating and drinking, but there is no nutrition-specific module to assess the relationship between QoL, nutritional status, malnutrition and nutrition support in this patient group. Deficits in nutritional status may impair QoL and nutritional support should be adjusted to meet an individual's needs. This can be achieved with screening and assessment. The impact of having a feeding tube on the patient's QoL requires further evaluation.

60.21 Conclusion

- Nutrition has an important role in the management and treatment of head and neck cancer from diagnosis to end of life care.

N

- Screening and nutritional assessment is essential to ensure early identification of patients who are at risk of nutritional deficits and/or malnutrition to enable timely and appropriate nutritional support.
- Nutrition support should aim to enhance the beneficial effects of treatment, support activities of daily living and improve QoL.

Further Reading

Arends J, Bachmann P, Baracos V, et al. ESPEN guidelines on nutrition in cancer patients. Clin Nutr. 2017; 36(1):11–48

Bradley PT, Brown T, Paleri V. Gastrostomy in head and neck cancer: current literature, controversies and research. Curr Opin Otolaryngol Head Neck Surg. 2015; 23(2):162–170

Brown TE, Banks MD, Hughes BGM, Lin CY, Kenny LM, Bauer JD. Randomised controlled trial of early prophylactic feeding vs standard care in patients with head and neck cancer. Br J Cancer. 2017b; 117(1):15–24

Gourin CG, Couch ME, Johnson JT. Effect of weight loss on short-term outcomes and costs of care after head and neck cancer surgery. Ann Otol Rhinol Laryngol. 2014; 123(2):101–110

Head & Neck Guideline Steering Committee. Evidence-based practice guidelines for the nutritional management of adult patients with head and neck cancer. Sydney: Cancer Council Australia;2011. Clinical Society of Australia. Available at: http://wiki.cancer.org.au/australia/COSA:Head_and_neck_cancer_nutrition_guidelines. Accessed January 8, 2018

National Collaborating Centre for Acute Care. Nutrition support in adults oral nutrition support, enteral tube feeding and parenteral nutrition. National Collaborating Centre for Acute Care, London. 2006. Available at: http://www.nice.org.uk/CG32. Accessed January 5, 2018

NICE. 2016 Cancer of the Upper Aerodigestive Tract: Assessment and Management in People Aged 16 and Over. Available at: https://www.nice.org.uk/guidance/ng36. Accessed January 27, 2017

Paleri V, Roland N. Introduction to the United Kingdom national multidisciplinary guidelines for head and neck cancer. J Laryngol Otol. 2016; 130(Suppl 2):S3–S4

Talwar B, Findlay M. When is the optimal time for placing a gastrostomy in patients undergoing treatment for head and neck cancer? Curr Opin Support Palliat Care. 2012; 6(1):41–53

Weimann A, Braga M, Carli F, et al. ESPEN guideline: Clinical nutrition in surgery. Clin Nutr. 2017; 36(3):623–650

Related Topics of Interest

Hypopharyngeal carcinoma
Laryngeal carcinoma
Neck dissection
Oral cavity carcinoma
Oropharyngeal carcinoma

N

61   Oral Cavity Carcinoma

The lips are comprised of an external upper lip (vermilion border) and external lower lip (vermilion border) and the commissures. The oral cavity begins at the vermillion border of lips anteriorly and consists of the buccal mucosa, the upper and lower alveoli, the hard palate, the anterior two-thirds of the tongue (up to the circumvallate papillae) and the floor of the mouth to the anterior tonsillar pillars. It does not include the posterior third of the tongue, soft palate or tonsils, which are in the oropharynx.

61.1   Pathology

Although benign tumours of epithelial, salivary gland and connective tissue origin occur in the oral cavity, the majority are malignant. Over 90% of the malignant tumours are squamous cell carcinomas. Most of the remaining malignant tumours are salivary gland tumours (adenoid cystic carcinoma, mucoepidermoid tumours), or sarcomas and melanomas.

Risk factors The incidence of squamous cell carcinoma of the oral cavity varies worldwide. In the United Kingdom, it accounts for less than 2% of all malignancies, but in India it accounts for more than 40% because of the common practice of chewing betel quid or paan containing tobacco. Other aetiological factors include smoking tobacco, particularly in a pipe, and high alcohol consumption. There is also an increased incidence in patients with cirrhosis of the liver. Patients with Fanconi's anaemia have an estimated 500-fold increased risk of developing oral cavity cancer. Carcinoma of the oral cavity may develop de novo or from a pre-malignant dysplastic lesion that appears clinically as leukoplakia, erythroplakia or a combination of the two. The presence of human papilloma virus (HPV) in oral cavity carcinoma in non-smokers tends to occur in younger patients. However, HPV-related disease does not appear as frequently in the oral cavity as it does in the oropharynx and does not proffer an improvement in prognosis.

Subsites Most patients are over the age of 40 years with a peak incidence in the sixth and seventh decades. The male to female ratio is 2:1. Malignant tumours of the oral cavity affect the anterior two-thirds of the tongue (35%), floor of mouth (35%),

and less frequently the buccal mucosa, retromolar trigone, hard palate and gingivae.

Macroscopic presentation Oral cavity tumours usually present as an ulcer but may protrude as an exophytic-type lesion. Tumours of the anterior floor of mouth and alveoli tend to spread to the submandibular nodes, and those from the posterior oral cavity tend to metastasise to the jugulodigastric nodes. The tongue has a well-developed lymphatic drainage. Tongue tip tumours spread to the submental lymph nodes first, tumours of the lateral border of the tongue spread to the jugulodigastric nodes, but some anterior tumours may spread directly to the jugulo-omohyoid nodes. Some tumours present with no nodes palpable (N0), but the incidence of occult metastases is high, greater than 20%. In addition, second primary tumours occur in up to 30% of patients with oral cavity carcinoma. They are most commonly found in the oral cavity, but also occur in other sites in the head and neck, the oesophagus and in the lungs.

Microscopic factors Several histological subtypes exist with different prognoses such as verrucous (better prognosis) and basaloid (worse prognosis) carcinomas. Other histopathological factors that have been shown to be of prognostic importance are tumour thickness, extracapsular spread (ECS) of nodal metastasis and patterns of invasion (those cancers that have a non-cohesive invasive front and/or perineural invasion appear to be associated with an increased risk of locoregional relapse). Oral cavity tongue squamous cell carcinoma (SCC) of greater than 4-mm tumour thickness is considered to represent a greater than 20% risk of cervical lymph node metastatic involvement. ECS in cervical lymph nodes is associated with an increased risk of locoregional recurrence, distant metastasis and decreased survival.

Lip cancer Cancer of the lip is similar to that of skin cancer in its clinical behaviour. Incidence rates are around 12.7 per 100,000 in North America. It is caused by ultraviolet (UV) radiation, tobacco smoking and viruses. About 90% of tumours arise in the lower lip with 7% occurring in the upper lip and 3% at the oral commissure. SCC is the commonest histological tumour type in lip cancers, followed by basal cell carcinoma. The most common non-mucosal form of lip cancer arises from tumours of the minor salivary glands, with the upper lip being more commonly involved than the lower, in contradistinction to mucosal lip cancer.

61.2 Clinical Features

The patient may have a painful ulcer, a warty growth, halitosis and, later, trismus, difficulty in eating and speaking and referred otalgia. Alveolar tumours may interfere with denture fit. On examination, the site, size and extent of the tumour should be assessed. Tongue mobility and dental hygiene should also be noted. The neck should be examined for nodal metastases, which are present in nearly a third of patients at the time of presentation. Lip cancer usually presents with an exophytic crusted lesion and actinic damage of the surrounding lip. In all cases, the patient's general health, comorbidity and social circumstances should be documented.

61.3 Investigations

An orthopantomogram (OPG) may demonstrate involvement of the lower alveolus by the appearance of a moth-eaten rim or an opacity of the normally lucent dental canal. It is also mandatory to have a pre-treatment dental assessment when carious teeth should be appropriately managed.

Ultrasound scan (USS) with USS-guided fine-needle aspiration biopsy is the investigation of choice in confirming the presence of nodal metastases in patients who present with an enlarged neck node.

Magnetic resonance imaging (MRI) scans are particularly useful in the soft tissue delineation of tongue tumours and depth of tumour invasion. A computed tomography (CT) scan is also useful to delineate mandibular invasion of these tumours. A chest CT scan is mandatory to exclude lung metastases.

All patients should have an examination under anaesthetic to obtain an incisional biopsy, evaluate the tumour, exclude a second primary, check the neck for nodes and stage the disease. Treatment, including the feasibility and nature of a surgical resection and reconstruction, can then be planned. A biopsy should only be performed following imaging to avoid oedema artefact.

Sentinel node lymph node biopsy is now indicated (as advocated by NICE) for small (T1 and T2)

▶ **Table 61.1** The eighth edition of the UICC/AJCC TNM staging system

TX	Primary tumour cannot be assessed
T0	No evidence of primary tumour
Tis	Carcinoma in situ
T1	Tumour ≤ 2 cm in greatest dimension and ≤ 5 mm depth of invasion[a]
T2	Tumour ≤ 2 cm in greatest dimension and > 5 mm but ≤ 10-mm depth of invasion or Tumour > 2 cm but ≤ 4 cm in greatest dimension and depth of invasion ≤ 10 mm
T3	Tumour > 4 cm in greatest dimension or > 10-mm depth of invasion
T4a	(Lip) Tumour invades through cortical bone, inferior alveolar nerve, floor of mouth or skin (of the chin or the nose)
T4a	(Oral cavity) Tumour invades through the cortical bone of the mandible or maxillary sinus, or invades the skin of the face
T4b	(Lip and oral cavity) Tumour invades masticator space, pterygoid plates or skull base, or encases internal carotid artery

[a]Superficial erosion alone of bone/tooth socket by gingival primary is not sufficient to classify a tumour as T4a.

cancers since a negative sentinel node biopsy can avoid the morbidity of neck dissection and is considered to be more cost-effective.

61.4 TNM Classification

The eighth edition of the UICC/AJCC TNM staging system has altered for oral cavity staging as it now takes into consideration the prognostic importance of depth of invasion (▶ Table 61.1).

The eighth UICC/AJCC staging system also submits a 'prognostic grid' for the oral cavity taking into consideration tumour-related factors (tumour node metastasis [TNM], ECS, margin, tumour volume, epidermal growth factor [eGFR], Bcl-2 and p53 expression), host factors (performance status, tobacco addiction, age and comorbidity) and environment-related factors (radiotherapy [RT]/chemoradiotherapy [CRT] regime).

61.5 Oral Cavity Cancer Management

The management of all patients depends on the site and size of their tumour, the extent of local

O

and distant spread, the presence of any inter-current disease and their general condition.

Surgery is the mainstay of management for oral cavity carcinomas. The aim of surgery is to resect the disease while maintaining maximal function and cosmesis. The tumour resection should have a clinical clearance of ideally 1 cm, vital structures permitting. Close margins are defined as a histo-pathological margin of less than 5 mm and mean further surgery or adjuvant radiotherapy. Such cases should be discussed by the multidisciplinary team (MDT).

It is important to remember that the surgery required can impair the functions of swallowing and speech besides its effect on the appearance of the patient. Prior to treatment all patients should have an orthopantomogram (OPG) and see a dentist/prosthodontist to assess the sta-tus of their teeth. They should also be referred to a speech therapist for counselling in respect of their post-operative speech and swallowing reha-bilitation. Nutritional status and the need for a percutaneous gastrostomy should be assessed.

T1 and T2 tumours Surgery or brachytherapy can be used in the treatment of early-stage tumours. Small tumours can be resected transorally using a cutting diathermy or CO2 or KTP laser with primary closure or closure with a quilted split-skin graft. Some of the larger T2 tumours require reconstruction with a radial forearm free flap. Radiotherapy can also be used for T1 and small T2 tumours, but external beam RT is not recom-mended because of the significant morbidity of treatment including mucositis, xerostomia, loss of taste, pain and the spectre of developing osteoradionecrosis of the mandible. Brachytherapy concentrates radiation in the tumour tissue more effectively than with RT, and so higher doses and fewer long-term side effects can be achieved. Brachytherapy requires specific expertise which is not always widely available.

T3 and T4 tumours Advanced disease is usually treated by surgical resection, neck dissection, reconstruction and post-operative radiotherapy. Larger tumours of the tongue need a partial or total glossectomy. A partial glossectomy, remov-ing up to half of the tongue, can be repaired with a radial forearm free flap. If more than half of the tongue is removed, it should be reconstructed by a rectus abdominus free flap. Small tumours of the alveolar margin can be treated by a rim or marginal mandibulectomy, preserving the outer cortex of the mandible, but a partial mandibulectomy may be required. If much of the anterior segment of the mandible is removed, the soft tissue and bony defect should be reconstructed with a composite osteocutaneous free flap. The radial forearm, com-posite fibula flap, iliac crest flap or scapula flap are usually used.

Neck nodes In some cases, no nodes are palpable (N0), but the incidence of occult metastases is high (> 20%). An elective selective neck dissection (levels I–IV) offers an improved overall and dis-ease-free survival compared with a therapeutic neck dissection. Sentinel node lymph node biopsy is advocated for small (T1 and T2) cancers since a negative sentinel node biopsy can avoid the mor-bidity of a neck dissection. Anterior oral cavity lesions and those located in the midline have an increased risk of bilateral disease, so consideration should be given to treatment of both sides of the neck. If the patient has palpable neck node metas-tases, surgical excision of the primary tumour and an appropriate selective neck or modified radical neck dissection is the treatment of choice.

Post-operative radiotherapy Adjuvant radiotherapy after surgery improves local control and over-all survival compared to surgery alone in locally advanced cancers. RT and CRT should be considered in all patients with larger T3 or T4 tumours, where there is extracapsular spread (ECS) or N2/N3 neck disease, when there are positive margins, poor histological differentiation, two or more positive nodes and perineural invasion. Most surgeons advocate the use of post-operative radiotherapy, to be given within 6 weeks of surgery.

Palliative treatment Some patients who have a large tumour with advanced local spread or with distant metastases will not be suitable for curative treatment. In addition, it may be inappropriate to subject elderly, infirm patients who are in poor general condition or who have major or multiple comorbidities, to radical treatment. These patients should have supportive nursing care and when necessary, adequate analgesia for pain relief.

61.6 Follow-Up and Aftercare

For oral cavity cancer, 2-year crude survival rates are around 85% for stage I disease, 70% for stage II disease, 50% for stage III disease and 40% for stage

IV disease. See Chapter 9, Cervical Lymphadenopathy for more details.

The highest mortality is in the first 2 years after diagnosis. If there is going to be a recurrence, it is likely to be in the first year. Patients should have a monthly outpatient review for the first 6 months and then every 2 months for 6 months, then 3 monthly for the second year. The oral cavity and neck should be carefully examined for signs of recurrent disease. The risk of a second primary tumour should be remembered. The donor sites of grafts and flaps should be checked until they have healed. The nutritional status and weight of the patient should be monitored, and speech therapy may be appropriate in some cases. Intense prosthodontic rehabilitation should be given where appropriate.

61.7 Lip Cancer Management

Early-stage lip cancer can be treated by surgery or radiation therapy. In contrast to mucosal oral cavity tumours, neck dissection is not required in the N0 neck. Small lesions are managed by simple surgical excision and primary closure. Similarly good results can be achieved with external beam radiotherapy or brachytherapy. RT using electrons or orthovoltage photons minimises the radiation dose to the oral cavity so that mucositis only affects the treated lip.

Larger lesions of the lip require more consideration regarding reconstruction techniques. The functional outcome of the repair with respect to lip sensitivity and muscle function also needs to be taken into consideration. Whenever possible, full-thickness skin flaps (skin, muscle and mucosa) should be used. The repair should provide sufficient mucosa to the commissure to avoid contracture.

Superficial field change lesions affecting the external vermilion of the lip such as leukoplakia or actinic keratosis are best managed via a lip shave and mucosal advancement.

The 5-year crude survival rates for surgical treatment are around 75 to 80% for T1 to T2 tumours, dropping to 40 to 50% for T3 and T4 tumours.

Further Reading

D'Cruz AK, Vaish R, Kapre N, et al; Head and Neck Disease Management Group. Elective versus therapeutic neck dissection in node-negative oral cancer. N Engl J Med. 2015; 373(6):521–529

Ganly I, Goldstein D, Carlson DL, et al. Long-term regional control and survival in patients with "low-risk," early stage oral tongue cancer managed by partial glossectomy and neck dissection without postoperative radiation: the importance of tumor thickness. Cancer. 2013; 119(6):1168–1176

Govers TM, Hannink G, Merkx MA, Takes RP, Rovers MM. Sentinel node biopsy for squamous cell carcinoma of the oral cavity and oropharynx: a diagnostic meta-analysis. Oral Oncol. 2013; 49(8):726–732

Kerawala C, Roques T, Jeannon J-P, Bisase B. Oral cavity and lip cancer: United Kingdom National Multidisciplinary Guidelines. J Laryngol Otol. 2016; 130(S2):S83–S89

Ragbir M, Brown JS, Mehanna H. Reconstructive considerations in head and neck surgical oncology: United Kingdom National Multidisciplinary Guidelines. J Laryngol Otol. 2016; 130(S2):S191–S197

Related Topics of Interest

Oropharyngeal carcinoma
Reconstructive surgery
Radiotherapy and chemotherapy for head and neck cancer

62 Oral Lesions

62.1 Oral Ulcers

Oral ulceration is the most common complaint presenting to both primary and specialist care and the aetiology includes a wide variety of both trivial and serious conditions. Management is informed by careful history and examination and selective use of biopsy where indicated. The four commonest causes of oral ulceration are trauma, aphthae, oral lichen planus (OLP) and oral squamous cell carcinoma (OSCC) (▶Table 62.1).

62.2 Oral Squamous Cell Carcinoma

The majority of ulcers are painful, with the notable exception of OSCC, which is often painless. The lesion presents as a rolled everted margin with a sloughy base (▶Fig. 62.1). A persistent, painless ulcer found on routine examination, particularly in the elderly and in those who drink and smoke, should be considered an SCC.

62.3 Oral Lichen Planus

OLP is a common, often asymptomatic disease that may present with lesions which are typically reticular. It is common in middle-aged women (▶Fig. 62.2). Specifically, erosive, atrophic and bullous forms are painful and may present with oral ulceration. The cause is unknown and symptomatic treatment is usually reliant on topical or systemic steroids. Additionally, there is a small risk of malignant transformation, which is higher in conditions where OLP coexists with dysplastic change and other atypical lesions. OLP can coexist with extraoral lesions on genitalia, oesophagus, wrists or ankles. Lichenoid reactions may be local or systemic and bear some of the clinical and/or pathological characteristics of OLP.

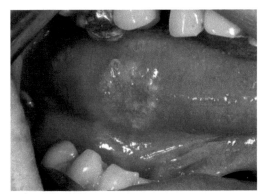

Fig. 62.1 OSCC cT1N0 lesion of the lateral tongue.

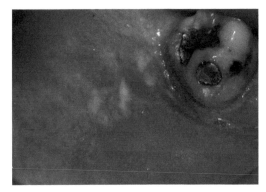

Fig. 62.2 Oral lichen planus of buccal mucosa— reticular appearance of oral mucosa.

▶ **Table 62.1** Causes of oral ulceration

Primary (lesions start as an ulcer)	
Malignancy	Oral squamous cell carcinoma (OSCC), minor salivary gland malignancies
Recurrent apthous stomatitis	Minor, major and herpetiform. May be associated with Fe/B12 deficiency, with GI conditions (Crohn's, UC) or other conditions
Trauma	Usually dental in origin
Infections	TB, syphilis and HIV
Drugs	Aspirin and other caustic burns, cytotoxic drugs Drugs causing neutropenia, nicorandil and lichenoid reactions
Secondary (bullous lesions that break down to cause an ulcer)	
Viral	Herpetic gingivostomatits
Dermatoses	Pemphigus, pemphigoid and epidermolysis bullosa
Angina bullosa haemorrhagica	Idiopathic

Abbreviations: GI, gastrointestinal; TB, tuberculosis; UC, ulcerative colitis.

62.4 Recurrent Apthous Stomatitis

Recurrent apthous stomatitis (RAS) is a common condition, affecting up to 10% of the teenage and young adult population. The diagnosis is clinical and there are three variants: minor, major and herpetiform. For most patients, the management is symptomatic and conservative although it is important to consider any serious underlying systemic cause, particularly if RAS is newly diagnosed in an adult. The ulcers are frequent, painful, with a yellow–white sloughing base and inflammatory erythematous halo; the ulcers are not indurated and heal spontaneously within 2 weeks (unless major aphthae, which can take longer, are sometimes hard to distinguish from OSCC and may require biopsy).

Guidance on 'red flag' symptoms dictates that any ulcer present for more than 3 weeks should be referred to a head and neck clinic within 2 weeks (NICE).

62.5 White and Red Lesions in the Mouth

Oral white lesions are relatively common and most frequently reactive, for example, related to friction or associated with OLP (▶Table 62.2). History and examination are helpful, but biopsy is frequently required to confirm diagnosis. Leukoplakia is a specific term used for a white lesion that cannot be rubbed off or otherwise attributed to another cause. It is important to diagnose leukoplakia because of its association with oral epithelial dysplasia and associated risk of malignant transformation.

▶ **Table 62.2** White lesions of the mouth

Developmental (rare)	White sponge naevus
Reactive or frictional	Frictional keratosis, smoker's keratosis
Infective	*Candida* (thrush), hairy leukoplakia associated with EBV
Dematoses	OLP, geographic tongue
Oral potentially malignant disorders	Leukoplakia, erythroleukoplakia and OSCC Proliferative verrucous leukoplakia

Abbreviations: EBV, Epstein–Barr virus; OLP, oral lichen planus; OSCC, oral squamous cell carcinoma.

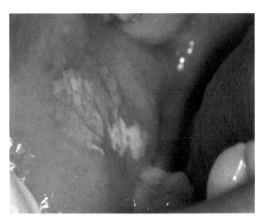

Fig. 62.3 Leukoplakia of the buccal mucosa.

62.6 Leukoplakia

Leukoplakia (▶Fig. 62.3) is a common lesion, but oral epithelial dysplasia (OED) is demonstrated in 25% of biopsies of leukoplakia. The risk of malignant transformation has been found to correlate with the severity of OED, larger lesions, lateral tongue site, non-smoking status and non-homogeneous appearance. Management usually involves long-term review and sometimes surgical excision and is informed by the risk of malignant transformation which over a long period is around 10 to 20% if OED is present. It is apparently paradoxical that smoking is associated with a slightly lower risk of cancer than non-smoking, but this only pertains to a situation where leukoplakia with histologically proven OED has been found. A more rare form, proliferative verrucous leukoplakia, usually has no risk factors, has a more verrucous appearance and is often widespread in multiple oral sites with a very high risk for OSCC. In oral leukoplakia, without OED the risks of malignancy are much lower, 40 to 50% regress spontaneously and less than 1% transform.

62.7 Erythroplakia

Erythroplakia has a velvety red appearance that is not diagnosed as any other lesion. It is rare and frequently associated with higher grade of OED or OSCC and therefore biopsy is usually indicated. Where red and white lesions coexisit, the term speckled leukoplakia or erythroleukoplakia is used, and this also has high risk for transformation.

O

62.8 Lumps in the Mouth

The most common lumps in the mouth are listed in ▶Table 62.3. The most frequent lesions are mucocele or fibroepithelial polyp and the clinical characteristics of many lumps will generally exclude more serious pathology. Where doubt arises, biopsy is indicated.

▶ **Table 62.3** Lumps in the mouth

Salivary	Mucocele lower lip, benign salivary gland tumour in upper lip and in palate
Trauma	Fibroepithelial polyp
Infection	Dental abcess, pyogenic granuloma and viral papilloma
Malignant	OSCC, salivary, sarcoma, odontogenic and haematological
Congenital/anatomy	Torus of mandible or maxilla, osteoma

Abbreviation: OSCC, oral squamous cell carcinoma.

Further Reading

Field EA, McCarthy CE, Ho MW, et al. The management of oral epithelial dysplasia: The Liverpool algorithm. Oral Oncol. 2015; 51(10):883–887

Fitzpatrick SG, Hirsch SA, Gordon SC. The malignant transformation of oral lichen planus and oral lichenoid lesions: a systematic review. J Am Dent Assoc. 2014; 145(1):45–56

Flint S. Oral Ulceration; GP guide to diagnosis and treatment. Prescriber. 2006:34–48

Ho MW, Risk JM, Woolgar JA, et al. The clinical determinants of malignant transformation in oral epithelial dysplasia. Oral Oncol. 2012; 48(10):969–976

Roosaar A, Yin L, Johansson AL, Sandborgh-Englund G, Nyrén O, Axéll T. A long-term follow-up study on the natural course of oral leukoplakia in a Swedish population-based sample. J Oral Pathol Med. 2007; 36(2):78–82

Villa A, Woo SB. Leukoplakia—a diagnostic and management algorithm. J Oral Maxillofac Surg. 2017; 75(4):723–734

Related Topic of Interest

Oral cavity carcinoma

63 Oropharyngeal Carcinoma

O

There has been significant debate in the manage-ment of oropharyngeal cancer in the last decade, especially considering the increased incidence, clarification of the role of the human papilloma virus (HPV) and the treatment responsiveness of HPV-positive cancers. This is reflected in changes on assessment, staging and treatment paradigms.

63.1 Anatomical Boundaries of the Oropharynx

1. Anterior wall (glossoepiglottic area):
   a. Base of tongue (posterior to the circumvalla-te papillae or posterior third).
   b. Vallecula.
2. Lateral wall:
   a. Tonsil.
   b. Tonsillar fossa and tonsillar (faucial) pillars.
   c. Glossotonsillar sulci (tonsillar pillars).
3. Posterior wall (from the level of the hard palate to the hyoid bone or floor of vallecula).
4. Superior wall:
   a. Inferior surface of soft palate.
   b. Uvula.

63.2 Pathology

Oropharyngeal squamous cell carcinoma (OPSCC) will dominate this chapter, but there are other oro-pharyngeal tumours which are noteworthy as they are seen in clinical practice and asked about in examinations. Oropharyngeal tumour pathology is as follows:

- Oropharyngeal squamous cell carcinoma: 85%.
- Non-Hodgkin's lymphoma (NHL): 10%.
- Minor salivary gland carcinoma (MSGC): 2%.
- Others, for example, rhabdomyosarcoma, mela-noma: 3%.

Ninety-five percent of NHL involves the palatine or lingual tonsil. Most MSGC arises from the lateral wall, of these 50% are adenoid cystic. Most soft palate MSG tumours are pleomorphic adenomas. The majority of OPSCC affects the tonsil (45%) or the tongue base (40%) with the soft palate (15%) and posterior pharyngeal wall (5%) less common. Thirty percent of SCC patients will have either a synchronous second primary or will develop a

metachronous second primary within 10 years of presentation. There is a male: female ratio of 5:1 for SCC. Betel nut chewing, smoking tobacco and alcohol are risk factors. Leukoplakia and erythro-plakia are premalignant. The incidence of OPSCC is increasing significantly in developed countries. This is due to HPV infection, with HPV 16 being the predominant subtype responsible. The proportion of cases with evidence of HPV infection has risen rapidly and HPV is now responsible for over 70% of OPSCCs in Europe and the United States.

63.3 Clinical Features

Many patients present with a neck lump as the only symptom. Sore throat, referred otalgia, odynophagia and muffled speech (hot potato voice) are common. Trismus is a late symptom and suggests pterygoid involvement. A full head and neck examination is mandatory because of the high incidence of a second primary. OPSCC is either exophytic or ulcerative, but with NHL the tonsil is usually large, vascular and asymmetrical compared to its contralateral partner. Fibre-optic examination should be undertaken to define the superior extent (and any nasopharynx and skull base extension) and inferior limits of the tumour. Palpating the tumour and the neck is important to assess the extent of infiltration of the primary and to assess the size, level, number and fixation of any palpable neck lump. NHL requires early referral and assessment by a haematology oncologist to properly stage and manage the disease.

63.4 Investigations

A magnetic resonance imaging (MRI) scan with gadolinium enhancement will accurately define the extent of soft tissue invasion, such as tongue base spread, and neck node involvement. It is pre-ferred to computed tomography (CT) scanning, but this can be useful to assess bony extent if there is mandibular or skull base invasion. A chest and upper abdomen CT scan is performed for exclusion of distant metastases.

Ultrasound-guided fine-needle aspiration cytol-ogy (USSgFNAC) of any palpable neck lump is an accurate method of confirming and staging nodal disease.

Positron emission tomography combined with computed tomography (PET-CT) is useful if there is uncertainty on clinical findings or other imaging results. PET-CT can be used for staging purposes in cases of lymphoma. PET-CT scanning is now also recommended for the assessment of treatment response in OPSCC approximately 3 months post-chemoradiotherapy, particularly in patients with advanced nodal disease. In the United Kingdom, PET-Neck trial, PET-CT–guided active surveillance showed similar survival outcomes to the planned neck dissection arm, but resulted in considerably fewer neck dissections, and fewer complications, and was cost-effective, supporting its use in routine practice. PET-CT is also useful in surveillance for recurrent disease.

Panendoscopy under general anaesthesia is necessary to properly assess the extent of the primary tumour and whether it is resectable and to check the hypopharynx, oesophagus, trachea and bronchi for synchronous disease. If disease is limited to the tonsil, an intra-lesional tonsil biopsy is preferred to a tonsillectomy as transoral laser resection may be subsequently used as a definitive treatment. Suspicious tongue base lesions will require a deep biopsy as the cancer can be submucosal.

HPV testing in OPSCC aids stratification of treatment outcomes. The immunohistochemical identification of overexpression of p16 protein is a useful screening method for HPV infection as HPV-associated carcinomas show strong nuclear and cytoplasmic expression of p16 in over 70% of malignant cells and p16-negative cases are almost certainly not HPV associated. Carcinomas showing p16 overexpression should have the presence of HPV confirmed by high-risk HPV DNA in situ hybridisation.

63.5 Staging Summary

The eighth edition of the UICC/AJCC TNM staging system now reflects the importance of HPV-associated oropharyngeal cancer and has a separate classification for p16-positive disease. Essentially it is recognised that T4a stage has similar outcome in p16-positive disease with T4b (i.e., the outcome is similar even if tumour invades pterygoids, lateral nasopharynx and skull base, or encases carotid artery), so there is no separation of these. In respect of N stage, it is recognised that nodal extension (extracapsular spread [ECS])

will not be a significant factor if the tumour is p16 positive. Prognosis is dependent on stage at presentation as well as HPV status. HPV-positive OPSCC has a 58% reduction in the risk of death compared with HPV-negative OPSCC with 3-year overall survival rates of over 80% for HPV-positive disease compared with approximately 55% for HPV-negative disease.

63.5.1 Oropharynx p16–Negative Cancers

(Or oropharyngeal cancers without a p16 immunohistochemistry performed)

T1	Tumour 2 cm or less in greatest dimension.
T2	Tumour more than 2 cm but not more than 4 cm in greatest dimension.
T3	Tumour more than 4 cm in greatest dimension or extension to lingual surface of epiglottis.
T4a	Tumour invades any of the following: larynx*, deep/extrinsic muscle of tongue (genioglossus, hyoglossus, palatoglossus and styloglossus), medial pterygoid, hard palate or mandible.
T4b	Tumour invades any of the following: lateral pterygoid muscle, pterygoid plates, lateral nasopharynx and skull base, or encases carotid artery.

63.5.2 Oropharynx p16–Positive Tumours

Tumours that have positive p16 immunohistochemistry overexpression.

T1	Tumour 2 cm or less in greatest dimension.
T2	Tumour more than 2 cm but not more than 4 cm in greatest dimension.
T3	Tumour more than 4 cm in greatest dimension or extension to lingual surface of epiglottis.
T4	Tumour invades any of the following: larynx*, deep/extrinsic muscle of tongue (genioglossus, hyoglossus, palatoglossus and styloglossus), medial pterygoid, hard palate, mandible*, lateral pterygoid muscle, pterygoid plates, lateral nasopharynx skull base, or encases carotid artery.

*Mucosal extension to lingual surface of epiglottis from primary tumours of the base of the tongue and vallecula does not constitute invasion of the larynx.

63.5.3 Oropharynx p16 Negative

NX Regional lymph nodes cannot be assessed.

N0 No regional lymph node metastasis.

N1 Metastasis in a single ipsilateral lymph node, 3 cm or less in greatest dimension without extranodal extension.

N2 Metastasis described as follows:

N2a Metastasis in a single ipsilateral lymph node more than 3 cm but not more than 6 cm in greatest dimension without extranodal extension.

N2b Metastasis in multiple ipsilateral lymph nodes, none more than 6 cm in greatest dimension, without extranodal extension.

N2c Metastasis in bilateral or contralateral lymph nodes, none more than 6 cm in greatest dimension, without extranodal extension.

N3a Metastasis in a lymph node more than 6 cm in greatest dimension without extranodal extension.

N3b Metastasis in a lymph node more than 3 cm in greatest dimension with extranodal extension or multiple ipsilateral, contralateral or bilateral, with extranodal extension*.

*The presence of skin involvement or soft tissue invasion with deep fixation/tethering to underlying muscle or adjacent structures or clinical signs of nerve involvement is classified as clinical extranodal extension.

63.5.4 Oropharynx p16 Positive

NX Regional lymph nodes cannot be assessed.

N0 No regional lymph node metastasis.

N1 Unilateral metastasis, in lymph node(s), all 6 cm or less in greatest dimension.

N2 Contralateral or bilateral metastasis in lymph node(s), all 6 cm or less in greatest dimension.

N3 Metastasis in lymph node(s) greater than 6 cm in dimension.

63.6 Management

Lymphoma Most oncologists treat medium- and high-grade NHL as a disseminated disease and the CHOP regime (cyclophosphamide, hydroxydaunorubicin, Oncovin [vincristine] and prednisolone) is the most commonly favoured. VAPEL-B (vincristine, adriamycin, prednisolone, etoposide, cyclophosphamide and bleomycin) is a more recent regime favoured by some oncologists. In the relatively unusual event that the lymphoma is very localised, radiotherapy may be used.

Squamous cell carcinoma The association of HPV infection has allowed targeted vaccination to prevent OPSCC. Cervarix targets HPV 16 and 18 and the quadrivalent Gardasil targets HPV 6, 11, 16 and 18. Vaccination programmes usually target girls age 12 to 22, but it has been recently agreed in the UK that boys will be vaccinated too.

Although there are no specific studies that compare primary surgical versus non-surgical management for OPSCC, similar survival outcomes have been reported in studies of primary chemoradiotherapy (CRT) and of surgery followed by post-operative radiotherapy (RT) and/or CRT. Treatment decisions are made based on the size and position of the tumour and potential functional deficit. Prior to treatment, patients should undergo dietetic, speech and language therapy and dental review.

63.7 Early OPSCC (T1–T2, Node-Negative Disease)

Early-stage OPSCC should ideally be treated with single-modality therapy, and either primary surgery or RT can be used.

- Primary RT is usually given at 70 Gy in 35 fractions. Planning can be carried out using three-dimensional conformal planning (typically using a 'wedged pair' of RT fields) or intensity-modulated radiotherapy (IMRT). IMRT has been shown to reduce toxicity.

- Surgery for T1–T2 N0 OPSCC can be carried out transorally, either by transoral laser microsurgery (TLM) or transoral robotic surgery (TORS). TLM removes tumours in several pieces and this can cause difficulty in pathological scrutiny of the resected tissue to determine margins. Representative marginal biopsies, taken from the peripheral mucosal resection margins and tumour bed are therefore essential to help rule out the presence of residual microscopic disease. TORS involves en bloc removal of the tumour and as a result, surgical margins are easier to interpret. Although single modality is the ideal, adjuvant RT and/or CRT may be required due to adverse pathological features following surgery (e.g., positive margins). Post-operative RT is usually in a dose of 60 Gy in 30 fractions. It is important to appreciate that adjuvant treatment may affect functional outcomes following surgery.

In early disease patients who are clinically N0 there is a high risk of occult nodal disease (up to 30%). Therefore, patients having surgery to the primary should also undergo ipsilateral selective neck dissection (levels II–IV). Level IIb does not need to be dissected, if there are no findings pre-operatively of level IIa disease, which helps reduce morbidity from accessory nerve damage. Patients having RT should have elective RT to the ipsilateral cervical lymph nodes (levels II–IV is recommended; level Ib may also be included in cases with anterior extension of tumour and/or involvement of the anterior tonsillar pillar). Prophylactic treatment to the contralateral neck may also be considered in tumours arising at or very near the midline (in the soft palate, tongue base or posterior pharyngeal wall).

63.8 Advanced OPSCC (T3–T4 and Node-Positive Disease)

- Primary RT or CRT for advanced OPSCC, as part of an 'organ preservation' strategy, is now considered to be the treatment of choice. IMRT reduces toxicity in patients treated with radical radiotherapy, compared with conventional radiotherapy. A RT dose equivalent of 70 Gy in 35 fractions with concurrent cisplatin chemotherapy is recommended for stage III and IV disease. If there is a contraindication to platinum chemotherapy (e.g., renal dysfunction or hearing impairment), concurrent cetuximab (a monoclonal antibody targeting the epidermal growth factor receptor) was used as an alternative. However, the De-ESCALate trial revealed that cetuximab showed no benefit in terms of reduced toxicity, but instead caused significant detriment in terms of tumour control. It was concluded that Cisplatin and radiotherapy should be used as the standard of care for HPV-positive low-risk patients who are able to tolerate cisplatin. RT alone may be given to patients with advanced disease who are not fit for concurrent treatment. In patients over 70 years of age the benefits from concurrent chemotherapy are reduced and it is not recommended.

- Transoral resection by TLM or TORS of some T3 tumours may be considered if it is anticipated

that negative margins can be achieved. It is rarely appropriate for T4 primary tumours. Also, where a larger resection of the soft palate is required, the consensus is that surgery gives a poor functional outcome. Open surgical procedures may be considered, which usually require paramedian mandibulotomy for access and reconstruction with a reconstruction performed using radial artery free flaps or anterolateral thigh free flaps. It should also be noted that approximately 80% of patients who undergo primary surgery will also receive post-operative RT or CRT. Indications for post-operative RT alone include multiple nodal metastasis, T3 or T4 tumours and tumours with other adverse features, including perineural or lymphovascular invasion. Patients with extracapsular invasion and/or microscopically involved (< 1 mm) surgical resection margins around the primary tumour experience significant benefit in terms of overall and disease-free survival from post-operative CRT compared with RT alone.

The likelihood of nodal metastasis for advanced oropharyngeal carcinoma is over 50%. Therefore, the N0 neck should be treated electively either by surgery or RT. When surgery is used, a selective neck dissection (level II–IV) is generally recommended, and in some cases level I may be included. All patients with node-positive disease who are being treated by surgery should have a modified neck dissection or at least a level I–IV selective neck dissection. For transoral resections, the neck dissection may be performed at the same time, or as a staged procedure, around 2 weeks before transoral resection of the primary. A staged approach may help prevent the development of a fistula if there is lateral pharyngeal wall transoral resection. For any transoral resection of the oropharynx, ligation of the individual feeding vessels from the external carotid artery should be performed (ascending pharyngeal, lingual and facial branches) to limit the risk of post-operative haemorrhage. Patients with advanced nodal (N2 or N3) disease receiving radical CRT should have a PET-CT scan 10 to 12 weeks after treatment, with a subsequent neck dissection within 4 weeks if residual abnormal or equivocal nodal disease is detected. This has been shown to produce similar survival rates to a planned neck dissection, with less morbidity and higher cost-effectiveness.

63.9 Follow-Up and Aftercare

After surgery for advanced disease, swallowing is frequently seriously impaired. CRT is associated with greater toxicity than RT alone and late toxicity, particularly swallowing dysfunction, can have a significant impact on quality of life. Gastrostomy dependence rates of over 10% have been reported. Swallowing rehabilitation should be instituted by a speech therapist with a special interest in swallowing as soon as possible during treatment.

Further Reading

Brierley JD, Gospodarowicz MK, Wittekind C, eds. The TNM Classification of Malignant Tumours. 8th ed. Chicester: Wiley Blackwell; 2016

Mehanna H, Beech T, Nicholson T, et al. Prevalence of human papillomavirus in oropharyngeal and nonoropharyngeal head and neck cancer—systematic review and meta-analysis of trends by time and region. Head Neck. 2013; 35(5):747–755

Mehanna H, Evans M, Beasley M, et al. Oropharyngeal cancer: United Kingdom National Multidisciplinary Guidelines. J Laryngol Otol. 2016; 130(S2):S90–S96

Mehanna H, Wong WL, McConkey CC, et al; PET-NECK Trial Management Group. PET-CT surveillance versus neck dissection in advanced head and neck cancer. N Engl J Med. 2016; 374(15):1444–1454

Moore EJ, Hinni ML. Critical review: transoral laser microsurgery and robotic-assisted surgery for oropharynx cancer including human papillomavirus-related cancer. Int J Radiat Oncol Biol Phys. 2013; 85(5):1163–1167

Mirghania H, Blanchard P.. Treatment de-escalation for HPV-driven oropharyngeal cancer: Where do we stand? Clin Transl Radiat Oncol. 2018; 8:4–11

Mehanna H, Robinson M, Hartley A, et al. Radiotherapy plus cisplatin or cetuximab in low-risk human papillomavirus-positive oropharyngeal cancer (De-ESCALaTE HPV): an open-label randomised controlled phase 3 trial. The Lancet. November 15, 2018

Related Topics of Interest

Hypopharyngeal carcinoma
Laryngeal carcinoma
Oral cavity carcinoma
Radiotherapy and chemotherapy for head and neck cancer
Reconstructive surgery

64 Otalgia

Otalgia is pain in the ear (earache). It is a symptom not a diagnosis. It may be caused by primary disorders of the ear (otological in origin) or may be secondary to disease from other sites in the head and neck, which share the same sensory innervation (referred pain). Otalgia is a common symptom presenting to the ENT clinic. It is therefore vital that one has a good understanding of the causes, a thorough method of assessment and a knowledge of the appropriate management of these patients.

64.1 Anatomy

The sensory nerve supply of the external and middle ears arises from several sources:

- The lower half of the pinna receives its sensory supply from the great auricular nerve via the cervical plexus, predominantly C2 and C3.
- The upper half receives its supply from the lesser occipital nerve (C2) medially and the auriculotemporal nerve laterally (mandibular branch of fifth cranial nerve).
- The external auditory meatus and lateral tympanic membrane receive their supply from the auriculotemporal nerve and auricular branches of the facial and vagus nerves (Arnold's nerve, named after Friedrich Arnold, 1803–1890, Professor of Anatomy at University of Heidelberg).
- The medial aspect of the tympanic membrane and middle ear is supplied through the tympanic plexus by the facial nerve (nervus intermedius, which contains a sensory branch from the geniculate ganglion and also parasympathetic fibres from the superior salivary nucleus) and glossopharyngeal nerve (Jacobsen's nerve, which contains not only sensory fibres from cranial nerve [CN] IX but also parasympathetic fibres from the inferior salivary nucleus). Remember that the lesser (sometimes and equally correctly called the superficial) petrosal nerve is a branch of the tympanic plexus which collects all the parasympathetic (secretomotor) fibres of the tympanic branches of the facial nerve (nervus intermedius) and Jacobsen's nerve to relay in the otic ganglion for the secretomotor supply of the parotid gland and minor salivary glands of the vestibule of the mouth.

64.2 Primary Otalgia

Primary otalgia arises because of direct stimulation of the sensory nerves due to otogenic pathology. The pain may emanate from the pinna, the external meatus or middle ear.

- Pinna: haematoma, perichondritis, lacerations, neoplasms and chondrodermatitis nodularis helicis.
- External auditory meatus: trauma from ear cleaning, otitis externa, furuncles and shingles. Malignant otitis externa (*Pseudomonas* infection) and tumours, by involving bone, are characterised by severe pain.
- Middle ear: traumatic perforation of the tympanic membrane, acute otitis media, myringitis bullosa (Coxsackie B virus infection), acute mastoiditis and neoplasms.

64.3 Secondary (Referred) Otalgia

Referred otalgia may arise from disease in any peripheral territory supplied by the nerves. It is important to remember that otalgia may arise from a primary neuralgia of any of the sensory nerves that supply the ear, although it is most commonly the glossopharyngeal nerve. This condition gives rise to severe lancinating pain arising in the tonsillar fossa or tongue base and radiating deeply in the ear, often induced by talking or swallowing. Less commonly the pain may be centred in the external auditory meatus and not be induced by throat movement. Shingles of the ear (herpes zoster oticus from sensory branches of eighth, ninth and tenth cranial nerves) also causes neuralgic type pain.

A brief list and system of classification for the commoner causes of referred otalgia is given below.

1. Second and third cervical nerves (C2 and C3):
   a. Arthritis/cervical spondylosis. In non-smoking patients over 50 years, this is the commonest cause of referred otalgia.
   b. Soft tissue injury.
2. Trigeminal nerve (fifth cranial nerve):
   a. Dental disease such as tooth impaction, caries and abscess, particularly of posterior teeth,

and temporomandibular joint dysfunction (common in young people).

b. Nasopharyngeal disease such as viral infection, tumour or post-adenoidectomy.

c. Sinonasal disease and salivary gland disease are uncommon causes of referred otalgia.

3. Glossopharyngeal nerve (ninth cranial nerve):

a. Almost any oropharyngeal infective process may lead to otalgia, such as pharyngitis, tonsillitis and quinsy. Otalgia is common following tonsillectomy.

b. Tumours of the tongue base or tonsil.

4. Vagus (tenth cranial nerve):

a. Carcinoma of the larynx and hypopharynx. Otalgia in the presence of a laryngeal carcinoma often suggests cartilage invasion.

64.4 Assessment

A full history and examination will normally facilitate a differentiation between primary otological pathology and secondary, referred, otalgia. However, given the wide range of possible causative pathologies for secondary otalgia, it is extremely important to be open minded, vigilant and thorough in one's assessment.

The examination should include the ears, the temporomandibular joints, the neck and the oral cavity. Particular attention should be paid to the tongue base, pharynx and larynx, as pathology here can be catastrophic if overlooked. In cases where the clinical examination is unrevealing and suspicion exists, particularly in older patients, smokers and those with a high alcohol intake, magnetic resonance imaging (MRI) scanning may be appropriate to identify small tumours of the tongue base, nasopharynx and hypopharynx.

64.5 Management

Appropriate treatment should then be directed at the underlying cause, and the reader is directed to the specific chapter for each condition.

Occasionally, no abnormality can be found even after a thorough examination and further investigation. A few patients with otalgia may shuttle back and forth between ENT and oral surgeons, with both claiming the symptom is in the other's remit. Cervical spondylosis or a neuralgia (e.g., glossopharyngeal neuralgia) should be reconsidered in such cases and an empirical trial of or amitriptyline may be beneficial in both diagnoses. Referral to a pain clinic, rheumatologist or a neurologist should be considered if such a trial fails. In intractable cases, division of the tympanic plexus (tympanic neurectomy) has been suggested, but this plexus only contains fibres from the vagus and glossopharyngeal nerves. It is therefore highly controversial as it will not help patients with a cervical nerve or trigeminal nerve aetiology.

Further Reading

Charlett SD, Coatesworth AP. Referred otalgia: a structured approach to diagnosis and treatment. Int J Clin Pract. 2007; 61(6):1015–1021

Cook JA, Irving RM. Role of tympanic neurectomy in otalgia. J Laryngol Otol. 1990; 104(2):114–117

Roberts DS, Yamasaki A, Sedaghat AR, Lee DJ, Reardon E. Tympanic plexus neurectomy for intractable otalgia. Laryngoscope Investig Otolaryngol. 2016; 1(5):135–139

Visvanathan V, Kelly G. 12 minute consultation: an evidence-based management of referred otalgia. Clin Otolaryngol. 2010; 35(5):409–414

Related Topics of Interest

Suppurative otitis media—acute
Headache and facial pain
Otitis externa

65 Otitis Externa

Otitis externa is an inflammation of the skin of the external auditory meatus (EAM). The commonest symptoms are otalgia, itching and otorrhoea. The mainstay of treatment is aural toilet with topical antibiotic/steroid preparations. The specific medical content of these preparations is an often-asked question in ENT examinations.

65.1 Pathology

The skin of the EAM is comprised, in the outer third, of an epithelial layer containing hair follicles, ceruminous glands and sebaceous glands, lying on a thin dermal bed containing sweat glands. The skin of the medial bony ear canal lacks appendages and thins from lateral to medial. The secretions of the sebaceous glands keep the stratum corneum watertight and supple. Sweat gland secretions keep the secretion at a pH between 3 and 5 which is lethal for most human pathogens. Usually, the EAM is sterile or contains *Staphylococcus albus* commensals. *Staphylococcus aureus* and non-haemolytic streptococci are unusual.

In the acute phase of otitis externa, there are dilated dermal blood vessels of increased permeability which cause signs of a red, hot, oedematous and tender ear canal. The epithelial reaction consists of vesication, parakeratosis and spongiosis. It is usually a diffuse process but may be more localised such as in bullous myringitis or, the most extreme example, a furuncle, usually arising from a single hair follicle.

65.2 Predisposing Factors

1. Heat, humidity, bathing, swimming.
2. Trauma, especially from dirty fingernails, cotton buds and hairgrips.
3. Inherited—narrow ear canals.
4. Skin conditions—non-atopic eczema, psoriasis.

65.2.1 Classification

1. Infective
   a. Bacterial diffuse otitis externa commonly caused by *Pseudomonas aeruginosa*, *S. aureus* and *Bacillu sproteus*.

Furunculosis, usually caused by *S. aureus*.

Malignant otitis externa, usually caused by *P. aeruginosa* or occasionally *S. aureus*.

Erysipelas caused by *Streptococcus pyogenes*. Perichondritis caused by *P. aeruginosa* (not, as is often thought, *S. aureus*).

Impetigo, an infection of the superficial layers of the epidermis, usually caused by *S. aureus* or occasionally *S. pyogenes*.

2. Fungal
Aspergillus niger
Aspergillus fumigatus
Candida albicans

3. Viral herpes simplex
Herpes zoster

Presumptive in otitis externa haemorrhagica and bullous myringitis.

   b. Reactive
      – Eczema.
      – Seborrhoeic dermatitis.
      – Neuro dermatitis.
      – Keratosis obturans.
      – Psoriasis.
      – Secondary to discharge from an acute or chronic otitis media.

65.3 Clinical Features

The cardinal symptom of this condition is pain, often preceded by itching and/or a sense of blockage. Other symptoms include otorrhoea (the discharge may be waxy, watery or serosanguineous) and hearing loss, although this is usually a secondary symptom.

Otitis externa may be confined to a relatively small area of the meatus (localised) but is more commonly widespread (generalised). Localised infection can be circumscribed or diffuse while generalised infection can be either primary otological or primarily dermatological.

A targeted history regarding direct trauma to the ear canal, swimming habits, atopic tendency and previous otological problems should be made. Symptoms of infection elsewhere in the head and neck, for example, tonsillitis and sinusitis and preceding symptoms of otitis media should be sought. A general medical history should specifically enquire about diabetes and skin diseases (eczema, psoriasis). The history may provide a pointer towards the diagnosis, severe itching suggests eczema, neurodermatitis or mycotic infection. Severe otalgia occurs with furunculosis and herpes infections.

Conditions affecting the ear canal are limited and a diagnosis can usually be made on examination. The skin of the ear canal will usually exhibit widespread erythema and oedema. Frequently, there will be waxy or keratinous debris and in fungal infections, mycotic debris. This can often be recognised by its 'wet cotton wool' appearance or the presence of fungal hyphae. It is not uncommon to find the ear canal occluded by oedema in the acute phase.

65.4 Investigations

An ear swab for microbiological culture, including fungal culture, and antibiotic/antimycotic sensitivity may be helpful, although many clinicians will only undertake this if the condition fails to respond as expected to standard first-line treatment.

65.5 Management

1. Meticulous and regular aural toilet, to clean inflammatory debris, paying particular attention to the anteroinferior meatal recess.
2. Topical anti-infective treatment. Combined antibiotic and steroid drops are most commonly prescribed, to be taken two or three times daily. These are also used for reactive otitis externa to prevent bacterial infection of the inflamed ear canal skin. If a fungal infection is suspected or confirmed, a topical antifungal (e.g., 1% clotrimazole solution or clioquinol) will be used.
3. Ear canal dressing. In severe cases, particularly when there is a lot of pain and oedema, an ear dressing can be very useful. It not only allows continuous and persistent direct contact for any topical treatment, but also splints the ear canal and helps with pain relief. Most commonly, and easily, an expandable otowick can be used.

An alternative strategy, particularly in resistant cases, is 12-mm ribbon gauze, impregnated with a suitable agent. Options include an antibiotic and steroid cream or ointment, 10% ichthammol in glycerine, the hygroscopic action of which reduces meatal swelling

or 8% aluminium acetate eardrops which act as an astringent. (Its low pH is lethal for many bacteria including *Pseudomonas*.) The dressing should be changed at least every 48 hours until the canal swelling has settled sufficiently to allow any applied drops to reach the anteroinferior recess directly.

4. Systemic antibiotics may be required if there is adjacent cellulitis involving the skin of the pinna or cheek. These may be oral or intravenous depending on the severity of the condition and the condition of the patient. Herpes zoster oticus should be treated with prednisolone and antivirals such as acyclovir; in adults, the dose is 800 mg five times daily for at least 7 days or in the i mmunocompromised for 2 days after all vesicles have turned to crusts.
5. General supportive measures including explanation, appropriate analgesia and water advice. The ears should be kept scrupulously dry until resolution. Swimming is inadvisable and precautions are taken when bathing to prevent water entering the ear canal.

65.6 Complications

65.6.1 Cellulitis

In severe cases, the inflammation may extend beyond the confines of the external canal to involve the pinna or facial skin, causing cellulitis, and even perichondritis. In such cases, there may be additional systemic upset and fever. Such cases will require systemic antibiotics which may be given orally in mild cases but may demand admission and intravenous treatment, if severe. (See also Chapter 28, External Ear Conditions.)

65.6.2 Canal Stenosis

In some cases, the chronicity or the severity of the condition may create sufficient fibrosis within the skin of the canal to cause a stenosis of the canal, or in extreme cases to a complete closing of the canal and a so-called 'false fundus'. This may be thin and membranous, or thick and fibrous. The inflammation and discharge may settle as a result, but often at the price of a significant conductive hearing loss. The treatment options for an EAM stenosis are no treatment, a bone-anchored hearing aid or surgery to reconstruct the EAM with a split-skin graft taken from the hairless upper inner arm to reestablish a patent external canal. The key to surgery is to use a very thin graft with the dermatome set at 0.2 to 0.3 mm.

65.7 Follow-Up and Aftercare

Treatment should continue for at least 1 week after resolution because of the tendency to recurrence, particularly in otomycosis. Itchy reactive conditions may benefit from a course of beclomethasone eardrops. An 8% solution of aluminium acetate or acetic acid is recommended in patients with chronic otitis externa after the acute infection has been eradicated. Periodic use of something like Betnovate scalp application can be very helpful in addressing any underlying dermatological issues.

65.8 Malignant (or Necrotising) Otitis Externa

This condition describes otitis externa which progresses to an osteomyelitis initially of the tympanic plate which then may spread to involve the skull base and petrous portion of the temporal bone. It is usually caused by *P. aeruginosa*, most common in elderly patients with diabetes or those who are immunocompromised. It should be suspected when such patients present with a constant, deep and severe otalgia. Patients have signs of otitis externa and may have granulations over the deep ear canal. It may cause 7th to 12th cranial nerve palsies, meningitis, sigmoid sinus thrombosis, brain abscess and death.

The diagnosis is clinical but may be supported by high-definition computed tomography (CT) or magnetic resonance imaging (MRI) scans of the skull base, which are helpful to assess the disease extent but not for length of treatment required. This is because the scan signs of osteomyelitis with soft tissue inflammation persist for many months after all infection has been eradicated. Histological and microbiological examination of granulation tissue may be required to exclude malignancy and confirm the organism responsible. These patients are unwell and will need surveillance of their blood sugar, C-reactive protein (CRP), erythrocyte sedimentation rate (ESR) and full blood count.

65.9 Treatment

Controlling diabetes and treatment with anti-pseudomonal antibiotics such as ciprofloxacin, meropenem and Tazocin are fundamental. The dose and duration of treatment should be decided after discussion with a senior microbiologist and by monitoring clinical response. Often therapy has to be continued for 6 to 12 weeks and monitored by the improving CRP and ESR. A Tc99 scan can also be used for monitoring response to therapy. Even with aggressive treatment there is a mortality rate which is usually quoted as 10% although the author can find no evidence of this figure in the literature. Regular aural toilet and opiate analgesia may be required to control the deep otalgia. Hyperbaric oxygen may be helpful, if available. In cases that are slow to improve, surgical debridement of the retromandibular space, infratemporal and pterygopalatine fossae and external meatus has been proposed but is controversial. The authors' experience is that the CRP and ESR start to significantly improve before the deep otalgia improves and therefore the key is to hold one's nerve in this circumstance and continue with conservative treatment.

Further Reading

Carney AS. Otitis externa and otomycosis. Chapter 78 in Scott-Browns Otolaryngology, Head and Neck Surgery, 8th Edition, Volume 2. Editors-in-Chief Watkinson JC & Clarke R. Published by CRC Press, Taylor & Francis group, Boca Raton, London, New York, 2018

Hobson CE, Moy JD, Byers KE, Raz Y, Hirsch BE, McCall AA. Malignant otitis externa: evolving pathogens and implications for diagnosis and treatment. Otolaryngol Head Neck Surg. 2014; 151(1):112–116

Kaushik V, Malik T, Saeed SR. Interventions to treat acute otitis externa. Cochrane Database of systematic reviews, 2010. http://onlinelibrary.wiley.com/doi/10.1002/14651858.CD004740.pub2/abstract Accessed June 22, 2018

Sylvester MJ, Sanghvi S, Patel VM, Eloy JA, Ying YM. Malignant otitis externa hospitalizations: analysis of patient characteristics. Laryngoscope. 2017; 127(10):2328–2336

Related Topics of Interest

External ear conditions
Suppurative otitis media—acute
Suppurative otitis media—chronic

66 Otitis Media with Effusion

Otitis media with effusion (OME) is the presence of fluid or an effusion in the middle ear space caused by inflammation of the middle ear cleft mucosa, but symptoms of infection are absent and there is no tympanic membrane perforation or otorrhoea.

66.1 Aetiology

The aetiology of OME (glue ear) is multifactorial, but there are two main theories regarding the same. These are the classic theory and the primary inflammation theory.

66.1.1 Classic Theory

The classic theory proposes that OME arises from Eustachian tube (ET) dysfunction. As a point of interest, the Eustachian tube is named after Bartholomeo Eustachi (1513–1574) who was the Professor of Anatomy in Rome and Physician to the Pope. He was one of the founders of the science of Human Anatomy and the first to describe the eustachian tube. Therefore, Eustachian has an upper case first letter.

Physiologically, between swallows, oxygen and nitrogen are absorbed/diffuse into the middle ear mucosa. A smaller volume of carbon dioxide is released from the mucosal cells into the middle ear cleft so that there is a net reduction in middle ear gas volume and therefore a negative middle ear pressure results. On swallowing or yawning, the Eustachian tube is pulled open so that air passes up the tube, equalising middle ear pressure to atmospheric pressure.

Eustachian tube dysfunction refers to the inadequate physiological opening of the tube. This can be caused by blockage of the mouth of the tube from enlarged adenoids, from swelling of the tube mucosa due to infection (perhaps from a upper respiratory tract infection [URTI] or from a source within the adenoids) or allergy, from weak palatal muscles that are unable to contract sufficiently strongly on swallowing to pull open the tube (the young and the elderly, and those with cleft palates) or from the angle of muscle pull being disadvantageous because the angle of the tube is more horizontally placed (young children).

When there is Eustachian tube dysfunction, middle ear pressure equalisation does not occur. If middle ear pressure becomes sufficiently negative, and for a long enough period, then a transudate from the middle ear mucosa will result, and a sterile middle ear effusion is therefore formed. This effusion is protein rich and attracts bacteria.

66.1.2 Inflammation Theory

This theory suggests that the middle ear mucosa becomes inflamed from bacteria already present in the middle ear or possibly from reflux of saliva containing URTI viruses or bacteria into the ET.

These microbes can then stimulate an immune response, with release of cytokines. Respiratory viruses may predispose to bacterial superinfection, or may stimulate an immune response themselves. Cytokines cause upregulation of mucin genes via a cyclic GMP-mediated pathway, leading to a secretion of mucin-rich fluid in the middle ear. The viscosity of the fluid impairs mucociliary clearance and the presence of subclinical bacterial infection causes prolonged stimulation of inflammation. The effusion persists, to be manifest clinically as OME.

Pepsin is found in the effusion of 60% of children with OME raising the possibility of a contribution to OME from gastro-oesophageal reflux too. Pepsin is thought to encourage mucin production.

It is likely that there is a contribution to OME from both models and neither is mutually exclusive. There is strong association of OME with recurrent URTIs, parental smoking, allergy and reduced overall nasopharyngeal dimensions. The adenoids are recognised as important contributors to OME, both as a source of pathological bacteria, but the contribution from obstruction of the orifice of the ET is probably less important. This is because we know that an adenoidectomy confers a significant reduction in the likelihood of recurrent OME when performed with grommet insertion regardless of the size of the adenoid pad.

66.2 Pathology

The prevalence of OME is highest in young children (point prevalence 20% at 2 years), with a second peak at around 5 years of age (point prevalence 16%) and thereafter decreases with age so that it is uncommon in teenagers (< 1% after 11 years). The prevalence is also higher in the winter months, in boys, in children with cleft palate or Down's

O

syndrome, in those with allergy and in the children of parents who smoke.

The underlying Eustachian tube dysfunction leads to a chronic reduction in middle ear pressure. This ultimately causes an inflammatory response in the middle ear mucosa and the production of 'glue': thick, tenacious mucus rich in glyco- and mucoproteins and containing inflammatory cells which fill the middle ear cleft.

In most cases (90%), spontaneous resolution occurs, punctuated by numerous remissions and relapses. In a small number of cases, there is progressive atrophy of the fibrous middle layer of the tympanic membrane leading to a pars tensa retraction pocket or sometimes generalised tympanic membrane atelectasis. In others, the upper third of the tympanic membrane, which lacks a fibrous layer (the pars flaccida), may retract. If the squamous epithelium lining, the pocket subsequently loses its migratory property, then cholesteatoma can result.

66.3 Clinical Features

The presence of fluid in the middle ear cleft leads to a conductive hearing loss of variable severity and is responsible for most of the clinical features. Hearing impairment, whether persistent or intermittent, noticed by parents, relatives or teachers or picked up at routine screening, is the presenting symptom in over 80% of cases. Learning difficulties due to being unable to hear the teacher above the classroom noise, poor concentration, behavioural problems and speech delay account for the bulk of the remainder. Parents often notice their child seems withdrawn and is not socialising. Sometimes parents report clumsiness or balance problems. Recurrent infections and otalgia are uncommon features of this condition (1–2%), although they are common complaints in childhood.

Presentation is commonest between the age of 3 and 6 years, with the more severe cases tending to present earlier. Examination may or may not reveal a middle ear effusion depending on the activity of the process at consultation. The otoscopic appearance of the effusion varies. The tympanic membrane can look dull red, blue, grey or an amber yellow colour. It can bulge forward or be retracted. Attic and posterior retraction pockets may occur and if the tympanic membrane retracts onto the long process of the incus (LPI), then erosion of the LPI may occur. Air bubbles or a fluid level can occasionally be seen.

The presence of nasal obstruction and mouth breathing should be noted and the nose and throat should be examined to identify any contributing factors.

66.4 Investigation

An audiogram appropriate to age and impedance audiometry is required. Pure-tone audiometry, if feasible, will show a conductive hearing loss. During a period of good health and of avoiding URTIs, a child with persistent OME may have hearing within the normal range. At other times, it may be as poor as 45 dB in the low frequencies or 40 dB in the middle- or high-frequency range. If hearing is poorer than this, then a coexistent cause of hearing loss should be considered. Impedance audiometry will show a flat tympanogram (type B) in OME.

66.5 Management

Management should be appropriate to the severity of the symptoms and should take account of the natural history of the condition towards spontaneous resolution. For many children, explanation of the condition to the parents and reassurance that natural resolution may occur with time, may suffice. A review visit after 3 months is necessary to establish if OME is persistent and to repeat a paediatric hearing assessment.

Medical treatment has little role to play in this condition: antihistamines and decongestants have no useful effects and antibiotics produce short-term improvements, but do not affect the long-term course. Autoinflation of the Eustachian tube using the Otovent balloon device may help some children, but it is significantly less effective than grommets. Many children do not like using it so that there may be poor compliance. A 2015 study in a primary care setting, however, showed that at 1 and 6 months the incidence of normal tympanograms was significantly larger in the group using the Otovent device (at 6 months 50% with Otovent, 40% without). There is a concern that uncontrolled autoinflation of the middle ear may push infected nasopharyngeal mucous into the middle ear cleft and a sudden excessive increase in middle ear pressure could cause barotrauma but studies do not seem to have borne this out.

In more severe cases, with a persistent and significant hearing loss (current NICE guidance suggests ~ 25-dB hearing loss for a minimum of 3 months), the insertion of ventilation tubes improves hearing and shortens the overall duration of the condition. The benefits of ventilation tubes may be augmented by combination with an adenoidectomy. The benefits of an adenoidectomy are greatest between the ages of 4 and 8 years, and if upper airway symptoms coexist. Tonsillectomy does not seem to influence the condition.

Grommets are preferred to T tubes, which are associated with a high rate of residual perforation (papers report a wide range of between 15 and 40%). The main complications of grommets are infection, perforation (1–2% with evidence that the perforation rate increases the longer the grommet is in situ, and it is why some clinicians will remove grommets that have been in place for more than 2 years) and the development of tympanosclerosis (which is found in 30–40% of children 1 year after grommet insertion). Tympanosclerosis is associated with multiple episodes of grommet insertion and intratympanic bleeding at myringotomy; mini-grommets seem to cause less morbidity but tend to extrude sooner. Infections should be treated by aural toilet and antibiotic/steroid eardrops in the first instance. Grommet removal may be required if the condition fails to settle because it is felt that in such children, the grommet has become the source of infection.

Hearing aids are a useful alternative where surgery is not preferred, or relatively contraindicated, such as in children with Down's syndrome, cystic fibrosis or Kartagener's syndrome (in the latter two conditions, the grommets usually rapidly block with inspissated glue and the ears will often then become infected).

66.6 Follow-Up and Aftercare

Grommets require little aftercare. There is no good-quality evidence that swimming with unoccluded ears increases the risk of infection in swimming pool water. Children should be advised not to dive beneath the water or to dive from the side into the pool due to these increasing intra-canal pressure. Swimming in the sea probably increases the risk of infection even with earplugs due to the increased bacterial concentration of sea water close to shore. Earplugs should be worn when shampooing (soap reduces the surface tension of the water). Grommets extrude after approximately 6 to 24 months. Following extrusion, review is required to determine if OME has recurred and to recheck the hearing. Forty percent of children will require further subsequent grommet insertion with 10% of children requiring three or more sets of grommets.

Further Reading

Atkinson H, Wallis S, Coatesworth AP. Otitis media with effusion. Postgrad Med. 2015; 127(4):381–385

Maw R, Bawden R. Spontaneous resolution of severe chronic glue ear in children and the effect of adenoidectomy, tonsillectomy, and insertion of ventilation tubes (grommets). BMJ. 1993; 306(6880):756–760

NICE CG 60 Surgical management of otitis media with effusion, 2008. http://guidance.nice.org.uk/CG60/. Accessed December 17, 2018

Williamson I, Benge S, Barton S, et al. A double-blind randomised placebo-controlled trial of topical intranasal corticosteroids in 4- to 11-year-old children with persistent bilateral otitis media with effusion in primary care. Health Technol Assess. 2009; 13(37):1–144

Related Topics of Interest

Impedance audiometry
Paediatric hearing assessment
Tympanosclerosis
Adenoids

67 Otoacoustic Emissions

Using modern computing technology and processing, signal averaging techniques and miniature microphones, cochlear outer hair cell vibrations can be detected in the external auditory meatus as otoacoustic emissions (OAEs). They were first described by David Kemp in 1978, in response to sound stimulation, and represent an objective measure of cochlear function.

67.1 Physiology

The cochlea provides an elegant mechanism for transforming the physical properties of sound into electrical neural impulses. Sound vibrations pass from the environment through the external and middle-ear systems to cause vibrations of the cochlear perilymph. These vibrations produce travelling waves in the basilar membrane. As a result of the gradient of width, thickness and consequently stiffness, of the basilar membrane, these travelling waves reach maximal amplitude at specific points along the cochlea. High frequencies are represented at the basal turn and low frequencies at the apical portion. These traveling waves are detected as a result of shearing forces on two separate hair cell systems in the organ of Corti: the inner (IHCs) and outer (OHCs) hair cells. The inner hair cells are purely sensory and are responsible for detecting these vibrations and producing neural impulses to allow them to be perceived by the central nervous system as sound. The outer hair cells also detect these vibrations but, in contrast, have a motor function. The outer hair cells at the region of maximal travelling wave amplitude vibrate in synchrony with the stimulating signal whilst the OHCs on either side of this region suppress vibration of the basilar membrane. This mechanism allows the fine-tuning, and non-linear response, found in the healthy cochlea. These outer hair cell vibrations can be detected in the external auditory meatus as sounds and have been labelled: otoacoustic emissions (originally described as "cochlear echoes").

67.2 Types of Otoacoustic Emissions

Four classes of OAE exist:

1. Spontaneous OAEs (SOAEs). These are low- level signals that occur without external acoustic stimulation in about 40 to 50% of the normal hearing population. Although they are relatively constant in frequency, they vary in terms of occurrence and intensity and consequently have little use in clinical monitoring.

2. Stimulus-frequency OAEs (SFOAEs). These are recorded at the same frequency and at the same time as a stimulating pure tone. They appear to have found little clinical or research use.

3. Transient-evoked OAEs (TEOAEs). These signals, usually between 0.7 and 4 kHz, occur in response to short-lasting stimulatory acoustic signals (usually clicks or tone bursts). High frequency responses tend to have a shorter latency of onset, arising from the basal turn of the cochlea, whilst lower frequency responses, arising from the apical portion of the cochlea, have a longer latency. The signal is very different for each individual but remains fairly constant for any given ear. TE OAEs occur in almost all human ears with hearing levels better than 40 dB but are of greater amplitude (up to 20 dB SPL) and wider frequency range in children. Broadband clicks will tend to produce a broadband response whereas tone burst will tend to produce a more frequency specific response, closely related to the stimulating tone-burst frequency. Not surprisingly, a louder stimulating sound will tend to produce larger amplitude of response, up to about 70 dB SPL, where the system seems to reach saturation. As they are relatively quick and easy to measure, they are finding widespread use for clinical screening and research.

4. Distortion-product OAE (DPOAE). Stimulation with two pure tones of specific frequency and intensity ratios gives rise to DPOAEs. They are

nearly always present in normal hearing ears and can be measured across a wide frequency range. These characteristics make them an ideal tool for investigating frequency-specific cochlear function. The cochlea will produce multiple responses to such a signal, but it has been found that the largest response consistently occurs at a frequency of 2f1 –to f2, and when the two stimulating tones have a ratio of 1:2. In other words, f2 = 1.2 × f1 (and by convention f1 < f2). Clinical practice has found optimal results with a volume level of 65 dB for f1 and 55 dB for f2.

67.3 Otoacoustic Emission Measurement

An OAE analyser consists of a mobile probe, or earplug, which contains one (TEOAE) or two (DPOAE) sound emitters and a microphone for recording. Unlike a tympanometer, an airtight seal is not required. However, OAEs are typically in the range of 5 to 15 dB SPL and so a good seal is helpful to reduce extraneous noise. It is helpful to clear debris from the external canal and assess middle ear function prior to testing. Although OAEs can still be recorded in the presence of middle ear effusions, their magnitude and reliability may be compromised.

The acoustic stimuli are usually broadband clicks, at a maximal rate of 50 per second. The microphone will record both the stimulus sound, and the stimulated signals. This collective sound is then fed to a signal processor where, by the use of appropriate frequency filters and time window averaging, OAEs can be demonstrated on either a visual or print-out display. These can be measured as absolute values for the OAE amplitude, or a ratio

of signal to background noise, in the canal. The results are then compared to normative data values to indicate the presence of normal hearing, or some degree of hearing loss. In general, individuals with hearing loss demonstrate absent or very low volume (< 5dB SPL) OAEs. Contra-lateral sound stimulation can also affect OAE production.

67.4 Clinical Uses

Although still a research tool for the investigation of cochlear function, the use of evoked OAEs has found a well-established place in clinical practice in the screening of neonates and high-risk infants for hearing loss. Evoked OAEs are quick, easy to test and do not require an anaesthetic, in contrast to electrical evoked response audiometry. The sensitivity and specificity of the test is sufficiently good that there are now widespread programmes for screening all newborn infants for hearing loss by OAE prior to, or soon after, discharge from hospital. They can also be used as part of a test battery for assessment of known hearing loss; normal OAEs suggest a functioning cochlea and therefore may indicate some defect in another part of the auditory system.

Further Reading

Katx J, ed. Handbook of Clinical Audiology, 7th ed. New York, NY: Wolters Kluwer; 2015

Akinpelu OV, Peleva E, Funnell WR, Daniel SJ. Otoacoustic emissions in newborn hearing screening: a systematic review of the effects of different protocols on test outcomes. Int J Pediatr Otorhinolaryngol. 2014; 78(5):711–717

Related Topics of Interest

Evoked response audiometry
Paediatric hearing assessment

68 Otorrhoea

68.1 Definition

Otorrhoea is the discharge of material from the external auditory meatus. It is both a symptom and a sign. It is not a diagnosis. Otorrhoea may arise from a source in the external ear canal, middle ear cleft, mastoid air cells or intra-cranial cavity.

68.2 Causes

Otitis externa and active chronic otitis media are the commonest conditions causing otorrhoea. Malignancy is uncommon. The discharge may contain wax, squamous debris, blood (acute otitis media, trauma, neoplasm) and cerebrospinal fluid (CSF), which usually follows a petrous temporal bone fracture.

68.3 Clinical Features

The character of the discharge depends on, and gives clues to, its source.

1. *External ear* The cardinal symptoms of otitis externa are itch, pain and discharge. There are no mucinous glands in the external canal. Acute inflammatory conditions of the external meatus therefore tend to produce a watery, serous exudate or transudate. In addition, they tend to provoke a hyperkeratosis. This combination leads to soggy white debris collecting in the canal and a thin white, cloudy discharge from the ear. The external canal may also be the subject of trauma, or the site of a furuncle, either of which may lead to bleeding from the ear. A waxy ear discharge is common in children with a pyrexia because of the raised external ear canal temperature creating a more liquefied wax.

2. *Middle ear* The middle ear cleft is lined by mucosa. Mucosa is, by definition, a lining of one or more layers of non-keratinising squamous epithelium which produces mucous from mucous glands contained within. Thus, if there is a mucoid component to the discharge, it usually arises from the middle ear via a perforation of the tympanic membrane. Trapped keratin is offensive; if a cholesteatoma should become infected, the discharge tends to be particularly unpleasant and once smelt, it is never forgotten. A serosanguineous discharge is common

with chronic otitis media should the middle ear mucosa has become granular and polypoid. A sanguineous (meaning blood-stained) discharge is also a feature of carcinoma of the middle or external ear. Chronic otitis media is not typically characterised by pain. Therefore, in patients who have chronic otorrhoea with otalgia that fails to respond to the usual conservative measures, it is wise to consider either bone infection from a localised osteitis or a spreading skull base osteomyelitis (malignant otitis externa) or carcinoma.

3. *Cerebrospinal fluid* CSF rarely discharges from the ears spontaneously but may do so if there is a congenital defect in the tegmen that may allow, over many years, the formation of a meningocele or even an encephalocele. This may rupture spontaneously, but a minor head injury (one that has not caused loss of consciousness or a temporal bone fracture) may be sufficient to cause a tear in the thin dura lining the meningocele. More commonly CSF otorrhoea occurs because of skull base surgery or head trauma that has caused a temporal bone fracture. It will develop in 21% of temporal bone fractures. In such cases, the fluid may initially be mixed with blood and may be recognised by the halo sign in which there is a clear ring of moisture surrounding the blood after absorption onto blotting paper. This is due to the faster diffusion of the less viscous CSF. Differentiation of CSF from thin, watery, serous discharge from a middle ear cavity may be more difficult but can be done by estimation of the glucose content or by confirming the presence of β_2-transferrin in CSF.

If the tympanic membrane is intact, CSF may still leak from the ear should there be a fracture in the roof of the ear canal. Otherwise it may pass down the eustachian tube and become evident as rhinorrhoea or post-nasal drip. Therefore, remember that CSF rhinorrhoea may arise from both an anterior and a lateral skull base cause. Examination of the ears is mandatory in all such patients. It is also important to be cognisant of a further pitfall. Some patients with a spontaneous CSF leak into the middle ear cleft in the presence of an intact tympanic membrane will present with a gin clear middle ear effusion and not CSF rhinorrhoea. Many of these patients will have a grommet inserted to reverse a conductive hearing loss and if the clinician does not recognise that there is a pulsatile gin-clear discharge through the myringotomy or the inserted grommet, the diagnosis will be missed. Such patients will soon present with a persistent watery otorrhoea, but at this stage the diagnosis may still be overlooked because the clinician may feel that the now soggy, waterlogged skin of the external ear canal represents an otitis externa.

68.4 Management

Optimum management of otorrhoea depends on making an accurate diagnosis. Although the history may give many clues, the diagnosis may not be made until the external ear canal and tympanic membrane have been fully examined. This may not be possible at the initial consultation owing to swelling and debris in the external auditory meatus. A swab should be taken for culture and sensitivity (bacteria/fungi) in patients who have already been on treatments, which have not dried the ear. Any granulation tissue removed should be sent for histology. The mainstay of therapy is clearance of canal debris by microsuction clearance. This enables a thorough assessment, diagnosis of cause and allows better penetration of any topical treatments. An otowick may need to be inserted in very narrow external ear canals to allow penetration of antibiotic/steroid eardrops to the full length of the ear canal.

Treatment of the otitis externa will be sufficient if this is the diagnosis. Middle ear disease will demand treatment on its own merits (please see the chapters on Chronic Otitis Media, Chapters 66 and 107).

Patients with acute CSF otorrhoea from trauma should be initially given prophylactic antibiotics to reduce the risk of meningitis. Spontaneous CSF leaks with no history of trauma do not need antibiotic cover. Most post-traumatic leaks resolve spontaneously within a short period, but a temporal bone fracture causing a CSF leak means that there has been both a bone fracture and a tear of the dura lining the fracture site. A high-resolution computed tomography (CT) scan of the petrous temporal bone complemented by a magnetic resonance imaging (MRI) of the head will accurately show the length of the fracture line, the presence or absence of a displaced bone fragment that might tent the dura and whether there is soft tissue

protruding through the defect, indicating possibly brain. These factors will determine if a period of conservative management is appropriate and how long it is reasonable to wait for spontaneous resolution, if this is the initial plan. Some surgeons will wait a fortnight, others a month or two. Iatrogenic leaks should hopefully be recognised and repaired at the time of surgery. If not, conservative management may be reasonable for the first few post-operative days but surgical repair will be required if the leak fails to settle. Spontaneous CSF leaks from a lateral skull base source always require repairing.

Referral to a tertiary centre should occur if surgery is being considered because these patients will require discussion at a skull base multidisciplinary team (MDT). There may be the need for a neurosurgeon to be available for a middle fossa approach in some instances.

Conservative management includes sitting upright in bed and avoidance of manoeuvres that raise intra-cranial pressure (e.g., coughing, straining, etc.). Prior to any surgical intervention, a thorough radiological assessment of the temporal bone should be undertaken to try to establish the site of the leak. This is best achieved with high-resolution CT scanning and a complementary head MRI. Coronal sections are particularly useful in identifying the site and extent of the skull base defect. In the minority of cases where a source of the CSF otorrhoea cannot be identified, fluorescein injected by lumbar puncture may be helpful in finding the site of the leak at the time of surgery.

The type and method of repair employed will depend on the site and cause of the leak and to some extent the state of the middle ear and the patient's hearing; it would be inappropriate to obliterate the middle ear of an individual with normal hearing, for instance.

Further Reading

Applebaum EL, Chow JM, Leaks CSF. Otolaryngology. In: Cummings CW, ed. Head and Neck Surgery. 2nd ed. St. Louis, MO: Mosby; 1993:965–974

Related Topics of Interest

Suppurative otitis media—acute
Cholesteatoma
Suppurative otitis media—chronic
Otitis externa

69 Otosclerosis

Otosclerosis is an autosomal dominant disease of incomplete penetrance affecting otic capsule bone. Mature lamellar bone is replaced by less dense woven bone of greater cellularity and vascularity that features large haversian canals, lacunae, canaliculi and marrow spaces. It presents with a conductive hearing loss, usually starting at the age of 30 to 40 years but may initially present from teenage years to old age. The tympanic membrane is normal provided the patient has no prior history of tympanomastoid disease. Informed consent in its management is pivotal. It should involve the patients reflecting on all the treatment options and risks and particularly how a poor surgical outcome may affect their quality of life. The decision to proceed with surgery must be the patients'.

69.1 Pathogenesis

Otosclerotic foci are most commonly located just anterior to the oval window in the region of the fissula ante fenestram. Symptoms occur when these foci fix the stapedial footplate and encroach upon the labyrinth. It is uncertain whether vestibulocochlear symptoms arise directly from this encroachment or from factors released by the otosclerotic plaque or from both. Foci have also been noted in the region of the fossula post fenestram, the semicircular canals, the round window, the base of the styloid process, the petrosquamous suture and in the cochlea. Labyrinthitis ossificans is a rare end-stage finding in severe otosclerosis.

The three main theories of pathogenesis are as follows:

1. It is an expression of a genetic mutation in collagen metabolism which is only phenotypically expressed in bone derived from the otic capsule.
2. It is an expression of humoral autoimmunity to type II collagen.
3. It is an expression of persistent measles virus infection of otic capsule-derived bone. Electron microscopy has demonstrated viral nucleocapsids in otosclerotic bone cells as have immunohistochemical and polymerase chain reaction studies. Anti-measles immunoglobulin G (IgG) has also been found in the perilymph of patients with otosclerosis.

69.2 Prevalence and Incidence

The clinical disease has been estimated to affect 0.3% of the population (the prevalence). Postmortem temporal bone studies have shown that there are otosclerotic foci within the otic capsule bone in 10% of the population but in only about 10% of such cases (i.e., 1% of the population) does the otosclerosis encroach upon the stapes footplate. Therefore, only 30% of such cases present clinically, presumably because some patients have only mild disease and do not seek advice or have just a mild conductive loss when self-presenting to audiology and remain undiagnosed. The incidence of clinical disease (number of new cases per year) is, of course, much lower than 0.3% as the 0.3% with clinical disease may present from teenage years to late middle age. Seventy-five percent of patients have bilateral disease.

Otosclerosis is more common in Caucasians. A female: male ratio of 2:1 has been noted, perhaps because women are more likely to seek advice because pregnancy, menstruation and the menopause may cause the disease to progress rapidly. Women are more likely to have bilateral clinical disease.

69.3 Clinical Features

The main symptoms are as follows:

- *Deafness* Noticed in most cases before the age of 30. Better hearing in noisy surroundings may be described—paracusis Willisii.
- *Tinnitus* Present in 75% of patients especially when there is a cochlear element to the deafness.
- *Vertigo* Mild and usually transient. Symptoms may mimic benign paroxysmal positional vertigo.

Ten percent of ears display Schwartz's sign, a pink tinge of the tympanic membrane imparted from dilated blood vessels on the mucus membrane of the promontory. Otosclerosis causes no other otoscopy signs. Rinne's test usually suggests a conductive hearing loss. The Weber disease may be referred to either ear depending on whether disease is unilateral or bilateral, and on the cochlear function.

69.4 Investigations

Pure-tone audiometry (PTA) In addition to a conductive hearing loss, there may be cochlear impairment. Masked air conduction typically shows a loss which is greater at low frequencies when there is minimal cochlear impairment, but the frequency response curve flattens and then shows a predominantly high-frequency loss as cochlear impairment progresses. The masked bone conduction curve typically shows a dip at 2,000 Hz, particularly when there is only a slight cochlear loss (Carhart's notch due to the Carhart effect). The bone conduction curve shows a predominately high tone loss when there is severe cochlear impairment.

Speech audiometry With amplification, the score approaches 100 with normal cochlear function, but the score falls according to the severity of the cochlear loss.

Impedance audiometry Unreliable as a diagnostic aid although it may be useful in selecting the more suitable ear for surgery in bilateral otosclerosis with a symmetrical PTA by suggesting the more rigid stapes.

69.5 Differential Diagnosis

- Fibro-osseous footplate fixation.
- Congenital footplate fixation.
- Ossicular discontinuity.
- Fixed malleous–incus syndrome.
- Crural atrophy from a persistent stapedial artery.
- Congenital cholesteatoma.
- Paget's disease (usually produces a mixed hearing loss).
- Osteogenesis imperfecta.

69.6 Management

1. *Sodium fluoride* Its use remains controversial as there is only level IV evidence of the benefit.
2. *A hearing aid* The options include in-the-ear aids, behind-the-ear aids, bone-anchored hearing aids and middle ear implantable devices (see Chapter 36, Hearing Aids).
3. *Stapedectomy* The minimum requirements are at least a 15-dB conductive hearing loss with 60% speech discrimination. The ear including the external ear canal should be free of signs of infection. It is contraindicated in pregnancy. If both ears are suitable for surgery, in bilateral disease, the poorer hearing ear should be chosen. Second ear stapedectomy is advocated by many who perform the small fenestra procedure once the first ear has fully settled from surgery.

69.7 Pre-Operative Counselling

When counselling patients with otosclerosis, it is important to discuss all treatment options. This includes no treatment, that is, just monitoring, a hearing aid or a stapedectomy. Surgery, in a minority of cases, can cause harm to a patient. Therefore, when discussing stapedectomy, the surgeon should present sufficient information to the patient, including the surgeon's own success and complication rates, so that the patient can make an informed decision regarding treatment. It is not sufficient to just list possible complications; the patient should be asked to reflect on his or her likelihood and how those complications would impact on his or her life. It is emphasised that treatment should be the patient's own decision.

- A hearing aid is an alternative method of treatment.
- A dead ear may occur with stapedectomy. The incidence reported by expert otologists varies from less than 0.1 to 4% and a further 10% may have no better, or worse hearing, than pre-operatively.
- Tinnitus may not improve and may be more intense after surgery if there is a poor hearing result. With successful surgery (an improvement in hearing with an air–bone gap of < 10%), tinnitus usually reduces or resolves.
- Mild vertigo is usually present immediately post-operatively for a few days and occasionaly for a few weeks. In a minority, there may be a permanent sense of imbalance.
- Taste may alter if there is traction or an injury to the chorda tympani during surgery. This is usually a metallic taste and settles after a number of weeks but may be permanent. Dividing the nerve causes taste to be lost on one side of the tongue, but the majority of such patients soon report the taste returning to normal, presumably because they have become used to the new level of taste.
- There is a very small chance that the facial nerve will run an anomalous course either splitting around or coursing inferior to the oval window and may be injured. Laser injury to a dehiscent facial nerve has also been reported. Local

anaesthetic injection to the external ear canal may cause a transient facial nerve palsy as may traction on the chorda tympani during surgery.

- After an initial successful operation, there is occasionally late erosion of the long process of the incus from pressure necrosis of the prosthesis and a recurrent hearing loss.

69.8 Post-Operative Advice

- Avoid diving when swimming, lifting objects of more than 30 kg and aggressive nose blowing.
- Open the mouth on coughing or sneezing.
- Each surgeon will have his or her own post-operative advice on flying. Some advise that it is okay to fly immediately post-operatively, particularly if a vein graft is used to seal the stapedotomy prior to prosthesis insertion. Some surgeons who do not seal the stapedotomy and rely on the prosthesis and natural healing to form a stapedotomy seal, advise no flying for a month.

69.9 Technique

1. *Small fenestra* A micro drill, a stapedotomy needle or laser (argon or KTP) can be used to create the fenestra in the stapes footplate. The smaller the fenestra, the smaller is the risk of a high-tone cochlear hearing loss. A 0.6-mm fenestra drill piece and 0.4-mm prosthesis are popular. The Causse technique comprises a 0.8-mm fenestra over which a vein graft is placed and a 0.4-mm prosthesis.
2. *Large fenestra* A portion of the footplate is removed with picks and fine right angle hooks. An attempt is usually made to seal the oval window with a vein or fat graft prior to prosthesis insertion.

The otologist aims to get complete or overclosure of the air–bone gap. Overclosure is possible because of the Carhart effect and is greatest at 2,000 Hz (see Chapter 102, Speech Audiometry).

69.10 Complications of Stapedectomy

1. Peroperative
- Tympanic membrane tear.
- Chorda tympani injury.

- An overhanging facial nerve or a persistent stapedial artery may be encountered and may result in the procedure being abandoned.
- Tympanosclerosis arthrodesing the incudostapedial joint.
- Loose attachment of the prosthesis to the long process of incus due to inadequate crimping. Too aggressive crimping may also fracture the long process. Innovative piston designs such as the titanium CliP Piston a Wengen or the Olympus nitinol Smart self-crimping piston have helped to reduce these complications.
- Perilymph flooding. Teenagers with fluctuating hearing may have a patent vestibular aqueduct which, if not diagnosed pre-operatively, may result in perilymph, under high pressure, flooding the middle ear at stapedotomy. Immediate closure of the stapedotomy with a vein graft or fat, and prosthesis insertion should be performed. The risk of a severe hearing loss or a dead ear is high.
- Floating or partially detached footplate. Here the footplate or a portion of footplate is angled into the labyrinth. It may be possible with a 0.2- to 0.6-mm hook such as a Fisch hook to place the hook under the depressed segment and elevate and remove it. Injury to the saccule from leaving the depressed segment and from the attempted removal must be balanced, but most surgeons would attempt to remove a floating footplate or an attached angled segment.
- Depressed footplate. Here the footplate detaches and sinks into the labyrinth. A decision on whether to try to remove the footplate or just seal the oval window with a vein graft and prosthesis must be made. Most surgeons would not 'fish' for the footplate.
- Injury to the saccule. This lies as close as 0.4 mm beneath the footplate, but is usually 1 to 2 mm beneath. It is easily disturbed when performing the stapedotomy or inserting the prosthesis. It may be the cause of a dead ear from an apparently uncomplicated procedure.

2. Early
- Displacement of the prosthesis from the oval window.
- Detachment of the prosthesis from the long process of incus.
- Footplate granuloma.
- Persisting primary perilymph fistula.

- Sudden-onset vertigo and/or sensorineural hearing loss. While this may be an immediate post-operative complication, this may happen days or several weeks after surgery. In an uncomplicated operation, re-exploration of the ear is controversial. It is thought that in some cases, the acute vestibulocochlear injury causing such acute symptoms after an apparently successful operation may be due to a virus or bacteria entering the vestibule through an unsealed footplate. This is the reason why some surgeons advocate a peri-operative intravenous (IV) dose of a broad-spectrum antibiotic which is continued for a week or two PO post-operatively. Some surgeons advocate post-operative oral steroids for a week too, believing that their anti-inflammatory effect provides some immediate protection from the 'injury' of surgery and from a peri-operative infective insult.

3. Late
- Secondary perilymph fistula.
- Necrosis of the long process of the incus.
- Late detachment or displacement of the prosthesis.

69.11 Cochlear Otosclerosis

Consider when there is a family history of otosclerosis and progressive sensorineural hearing loss in early adult life of no apparent cause. Look for Schwartz's sign on otoscopy. A high-definition computed tomography (CT) scan may detect that the otic capsule has been replaced by less dense woven bone. This is seen radiologically as a lucent halo surrounding the labyrinth.

69.12 Revision Stapedectomy

There are three main group of patients who should be considered for revision stapedectomy:

a. Patients who have redeveloped a conductive hearing loss after stapedectomy. The commonest causes are a dislocated prosthesis (from either the oval window or from the incus), or erosion of the long process of the incus due to pressure necrosis from the loop of the prosthesis.
b. Patients who have had no closure of the air–bone gap following stapedectomy. The commonest causes of a persistent conductive hearing loss are a dislocated prosthesis, a prosthesis which is too short or a dislocated malleoincudal joint.
c. If vertigo persists or develops several weeks after stapedectomy, particularly if associated with loud noises or with applying pressure to the external ear canal. This may be due to too long a prosthesis irritating the saccule. An immediate dead ear may occur if too long a prosthesis injures the saccule.

The overall results of revision surgery are not as good as primary surgery. Reported post-operative sensorineural loss in several series varies from 0.7 to 20%.

Further Reading

Kishimoto M, Ueda H, Uchida Y, Sone M. Factors affecting post-operative outcome in otosclerosis patients: predictive role of audiological and clinical features. Auris Nasus Larynx. 2015; 42(5):369–373

Shea JJ Jr. A personal history of stapedectomy. Am J Otol. 1998; 19(5, Suppl):S2–S12

Virk JS, Singh A, Lingam RK. The role of imaging in the diagnosis and management of otosclerosis. Otol Neurotol. 2013; 34(7):e55–e60

Related Topics of Interest

Labyrinthitis
Perilymph and labyrinthine fistula
Speech audiometry

70 Ototoxicity

Ototoxicity is the term used to describe damage to the vestibulocochlear apparatus reducing function and caused by the interaction of chemicals, most commonly pharmacotherapeutic agents, with the sensory structures of the vestibule and/or cochlea.

Although there are many ototoxic substances, only a small group of drugs, in common therapeutic use, are regularly associated with ototoxicity:

- Aminoglycoside antibiotics (e.g., gentamicin).
- Chemotherapy agents (e.g., cisplatin).
- Loop diuretics (e.g., frusemide).
- β-Blockers (e.g., propranolol).
- Salicylates (e.g., aspirin).
- Quinine.
- Anticonvulsants (e.g., phenytoin and ethosuximide).

The most frequent agents causing permanent damage are the aminoglycoside antibiotics and the chemotherapeutic agent, cisplatin. Rates of ototoxicity vary from 20 to 50% depending on definitions (particularly the frequencies affected and the amount of hearing loss), duration of use, dose used and the agent in question, with some series quoting a prevalence of 90% for some degree of hearing loss with cisplatin use! This chapter will therefore focus primarily on these agents.

70.1 Aminoglycosides

Since their discovery in the late 1940s, aminoglycoside antibiotics have found widespread use in medicine because of their effectiveness against gram-negative bacteria and mycobacteria, relatively low incidence of bacterial resistance and cost. They exert their antibacterial effect by binding with the 30S ribosomal subunit of prokaryotic cells causing a misreading of the genetic code and an interruption of bacterial protein synthesis. Cell death follows. They are poorly absorbed by the gut and so are usually administered parenterally, or topically as eardrops.

The severity of ototoxicity varies amongst the aminoglycosides: neomycin is considered highly toxic; gentamicin, kanamycin and tobramycin somewhat less; and amikacin and netilmicin are regarded as the least toxic. Aminoglycoside antibiotics tend to be either predominantly cochleotoxic (e.g., neomycin and amikacin) or vestibulotoxic (e.g., gentamicin and tobramycin). The former

may relate to the number of free amino groups ($-NH_2$), the latter to the number of free methylamine groups ($-NHCH_3$). It is not related to any site-specific uptake mechanism or to drug levels in the cochlear and vestibular tissues. Indeed, the severity of gentamicin-induced vestibulotoxicity is the basis of vestibular ablation therapy for the treatment of Ménière's disease.

Aminoglycosides are excreted by the kidney and the administered dose must be reduced in renal failure. Hypoproteinemia, anaemia, pyrexia and increasing age all increase the chances of ototoxicity. The risk of aminoglycoside ototoxicity is greatly enhanced by the synchronous use of a loop diuretic.

Mutations in the mitochondrial genome are also well-defined risk factors; quite striking is the effect on aminoglycoside ototoxicity of the A1555G mutation in the 12S ribosomal RNA whose carriers may sustain profound deafness after a single injection. This mutation, which is passed on by the mother, pervades all geographic and ethnic groups and may account for deafness in about 20% of patients with aminoglycoside ototoxicity.

70.2 Cisplatin

Cisplatin is a chemotherapeutic agent effective in treating many solid tumours including head and neck cancer. Its anti-tumour effects were discovered serendipitously in the 1960s and appear to be due to its ability to bind to cellular DNA, thereby blocking transcription and cell replication. Cell death usually follows. Unlike the aminoglycosides, cisplatin appears to be exclusively cochleotoxic. Its ototoxic effects are potentiated by hypoproteinemia and anaemia.

70.3 Mechanism of Damage

These agents both enter the inner ear fluids via diffusion from the bloodstream, or by direct diffusion through the round or oval window membranes for topically applied drops. From there, a process of cellular uptake occurs. For cisplatin, cellular uptake seems to be tied to the active regulation of intra-cellular copper and platinum concentrations. Tumour cells with mutations or deletions in copper transport genes are resistant to cisplatin treatment. Moreover, copper and cisplatin uptake are mutually inhibitory. Studies of the mechanism of aminoglycoside uptake point to the possibility of multiple modes of entry, perhaps in a cell-dependent manner.

Regardless of the mode of uptake, once inside the cell, these agents interfere with various metabolic pathways resulting in the production of reactive oxygen species (ROS) and free radicals. For gentamicin, this may involve binding with iron to form a toxic metabolite which then generates these damaging compounds. The consequent oxidative stress leads to cell necrosis and apoptosis.

In the organ of Corti, the ensuing histopathology of cisplatin and aminoglycoside ototoxicity is remarkably similar. Outer hair cells are generally the most susceptible to damage and are affected gradually from the base of the cochlea to its apex.

In addition, the drugs induce a lateral gradient of damage with hair cell death occurring in the first row (innermost) of outer hair cells first, followed by the second and third rows as the damage progresses. Inner hair cells are more resistant and they usually disappear only after outer hair cells in the vicinity have been completely ablated. Deficits in the vestibular organ are mostly due to loss of types I and II hair cells, with the semicircular canals being more sensitive than the utricle or saccule.

70.4 Prevention

Interventions to attenuate ototoxic side effects take one of two approaches: the augmentation of protective pathways or the inhibition of cell death pathways. An agent that shows promise for the clinical setting is cimetidine. It completely protected animals against cisplatin-induced auditory threshold shifts, although some evidence of nephrotoxicity persisted. Importantly, cimetidine did not change the therapeutic efficacy of cisplatin on a human acute lymphoblastic leukaemia T-cell line.

Studies with preloading with antioxidants (in particular glutathione and vitamin C) prior to aminoglycoside exposure have shown a significant protective effect. In addition, two compounds have already proven clinically successful: aspirin and N-acetylcysteine. Salicylate, the active principle of aspirin (acetyl salicylate), was first established as an effective protectant in guinea pigs in 1999, and subsequently aspirin was tested in a randomised double-blind placebo-controlled trial in patients receiving gentamicin for acute infections. Fourteen of 106 patients (13%) met the criterion of hearing loss in the placebo group compared to 3/89 (3%) in

the aspirin group, constituting a 75% reduction in risk. Aspirin did not influence gentamicin serum levels or the outcome of therapy. N-Acetylcysteine significantly reduced the incidence of hearing loss in a small trial involving patients receiving haemodialysis and gentamicin for bacteraemia. It is of note that two iron chelators, deferoxamine and 2,3-dihydroxybenzoate, reduce gentamicin ototoxicity in guinea pigs in vivo and iron chelators may have a clinical role to play in reducing aminoglycoside ototoxicity in the future.

70.5 Clinical Features

Hearing loss induced by cisplatin or aminoglycosides is generally bilateral and begins at high frequencies, extending to lower frequencies with prolonged treatment. Tinnitus may occur during or after withdrawing treatment and may become more intense and persistent despite drug withdrawal.

The vestibulotoxicity of aminoglycosides can manifest as loss of balance with or without vertigo. The vertigo is characteristically a bobbing oscillopsia whereby distant objects appear to jump about on head movement. This is typical of hair cell loss affecting the saccule and occasionally the superior semicircular canal. Nystagmus may not be demonstrable but caloric testing shows a bilateral decline in labyrinthine function.

Symptoms may be delayed days or weeks after commencement of therapy and can continue to progress even when treatment has been discontinued, although withdrawing therapy may prevent further significant deterioration provided renal function is adequate.

70.6 Investigations

Monitoring of patients taking aminoglycosides by regular enquiry for otological symptoms and by the regular measurement of serum peak and trough levels are necessary to reduce the incidence of ototoxicity and to allow early withdrawal of therapy should they arise. Pre- and post-dose audiometry can be helpful to monitor cochleotoxicity, as may extended high-frequency audiometry. This is because the initial damage to the cochlea affects the basal turn and therefore initially damages hearing receptors above the frequency range responsible for speech (which are those in the 300–3,000-Hz range). Otoacoustic emissions may also have a useful role in monitoring because the initial cochlear damage is typically to the outer hair cells. Caloric testing can be used to assess vestibular function but is not sufficiently sensitive to identify less than a 15% canal paresis.

70.7 Other Drugs Associated with Ototoxic Effects

70.7.1 Loop Diuretics

Furosemide, bumetanide and ethacrynic acid in high doses may produce a reversible high-tone sensorineural hearing loss. Light microscopy shows the stria vascularis to be grossly oedematous, but the organ of Corti remains essentially normal. This causes a loss of the endocochlear potential. A permanent hearing loss is unusual but has been described in renal dialysis and transplant patients. Since 5% of those on renal dialysis group become deaf because of their disease, the contribution of the diuretic to the deafness may be uncertain in many patients.

70.7.2 β-Blockers

A mixed deafness has been described, the conductive element being secondary to a middle ear effusion. The pathogenesis of both the cochleotoxicity and the effusion is unknown. The cochleotoxic effects are generally mild and reversible after withdrawal of the medication.

70.7.3 Salicylates

Aspirin in overdose may induce tinnitus and a flat pure-tone hearing loss of up to 60 dB. This is usually reversible on withdrawing the drug. The vestibular apparatus is undisturbed and recent work has suggested a direct effect of salicylates on ionic conductance of the outer hair cells of the cochlea. Aspirin is cleared rapidly by the kidney so that treatment comprises adequate hydration and the use of an H2 antagonist, for example, cimetidine or a proton pump inhibitor, for example, omeprazole to prevent upper gastrointestinal (GI) complications. It is interesting that aspirin and cimetidine have both been found to have a protective effect against the toxicity of aminoglycosides.

70.7.4 Quinine

Formerly used in the treatment of malaria and still used today to control night leg cramps, quinine has cochleotoxic effects by altering outer hair cell motility. The hearing loss may progress after withdrawing therapy and may be permanent. Hypersensitivity may occur whereby cochleotoxicity develops at therapeutic plasma levels. Most of the drug is bound to plasma proteins so that plasmapheresis is an effective therapy in massive overdose.

70.7.5 Anticonvulsants

Vestibulotoxicity has been described with phenytoin and ethosuximide. The vertigo may be either acute and reversible on withdrawing treatment or more commonly chronic. In those where phenytoin must be used to control the disorder, careful monitoring of the serum levels is necessary.

70.8 Follow-Up and Aftercare

Cochleotoxic symptoms require regular pure-tone audiometric monitoring until thresholds are stable or improve (temporary threshold shift) to quantify the disability. Hearing aids and auditory rehabilitation may be required depending on the severity of persisting symptoms and their handicap. Vestibulotoxic recovery can be symptomatically monitored by outpatient assessment and if necessary, quantified by electronystagmography (ENG) caloric measurements. Vestibulosedative medication and rehabilitation exercises, for example, Cooksey–Cawthorne exercises, minimise morbidity and may aid symptomatic recovery by accelerating compensation.

Further Reading

Forge A. Ototoxicity. Chapter 59 in Scott-Browns Otolaryngology, Head and Neck Surgery, 8th Edition, Volume 2. Editors-in-Chief - Watkinson JC & Clarke R. Published by CRC Press, Taylor & Francis group, Boca Raton, London, New York, 2018

Landier W. Ototoxicity and cancer therapy. Cancer. 2016; 122(11):1647–1658

Rizzi MD, Hirose K. Aminoglycoside ototoxicity. Curr Opin Otolaryngol Head Neck Surg. 2007; 15(5):352–357

Schacht J, Talaska AE, Rybak LP. Cisplatin and aminoglycoside antibiotics: hearing loss and its prevention. Anat Rec (Hoboken). 2012; 295(11):1837–1850

Related Topics of Interest

Sudden hearing loss
Vertigo
Tinnitus
Caloric tests
Otoacoustic emissions

71 Paediatric Airway Problems

Airway obstruction in children can be at the level of the nasal or pharyngeal airway causing a low-pitched snoring-like noise—'stertor'. Laryngotracheal obstruction is more likely to cause a 'higher-pitched stridor' although there is some overlap. Stertor is dealt with in Chapters 104 (Stertor and Stridor) and 75 (Paediatric Nasal Obstruction).

71.1 Larynx and Trachea

Laryngotracheal obstruction in a child can progress rapidly with devastating consequences. The narrowest point in the baby's airway is the cricoid ring. Poiseuille's law dictates that the fourth power of the radius affects airway resistance, so a small reduction in airway radius can produce a profound increase in resistance in an already very small lumen (2-mm radius in a newborn). As fluid (e.g., air) passes through a narrow point, the pressure at the point of narrowing reduces (Bernoulli's principle). As air passes through an already narrowed tube, the tube tends to narrow further (Venturi's effect). This reduced pressure plus increased flow rate causes vibration in the walls of the 'tube', in this case, the airway and in the column of air. Streamlined or 'laminar' flow becomes disordered and 'turbulent'. This vibration produces a sound which is recognised as 'stridor'. Clinical features of airway obstruction include stridor, tachypnoea, poor feeding, sternal recession as the baby works hard to breathe, and in the late stages, tiredness, exhaustion and cyanosis—a truly desperate sign. Stridor is typically inspiratory, but as obstruction progresses, it becomes biphasic. Biphasic stridor needs immediate attention. Aetiology may be congenital or acquired.

71.2 Congenital Causes of Laryngotracheal Obstruction

- Laryngomalacia.
- Laryngeal webs.
- Tracheomalacia.
- Vocal cord palsy.
- Subglottic haemangioma.
- Vascular ring.
- Congenital subglottic stenosis.

71.3 Acquired Causes of Laryngotracheal Obstruction

- Acute laryngotracheobronchitis (ALTB or croup).
- Epiglottitis (now rare as children are vaccinated against *Haemophilus influenzae* B [Hib]).
- Cysts.
- Subglottic stenosis (usually related to intubation).
- Inhaled foreign body.
- Recurrent respiratory papillomatosis.

71.3.1 Laryngomalacia

This condition (floppy larynx) may appear within an hour or two of birth, but more often becomes noticeable in the first few weeks. It is the commonest cause of stridor in infants. It is characterised by an intermittent stridor of varying severity due to an indrawing of floppy supraglottic structures (particularly the arytenoids and aryepiglottic folds) during inspiration. It may be very mild and require no intervention, or it can be severe with sternal recession, poor feeding and failure to thrive. If it is diagnosed by endoscopy, flexible endoscopy in clinic will show the characteristic indrawing of the epiglottis and the arytenoids. If severe or if there is diagnostic uncertainty, then a direct laryngoscopy confirms the diagnosis. Endoscopic features include a tightly curled 'omega'-shaped epiglottis, bulky tethered aryepiglottic folds and redundant arytenoid and supraglottic mucosa. The characteristic feature is stridor, typically presenting a few days after birth as the baby's oxygen requirements increase. Severe cases cause failure to thrive, as the baby uses so much of his or her caloric intake simply to maintain a normal breathing pattern, and often repeated respiratory infections. The diagnosis is a dynamic one and is confirmed at endoscopy—flexible (in clinic) or rigid (under general anaesthesia). A small number of babies with laryngomalacia will have additional airway pathology and a small number of babies with suspected laryngomalacia will have an alternative diagnosis—sometimes serious—to explain their airway obstruction.

Management consists of first making the diagnosis (endoscopy) and proceeding according to the severity of the symptoms. Mild cases can be managed expectantly in the knowledge that the condition gets better in time. Treatment of gastro-oesophageal reflux (GER) is usually recommended, but the evidence base for this is uncertain.

In severe cases, the aryepiglottic folds can be divided to expand the laryngeal introitus (aryepiglottoplasty or supraglottoplasty). Techniques vary, but most surgeons nowadays use cold steel and focus on dividing the tight aryepiglottic folds with minimal, if any, excision of mucosa.

71.3.2 Laryngeal Webs

Laryngeal webs (atresia) may be above (supraglottic), at the level of (glottic) or below the cords (subglottic). They tend to recur if divided and may require tracheostomy and major reconstructive surgery.

71.3.3 Tracheomalacia

Tracheomalacia is characterised by partial or complete tracheal collapse during respiration. It may be primary or idiopathic or occur as part of a spectrum of aerodigestive tract disorders (e.g., tracheo-oesophageal fistula). Often the airway obstruction is mainly expiratory as the airways collapse with changes in intra-thoracic pressure. Sudden episodes of collapse ('dying spells') when the child's oxygen saturation deteriorates, followed by an anoxic arousal response, can cause extreme parental anxiety. Mild case may be managed expectantly, but some children will require ventilatory support, for example, by continuous positive airway pressure (CPAP). In some cases, a tracheostomy will help bypass the obstruction or more commonly it can be used to facilitate CPAP. Surgery in the form of aortopexy to anchor the trachea to the mediastinal structures or in rare cases the use of indwelling stents may be needed.

71.3.4 Vocal Cord Palsy

Vocal cord palsy may be congenital or acquired (e.g., post-thoracotomy when the recurrent laryngeal nerve is damaged). It may cause airway issues, an abnormal cry and aspiration. Most cases can be managed conservatively. Tracheostomy is hardly ever needed except in some bilateral cases.

71.3.5 Subglottic Haemangioma

Subglottic haemangioma (SGH) presents with progressive stridor as the lesion grows—often at about 3 to 6 months of age. Most children with SGH can nowadays be managed with propranolol, avoiding surgery.

71.3.6 Vascular Rings

Vascular rings can compress the trachea causing a pulsatile swelling obvious at endoscopy, and if suspected, they are nowadays well demonstrated by magnetic resonance imaging (MRI).

71.3.7 ALTB (Croup)

ALTB is a common childhood infection, typically occurring between the ages of 6 months and 3 years. The respiratory syncytial virus (RSV) may be responsible. The child develops a barking cough and stridor can be severe. Mild cases can be managed expectantly at home, severe cases may need admission and occasionally endotracheal intubation. Humidification is often used in primary care, but the evidence base is weak. In the acute phase, nebulised adrenaline is helpful. Systemic steroids hasten resolution.

71.3.8 Cysts and Subglottic Stenosis

Cysts are nowadays often found in the subglottis of babies who have been intubated and looked after on the paediatric intensive care unit (PICU). They are probably an inflammatory mucosal reaction to the endotracheal tube. They may cause severe airway problems, including failure to extubate. They respond to surgery in the form of 'uncapping' at endoscopy under general anaesthesia.

More severe reactions give rise to subglottic stenosis (SGS) so that the baby remains dependent on an endotracheal tube (failure to extubate) or develops progressive stridor. Management is complex and specialised. A 'cricoid split' to permit the introduction of a larger endotracheal tube may suffice in a small number of cases. A tracheostomy may be needed, ideally as a temporary measure prior to definitive treatment. Laryngotracheal reconstruction (LTR) using a graft, often costal cartilage or in some cases a resection of the stenotic segment with anastomosis of the ends of the larynx and trachea (cricotracheal resection [CTR]) may be required. Balloon dilation is increasingly successful in helping to manage some cases of SGS.

71.3.9 Juvenile-Onset Recurrent Respiratory Papillomatosis

Juvenile-onset recurrent respiratory papillomatosis (JORRP) is caused by the human papilloma virus (HPV). The virus is transmitted to the baby via the mother at birth. JORRP is characterised by recurrent warty swellings in the larynx causing hoarseness and if severe, stridor. Presentation is with hoarseness, or very occasionally with airway obstruction. Multiple repeated procedures can be needed. Management is surgical most often nowadays using the microdebrider. There is a risk of malignant transformation and the development of squamous carcinomas of the respiratory tract. Now that girls—and in some countries boys—are vaccinated against HPV, we may see a dramatic reduction in the incidence of this condition.

71.3.10 Gastro-Oesophageal Reflux

Gastro-oesophageal reflux is often quoted as an important factor in all sorts of paediatric airway problems. As many as 80% of laryngomalacia babies are said to have GER and it is suggested that they be treated empirically with anti-reflux medication. GER can cause acute laryngeal inflammation and make for less than ideal conditions for laryngeal surgery, so it may be important to treat the GER before embarking on, for example, LTR.

71.4 Summary

- The narrowest part of the child's airway is the cricoid.
- A small reduction in the radius of a child's airway can cause severe airway obstruction.
- Stridor is caused by a vibrating air column and signifies significant obstruction.
- Biphasic stridor is an indication for urgent intervention.
- ALTB or croup is common, usually benign, and responsive to steroids.
- Laryngomalacia is usually benign and self-limiting. The diagnosis is a dynamic one.
- Subglottic haemangiomas are now best treated with systemic propranolol.
- Recurrent respiratory papillomatosis (RRP) is now best treated with the microdebrider.
- GO Reflux may be an important compounding pathology in many cases of airway obstruction in children.

Further Reading

Donne AJ, Rothera MP. Airway obstruction in children. In: Clarke RW, ed. Pediatric Otolaryngology: Practical Clinical Management. Stuttgart: Thieme; 2017:272–280

Sunders M, Clarke RW. Acquired disorders of the larynx, trachea, and bronchi. In: Clarke RW, ed. Pediatric Otolaryngology: Practical Clinical Management. Stuttgart: Thieme; 2017:303–319

Tweedie D, Hartley B. Congenital disorders of the larynx, trachea, and bronchi. In: Clarke RW, ed. Pediatric Otolaryngology: Practical Clinical Management. Stuttgart: Thieme; 2017: 281–302

Related Topics of Interest

Paediatric endoscopy
Paediatric nasal obstruction
Stertor and stridor
Tracheostomy

72 Paediatric Endoscopy

Paediatric airway endoscopy is commonly performed. The main indications are stridor, feeding problems and hoarseness. Airway assessment starts with a thorough history. Ask about the birth history, feeding, the nature of any noisy breathing (stridor, stertor and wheezing). Note the breathing pattern, whether the baby is working hard, any evidence of tracheal tug or sternal recession. Flexible endoscopy in clinic is often well tolerated by babies and toddlers if the child is gently but firmly held by the mother. The endoscope can be introduced per orally using the examiner's finger between the gums to protect the instrument, or transnasally. A good view of the adenoids, the nasopharynx and the upper larynx can be obtained.

Rigid laryngotracheobronchoscopy (LTB) nowadays means looking at the airway with a Hopkins rod lens, displaying the image on a monitor, and capturing still or video images which can be recorded and studied afterwards, sometimes combined with microscope examination (MLTB) to leave the surgeon's hands free for manipulation of instruments. This requires skilled paediatric anaesthesia. The fibre-optic scope can be used as an adjunct to assess vocal cord movement or to view the trachea via a laryngeal mask.

72.1 Laryngotracheobronchoscopy: Technique

The anaesthetist will make sure to have venous access. The cords are sprayed with local anaesthetic to reduce gagging and laryngospasm. Spontaneous breathing is nearly always preferred to paralysis. Endotracheal intubation can be avoided if the anaesthetist places the end of the endotracheal tube in the pharynx leaving the larynx free for inspection during spontaneous respiration.

Specialised children's instruments are used nowadays, for example, the Lindholm laryngoscope which has a blade that sits in the vallecula and provides a view of the cords, the arytenoids and the epiglottis. This is especially good to demonstrate the dynamic changes of laryngomalacia.

Be careful introducing the laryngoscope—it is easy to pinch the lips or bruise the gums. A swab can be useful to protect the gums or the teeth in an older child. Use suction gently and don't poke the

mucosa as it will swell up very quickly especially around the arytenoids. If there is a lot of mucosal swelling, an adrenaline-soaked patty can help to shrink the tissue to give you a better view but is not usually needed.

Check the dynamics of the supraglottis—the characteristic indrawing of the arytenoids and the epiglottis is easily seen in laryngomalacia. Check for a laryngeal cleft, assess the calibre of the subglottis and look at the carina and the orifices of the main stem bronchi. Look at the tracheal lumen. An extrinsic mass—often a vascular ring—will cause tracheal compression, and in tracheomalacia the lumen will be ellipsoid, sometimes closing completely during respiration. Pass the bronchoscope down to the carina and look at the posterior wall of the trachea to exclude a tracheo-oesophageal fistula. Check the mobility of the cords—best done when the child is waking up.

Record your findings—most surgeons will give the parents one set of prints and keep one as part of the child's medical records.

72.2 Bronchoscopy

You can get a really good view of the trachea and bronchi using a rigid telescope passed through the vocal cords while the child breathes spontaneously. You will rarely need a ventilating bronchoscope unless you need to introduce instruments, for example, the grasping forceps to remove a foreign body. Modern bronchoscopes are highly sophisticated with superb optics and permit ventilation and gas exchange during the procedure (ventilating bronchoscope). Optical forceps with an integrated telescope that fits through the lumen of the bronchoscope has made the removal of bronchial foreign bodies much easier and safer provided the surgeon, the anaesthetist and the theatre team are experienced in the use of these instruments.

For a bronchial foreign body introduce a bronchoscope of suitable size into the larynx using a McGill's anaesthetic laryngoscope, to guide the instrument through the cords. Get a good view and enter the main stem bronchus. Once you have identified the foreign body, remove secretions with gentle suction, shrink the mucosa with an adrenaline patty if needed and choose some suitable grasping forceps—with an integrated telescope, that is, optical forceps and introduce it through the lumen of the bronchoscope to engage and deliver the foreign body. An organic foreign body—for example, a peanut—or a foreign body which has been in for a few days—can cause a brisk inflammatory response and the child may need careful post-operative monitoring and long-term follow-up.

72.3 Paediatric Tracheostomy

Tracheostomy is covered in Chapter 116. Some features of tracheostomy in children are very different from the situation in adults. The child's neck is shorter and fatter, the cricoid is higher in the neck and the vital structures—including the carotid sheath—can be crowded very close together. The trachea itself is softer, more mobile and inclined to move from side to side with minimal manipulation so that it can be hard to identify and stabilise, especially if there is no endotracheal tube in place to guide the operator. Tracheostomy can be lifesaving, but with improved training and better endotracheal intubation techniques in children, an emergency tracheotomy is very rarely needed. Indications have changed over the years and many children now need tracheostomy to facilitate long-term ventilation rather than to bypass an obstruction.

72.3.1 Technique

Position the child on the table with the neck extended a little and the head gently stabilised in a head ring. Be careful not to overextend, as this will bring the apical pleura or the thoracic veins (brachiocephalic vein) into the operative field. Make a skin incision, remove a small piece of subcutaneous fat and keep your dissection to the midline. Stay well below the first tracheal ring to avoid the risk of stenosis. It is never wise to remove cartilage in a baby as this risks tracheal stenosis. Use well-secured stay sutures on either side of the tracheal incision to facilitate the entry of the tube and to make for easier access should the tube become dislodged. Make sure the lower end of the tube is well (at least 1–2 cm) above the carina as otherwise it may slip into a main stem bronchus in the early post-operative period so the child is ventilating on only one lung.

72.3.2 Post-Op Care

Regular suction and humidification are even more important than in an adult as the small-diameter tube can easily get blocked. Babies tend to produce quite brisk tissue inflammatory responses to foreign bodies, and granulation tissue often develops at the site of the stoma or above (suprastomal granulation), and at the distal end of the tracheostomy tube. Health care personnel looking after the child need to be appropriately trained, and parents usually manage to become very skilled at looking after suction, tube changes and humidification.

72.3.3 Tracheostomy Tubes

Inevitably these are smaller than in adults. The narrow calibre makes for a higher risk of obstruction with secretions. Typically, there is no outer tube as the small calibre doesn't permit this, and cuffs are far less useful for the same reason. Fenestrated tubes are rarely used as the fenestra is inclined to get blocked with granulation tissue.

72.3.4 Decannulation

A small number of children will be tracheostomy-dependent indefinitely, but the aim for most will be decannulation when circumstances permit, that is, when the condition that necessitated tracheostomy has resolved. Protocols and approaches differ but decannulation typically required several days in hospital under strict supervision while the child's progress is monitored until he or she is deemed safe to manage without a tracheostomy tube.

72.3.5 Tracheocutaneous Fistula

Following long-term tracheostomy and decannulation, the stoma may stay patent and produce a troublesome mucoid discharge. If this persists beyond 6 months, then surgical repair is usually considered.

72.4 Summary

- Airway endoscopy should be guided by a careful history and clinical examination.
- Babies will usually tolerate flexible endoscopy if the endoscopist is experienced.
- Rigid endoscopy with Hopkins' lenses and a high-quality monitor with good image capture

P

facilities provide the gold standard for airway endoscopy.

- Be careful to avoid trauma to the gums and lips.
- Use suction judiciously, especially around the arytenoid cartilages.
- Highly skilled paediatric anaesthesia and a good rapport between anaesthetist and endoscopist are essential to good paediatric airway endoscopy.

Further Reading

Donne AJ, Rothera MP. Airway obstruction in children. In: Clarke RW, ed. Pediatric Otolaryngology: Practical Clinical Management. Stuttgart: Thieme; 2017:272–280

Related Topics of Interest

Stertor and stridor

Tracheostomy

73 Paediatric Genetic Syndromes and Associations

73.1 Definitions

- A syndrome is a group of birth defects with a single (usually genetic) cause, for example, Down's syndrome (trisomy 21).
- In a sequence (Pierre Robin) the clinical features are due to a single anatomical abnormality—that is, it is the mandibular hypoplasia that causes micrognathia, tongue base prolapse and palatal defects.
- An association is a group of defects that commonly occur together, without a specific known cause, for example, VATER, CHARGE (see later).

73.2 Syndromes

- Down's syndrome.
- Turner's syndrome.
- Treacher Collins syndrome.
- Goldenhar's syndrome.
- Crouzon's syndrome.
- Apert's syndrome.
- 22Q11 deletion syndrome.
- Syndromes causing congenital deafness.

73.3 Sequences and Associations

- Pierre Robin sequence.
- VATER association.
- CHARGE association.

73.4 Down's Syndrome

Down's syndrome (trisomy 21) is a genetic disorder almost always associated with an extra partial or complete chromosome 21. Affected children have a variety of features, including somewhat flattened facies, a short neck, a protruding tongue, upward-slanting palpebral fissures (eyelids), small ears, hypotonia (floppy baby), short broad hands and short stature. They are prone to a variety of medical pathologies (▶Table 73.1) and a number of ENT pathologies (▶Table 73.2).

Children with Down's syndrome have a high incidence of obstructive sleep apnoea (OSA) due to muscle hypotonia, relative macroglossia due to a midfacial hypoplasia and large obstructing tonsils and adenoids. OSA can precipitate pulmonary hypertension, a serious and potentially devastating feature of Down's syndrome. Airway problems are common, for example, tracheo-oesophageal fistula, tracheomalacia and subglottic stenosis. Other ENT issues include deafness, both sensorineural and conductive. A small external ear canal, a high prevalence of otitis media with effusion (OME) and anatomical abnormalities of the ossicles, the cochlea and the facial nerve are all well documented. Thyroid pathology is also more common in these children. Children with Down's syndrome often feature on ENT operating lists and the surgeon and anaesthetist need to be aware of some particular issues relating to anaesthesia, for example, a child with Down's syndrome will often need a smaller-sized endotracheal tube than his or her age-matched peer and have a tendency towards atlantoaxial instability so the child's head has to be manipulated with special care.

▶ **Table 73.1** Medical issues in children with Down's syndrome

Cardiac: Congenital heart disease, pulmonary hypertension

Gastrointestinal (GI): Feeding problems, GO reflux and Hirschsprung's disease

Eyes: Cataracts, acuity issues

Haematological: Leukaemias

Endocrine: Thyroid disease, diabetes mellitus

Neurological: Epilepsy, learning disability, autistic spectrum disorders and premature dementia

▶ **Table 73.2** ENT issues in Down's syndrome

Airway: OSA due to small midfacial skeleton, hypotonia, prolapsing tongue base. Narrow subglottis, tracheomalacia and cleft palate

Ear problems: OME, sensorineural deafness, ossicular anomalies, facial nerve anomalies and external ear deformity

Nose and sinus: Rhinosinusitis

Abbreviations: OME, otitis media with effusion; OSA, obstructive sleep apnoea.

73.5 Turner's Syndrome

Girls with this syndrome have the sex chromosome makeup XO. ENT issues are common and include both sensorineural deafness and conductive deafness, a high incidence of cleft palate and abnormalities of the pinna.

73.6 Treacher Collins Syndrome

This is now known to be caused by a gene defect—most commonly in the *TOCF1* gene which codes for a protein known as 'treacle'. It is inherited as an autosomal dominant. ENT features include abnormalities of the pinna, microtia, conductive deafness, cleft palate, choanal atresia and mandibular and maxillary hypoplasia. Micrognathia can cause severe airway problems necessitating a tracheostomy.

73.7 Craniofacial Syndromes

Conditions such as *Goldenhar's, Crouzon's, Pfeiffer's* and *Apert's* syndrome are characterised by craniofacial dysmorphism, often with hemifacial microsomia, craniosynostosis (premature fusion of the skull sutures), microtia, mandibular and maxillary hypoplasia, cleft palate and often severe airway problems needing tracheostomy.

22Q11 deletion syndrome (formerly known as DiGeorge's syndrome) is increasingly recognised as a cause of sensorineural deafness. A number of specific syndromes—Waardenburg's, Pendred's, Alport's and Jervell/Lange–Nielsen syndrome are known causes of profound sensorineural hearing loss and are seen in cochlear implant clinics. Genetic testing is becoming increasingly sophisticated and more and more cases of hearing loss are now traced to a genetic aetiology.

Pierre Robin sequence is characterised by mandibular hypoplasia, cleft palate and micrognathia. Glossoptosis, a tendency of the tongue to prolapse back into the airway, contributes to airway obstruction. Feeding problems are common and these babies are best nursed prone in contrast with the usual advice to put babies on their backs—'back to sleep'. They may need a nasopharyngeal airway but the airway improves as the baby develops and the mandible grows, and the NPA can eventually be dispensed with. Some parents with appropriate training become very adept at managing their baby's NPA and these babies are best looked after at home. Tracheostomy is nowadays very rarely needed.

The *VATER (VACTERL)* association is characterised by vertebral, anorectal, cardiac, tracheal, oesophageal, renal and limb abnormalities, is not uncommon in paediatric practice and some of these babies may have ENT conditions as well, for example, tracheomalacia, subglottic stenosis.

CHARGE association is characterised by coloboma, heart defects, atresia of the choanae, renal abnormalities, growth defects (often genital hypoplasia) and ear defects. ENT surgeons most often diagnose the condition as it presents with severe airway obstruction in the newborn due to choanal atresia (see Chapter 75, Paediatric Nasal Obstruction).

73.8 Conclusions

Be sensitive with your language when dealing with the parents of children with syndromes. Refer to the child first and the condition later, for example, parents prefer the term 'a child with Down's syndrome' to 'a Down's syndrome child'. When comparing the progress of a child with a syndrome to another child, avoid the use of terms such as 'normal'. A child with Down's syndrome, for example, is more likely to have middle ear effusions than a 'typically developing child' rather than a 'normal' child. Attention to such subtleties makes for a far better rapport with parents. Children with syndromes usually need intensive multidisciplinary input but are increasingly seen in ENT clinics. Many will have cochlear implants, bone-anchored hearing aids (BAHAs) and tracheostomies. Parents are usually well versed in the features of their child's syndrome and may be members of one of a number of patient/parent support groups.

Further Reading

http://www.downs-syndrome.org.uk/for-new-parents Accessed June 26, 2018/

Kunanandam T, Kubba H. The child with a syndrome, Chapter 6 in Scott-Browns Otolaryngology, Head and Neck Surgery, 8th Edition, Volume 2. Editors-in-Chief–Watkinson JC & Clarke R. Published by CRC Press, Taylor & Francis group, Boca Raton, London, New York, 2018

Sheehan P. The child with special needs. In: Clarke RW, ed. Pediatric Otolaryngology: Practical Clinical Management. Stuttgart: Thieme; 2017:46–54

74 Paediatric Hearing Assessment

Assessing hearing in children requires experience, expertise and skill. It requires close teamwork as, under the age of 4 years, the assessment often requires two testers who must have good mutual understanding. The importance of assessment cannot be emphasised enough as early detection of hearing loss in children leads to more favourable management outcomes. This is because in pre-lingual children, the crucial window for speech acquisition is finite. It is important that the child with a hearing loss is managed by appropriate amplification as early as possible. This is the basis of the newborn hearing screening programme designed to pick up a hearing loss in a child soon after birth. In post-lingual children, a hearing loss may generate a negative emotional and behavioural reaction and early intervention is also recommended and helpful. Hearing assessment in children is performed by behavioural audiometry or objective audiometry. Universal newborn hearing screening (UNHS) employs automated objective audiometry.

74.1 Rationale for Hearing Assessment in Children

Epidemiologically, congenital hearing loss is a significant morbidity affecting 1.06:1,000 live births and for late-onset or acquired hearing loss the prevalence is 1.65 to 2.05:1,000 up to 9 years. Late-onset congenital hearing losses and acquired hearing losses are thus important and indeed one of the commonest conditions in childhood. In all cases, early intervention after diagnosis from a multidisciplinary team is essential as hearing loss is inexorably linked to the development and behaviour of the child. It has been shown that early intervention leads to better speech development in pre-lingual hearing losses and hastens positive social and mental development. For post-lingual children, early intervention can preclude many negative emotional reactions and improve worsening academic grades as a result of the hearing loss.

74.2 The Newborn Hearing Screening Programme

Many countries in the world have adopted a universal newborn hearing screening programme either mandated by federal government or by state. In the United Kingdom, this is a government initiative.

An automated transient otoacoustic emission test (AOAE) is carried out in all newborns which the machine scores as a pass or a fail in the form of a clear response (CR) or a no clear response (NCR). A pass is a discharge unless there are reasons for targeted surveillance. An initial failure leads to a second test. If the child fails the second test, it is referred for an automated auditory brainstem response test (AABR). A pass in this test is a discharge again, unless complicated by risk factors demanding subsequent targeted surveillance. A failure, however, necessitates full diagnostic auditory brainstem response (ABR) and otoacoustic emissions (OAEs) under natural sleep in the local audiology unit. The automated tests are neither 100% sensitive nor specific; subsequent normal hearing can still be found in some cases.

Some children who have passed their newborn hearing screening may still be reappointed for behavioural audiometry at 8 months after birth for targeted surveillance in the presence of a risk factor—examples include ototoxic medication, prematurity, some infections, meningitis and genetic syndromes.

The diagnostic ABR also establishes hearing thresholds for effective prescriptive fitting of digital amplification within a maximum of 6 months after birth for maximum outcome or in case of profound hearing losses referred for cochlear implantation. At the same time, the child is investigated thoroughly from an aetiological point of view. Detecting a cause is an important management process. The moment a child's hearing loss is diagnosed, a full multidisciplinary process is set in motion that involves the audiovestibular physician, the otologist, the audiologist, the speech and language therapist, the paediatricians, the sensory services and the parents.

The protocol for premature children or children admitted to the neonatal intensive care unit (NICU) is slightly different. They undergo both AOAE and AABR to pick up auditory neuropathy spectrum disorder (ANSD) which is a condition characterised by normal cochlear function with abnormal auditory brainstem responses and management instituted accordingly.

74.3 Behavioural Audiometry in Children

74.3.1 Under 6 Months

Under 6 months formal behavioural audiometry is impossible as children do not exhibit the cognitive ability to correlate a sound with a head turn. However, informal ways, for example, startling to sound, stilling to sound or visual tracking of sound can be observed. Parental identification of these behavioural responses is sensitive in about 50% cases. Another way of indirectly inferring that the hearing might be impaired is when the child does not vocalise.

74.3.2 From 6 to 18 Months

Distraction testing in the sound field with varieties of frequency-specific sounds including a high-frequency rattle, low-frequency domestic sounds like a cup and spoon, high-frequency sibilant sounds or even ordinary voice is presented in the sound field to the child from the back by the tester with a distractor in front holding the child's attention. The child turns the head as a reflex to the site and the source of the sound. In a controlled setting with trained professionals, this is a useful screening tool for further diagnostic work-up.

74.3.3 From 6 to 36 Months

The most widely used test in this age group is conditioned audiometry where the child is distracted by one tester in the front and presented with frequency-specific warble tones by the second tester behind while it sits on the carer's lap. It is 'conditioned' first with a visual reward from a monitor following a sound presented at the same time. After conditioning, a positive and a true response is when the child, after hearing a sound, turns to the visual monitor anticipating the visual reward. Thresholds thus can be obtained both in the sound field and importantly, with insert earphones, from each ear as well. This test is visual reinforcement audiometry (VRA) and can be as robust as a pure-tone audiogram (PTA). The test demands a high skill set and expertise and may be very difficult to perform in cognitively challenged children, for example, disabled children or autistic children.

74.3.4 From 24 to 48 Months

A different variety of conditioned audiometry is play or performance audiometry which can employ two testers or one. Here the child is conditioned so that in response to a sound, he or she will complete a playful action, for example, putting a man in a boat or banging the table with a spoon. This task needs a higher cognitive level than the VRA. The test can be done in a free sound field, that is, not ear specific.

74.3.5 From 36 Months Onwards

A PTA with a descending staircase adaptive method can be utilised with conditioning.

74.4 Important Considerations When Performing Behavioural Audiometry

The clinician must be fully versed with child development especially motor and cognitive development. For a well-child, the above suggested age ranges can be applied as a rough guide, but it should be remembered that choosing the right test for a child is not only dependent on age but also on the development of the child which should be assessed before undergoing the test.

74.4.1 Speech Tests

The best test to have an idea about functional hearing in a child is by speech testing with McCormick's toys. Here physical figurines with similar phonemes (man/lamb; plate/plane) are presented to the child through a loudspeaker or by live voice and the child is instructed to correctly identify these and scored according to correct responses. This test can be employed as soon the child acquires the appropriate vocabulary. This is a very useful test to assess efficacy of digital amplification. Another speech test is the Manchester picture test where instead of toys, pictures are used.

74.4.2 When Behavioural Audiometry Is Unreliable or Impossible

Occasionally, behavioural audiometry becomes difficult or impossible in behaviourally challenged children or children with multiple sensory issues.

These children are then subjected to objective audiometry under supervised sedation or melatonin-induced sleep or, in extreme cases, a general anaesthetic.

74.5 Objective Audiometry in Children

74.5.1 Impedance Audiometry

Tympanometry and stapedial reflex tests can be attempted at any age. In newborns, a high-frequency tympanometry tone should be used as the middle ear does not react to the standard 226-Hz probe tone. Stapedial reflexes are useful for screening ANSD and should be performed in every case, especially in children with behavioural problems. An abnormal stapedial reflex test may suggest the need for diagnostic ABR for ANSD.

74.5.2 Otoacoustic Emissions

The human cochlea is a biologically active organ where the outer hair cells expend energy to modify the acoustic signal incident on it. This activity generates cochlear emissions which can be measured to assess cochlear function. The transient OAE is in response to a broad-spectrum click and is not frequency specific. It is used in the newborn hearing screening programme. It is useful to obtain an overall picture of cochlear function but may also be compromised by middle ear disorders. The distortion product OAE uses pure tones and is frequency specific. Contralateral suppression of OAE assesses cochlear efferent activity and the medial olivocochlear bundle. Information is useful to assess auditory processing disorders, hyperacusis and tinnitus in children.

74.5.3 Cochlear Microphonics

The cochlear microphonic is believed to be a receptor potential from the outer hair cells which can be measured by ABR software. The measurement in some instances is more resistant to middle ear changes and therefore more specific than the OAE. Cochlear microphonics are frequently used to diagnose ANSD.

74.5.4 Auditory Brainstem Response

The auditory nerve, originating from synapses of spiral ganglion cells from the inner hair cells of the cochlea, traverses the internal auditory canal and enters the brainstem, relaying to a number of cochlear nuclei. Auditory nerve action potentials in this pathway can be recorded by surface electrodes in response to an ear-specific acoustic stimulus. Two different types of stimuli are used—a broadband click stimuli and a frequency-specific tone burst stimuli. The latter is the chosen method after newborn hearing screening failure as frequency-specific information is needed for digital amplification. Correlation is good when compared to pure-tone prescription thresholds. In addition, it can be used for non-organic hearing loss.

The child has to be still during the procedure and the test can be done in older children without any other intervention. However, in younger and in behaviourally challenged children, it must be done under natural sleep or with some sedation or even with a general anaesthetic.

74.5.5 Other Electrophysiological-Evoked Responses

Auditory steady-state response (ASSR) is an electrophysiological response to rapidly occurring auditory stimuli, faster than the ABR stimulus and is frequency specific. The objective is to obtain a PTA-like index of hearing sensitivity. Cortical response–evoked audiometry in children is a key topic for research where the action potential generated by an acoustic stimulus is measured in the cerebral cortex and can be a more robust indicator of auditory thresholds than the ABR.

74.5.6 Measurement of Non-Organic Hearing Loss in Children

Any abnormally measured threshold by conventional PTA in older children, in the absence of an organic pathology, or which is disproportionate to the functional hearing of the child, raises the possibility of non-organic hearing loss (NOHL). The aetiology is usually due to emotional and/

P

or behavioural issues such as school and social surroundings, attention seeking, bullying or domestic violence. Pure-tone audiometry is the screening test followed by special pure-tone audiometry, for example, Stenger's test. In difficult cases, objective audiometry may need to be performed. It is important to diagnose NOHL correctly due to its holistic ramifications.

Further Reading

McCormick B. Paediatric Audiology 0–5 Years. 3rd ed. London: Whuur; 2003

Parker G. Hearing tests in children, Chapter 9 in Scott-Browns Otolaryngology, Head and Neck Surgery, 8th Edition, Volume 2. Editors-in-Chief – Watkinson JC & Clarke R. Published by CRC Press, Taylor & Francis group, Boca Raton, London, New York, 2018

Related Topics of Interest

Evoked response audiometry
Otoacoustic emissions
Non-organic hearing loss
Hearing aids
Congenital hearing disorders

75 Paediatric Nasal Obstruction

Neonates and young children presenting with nasal obstruction are common in general practice and paediatric ENT clinics. A key point to consider is that neonatal rhinitis can mimic choanal atresia. Choanal atresia is a neonatal emergency and transfer for surgery should be arranged as soon as possible following diagnosis. Assessment with endoscopy using the 120-degree Hopkins rod has transformed the management of choanal atresia. Remember that some nasal masses may have an intra-cranial origin, so high-quality imaging should be requested. It is important to think of cystic fibrosis if presented with a child with nasal polyps. Beware angiofibroma in adolescent boys. These are important clinical precepts, and they are essential edicts for the examination.

75.1 Causes of Nasal Obstruction in the Newborn

- Rhinitis (common).
- Choanal atresia/pyriform aperture stenosis.
- Nasal/pharyngeal masses.

75.2 Causes of Nasal Obstruction in Older Children

- Adenoids.
- Rhinitis.
- Nasal polyps (consider cystic fibrosis).
- Osseocartilaginous deformity.
- Foreign body.
- Nasal masses.
- Fibrous dysplasia.
- Angiofibroma (adolescent boys).

75.3 Neonatal Rhinitis

Neonatal rhinitis is fairly common and can mimic choanal atresia. Treatment is expectant and mostly the condition is short-lived. Saline nose drops and in severe cases a short course of intra-nasal steroids will hasten resolution.

75.4 Choanal Atresia

Congenital choanal atresia is due to the embryological failure of the primitive bucconasal membrane to rupture before birth. This results in the persistence of either a bony plate (90%), a fibrous membrane or both, obstructing the choana. It occurs in about 1 in 10,000 births. Unilateral choanal atresia is twice as common as bilateral. Bilateral choanal atresia may cause respiratory distress and if not recognised, respiratory arrest and death shortly after birth. The choana means the posterior opening of the nose and therefore the frequent description of the choana as the 'posterior choana' when describing the posterior opening is incorrect.

75.5 Embryology

The mouth, palate, nose and paranasal sinuses develop from the cranial portion of the primitive foregut. The nose begins as two epithelial thickenings known as the nasal placodes, which appear above the stomatodeum about the fourth week in utero. The placodes deepen to form olfactory pits which lie between the medial and lateral nasal processes. The medial processes fuse to form the frontonasal process. This is compressed to form the nasal septum as the lateral nasal processes approach each other. The nasal septum will then grow posteriorly to divide the two nasal cavities. Each nasal cavity is closed posteriorly by the thinned out posterior wall of the nasal sac, called the bucconasal membrane. This usually breaks down around the sixth week in utero. Its persistence is thought to be the cause of choanal atresia.

75.6 Clinical Features

A unilateral obstruction may be asymptomatic at birth but will later cause unilateral nasal discharge and obstruction. Examination of the nose will show thick gelatinous secretions on the affected side, and no airway can be demonstrated when holding a cold-plated spatula below the nares. Only the patent side will steam the surface (mirror test). A unilateral choanal atresia may be treated electively and indeed some are only diagnosed after some years when a parent and/or GP becomes fed up with the child having a unilateral nasal discharge that does not respond to repeated courses of antibiotics and nasal decongestants.

Bilateral choanal atresia presents as a respiratory emergency at birth. The newborn is a near-obligate nasal breather and nasal obstruction will therefore produce difficulty in breathing. The alae nasi dilate and the accessory muscles of respiration are used, but to no avail. There is pallor and cyanosis until the mouth is opened. A few quick breaths are taken, the infant cries, the cyanosis resolves and then the baby becomes quiet again. This cycle of events continues. In some children mouth breathing appears to occur without too much distress at rest but cyanosis occurs when feeding. The diagnosis should be suspected as one of the differentials in a newborn who has cycles of cyanosis or who has a respiratory arrest. In such a baby, an oropharyngeal airway should be inserted to assist respiration.

About half of infants with choanal atresia display other abnormalities, including the CHARGE syndrome. This refers to an autosomal dominant genetic disorder of multiple congenital anomalies. It comprises the following:

C, coloboma of the iris, choroid and/or microphthalmus.
H, heart disease such as atrial septal defect (ASD).
A, atresia choanae.
R, retarded growth and development.
G, genitourinary anomalies such as cryptorchidism and hydronephrosis.
E, ear abnormalities that may be external, middle and/or vestibulocochlear and deafness.

Choanal atresia, either unilateral or bilateral, is found in all children with CHARGE syndrome, but only three of the remaining five anomalies are required to make the diagnosis. In addition, half exhibit facial nerve palsies and one-third of cases have laryngotracheal anomalies.

75.7 Investigations

Suspicion regarding the diagnosis can be increased by the mirror test or by not being able to pass a fine endobronchial suction catheter through the nose into the nasopharynx. If there is an obstruction, the catheter will not pass beyond 4 cm. Fibre-optic endoscopy using a 2.2-mm paediatric endoscope after gently suctioning the nose of secretions using a soft endobronchial suction catheter and then nasal decongestion, may confirm the diagnosis, provided that an adequate view of the choana is

obtained. Neonates with choanal atresia may have narrow or funnel-shaped posterior nares because the posterior vomer may widen medially, the lateral nasal wall may be medialised and inferiorly the height of the nasal cavity may be reduced by there being a highly arched hard palate. A high-resolution multislice computed tomography (CT) scan is required to accurately delineate the nature and thickness of the atresia before surgery is performed.

75.8 Management

Cases of unilateral atresia can initially be observed without treatment. In the case of the newborn with bilateral atresia, the priority is to insert and maintain an oropharyngeal airway. The treatment of choanal atresia is surgical. The challenge is to provide a nasal airway which has a mucosal lining, and to prevent granulation tissue formation and subsequent stenosis. Two approaches are in common use.

1. Combined transoral/transnasal approach. This is the usual approach in neonates. Using a 120-degree rigid endoscope placed in the oropharynx, the nasopharyngeal face of the choana is visualised. The nasal aspect of the choana is visualised endoscopically after nasal decongestion. If the CT shows just a membranous atresia, the patient may require no more than serial dilations after the initial rupture of the atresia is achieved. This can also be accomplished with electrocautery or laser. In the more common bony occlusions, it will be necessary to perform a trephine and remove the obstruction with a 1–2-mm diamond burr or use a 1–2-mm-tip diameter Kerrison's forceps. Some surgeons advocate stenting the choana with a modified Portex endotracheal tube that is bent around the choana. A fenestra is created in the tube at the choana to allow the infant to nose breath. Bending the tube places a lateral force on the tube in each naris which may cause alar rim ulceration and scarring. Regular examination of the anterior nares for ulceration is imperative after stent placement. The stent is left in situ for 4 to 6 weeks. The problem is that nasal mucosa may not grow over the exposed drilled bone around the circumference of the created aperture so that granulations form over the bone. This leads to scarring and restenosis.

Some surgeons therefore do not stent but try to preserve mucosa at the choana by scraping back mucosa before drilling and once a wide aperture has been created, this mucosa is draped over the exposed bone. Finally, some surgeons use this mucosa-preserving technique but insert a smaller-diameter stent so that there is not significant tube pressure on the aperture rim, in the hope that the stent does not cause pressure necrosis of the mucosa. A Cochrane review has not demonstrated that one method is superior to another, so it is important that paediatric ENT surgeons keep records of their results so that they are aware of their outcomes. Significantly better outcomes with their chosen technique can then be reported.

2. Transpalatal. This is preferred by some surgeons, especially when the atresia is bilateral, or if the nasal airway is particularly small or if a previous transnasal repair has not been successful. The palate is incised just in front of the posterior edge of the hard palate as a curved incision to allow the raising of a wide-based mucoperiosteal flap. The soft palate is retracted, and the occlusion removed together with part of the vomer and border of the hard palate.

75.9 Follow-Up and Aftercare

Presently, whatever the technique used to create an aperture at the choana, a series of dilations of the choana is advised every 4 to 8 weeks, to maintain an adequate lumen. An average of about five dilations are required.

75.10 Nasal Masses

Nasal masses in the newborn are uncommon but are reported in 1 in 4,000 children.

• Some originate in the cranial cavity; for example, meningocele, encephalocele and glioma. These are midline nasal masses, but they represent herniation of intra-cranial contents into the nose. A meningocele contains cerebrospinal fluid (CSF), and an encephalocele contains CSF, neural tissue and meninges. A glioma contains glial cells, with fibrous and vascular tissue. A glioma—despite its intra-cranial origin—is separated from the intra-cranial tissues but can be attached by a fibrous stalk. Glial heterotopia refers to the occurrence of glial tissue outside the cranial cavity, and it can be an extensive mass in, for example, the nose and nasopharynx. No nasal mass should be biopsied without detailed prior imaging and careful planning as the risk of a CSF leak and devastating meningitis is high with injudicious surgery.

• Cysts, polyps and tumours—including teratomas—also occur. Dermoid cysts are frequently evident on the dorsum of the nose, often with an associated external pit. Treatment is surgical, following thorough radiological investigations to exclude intra-cranial involvement. Brow incisions, an external rhinoplasty approach, and in some cases, endoscopic techniques have been advocated.

• Fibrous dysplasia is a dysplastic condition involving the craniofacial skeleton, usually occurring in adolescents or young adults. There may be facial deformity, and involvement of the nasal skeleton (the maxilla in particular) can cause both aesthetic issues and nasal obstruction. Diagnosis is radiological, and treatment is not always required.

• Nasal polyps are not common in children and should prompt concern regarding cystic fibrosis.

• Angiofibroma is very rare, but ENT surgeons should be aware that it needs to be considered in adolescent boys who present with nasal obstruction or unexplained epistaxis.

• Septal deformity, adenoids and allergic rhinitis are of course far more common.

Further Reading

Section 1, Paediatrics, in Scott-Browns Otolaryngology, Head and Neck Surgery, 8th Edition, Volume 2. Editors-in-Chief–Watkinson JC & Clarke R. Published by CRC Press, Taylor & Francis group, Boca Raton, London, New York, 2018

Kwong KM. Current updates on choanal atresia. Front Pediatr. 2015; 3:52

Newman JR, Harmon P, Shirley WP, et al. Operative management of choanal atresia: a 15-year experience. JAMA Otolaryngol Head Neck Surg. 2013; 139(1):71–75

Wyatt M. Nasal obstruction in children. In: Clarke RW, ed. Pediatric Otolaryngology: Practical Clinical Management. Stuttgart: Thieme; 2017:210–219

Related Topics of Interest

Paediatric airway problems
Paediatric endoscopy
Stertor and stridor

76 Papilloma of the Larynx

Squamous cell papilloma is by far the commonest benign tumour of the larynx. Adenomas, chondromas, fibromas, haemangiomas and other neurogenic and mesodermal benign tumours are all rare and will not be considered further.

76.1 Aetiology and Pathogenesis

The aetiology of laryngeal papillomas is now known to be infection of the epithelial cells with human papillomavirus (HPV), a DNA virus with over 170 subtypes. HPV subtypes 6 and 11 are responsible for over 90% of laryngeal papillomas. HPV 11 is associated with more aggressive and extensive disease. Laryngeal papillomatosis shows a bimodal distribution, affecting young children (typically ages 2–5) and young adults (typically in the third and fourth decades). It is thought that the disease is transmitted from infected secretions in the birth canal during delivery, although in a small proportion the virus is transmitted via the placenta prior to birth. In adults, HPV is spread through sexual contact. Electron microscopy and immunofluorescent techniques have shown that HPV DNA is incorporated into the host's cellular DNA. Polymerase chain reaction (PCR) and in situ hybridisation (ISH) are the most sensitive techniques available to show evidence of HPV infection. Apparently, normal mucosal cells adjacent to the papillomas also contain viral DNA, which may become activated to form a recurrent lesion. This partly explains the difficulty in curing the disease.

Squamous papillomas may grow anywhere in the respiratory tract from the lips to the lungs, but the vocal cords, anterior commissure and vestibular folds are the commonest sites of involvement. The lesions have a predilection for points of airway constriction, where there is increased airflow, drying, crusting and irritation. These areas of microtrauma allow HPV to infect the basal layer of the epithelium. Laryngeal mucus is thought to behave as a protective blanket in some sites, for example, the interarytenoid area. The growths may present as scattered single lesions or clusters or as a huge exuberant mass. They can be sessile or pedunculated and are characteristically non-keratinising with a connective tissue core.

76.2 Clinical Features

Hoarseness of voice or an abnormal cry is the usual presenting symptom. Respiratory obstruction and increasing stridor are late manifestations of the disease process.

76.3 Investigations

Laryngotracheobronchoscopy is required to establish the diagnosis, obtain tissue for confirmatory histology, and to assess the extent of the disease and potential risk to the patient's airway. Treatment can also then be initiated.

76.4 Treatment

The aim of treatment is to remove the papillomas as they appear, to maintain a safe patent airway and laryngeal function, without damaging the larynx in the process, and to wait for resolution of the condition.

76.4.1 Surgery

Surgical excision of the papillomas remains the mainstay of treatment. Multiple procedures are nearly always required because of the propensity of the papilloma to recur. The use of lasers to ablate laryngeal papillomas has been associated with complications such as laser burns, scarring and poor voice outcomes. Such complications can be greatly reduced, or prevented in experienced hands, by using a microspot micromanipulator. Microdebriders such as the Medtronic Skimmer blade allow for the precise excision of papillomas while limiting damage to underlying normal tissue and this is now the most popular surgical technique. If disease is found to involve the anterior commissure, staged excisions are required to avoid web formation, treating first one cord then the other. Tracheostomy should be avoided if possible as these sites of mucosal trauma can result in implantation of papillomas into the trachea and bronchi.

76.4.2 Medical Treatment

Medical treatments tend to be used in an adjuvant setting for papillomas recalcitrant to multiple surgical treatments.

One of the early medical treatments was interferon-α, which has been shown to significantly reduce the growth rate of papillomas in one-third of patients. The use of interferon is limited by multiple side effects and systemic toxicity, and is no longer commonly used.

Cidofovir, an antiviral medication that works by inhibiting viral DNA polymerases, has been administered as an intra-lesional injection into laryngeal papillomas. Although there is a theoretical risk of causing malignant transformation with the use of cidofovir, large international studies have not found any evidence of this.

Bevacizumab is a recombinant humanised monoclonal antibody that inhibits vascular endothelial growth factor A (VEGF-A). It has been used as systemic therapy for aggressive papillomatosis that has spread to the tracheobronchial tree some remarkable results. However, the current evidence is limited to isolated case reports.

HPV vaccines have an excellent safety profile with few side effects. Nonavalent HPV vaccines protect against subtypes 6, 11, 16, 18, 31, 33, 45, 52 and 58. It has been shown that adults with active laryngeal papillomas have lower anti-HPV antibody titres compared to adults without laryngeal papillomas. There are limited case series which demonstrate that HPV vaccination, when used as an adjunct to surgical excision, can prolong intersurgical intervals. It is hoped that national HPV vaccination programmes will offer the potential for significantly reducing the incidence of this disease.

76.5 Follow-Up and Aftercare

Surgical excision is repeated as often as necessary to preserve the airway and the voice in those cases which do recur.

Further Reading

Fortes HR, von Ranke FM, Escuissato DL, et al. Recurrent respiratory papillomatosis: a state-of-the-art review. Respir Med. 2017; 126(Suppl C):116–121

Sullivan C, Curtis S, Mouzakes J. Therapeutic use of the HPV vaccine in recurrent respiratory papillomatosis: a case report. Int J Pediatr Otorhinolaryngol. 2017; 93(Suppl C):103–106

Tjon Pian Gi RE, Ilmarinen T, van den Heuvel ER, et al. Safety of intralesional cidofovir in patients with recurrent respiratory papillomatosis: an international retrospective study on 635 RRP patients. Eur Arch Otorhinolaryngol. 2013; 270(5):1679–1687

Tjon Pian Gi RE, San Giorgi MR, Slagter-Menkema L, et al. Clinical course of recurrent respiratory papillomatosis: comparison between aggressiveness of human papillomavirus-6 and human papillomavirus-11. Head Neck. 2015; 37(11):1625–1632

Zur KB, Fox E. Bevacizumab chemotherapy for management of pulmonary and laryngotracheal papillomatosis in a child. Laryngoscope. 2017; 127(7):1538–1542

Related Topics of Interest

Examination of the head and neck
Laryngeal carcinoma
Lasers in ENT
Paediatric airway problems
Stertor and stridor

77 Parathyroid Disease

77.1 Introduction

The parathyroid gland is the last major endocrine gland to be discovered in the human body and was first described in 1862 by Richard Owen. Parathyroid hormone or parathormone (PTH) has the physiological effects of mobilising calcium from bone, enhancing absorption of calcium from the small intestine and suppressing excretion of calcium in the urine. Primary hyperparathyroidism (pHPT) results from excessive secretion of PTH and is the commonest cause of hypercalcemia in the outpatient population and second only to malignancy in the inpatient population. It is characterised by hypercalcemia with unsuppressed PTH levels.

Parathyroid neoplasia is the commonest cause of hypercalcemia and is benign in over 99% cases, and over 80% are single-gland adenomas. Over 80% are asymptomatic on presentation but may have complications of hypercalcemia as indications for surgery. High-frequency ultrasound and radioactive sestamibi scans are the main imaging modalities for localisation. Minimal access single-gland exploration is the procedure of choice for the majority of pHPT cases. Secondary hyperparathyroidism is usually due to chronic renal failure and may require subtotal/total parathyroidectomy. Parathyroid carcinoma is a rare occurrence and has an acute metabolic onset.

The incidence of pHPT is estimated to be between 0.5 and 5 per 1,000 and is commoner in patients over 45 years of age with a male to female ratio of 1:3. The incidence of pHPT is increasing due to the advent of more readily available blood tests showing up hypercalcemia in asymptomatic patients. In 80% of patients with pHPT, the symptoms of hypercalcemia are mild or absent at the time of diagnosis.

The vast majority of pHPT (95%) are sporadic of which 80 to 90% are solitary, 4 to 6% are double adenomas and 5 to 10% are due to four-gland hyperplasia. The remaining 5% are hereditary, associated with endocrine syndromes such as multiple endocrine neoplasia types 1 and 2A (MEN1 and MEN2A).

77.2 Surgical Anatomy

Normally there are two pairs of parathyroid glands, each about 5 to 7 mm in size, with an average weight of 30 to 40 mg. They are usually bean shaped and in younger patients the colour is reddish brown, while in the older patient it may be yellowish due to the increased fat content and of oxyphil cells. They are positioned as a superior and inferior pair on the posterolateral aspect of each thyroid lobe with the upper pair being more constant in position. Supernumerary fifth glands have been reported in 5% of cases and are often found in the thymus.

The inferior glands receive their blood supply from the inferior thyroid artery. In 50% of cases, the inferior glands are found within 1 cm of the lower pole of the thyroid lobe. They are superficial to the recurrent laryngeal nerve and caudal to the inferior thyroid artery. In 25% of cases, the inferior parathyroid gland may be found within the thymic tissue. In the remaining 25% of cases, their position is variable, lateral to the thyroid (12%), ectopically in the mediastinum or at the carotid bifurcation, and rarely it may be intra-thyroidal (0.5–4%).

The superior parathyroid gland is deeper to the recurrent laryngeal nerve in the coronal plane and is more symmetrical in position and shape. In 80% of cases, the superior parathyroid gland is found adjacent to the cricothyroid junction, 1 cm cephalic to the junction of the recurrent laryngeal nerve and the inferior thyroid artery. The main blood supply is from the inferior thyroid artery while in some cases it may also be from the superior thyroid artery. In 3% of cases, the superior parathyroid glands may be ectopic in a retropharyngeal, retrolaryngeal or tracheo-oesophageal position.

77.3 Histopathology

Parathyroid glands have a fine capsule with multiple septa that divide them into lobules. The stroma consists of islands of secretory cells interspersed with fat cells and a rich sinusoidal capillary network.

There are two cell types:
1. Chief cells are the predominant cell type in children and synthesise PTH.
2. Oxyphil cells are larger and their number increases with age, their actual function is not known.

The adenomatous portion of the parathyroid may consist predominantly of chief cells with a suppressed rim of normal parathyroid tissue differentiating it from a hyperplastic gland.

77.4 Pathophysiology

- *Primary hyperparathyroidism* (high PTH, high calcium)
  The excess PTH is produced by either neoplastic or hyperplastic parathyroid parenchymal cells.

- *Secondary hyperparathyroidism* (high PTH, low calcium)
  The chronic stimulation of the parathyroid gland leads to parathyroid cell proliferation and usually reverts to normal once the stimulus is removed. In chronic renal failure, low-calcium and a high-phosphate burden causes parathyroid proliferation. There is also reduced responsiveness of calcium receptors to PTH secretion due to metabolic acidosis during renal failure. Prolonged use of lithium and vitamin D deficiency are also related to secondary hyperparathyroidism.

- *Tertiary hyperparathyroidism* (high PTH, high calcium)
  Follows prolonged stimulus in chronic renal failure. The hyperplastic gland may become autonomous and may not revert to its normal state after the stimulus ceases.

77.5 Clinical Assessment

Usually the referring endocrinologists will have identified patients with pHPT from other causes of hypercalcemia. It is important to ask about risk factors for hyperparathyroidism (such as lithium therapy and neck irradiation). The majority of patients with pHPT are asymptomatic (80%) and their hypercalcemia is picked up incidentally on biochemical screening for other reasons. Most symptomatic patients have non-specific complaints such as fatigue, lethargy, depression, lack of concentration and joint and bone pain. The neurocognitive symptoms can mimic dementia in the elderly population. Gastrointestinal symptoms may include abdominal pain, chronic constipation, peptic ulceration and pancreatitis. Renal involvement includes nephrolithiasis and hypercalciuria and occurs in 20% and 40% respectively of all patients with pHPT. These patients are then further evaluated with PTH assay, 24-hour urinary collection for calcium level

and creatinine clearance/glomerular filtration rate (GFR). A raised PTH assay, hypercalcemia and hypercalciuria confirm the diagnosis of pHPT. In young patients with pHPT, family history of MEN should be investigated. The surgical mnemonic to help aid memory of these symptoms is 'Bones, Stones, Groans and psychic Moans'.

77.6 Examination

In the majority of patients, there are no specific physical signs. The occasional giant adenoma may present as neck fullness. In suspected cases of parathyroid malignancy, patients may present with palpable nodes or vocal cord paresis.

77.7 Investigations

77.7.1 Biochemical Variations

A small number of primary hyperparathyroid patients may present with normocalcemia and elevated PTH. As part of the investigations, these patients should be assessed for vitamin D deficiency, low calcium intake and gastrointestinal and renal disorders, which lead to secondary hyperparathyroidism. An elevated parathyroid hormone level with an elevated ionised serum calcium level is diagnostic of primary hyperparathyroidism and must be repeated. A 24-hour urine calcium measurement is necessary to rule out familial benign (hypocalciuric) hypercalcemia.

77.7.2 Localisation Studies

This is the key to reducing complications and allowing focused minimal access parathyroidectomy.

Ultrasound Scan

In experienced hands, preferably a dedicated radiologist, high-frequency (7.5–15 MHz) ultrasound scan (USS) has an overall sensitivity of 89% and positive predictive value (PPV) of 98% for localising solitary adenomas. The gland is identified by its appropriate anatomical location, shape, size and hypoechoic texture. Color-flow Doppler (CFD) helps differentiate it from a lymph gland by demonstrating peripheral blood flow of the abnormal parathyroid gland. Deeply placed, retropharyngeal and retrolaryngeal adenomas are difficult to identify on ultrasonography and may also be challenging in a background of a multinodular goitre. Surgeon-performed ultrasound is increasingly popular in North America.

Sestamibi Scintigraphy

Technetium-99m methoxyisobutylisonitrile (MIBI) (sestamibi) is the radioisotope used in this metabolic scan and accumulates almost exclusively within the mitochondria. Parathyroid tissue has higher mitochondrial activity compared to normal thyroid tissue, which explains its high uptake of sestamibi. It has a sensitivity of around 85% and PPV of between 91 and 96%. The sensitivity and PPV decrease in the presence of thyroid nodules and parathyroid hyperplasia. The sestamibi scan is good at detecting ectopic adenomas and deeply placed glands, which may not be identified by ultrasound. Parathyroid images are taken 20 minutes (early phase) and 2 hours (late phase) after administration of sestamibi. The localisation can be made on multiple dimensions by single-photon emission computed tomography (SPECT) which gives more accurate anatomical information. One way of trying to improve the localisation accuracy of scintigraphy is to employ dual-phase imaging with double tracer (99m-sestamibi and iodine-123) subtraction scanning.

Ultrasound Scan or MIBI or Both

Opinion varies as to which is more helpful and whether ultrasound should be the first localisation investigation. The common practice is to have both USS and MIBI scans to help localise solitary adenomas. Parathyroidectomy in cases with concordant USS and MIBI scans have been reported to have up to 95 to 99% success rate, defined by normocalcemia.

CT Scan, MRI Scan and PET Scan

They are less sensitive compared to MIBI or USS but are useful before revision surgery or for ectopic adenomas and are usually not the first line of imaging.

With high-resolution CT scans at 2.5- to 3-mm slices with rapid contrast enhancement (4D-CT), the sensitivity for localising parathyroid adenomas ranges from 46 to 87%. Magnetic resonance imaging (MRI) scans may be able to help localise ectopic or mediastinal glands (up to 71–88% sensitivity). Fluorodeoxyglucose–positron

emission tomography (FDG-PET) scans have very good sensitivity (86%) and acceptable specificity (78%) for solitary adenomas.

Fine-Needle Aspiration

Ultrasound- or CT-guided fine-needle aspiration (FNA) to test for PTH assay is generally recommended in revision surgery to differentiate from non-parathyroid tissue. Cytology is less sensitive as follicular thyroid neoplastic cells may mimic parathyroid tissue.

Venous Sampling

This can help regionalise (neck/mediastinum) and lateralise (right/left) the abnormal parathyroid gland when imaging studies have been conflicting, negative or in a reoperative situation. Selective venous sampling has a high overall sensitivity (87–95%).

Intra-Operative Localisation Techniques

The intra-operative localisation techniques commonly include the use of intra-operative PTH monitoring (IOPTH), radio-guided parathyroidectomy (RGP), frozen-section histology and methylene blue injections. These can be employed in various situations to improve surgical outcomes such as in non-concordant scans or revision surgery.

77.7.3 Intra-Operative PTH Monitoring

IOPTH can be performed from a central or peripheral site but should be consistent for any whole procedure. IOPTH may be helpful in deciding intra-operatively if a biochemical cure has been achieved following surgery for pHPT. Cure is defined as greater than or equal to 50% decay from the highest (pre-incision or pre-excision) value within 10 minutes of removing the hyperfunctioning gland(s).

77.7.4 Radio-Guided Parathyroidectomy

This is intra-operative localisation of parathyroid tissue with a gamma probe after pre-operative sestamibi (MIBI) administration and is contraindicated in pregnancy or MIBI allergy/sensitivity.

77.7.5 Frozen Section

This helps in differentiating parathyroid from non-parathyroid tissue (e.g., lymph node, thyroid tissue), but does not provide a definitive diagnosis of an adenoma.

77.7.6 Methylene Blue

Methylene blue (MB) selectively stains parathyroid tissue and can therefore facilitate surgery. This is administered pre-operatively via intravenous infusion of MB 5 mg/kg body weight, diluted in 100-mL normal saline. Its use may be limited due to the fact that it may interfere with pulse oximetry and recent reports of toxic encephalopathy.

77.8 Management Options

77.8.1 Primary Hyperparathyroidism

The treatment modality may range from watchful waiting to surgical intervention. The symptomatic patient should be offered surgery for a curative outcome. The asymptomatic patients may be managed conservatively with adequate hydration, avoidance of thiazide diuretics and control of calcium and PTH levels by treating with bisphosphonates. Calcimimetic drugs are being used to control serum PTH levels, mostly in secondary hyperparathyroidism. They work by mimicking calcium at the parathyroid receptors. In asymptomatic patients, if a conservative management option is chosen, annual calcium, PTH, bone mineral density and renal functions should be assessed. The indications for surgery in asymptomatic patients are given in ▸ Table 77.1.

77.8.2 Surgical Approaches to Primary Hyperparathyroidism

Surgical treatment for single-gland adenoma in sporadic pHPT in experienced hands carries a success rate of more than 95% with morbidity of less than 1%. Minimally invasive parathyroidectomy (MIP) under local or general anaesthesia is the recommended choice for single-gland adenomas following the current imaging modalities in

▸ **Table 77.1** Guidelines for parathyroid surgery in asymptomatic primary hyperparathyroidism

Serum calcium	> 1 mg/dL above normal range
24-Hour urine for calcium	Not indicated in the absence of renal stones/nephrolithiasis[a]
Creatinine clearance	< 60 mL/min
Bone mineral density	T score < −2.5 at any site and/or previous fracture
Age	< 50 years
Patients for whom effective medical surveillance/follow-up is not possible	

[a]Some centres consider 24-hour urinary calcium greater than 400 mg as an indication.

▸ **Table 77.2** Surgical techniques for minimally invasive parathyroidectomy general or local anaesthesia

Surgical access for MIP	Technique
Open mini-incision MIP (OMIP)	Small horizontal cervical skin incision (~ ≤2.5 cm) on neck as positioned as per pre-operative image localisation.
Video and endoscopic MIP	Rigid endoscope with or without gas insufflation. Magnified view with optimal lighting. Access via midline between the strap muscles or lateral access via the paracarotid gutter.

Abbreviation: MIP, minimally invasive parathyroidectomy.

accurately localising the adenomas (▸Table 77.2). It has less morbidity, reduced cost and shorter operating time with comparable success rates. Bilateral neck exploration (BNE) is useful in multigland disease, recurrent/residual disease or when there is inconclusive pre-operative localisation imaging. Some use nerve monitoring if general anaesthesia is being administered while others use it only for selected cases such as revision surgery or if the suspected adenoma is more deeply placed. Single-gland exploration is performed as a day-case procedure unless patient factors do not allow it. The final decision on the technique would depend on patient factors and the experience of the operating surgeon.

77.8.3 Four-Gland Exploration (Bilateral Neck Exploration)

Ideally all four glands are exposed via bilateral dissection and the macroscopically abnormal gland is excised (▶ Table 77.3). The gland may then be sent for frozen-section tissue analysis and IOPTH is performed to confirm biochemical cure. If it is negative, then further glands may be dissected out (▶ Table 77.4).

▶ **Table 77.3** Management of non-primary hyperparathyroidism

	Surgical options	Indication for operation
MEN1	Subtotal (3.5 gland) parathyroidectomy	Osteoporosis Zollinger–Ellison syndrome
	Total (4 gland) parathyroidecto-my and forearm autotransplantation	Significant 4-gland enlargement
MEN2A	Total thyroidecto-my ± removal of en-larged parathyroids	*Medullary carcinoma*
Secondary and tertiary hyperparathy-roidism	Total (4 gland) parathyroidectomy and forearm autotransplantation	Failure of med-ical therapy (as decided by renal physicians). Marked 4-gland enlargement

▶ **Table 77.4** Main indications for four-gland exploration as the initial procedure

Secondary or tertiary hyperparathyroidism with renal failure

Suspected MEN syndromes

As extension of single-gland surgery when PTH levels do not fall

Negative imaging localisation studies

Surgeon preference

Abbreviations: MEN, multiple endocrine neoplasia; PTH, parathyroid hormone.

77.8.4 Failed Initial Exploration, Persistent and Recurrent Hyperparathyroidism and Re-Exploration

The most common cause of persistent sporadic pHPT has been shown to be inadequate neck exploration in up to 80% of cases. This is followed by failure to locate or remove an ectopic adenoma located at various sites in the neck, superior or middle mediastinum (25%), supernumerary parathyroid glands (5%) and multigland disease (MGD) (10–15%). Re-exploration should be performed preferably in a tertiary referral centre adopting a systematic approach. Normocalcemia after reoperative surgery in expert centres is achieved in 84 to 98% of patients. If the hyperparathyroidism is diagnosed 6 months after initial surgery, it is classified as a recurrent disease.

77.9 Parathyroid Carcinoma

Carcinoma of the parathyroid is a rare condition occurring in 0.5 to 5% of patients with primary hyperparathyroidism. It tends to occur after the fourth decade and has an equal sex incidence. It usually has a rapid-onset warranting surgical exploration. The presenting symptoms are usually related to severe hypercalcemia and examination may reveal a palpable neck mass and vocal cord paresis. The PTH levels may be 5 to 50 times the normal level. It usually runs an indolent course because the tumour has a rather low malignant potential and may invade the thyroid gland, muscles, recurrent laryngeal nerve, trachea or oesophagus.

Initial management is geared towards management of the, often severe, hypercalcemia. Failure to control the calcium medically is the eventual cause of death.

If surgery is performed, en bloc removal is the procedure of choice (hemithyroidectomy, paratracheal nodes and fat and thymic tissue ± modified/radical neck dissection in gross nodal involvement). Data from the U.S. National Cancer Database showed a 5-year survival of 88.5% and a 10-year survival of 49.1%.

Further Reading

Bilezikian JP, Potts JT Jr, Fuleihan Gel-H, et al. Summary statement from a workshop on asymptomatic primary hyperparathyroidism: a perspective for the 21st century. J Bone Miner Res. 2002; 17(Suppl 2):N2–N11

Fraser WD. Hyperparathyroidism. Lancet. 2009; 374 (9684): 145–158

Kelly CW, Eng CY, Quraishi MS. Open mini-incision parathyroidectomy for solitary parathyroid adenoma. Eur Arch Otorhinolaryngol. 2014; 271(3):555–560

Mihai R, Simon D, Hellman P. Imaging for primary hyperparathyroidism—an evidence-based analysis. Langenbecks Arch Surg. 2009; 394(5):765–784

Stack B. Minimally invasive radioguided parathyroidectomy. Operative Techniques in Otolaryngology. 2009; 20:54–59

Related Topics of Interest

Thyroid disease—malignant
Thyroid disease—benign
Imaging in ENT

P

78 Perilymph and Labyrinthine Fistula

Patients with perilymph and labyrinthine fistula may present with Ménière's syndrome and be incorrectly diagnosed with Ménière's disease.

78.1 Definitions

Labyrinthine fistula This is a defect or abnormal opening in the bony labyrinth, including the bone or membranes of the medial wall of the middle ear and semicircular canals, that either exposes or ruptures the endosteum. An example is a lateral semicircular canal fistula and a perilymph fistula (PLF). If rupture occurs, a perilymph leak occurs.

Perilymph fistula This is a perilymph leak from the bone or membranes of the medial wall of the middle ear into the middle ear cavity. Usually, it arises from a defect in the oval or round window. A PLF has also been described arising from the fissula ante fenestram, a small connective tissue–filled cleft sited immediately anterior to the anterior margin of the oval window but posterior to the processus cochleariformis. Microfissures extending from the ampulla of the posterior semicircular canal to the round window have also been described as a site of a PLF.

One should also be aware of two other entities, namely, the cochlear aqueduct and the vestibular aqueduct.

Cochlear aqueduct It is a tiny bony passage arising from the basal turn of the cochlea and opening just behind and medial to the carotid canal at the skull base. It is lined on the cochlea side by endosteum and on the skull base side by a prolongation of dura. There is therefore a direct communication between the perilymph of the cochlear aqueduct and the subarachnoid space. Usually the aqueduct is occluded with arachnoid tissue and this tissue becomes denser with age. Therefore, raised intra-cranial pressure does not usually cause raised perilymph pressure but the density of the arachnoid tissue is thought to be a factor in the risk of developing a sensorineural hearing loss with meningitis and why some drugs that enter the cerebrospinal fluid (CSF) may cause ototoxicity. Sometimes, however, the cochlear aqueduct is thought to be patent and a patent cochlear aqueduct will allow direct transmission of CSF pressure to the cochlea and to the adjacent vestibule. Over time, this can dilate the vestibular aqueduct. Most patients with an enlarged vestibular aqueduct have a normal-sized cochlear aqueduct, so it is the patency of the cochlear aqueduct that is the important factor and not the size. That said, it is thought that an enlarged cochlear aqueduct is a risk factor for developing a patent cochlear aqueduct.

Of further interest, a patent cochlear aqueduct is not inevitably associated with an enlarged vestibular aqueduct, perhaps because fibrous tissue can occlude the ductus endolymphaticus. Such cases, one might presume, should be associated with fluctuating hearing loss and indeed there have been several case reports of an enlarged cochlear aqueduct, without a coexisting enlarged vestibular aqueduct, in children with a progressive sensorineural hearing loss.

Vestibular aqueduct It is a tiny bony passage arising from the posteromedial wall of the vestibule and extends to open on the posterior surface of the petrous temporal bone. It is lined by endosteum forming the ductus endolymphaticus. On reaching the posterior surface of the petrous temporal bone the ductus expands to form a blind ending sac, the saccus endolymphaticus. Enlargement of the vestibular aqueduct is often stated to be an aqueduct that is greater than 1.5 mm at its widest point, but recent studies have suggested the correct definition should be a vestibular aqueduct that is greater than 1 mm at the midpoint of the aqueduct and 2 mm at the operculum.

Enlargement of the vestibular aqueduct is associated with enlarged vestibular aqueduct syndrome, where there is fluctuating and often progressive sensorineural hearing loss and sometimes vertigo, usually in both ears. It may be associated with Pendred's syndrome. The diagnosis is made by high-resolution computed tomography (HRCT) or magnetic resonance imaging (MRI) scanning of the petrous temporal bone. As a guide, the membranous labyrinth in the adjacent posterior semicircular canal (PSSC) is 1 mm in width.

When the diagnosis is made in young patients, the avoidance of contact sports is important because the evidence is that even minor head trauma, such as heading a football or playing rugby, may be associated with a progression of hearing loss. One of the hypotheses of this is that, in such patients, there is a patent cochlear aqueduct that allows direct transmission of CSF pressure to the perilymph and which, over time, may dilate the vestibular aqueduct. Minor head trauma, in such patients, can cause a momentary increase in intra-cranial pressure which is directly transmitted to the cochlear perilymph through the patent cochlear aqueduct. This may injure cochlear receptors. In such cases, an enlarged vestibular aqueduct is merely evidence of a pre-existing patent cochlear aqueduct.

78.2 Perilymph Fistula

78.2.1 Aetiology

1. Congenital
   Middle and inner ear deformities, in particular, Mondini's dysplasia, where there is incomplete partitioning of the cochlea and often an associated malformed stapes footplate.

2. Spontaneous perilymph fistula
   In PLF, loss of perilymph alters the pressure gradient of perilymph within the scala vestibule and scala tympani. It also alters the pressure gradient of the endolymph within the scala media. The pressure in the scala media therefore becomes relatively higher, a similar situation to that which occurs in Ménière's disease (when the endolymph volume increases to increase endolymph pressure). The presenting symptoms of PLF are aural fullness or pressure, acute hearing loss, acute vertigo and tinnitus. They are similar to Ménière's disease. If PLF is intermittent, then these acute symptoms settle when the PLF temporarily seals, again mimicking the resolution of acute symptoms occurring in Ménière's disease. One can therefore see the reason why there is no consensus on the incidence of PLF, how it should be diagnosed, or how it should be treated when suspected. Indeed, in the past, many giants of otology have doubted its spontaneous occurrence and claimed the proposed entity was being used as an excuse to develop a lucrative tympanotomy practice. Shea's series of iatrogenic post-stapedectomy PLFs presented with usually mild but sometimes profound vertigo and a mixed hearing loss but in over 36,000 otological operations he had not visualised a spontaneous PLF. Schuknecht had never seen temporal bone evidence of a spontaneous PLF including the review of the temporal bones of patients reported by Kohut as having a PLF. There is currently no consensus view on whether a spontaneous PLF may occur in an otherwise normal ear without the risk factors of barotrauma, head injury or iatrogenesis.

3. Barotrauma
   Heavy lifting, straining, coughing and sneezing are associated with an increase in CSF pressure which may be transmitted to the perilymph through a cochlear aqueduct that is patent or lightly filled with arachnoid tissue. Such an increase in perilymph pressure may result in a tear of the oval window annulus or round window membrane or membranes protecting the fissula ante fenestram and a PLF occurs.
   A rapid true or relative increase in middle ear pressure may also cause a PLF from the same sites. A rapid relative increase may occur in reverse squeeze when ascending from scuba or free diving or ascending with reverse squeeze in an aircraft. A Valsalva manoeuvre and a stifled sneeze may cause a rapid increase of middle ear pressure. Conversely, a rapid relative reduction in middle ear pressure such as barometric pressure change in an aircraft during descent or descending during a scuba or free dive may do the same.

4. Head injury
   A fracture of the bony labyrinth may cause either a labyrinthine fistula or PLF. A slap to the ear may cause a sudden increase in external ear canal pressure which may be transmitted by the ossicular chain to the stapes footplate causing a tear of the oval window annulus or round window rupture. A rupture of the tympanic membrane may also occur. A sensorineural, conductive or mixed hearing loss can therefore arise from such trauma.

5. Iatrogenic
   PLF is a risk following stapedectomy surgery.

78.3 Clinical Features

A congenital PLF or enlarged vestibular aqueduct should be suspected in children with an unexplained fluctuating or progressive sensorineural hearing loss with or without vertiginous symptoms. Sudden and profound permanent sensorineural hearing loss may also arise. Older children and adults will often complain of ear

P

pressure and tinnitus that increases when there is hearing loss and reduces when the hearing improves. In other words, they describe Ménière's syndrome of which the commonest cause is Ménière's disease, but may be due to PLF. The patients may have the Tullio phenomenon (vertigo when exposed to loud sounds) and a positive fistula or Hennebert's sign (vertigo when there is a change in external ear canal pressure) and these signs are not seen in Ménière's disease. An external ear deformity may occur with the middle and inner ear malformation. It is reasonable to assume that a similar history following a head injury, barotrauma or middle ear surgery is due to a PLF until proven otherwise.

78.4 Investigations

A HRCT scan of the petrous temporal bone is mandatory in suspected congenital PLF. A minor or major aplasia (see Chapter 13, Congenital Hearing Disorders) and in particular, an enlarged vestibular aqueduct or Mondini's dysplasia, may be displayed. Eighty-five percent of congenital PLFs will have anomalies of the stapes superstructure, incus, promontory or round window demonstrable on CT. β-Transferrin is found in all human CSF and perilymph but in the serum of only 1 in 100 subjects. In those where a PLF is suspected from the history but not confirmed by a tympanotomy, washings of the middle ear for β_2-transferrin can be made. Difficulty arises in deciding whether CSF or perilymph is the responsible agent in head injury patients with a positive β_2-transferrin test. Positioning a patient with a suspected PLF with the affected ear uppermost often improves hearing thresholds presumably because little perilymph escapes due to gravity.

78.5 Management

The indications for exploratory tympanotomy are controversial, because the history may not be classic of PLF and the history of a patient with Ménière's disease is often indistinguishable from PLF. Of the children explored, the two main series showed a PLF in 42% of 244 children and 66% of 335 (in the latter the tympanotomy criteria were stricter) and Pullen reported that 48 of 62 patients with symptoms suggestive of PLF after scuba or free diving had round window membrane rupture, in some after a depth of only 4 ft. Weber showed

that surgical repair of a PLF does not result in a significant post-operative hearing gain, but fistula repair may prevent further hearing loss. The diagnosis of PLF can only be made at tympanotomy and to perform a tympanotomy, the history should be highly suggestive of PLF. There should be fluctuating sensorineural hearing loss shown on serial air and bone conduction pure-tone audiograms, and a judgement made that the likelihood of additional hearing loss is greater without surgery than with surgery. Sixty percent of congenital PLFs arise from the oval window, 20% from the round window, 20% from both windows and 20% are bilateral. The oval or round window should be plugged with a fat graft, temporalis fascia or a vein graft. Fibrin glue and the KTP laser have been suggested to properly anchor an oval or round window graft in position. Temporalis muscle may be used to splint a round window graft reinforced by fibrin glue.

78.6 Follow-Up and Aftercare

Bed rest in the sitting up position for a fortnight is suggested as is avoiding straining or flying for 3 months. Diving is contraindicated. The patient is advised to cough or sneeze with the mouth open and not to lift a weight of more than 30 kg to reduce the risk of recurrent PLF. One week of antibiotic cover is recommended.

78.7 Labyrinthine Fistula

The commonest cause is erosion of the otic capsule by cholesteatoma. A head injury may also fracture the otic capsule. The symptoms and signs are similar to PLF. It has been argued that when these symptoms (ear pressure, fluctuating sensorineural hearing loss and tinnitus associated with vertigo at the time of hearing loss, i.e., Ménière's syndrome) and signs (Tullio's phenomenon and positive fistula sign) occur after head injury, a PLF is much more likely than a labyrinthine fistula because a fracture of the otic capsule more frequently causes either an acute and often profound vertigo from vestibular injury or an acute and profound sensorineural hearing loss, or both.

Superior semicircular canal dehiscence syndrome (SCDS) describes symptoms from an important type of labyrinthine fistula. The cause is deficient bone exposing the endosteum over the arcuate eminence of the superior semicircular canal. The incidence increases with age, but the cause is unknown. It may be that thin labyrinthine bone covering the otic capsule becomes further thinned with time, perhaps from contact with dura.

Patients may present with vertigo when exposed to loud noise (Tullio's phenomenon) or altered ear canal pressure. Some patients have autophony— the unusually loud hearing of their own voice. They may be aware or hear their own eye movement and have hyperacusis (hypersensitivity to everyday sounds). On examination, patients may have a positive fistula sign, a conductive hearing loss but a negative Hallpike and Romberg's test. The diagnosis is confirmed by HRCT and/or MRI. It is best seen on HRCT in the coronal plane and with a 0.5-mm slice thickness, or MRI. An MRI does not define bone anatomy but may be at least as good as CT in diagnosing the condition as it will allow an assessment of the integrity of bone covering the arcuate eminence.

Treatment depends on how the patients' symptoms affect their functioning but for most patients, the avoidance of loud sounds is sufficient to manage the condition. Surgical treatment is invasive and involves occluding the dehiscent arcuate eminence with bone pâté and temporalis fascia (not bone cement as this causes a local inflammatory reaction) via a middle fossa craniotomy. The risks of surgery include facial nerve injury, stroke and death. Minimally invasive endoscopic middle fossa craniotomy, where a 2-cm craniotomy is made and the arcuate eminence approached endoscopically, may be associated with lower complications while maintaining a high percentage (90% in some series) of symptom improvement. Sensorineural hearing loss is the symptom least likely to improve indicating that any pre-operative sensorineural element of hearing loss is likely to be due to a permanent injury of the affected hearing receptors.

Further Reading

Kohut RI, Hinojosa R, Ryu JH. Perilymphatic fistulae: a single-blind clinical histopathologic study. Adv Otorhinolaryngol. 1988; 42:148–152

Patnaik U, Srivastava A, Sikka K, Thakar A. Surgery for vertigo: 10-year audit from a contemporary vertigo clinic. J Laryngol Otol. 2015; 129(12):1182–1187

Schuknecht HF. Myths in neurotology. Am J Otol. 1992; 13(2):124–126

Shea JJ. The myth of spontaneous perilymph fistula. Otolaryngol Head Neck Surg. 1992; 107(5):613–616

Related Topics of Interest

79 Pharyngeal Pouch

The term pharyngeal pouch refers to a pseudo-diverticulum of the pharyngeal wall. Pharyngeal pouches are uncommon, with an incidence of approximately 1 case per 100,000 population per year. Zenker's diverticula are located superior to cricopharyngeus and are the most common pharyngeal pouch. An oesophagoscopy should be performed prior to treatment as rarely a squamous cell carcinoma can develop in the lining of the pouch. Rigid endoscopic stapling is the treatment of choice in most units. Patients must be fully informed of the risks of perforation which may necessitate an open procedure to close the perforation.

79.1 Aetiology and Pathogenesis

The precise mechanism for the development of pharyngeal pouches is not known. The current understanding is that pharyngeal pouches develop due to high intra-luminal pressure within the pharynx as a result of incoordination of swallowing. The pharyngeal wall then herniates through a weak area of the pharynx. As the diverticula involve only the submucosa and mucosa, and not the muscle, they are more correctly classified as pseudodiverticula. Zenker's diverticula are the most common of the pharyngeal pouches. These arise posteriorly by herniation of the pharyngeal mucosa through a relatively weak part of the posterior pharyngeal wall bounded by thyropharyngeus superiorly and cricopharyngeus inferiorly. Other types of pharyngeal pouches are Killian's diverticula, which arise inferior to cricopharyngeus laterally, and Laimer's diverticula, which arise inferior to cricopharyngeus in the posterior midline. Once a pouch is formed, food enters it and stretches it further, so that it enlarges. When the pouch reaches a moderate size, food may enter it preferentially. Pressure from the pouch may then be exerted on the oesophagus to cause dysphagia.

79.2 Staging

Various ways of staging pharyngeal pouches have been suggested over the years. Lahey (1930) described stages depending on the shape of the pouch seen on contrast radiography. Brombart (1964) described changes seen on contraction of the upper oesophageal sphincter, Morton (1993) classified stages on direct measurement of pouch size and van Overbeek (1994) classified stages depending on the number of vertebral bodies counted beside the pouch.

79.3 Clinical Features

Pharyngeal pouches are most frequently seen in the elderly. Presenting symptoms include a sensation of a lump in the throat, dysphagia, regurgitation of undigested food, halitosis, weight loss, chronic cough and recurrent chest infections due to aspiration. Hoarseness may occur as a result of irritation of the vocal cords from repeated aspiration. Swelling in the neck may be present which may gurgle on palpation (Boyce's sign) and empty on external pressure. Rarely, a pouch may have an invasive squamous cell carcinoma in its wall.

79.4 Diagnosis

Pharyngeal pouches are sometimes diagnosed incidentally during flexible oesophagogastroduodenoscopy (OGD). In these cases, it may be difficult to advance the flexible endoscope past the pharyngeal pouch and into the oesophagus. The definitive investigation is a barium swallow, which demonstrates the pouch.

Oesophagoscopy should be carried out to exclude the presence of carcinoma. The instrument usually enters the pouch and a septum may be seen anteriorly separating it from the oesophagus.

79.5 Management

No treatment

Pharyngeal pouches that are asymptomatic do not require treatment.

79.5.1 Endoscopic Techniques

Rigid Endoscopic Stapling

This is the first-line treatment of choice in many units. Under general anaesthesia, a split-beak rigid endoscope, such as the Weerda distending diverticuloscope, is inserted, with the lower beak in the pouch and the upper beak in the oesophagus. The pouch is inspected with a Hopkins rod and food debris removed. Under vision, an endoscopic linear cutting stapler is introduced and the septum of the pouch is simultaneously stapled and divided. With this technique, results are good, morbidity is low and hospital stay is short.

Rigid Endoscopy with Diathermy/ Laser

The initial setup is as for rigid endoscopic stapling. However, instead of using an endoscopic linear cutting stapler, cricopharyngeus and the septum of the pouch are divided using diathermy or laser. This may be more suitable for smaller pouches, as current stapling devices do not cut all the way to the tip, leaving a small residual pouch. There may be an increased risk of perforation and mediastinitis with these techniques as the mucosal edges may not be as robustly sealed compared with endoscopic stapling.

The major risks of rigid endoscopy with stapling, diathermy or laser are haemorrhage and perforation leading to surgical emphysema and mediastinitis. As such, patients should be fully informed and consented for the need for open surgery to deal with these complications.

Flexible Endoscopy with Diathermy

Flexible endoscopic treatment for pharyngeal pouches is a more recent development. Initially this technique was reserved for patients deemed to be poor surgical candidates, primarily due to anatomical difficulties or anaesthetic risks. The flexible endoscope is used with a hood, clear cap or soft overtube to aid visualisation of the pouch and septum. The septum is then divided using monopolar diathermy. As this is a relatively new treatment for pharyngeal pouches, it should only be done by experienced interventional endoscopists with training in the procedure.

79.5.2 Open Techniques

Open surgery for pharyngeal pouches tends to be reserved for cases when endoscopic techniques are not suitable or have failed.

An oesophagoscopy is first performed, the pouch inspected and food debris cleared. It is helpful to then place a wide-bore nasogastric tube in the oesophagus and to pack the pouch with ribbon gauze. A left-sided transcervical approach is used which minimises the risk to the recurrent laryngeal nerve. The pouch is identified and mobilised. The ribbon gauze is then removed transorally and a cricopharyngeal myotomy is performed. For small pharyngeal pouches, this may be all that is required.

For larger pouches, the pouch is invaginated into the oesophagus and its neck closed with a purse-string suture. This reduces the risk of perforation as the mucosa is not breached. Alternatively, a diverticulectomy may be performed where the neck of the pouch is transected and sealed, either with handsewn sutures or a stapling gun. The commencement of oral intake is usually delayed when a diverticulectomy is performed, resulting in a longer hospital stay.

79.6 Complications

1. Early
   - Dental injury.
   - Haemorrhage.
   - Perforation leading to surgical emphysema or mediastinitis.
   - Hoarseness (recurrent laryngeal nerve injury).
   - Wound infection.

2. Late
   - Stricture (too much mucosa excised when dividing the neck of the sac).
   - Recurrence (repeated endoscopic treatment usually possible).

79.7 Perforation of the Oesophagus

This is perhaps the most feared complication of endoscopic pharyngeal pouch surgery and oesophagoscopy. The management will depend on the following:

- The site of the perforation (whether the perforation is located in the cervical or thoracic oesophagus).
- When the perforation was recognised (in the intraoperative or postoperative period).
- Whether contamination has occurred.
- General health and intercurrent diseases of the patient.

P

P

79.7.1 Intra-Operative Identification of Perforation

In these cases, a nasogastric tube should be inserted under vision. A left-sided transcervical approach is used as described in the previous section. The perforation is closed using interrupted inverting sutures and a drain in inserted. The patient should be kept nil by mouth, with oral intake only recommended when a contrast swallow demonstrates no leak.

79.7.2 Post-Operative Identification of Perforation

Early diagnosis within 24 hours is associated with much lower mortality (10%) compared to late diagnosis (50%). Symptoms and signs of oesophageal perforation include neck, chest or back pain (typically between the shoulder blades), dysphonia, dyspnoea, pyrexia, surgical emphysema and shock. The patient should have a contrast swallow as soon as possible. The most sensitive radiological investigation is a computed tomography (CT) of the neck and chest with oral contrast.

Small localised perforations can usually be managed conservatively. These measures include nasogastric tube insertion, nil by mouth, broad-spectrum intravenous antibiotics and proton pump inhibitors.

It is unusual for patients to have a perforation of the thoracic oesophagus (but can occur with a lower tear or pre-procedural oesophagoscopy). These patients should be commenced on total parenteral nutrition and may require a chest drain. Early liaison with the thoracic surgery team is essential. Patients with clinical or radiological deterioration during conservative management (e.g., sepsis, hydropneumothorax) should be considered for endoscopic treatment with clips or stents, or open surgery.

Further Reading

Patel NN, Singh T. Cricopharyngeal dysphagia, Chapter 52 in Scott-Browns Otolaryngology, Head and Neck Surgery, 8th Edition, Volume 3. Editors-in-Chief - Watkinson JC & Clarke R. Published by CRC Press, Taylor & Francis group, Boca Raton, London, New York, 2018

National Institute for Health and Care Excellence (2003) Endoscopic stapling of pharyngeal pouch. NICE Guidance (IPG22); https://www.nice.org.uk/guidance/ipg513#.W-V3BQ7q_z8.email

National Institute for Health and Care Excellence (2015) Flexible endoscopic treatment of a pharyngeal pouch. NICE Guidance (IPG513); https://www.nice.org.uk/guidance/ipg22#.W-V21ph0ebk.email

Related Topics of Interest

Hypopharyngeal carcinoma
Globus pharyngeus

80 Pure-Tone Audiometry

Pure-tone audiometry is the cornerstone of clinical auditory assessment. It is a psychoacoustical test which aims to establish the subject's pure-tone hearing threshold levels at specific frequencies, that is, the minimum sound level at which a specific response can be obtained. It is used for the diagnosis, remedial action and rehabilitation of hearing loss.

80.1 Introduction

The ear responds equally, not to equal increments, but to equal multiples of sound intensity. In other words, intensity is exponentially related to loudness perception. Therefore, a logarithmic scale to measure loudness is necessary. The bel is the log to the base 10 of the ratio of the sound intensity being measured to a reference intensity which is constant and is measured in W/m^2. The decibel is 10 times this ratio. Therefore,

Sound intensity (Ix) in dB = $10\log_{10} Ix/Io$
where $Io = 10^{-12} W/m^2$

It is more usual to measure sound pressure rather than intensity, and since sound intensity is proportional to the square of sound pressure then:

Sound intensity in dB = $10\log_{10}$ sound pressure$_n^2$/sound pressure$_0^2$ which can be converted to:

$20\log_{10}$ sound pressure$_n$/sound pressure$_0$

Log_{10} 2 is about 0.3, so doubling sound intensity corresponds to a 3 dB increase. Each 10-dB increase represents a 10-fold increase in the intensity of the sound ($\log_{10}10 = 1$), a 3.3-fold increase in sound pressure, but to the ear, the perception of doubling the loudness.

80.2 Decibel Scales

1. *Sound pressure level* (dB SPL) In terms of sound pressure, the threshold of hearing corresponds (approximately) to a sound pressure level (dB SPL) of 20×10^{-6} pascals and the threshold of pain to a level of 200 pascals. The auditory system is less efficient at detecting sounds at the upper and lower ends of the frequency spectrum than in the middle regions. The detection of sounds in decibels of sound pressure level (dB SPL) produces a pure-tone audiogram which in normal circumstances would be flat, but dome shaped. It was considered that the use of a dB SPL scale in pure-tone audiometry would make abnormalities difficult to identify.

2. *Hearing level* (dB HL or dB ISO) A decibel scale of human hearing was designed so that 0-dB hearing level (HL) would be the expected threshold of detection of a pure tone irrespective of its frequency. The amount of energy at 0 dB HL at each frequency is not the same. It is measured in relative terms (dB ISO), where the reference zero is an internationally agreed standard. This standard represents the thresholds at each test frequency for a group of presumed otologically normal young adults. In the dB HL scale, normal hearing individuals would be expected to have a flat audiogram, the mean level being 0 dB HL. The clinical audiogram therefore gives an estimate of the subject's hearing relative to normal.

3. *The A-weighted scale* (dB A) The ear is not equally sensitive to sounds of different frequencies. It is particularly sensitive to sounds in the 'speech frequencies' (500–4,000 Hz) and progressively less so to sounds of lower and higher frequencies. In addition, it appears that the ear is less easily damaged by the sound frequencies to which it is less sensitive. To take account of this an 'A-weighting' is used, which reduces the contribution of very low and very high frequencies to the overall noise level measurement. This dB A scale is used in industrial and other noise exposure settings.

80.3 Background

Pure tones at several different frequencies are tested, usually 250, 500, 1,000, 2,000, 4,000 and 8,000 Hz for air conduction (although 3,000 and 6,000 Hz will be required for noise-induced hearing loss claims and can offer useful diagnostic indicators in routine clinics) and 500, 1,000, 2,000 and 4,000 Hz for bone conduction. The results of bone conduction become less reliable at and above 4,000 Hz, and at 250 Hz are often not representative as they may be felt rather than heard. Bone conduction is taken to give an indication of cochlea function, but because a variety of routes for the transmission of sound to the cochlea exist for bone conduction, it is not an absolute representation of inner ear threshold. When the skull is set in vibration by a bone conduction vibrator, the sounds reach the inner ear by the direct osseous route or via transmission across the middle ear. This causes an artificial depression of the bone conduction thresholds whenever a conductive defect is present. If the middle ear defect is corrected, then the bone conduction thresholds will appear to improve because of the addition of the middle ear component. This has become known as the 'Carhart effect' after he described it in patients who had successful fenestration surgery for otosclerosis.

80.4 Method

The subject is seated in a soundproof room and the procedure is carefully explained by the examiner. Earphones are used for air conduction (or if the canals are prone to collapse, insert earphones), and the subject is asked to signal by pressing a small handheld button as soon as the tone is heard and keep the button pressed for as long as the sound is heard (this enables the tester to check the

validity of the responses). Pure tones are produced by a calibrated audiometer (daily subjective listening tests should be performed by the tester and the maximum interval between objective calibration should not exceed 12 months) and are first presented to the subject's perceived better ear.

Thresholds are ascertained using a psychophysical method of limits and results are plotted on an audiogram form (▶ Fig. 80.1). Tones are first presented at an intensity above the patient's estimated threshold. The intensity is reduced in 10-dB steps until no sound is heard. The signal is then increased in 5-dB steps until half of the tone presentations are consistently heard. This continues in the following order: 1,000, 2,000, 4,000, 8,000, 500 and 250 Hz. Finally, 1,000 Hz is tested again to check on subject accuracy and should be within 0 to 10 dB of the initial result. The best result is plotted on the audiogram. Any gross differences require retesting. The second ear is then tested in identical fashion except for the 1-kHz retest. The timing and duration of signal presentation and gaps between the signals should

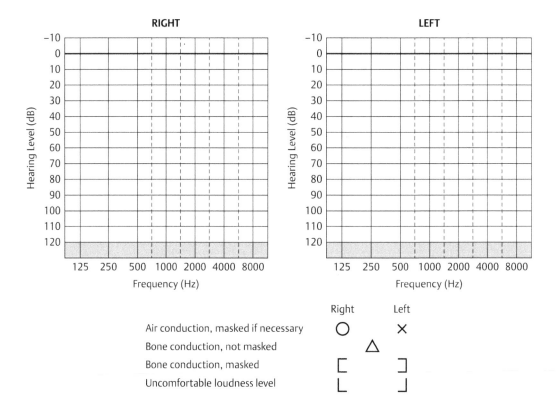

Fig. 80.1 Standard audiogram chart, format and symbols.

be varied, from 1 to 3 seconds, to avoid the patient pre-empting the stimulus and giving false-positive responses. No visual clues should be offered.

With any psychoacoustic test, there is a variation in the results obtained in any test–retest situation, with a standard error of 4 to 6 dB. For this reason, 5-dB steps are used for clinical audiometry. Smaller steps could be used (e.g., 2 or 3 dB) but the procedure would be markedly prolonged without significantly improving accuracy. Medicolegal audiometry requires more stringent control and it is usual to retest several or all air conduction frequencies, especially those around the diagnostic notches or bulges, after removal and replacement of the earphones.

80.5 Sources of Error

Physiological Competing somatosounds such as noisy breathing in children, murmurs and musculoskeletal sounds in older patients and recent noise exposure.

Psychological Mainly related to the subject's level of concentration, compliance and arousal.

Methodological Relating to tester's technique such as the predictability of tone presentation, and to the quality of his or her instructions to the subject.

Physical/acoustical Collapsing ear canals with headphones, poorly positioned or displaced headphones (jewellery, glasses), malfunctioning audiometer.

Age-related hearing loss is the commonest seen sensorineural deficit (▶ Fig. 80.2), but other disorders such as otosclerosis will have a conductive hearing loss and often a typical pattern (▶ Fig. 80.3).

80.6 Masking

When there are significant differences in thresholds between the two ears, masking is required to prevent cross-hearing (i.e., the better non-test ear picking up the sounds because of sound transmission through the skull from the worse side).

Masking is the phenomenon by which one sound impairs the perception of another. In the context of pure-tone audiometry, masking is used to raise the threshold in the non-test ear using air-conducted sound. This overcomes any cross-hearing (the interaural attenuation for air conduction is of the order of 40–60 dB when wearing headphones) and allows an accurate assessment of the true threshold of the test ear for either air or bone conduction. As masking is most effective when the frequency of the masking noise overlaps the test tone, narrow-band noise with a central frequency identical to

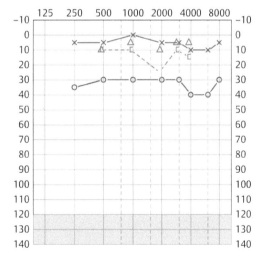

Fig. 80.3 Typical right conductive hearing loss with normal hearing thresholds on the left, as in otosclerosis. Note that the unmasked bone conduction from the right side is a shadow of the left ear due to cross-hearing, and the masked left bone conduction shows the typical Carhart notch at 2 kHz.

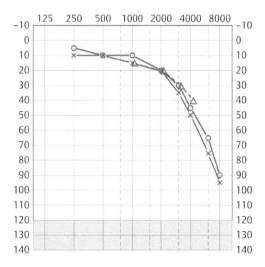

Fig. 80.2 Audiogram showing high-frequency loss as in age-associated hearing loss.

P

the test tone is used. The masking level in the non-test ear is determined by shadow masking and recording the thresholds on a masking chart. The masking noise is delivered by an ear insert for bone conduction and headphones for air conduction.

There are three scenarios where masking is essential:

1. Masking must be applied to the better ear when testing air conduction in the deafer ear if the difference in unmasked thresholds is found to be 40 dB or more (if using headphones, 55 dB or more if using insert earphones) to prevent interaural attenuation.

2. Air conduction studies whenever the unmasked bone conduction is 40 dB or more better than the worse air conduction.

3. Bone conduction testing whenever the unmasked bone conduction is 10 dB or more better than the worse air conduction.

80.7 Variations

1. Computerised pure-tone audiometry. In essence, this is identical to the above but a microprocessor presents the tones and analyses the responses against predetermined values. It is useful as a screening test and in very busy clinics, but if the result is unusual, it will require manual confirmation.

2. Bekesy's audiometry. This variant uses a special audiometer which automatically sweeps from low to high frequencies while presenting continuous or pulsed tones. The subject alters the intensity of the tone by pressing a button if the tone is heard which lowers the intensity of the signal. When the signal cannot be perceived, the button is released which increases the intensity again. Thus, a zigzag printout is obtained from which thresholds at each frequency can be estimated. As the test can be self-administered and provides an automatic printout, it is ideal for workforce screening. By varying the test technique (e.g., forward/backward sweeps, continuous/pulsed tones, etc.), additional diagnostic information about adaptation, recruitment and non-organic hearing loss can be provided. Although still used for screening industrial hearing loss, the method has fallen into disuse for most other problems because it is unreliable.

Further Reading

British Society of Audiology-Recommended procedure: Pure-tone air-conduction and bone-conduction threshold audiometry with and without masking. Date: August 2018, Due for review: 2023

On-line at www.thebsa.org.uk. Accessed December 19, 2018

Katx J, ed. Handbook of Clinical Audiology. 7th ed. Philadelphia, Baltimore, New York: Wolters Kluwer; 2015

Leijon A. Quantization error in clinical pure-tone audiometry. Scand Audiol. 1992; 21(2):103–108

Josephine E Marriage & Marina Salario-Corbetto, Psychoacoustic audiometry, Chapter 51 in Scott-Browns Otolaryngology, Head and Neck Surgery, 8th Edition, Volume 2. Editors in Chief–Watkinson JC & Clarke R. Published by CRC Press, Taylor & Francis group, Boca Raton, London, New York, 2018

Related Topics of Interest

Noise-induced hearing loss
Non-organic hearing loss

81 Radiotherapy and Chemotherapy for Head and Neck Cancer

81.1 Radiotherapy

Radiotherapy is treatment with ionising radiation. This may consist of high-energy electromagnetic radiation such as X-rays and gamma rays or particulate radiation such as electrons (beta particles) or protons.

- *X-rays* X-rays have a smaller wavelength (10^{-15} to 10^{-18} m) than ultraviolet light (between 4×10^{-12} and 10^{-13} m) and have high energy, from kilovolts (kV) to megavolts (MeV). The greater the energy, the greater its tissue penetration. They are produced when high-speed electrons expelled by thermionic emission from an electrically heated tungsten filament are arrested by a target anode of high atomic number, usually tungsten, converting their kinetic energy into heat and photons. The photon is simply a quantum or bundle of electromagnetic radiation. Megavoltage linear acceleration of the electrons produces X-rays in the energy range of 4 to 20 MeV. Orthovoltage machines produce X-rays with energy of about 300 kV. For the treatment of head and neck cancer, energy in the region of 4 to 6 MeV is used.

- *Gamma rays* Radioactive atoms disintegrate to form a more stable atom, releasing energy, which may be particulate (usually electrons) or uncharged electromagnetic radiation called gamma rays, having the same wavelength and energy as X-rays.

- *Electrons* External beam electrons produced by thermionic emission from an electrically heated tungsten filament in a linear accelerator can be used as an alternative to electromagnetic radiation. They give a uniform dose up to a certain depth which varies depending on the energy of the beam, with a rapid fall off in dose beyond this. They are used, in particular, to boost the dose to a neck lump lying in close approximation to the spinal cord. The technique is more skin sparing than orthovoltage radiotherapy and is the treatment of choice for irradiating the nose and pinna.

- *Protons* Protons are positively charged particles made by stripping an electron from a hydrogen atom. They are accelerated to high speed to form a proton beam. The difference between protons and photons is that protons deposit energy at a specific distance in tissue known as the Bragg peak. This means that there is very little energy passing into deeper tissues, allowing sparing of normal tissue structures deep to the tumour. Their exact role in head and neck cancer remains to be evaluated. The NHS has commissioned two proton centres in London and Manchester which should start treating patients in 2019 and 2020.

81.1.1 Biological Principles

Factors that affect the response of cells to a given dose of radiation include intrinsic radiosensitivity, cell repair, cellular oxygenation, linear energy transfer, relative biological effectiveness and position in the cell cycle.

- *Radiosensitivity* is an inherent characteristic of the cell (e.g., seminoma and leukaemia cells are exquisitely sensitive to radiation whereas glioma and melanoma cells are relatively radioresistant). This is to a certain extent dependent on cellular repair mechanisms, which are enhanced in melanoma cells. Squamous cell carcinoma is relatively sensitive to radiation.

- *Oxygen* is a potent sensitiser, due to its ability to form free radicals. Oxygen enhancement ratio (OER) is defined as the ratio between doses in hypoxic and euoxic cells to produce the same biological effect. OER for low energy X-rays is between 2.5 and 3, which means the dose required to kill hypoxic cells is three times greater than in oxygenated cells. Many head and neck tumours are thought to have necrotic and therefore hypoxic cores leading to radioresistance.

- *Linear energy transfer* (LET) is defined as the amount of energy deposited as the X-ray travels through matter. High LET radiation (e.g., neutrons) have a greater biological effect than low LET radiation (X-rays).

- *The position that the cell occupies in the cell cycle* also determines sensitivity to radiation. Cells in the S phase are relatively more resistant than cells in the G2 or M phase. DNA is most susceptible to lethal injury when the cell is dividing and is not able to repair DNA damage. Malignant cells have a greater proportion of actively dividing cells at any point in time (a larger growth fraction) and so a greater percentage of cells will die. Resting cells may also sustain DNA damage. Normal cells are better able to activate DNA repair factors such as p53 protein, which prolong the S phase (synthesis of DNA phase) of the cell cycle, allowing repair of damaged DNA before the next cell division. Resting malignant cells have much less capability to arrest in S phase, have a shorter cell cycle, are less likely to repair damaged DNA, and therefore more likely to undergo apoptosis before entering mitosis. A higher proportion of malignant cells will therefore die from radiotherapy compared to normal cells.

81.1.2 Clinical Principles

Radiotherapy should be defined in terms of type, method of application, number of fractions, fraction size, interval between fractions and volume treated. The principle is to provide a sufficient dose to the tumour to affect a cure or adequate palliation but deliver a minimal dose to the surrounding normal tissue to minimise complications. Each tissue has its own tolerance level beyond which radiation toxicity will occur, so that a small increase in dose may greatly increase tissue injury. Omission of one or two fractions of radiotherapy, perhaps because of concerns about acute side effects, can significantly reduce the chances of cure. Radiotherapy therefore should not be interrupted unless absolutely necessary.

Maximising the *therapeutic ratio* is the overriding principle of radiation therapy. This is the ratio between normal tissue complication rate and the tumour control rate. Many manoeuvres are utilised to maximise the ratio. These include the following:

- Fractionation of dose.
- Conformal (or focussed) radiotherapy.

81.1.3 Fractionation

Dose fractionation spares normal tissues because of cellular repair in between fractions and due to repopulation if the treatment time is sufficiently long. There are, however, more complex differences between various normal tissues and it is important to realise that prolonging treatment time has little effect on late effects, but a large sparing on early effects. This is because the dose–response curves for early- and late-responding tissues have different

shapes. As a result, fraction size is the dominant factor in determining late effects in normal tissue, while overall treatment time has little effect. In contrast, both fraction size and treatment time determine response of acutely responding tissues.

Studies have determined that for squamous cell carcinoma of the head and neck, sub-clinical (microscopic) disease can be controlled with doses of 45 to 50 Gy in 2 Gy fractions over 4 to 5 weeks in more than 90% of cases. However, for palpable disease (macroscopic, visible on imaging), doses of 60 to 70 Gy over 7 weeks are needed for local control. Conventional fractionation is defined as treating once daily at a dose of 1.8 to 2 Gy per fraction, five fractions per week over 5 to 7 weeks.

81.1.4 Altered Fractionation Schedules

Altered fractionations use more than one fraction per day and are essentially divided into two schedules of accelerated fractionation and hyperfractionation. Acceleration uses the same or slightly lower dose than conventional therapy with the same number of fractions delivered in a markedly reduced overall time. The intent is to reduce repopulation in tumours. The late effects are not reduced, as the fraction size is similar to conventional treatment. Hyperfractionation uses multiple fractions per day (usually two or three fractions), the total dose delivered is about 10 to 15% higher than conventional treatment.

In clinical trials, hyperfractionation and acceleration have shown improved tumour control but do not appear to improve overall survival. Because of the complexities of delivering these techniques (especially hyperfractionation), they are not commonly used in the United Kingdom, where chemoradiation is a more common approach.

81.1.5 Methods of Application of Radiotherapy

There are various methods of application in the head and neck:

1. External beam therapy using linear accelerators.

2. Interstitial brachytherapy, for example, iridium wires placed in flexible plastic tubes.

3. Systemic radioactive isotopes, for example, iodine-131 for thyroid cancer.

81.1.6 Treatment Planning

Modern radiotherapy is a highly technical treatment including computer-guided photon beams shaped to the patient's primary tumour and involved lymph nodes and elective irradiation to apparently uninvolved nodes where there is a greater than 20% risk of occult microscopic metastasis.

The patient's head and neck need to be immobilised during the delivery of treatment, so a customised thermoplastic shell is designed for each patient.

Contrast-enhanced computed tomography (CT), and sometimes also magnetic resonance imaging (MRI), is used to delineate the primary tumour and involved lymph nodes on each slice of the scan. This is known as the gross tumour volume (GTV). A variable margin (typically 5–10 mm) is added in three dimensions around the GTV to allow for microscopic involvement. This is called the clinical target volume (CTV). A further small margin (3–5 mm) is added to account for uncertainties in planning or treatment delivery to produce a planning target volume (PTV). Relevant critical organs such as the spinal cord, salivary glands, brain and optic structures are also delineated on each scan image.

For small tumours such as early-stage larynx cancer, the treatment technique may be very simple using two lateral opposed radiation beams. However, for most head and neck cancers which are locally advanced at presentation, or where significant elective nodal irradiation is indicated, then the best method of achieving coverage of the targets and avoiding radiosensitive normal tissues uses multiple radiation beams or arcing therapy where the linear accelerator passes through a 360-degree arc around the patient to utilise the best beam directions. Intensity-modulated radiotherapy (IMRT) uses multiple radiation beams or 360-degree arcs (volume-modulated arcing therapy) where the energy of the beam can be varied to maximise radiation dose to the tumour and minimise the dose to normal tissues. This has been shown to significantly reduce the side effects of radiotherapy.

For radical radiotherapy, doses of 65 to 70 Gy are delivered to the primary tumour and involved lymph nodes over a 6 to 7 week period treating once daily Monday to Friday. An elective nodal irradiation dose of 50 to 55 Gy is prescribed to lymph nodes at high risk of harbouring microscopic disease.

For patients requiring adjuvant post-operative radiotherapy, a dose of 60 Gy in 30 fractions is prescribed over a 6 week period treating once daily Monday to Friday.

81.1.7 Acute Radiotherapy Side Effects

1. General: Tiredness, lassitude and anorexia are common, nausea less so.

2. Skin: Erythema, dry or moist desquamation, epilation, atrophy of sweat glands and other skin appendages. This can be minimised by regular application of a simple moisturiser to the skin from the beginning of radiotherapy. Moist desquamation is treated by regular dressings and will usually heal within 2 weeks of completing radiotherapy.

3. Mucous membranes: Painful mucositis, comprising erythema and mucosal ulceration, is almost universal and requires aggressive treatment with analgesia up to and including opiates. Mucositis leads to painful dysphagia, loss of taste and mucous overproduction. Most patients will lose several kilograms in weight and some patients will require assisted feeding via a nasogastric or gastrostomy tube. Oral candidiasis is common and reduced saliva production from major and minor salivary glands occurs.

Radiotherapy side effects usually start in the second or third weeks of treatment and escalate in severity until the completion of treatment, taking 4 to 6 weeks to recover.

81.1.8 Long-Term Side Effects

Long-term side effects of radiotherapy include dryness in the mouth, tiredness, taste disturbance and swallowing difficulties. These will gradually improve during the first 2 years after radiotherapy, but can be permanent in a minority of patients.

Rare side effects of radiotherapy include necrosis of cartilage, bone or the brain. Osteoradionecrosis of the mandible is the most feared complication of treatment and is usually precipitated by tooth extraction, sometimes many years after treatment. Careful pre-radiotherapy dental assessment with selective dental extractions and ongoing dental rehabilitation can reduce this risk.

R

81.1.9 Assessment of Response

Assessment of response to radiotherapy should be made clinically at 4 to 6 weeks after completion of treatment. Positron emission tomography CT (PET-CT) is the most sensitive imaging modality and should be performed at approximately 3 months after the end of radiotherapy to allow sufficient time for the radiation side effects to settle and tumour response to complete.

81.2 Chemotherapy

Chemotherapy is used in two distinct indications in head and neck cancer. The most common is the use of chemotherapy during (concurrent) or prior (induction) to a radical course of radiation (chemoradiotherapy). Secondly, palliative chemotherapy can be used to control symptoms and prolong survival in patients with advanced or recurrent head and neck cancer which is incurable.

81.2.1 Concurrent Chemoradiotherapy

Concurrent chemoradiation is the most common treatment for locally advanced head and neck cancer. Typically a course of radiotherapy is delivered every weekday over 6 to 7 weeks, and chemotherapy with either cisplatin or cetuximab given concurrently.

Cisplatin is the most widely used drug for concurrent chemoradiotherapy in the United Kingdom. Cisplatin causes cross-links between purine bases on the tumour cell DNA. It interferes with DNA repair mechanisms, causing DNA damage, and subsequently inducing apoptosis in cancer cells. It is given as an intravenous infusion with pre- and post-hydration. Typically a dose of 100 mg/m^2 is administered every 3 to 4 weeks during radiation. Compared to patients receiving radiotherapy alone, the addition of concurrent chemotherapy confers a survival advantage of 6.5%. The survival benefit observed in this meta-analysis was confined to patients up to the age of 70 years.

The other drug commonly used is cetuximab, a monoclonal antibody which competitively binds to the epidermal growth factor receptor (EGFR). This blockage inhibits the binding of epidermal growth factors (EGFs) and reduces their effects on cell growth and metastatic spread. In a single randomised trial, the addition of cetuximab to radiation alone led to a similar survival benefit to cisplatin-based chemotherapy and prolonged survival. In the United Kingdom, NICE recommended that on cost-effectiveness grounds, cetuximab use should be limited to those patients who had a contraindication to cisplatin.

81.2.2 Induction Chemotherapy

The term induction (or neoadjuvant) chemotherapy refers to chemotherapy given prior to a radical course of treatment. The rationale is to shrink the tumour before radiotherapy in an attempt to make the radiation more effective. The most active chemotherapy combination uses docetaxel, cisplatin and 5-fluorouracil (TPF). Recently a number of randomised trials have failed to show a survival advantage for induction chemotherapy and so its use is now largely confined to the most advanced stages of locally advanced head and neck cancer.

81.2.3 Chemoradiotherapy

Chemotherapy is often combined with radiation due to its independent cytotoxic effects and the sensitisation of cancer cells to radiation-induced DNA damage by chemotherapy agents. There are two main indications for chemoradiation, the first is for curative treatment of stage III and IV cancers for patients up to the age of 70 without major surgical resection. The second is as an adjuvant therapy for high-risk patients (defined as major tumour resection with positive resection margins or lymph node metastasis with extracapsular spread). Compared to radiation alone, chemoradiation increases both the acute radiation reaction and the long-term complications such as fibrosis.

Chemotherapy with cisplatin commonly causes tiredness, nausea, vomiting and mucositis. Patients must be warned of the risk of neutropenia and neutropenic sepsis, which is an oncological emergency requiring rapid diagnosis and antibiotic treatment. Occasionally, peripheral neuropathy, auditory neuropathy and kidney injury may occur. Cetuximab, an anti-EGFR monoclonal antibody is used in patients in whom cisplatin is contraindicated, and has a different side effect profile dominated by skin rash. Recently immunotherapy agents have been shown to have activity against squamous cell carcinoma of the head and neck, but their optimal use is uncertain and is the subject of current trials.

81.2.4 Palliative Chemotherapy

For patients with locally recurrent or metastatic disease, chemotherapy can be used to relieve symptoms and may offer modest prolongation of life in some patients. Typically a platinum agent (cisplatin or carboplatin) is combined with 5-fluorouracil (5-FU). The addition of cetuximab to cisplatin and 5-FU was shown in a randomised trial to prolong overall survival from 7.4 to 10.1 months at the expense of additional side effects.

81.2.5 Side Effects

Common side effects of chemotherapy include tiredness, loss of appetite, altered sense of taste, indigestion, constipation or diarrhoea, sore mouth, vomiting, altered hearing/tinnitus, thinning of hair and peripheral neuropathy. Neutropenic sepsis is uncommon but a potentially life-threatening chemotherapy complication.

Further Reading

Bonner JA, Harari PM, Giralt J, et al. Radiotherapy plus cetuximab for squamous-cell carcinoma of the head and neck. N Engl J Med. 2006; 354(6):567–578

Cohen EE, Karrison TG, Kocherginsky M, et al. Phase III randomized trial of induction chemotherapy in patients with N2 or N3 locally advanced head and neck cancer. J Clin Oncol. 2014; 32(25):2735–2743

Haddad R, O'Neill A, Rabinowits G, et al. Induction chemotherapy followed by concurrent chemoradiotherapy (sequential chemoradiotherapy) versus concurrent chemoradiotherapy alone in locally advanced head and neck cancer (PARADIGM): a randomised phase 3 trial. Lancet Oncol. 2013; 14(3):257–264

Mehanna H, Wong WL, McConkey CC, et al; PET-NECK Trial Management Group. PET-CT surveillance versus neck dissection in advanced head and neck cancer. N Engl J Med. 2016; 374(15):1444–1454

Nutting CM, Morden JP, Harrington KJ, et al; PARSPORT trial management group. Parotid-sparing intensity modulated versus conventional radiotherapy in head and neck cancer (PARSPORT): a phase 3 multicentre randomised controlled trial. Lancet Oncol. 2011; 12(2):127–136

Pignon JP, le Maître A, Maillard E, Bourhis J; MACH-NC Collaborative Group. Meta-analysis of chemotherapy in head and neck cancer (MACH-NC): an update on 93 randomised trials and 17,346 patients. Radiother Oncol. 2009; 92(1):4–14

Vermorken JB, Remenar E, van Herpen C, et al; EORTC 24971/ TAX 323 Study Group. Cisplatin, fluorouracil, and docetaxel in unresectable head and neck cancer. N Engl J Med. 2007; 357(17):1695–1704

Related Topics of Interest

Hypopharyngeal carcinoma
Oral cavity carcinoma
Laryngeal carcinoma
Sinonasal tumours
Nasopharyngeal tumours

R

82   Reconstructive Surgery

Reconstructive surgery is the technique to replace tissue loss caused by trauma, tumours or congenital deformity. The advent of antibiotics, refined anaesthesia and microsurgery have allowed more major head and neck resection procedures to be developed. Manchot in 1889 studied the blood supply of the skin and introduced the concept of vascular territories, while in 1936 Salmon confirmed the distribution of the perforating branches from marginal arteries. Although skin cover could be achieved by staged transposition of tubed pedicled fasciocutaneous flaps from distant sites, cosmesis, retention of function and quality of life were usually poor. In addition, some procedures took over a year to complete. Such techniques are now essentially of historical interest. The development of one-stage pedicled myocutaneous flaps and microvascular free tissue transfer over the last 25 years has conferred enormous improvement in outcomes including morbidity, rehabilitation and the quality of life.

When considering reconstructive surgery, it is pertinent to reflect on the surgical ladder. We have classified reconstruction into four levels.

82.1   Level 1-Direct Closure

It may be desirable to close small defects directly. Excision of a lesion should be planned, so skin incisions are in the line of least tension as mapped out by Langer's lines. These lines are usually at right angles to the underlying muscle fibres. Following the excision, some limited undermining between tissue planes is usually necessary to reduce tension. The depth of plane varies according to site; for example, on the face, the level of undermining is very superficial, but on the scalp, it is deep to the galeoaponeurotica. On the trunk and limbs, it lies between the superficial and deep fascia. The skin is able to be stretched, but its tolerance varies according to site and age. Skin suturing should be without undue tension.

82.2   Level 2-Skin Grafts

Skin grafts are considered when the deflect is too large for primary closure, or where the aesthetic result is better than from other methods of closure such as rotation flaps as on the nasal tip. A skin graft is a segment of epidermis and dermis that has been completely separated from the donor site and thus has no blood supply. They may be classified into split-skin grafts (also called partial-thickness skin grafts) or full-thickness skin grafts (also called Wolfe's grafts). The graft has no blood supply and so needs a vascular bed. It will not take on bone without periosteum, cartilage without perichondrium or tendon without paratenon. A skin graft is less likely to take at sites of poor vascularity, for example, over fat, heavily irradiated tissue or on infected tissue. The contact between the graft and recipient site is maintained by a pressure dressing or by the exposed method. The pressure dressing could be a pressure bandage or dressing with foam or cotton wool sutured or stapled, in position. In exposed wounds, one needs to observe for a seroma, haematoma or a collection of pus between the graft and recipient site. If a haematoma or seroma develops, it can be promptly dispersed by making a small incision in the graft or drawing out the collection using a large-bore needle and syringe.

82.2.1   Split-Skin Grafts

Split-skin grafts (SSG) consist of epidermis and a thin layer of dermis, but the troughs of the rete pegs and epithelium lining the hair follicles are left in situ to allow reepithelialisation of the donor site. They are a very versatile and usually reliable graft and should be harvested using an electric dermatome set at 3 or 4 on the circular scale corresponding to a thickness of 0.3 to 0.4 mm. In the oral cavity, a thicker graft of 0.5 mm is often recommended. However, the take is liable to be poor in the presence of saliva and exposed intraoral defects can be allowed to heal by secondary intention such as following excision of a tumour using a CO_2 laser. It should be noted that the dermatome scale acts as a guide only: other factors such as angle of the dermatome to the skin and skin tension will alter the graft thickness. Immediate grafting with quilt suturing and cross-hatching of the graft is recommended so that blood and serum can escape and do not lift the graft from its bed. The donor site should be hairless and inconspicuous. The inner aspect of the upper arm or thigh is therefore recommended. With large surface areas, it is reasonable to harvest the split skin and place the graft keratin side down on tulle gras, which is rolled, placed in a sterile pot, and refrigerated at 4°C. After

3 to 5 days when all bleeding and serous ooze from the raw bed has stopped and vascular granulated tissue has started to form, the SSG can be unrolled and sutured to the donor site.

Indications

a. To cover donor sites, for example, radial forearm free flaps and deltopectoral flaps.
b. To cover excised conchal bowl, skin and cartilage defect after the excision of a basal cell carcinoma.
c. To line cavities, for example, the inner layer of a maxillectomy cheek flap, or to line the orbital cavity after exenteration.
d. Burns.
e. Other skin defects where primary closure is not possible.

82.2.2 Full-Thickness Skin Graft (Wolfe's Graft)

This consists of the epidermis and the whole of the dermis. Typical sites to harvest this graft are the abdomen, neck (supraclavicular), forehead or postauricular. If a large surface area is required, for example, to close over a radial donor site, then the abdomen is best. If thicker facial skin quality is needed, such as for nasal tip, the forehead skin works very well. The post-auricular donor site can be preferred following septodermoplasty because primary closure is easy and leaves an inconspicuous scar.

It is essential to adequately defat the graft to ensure successful take.

Indications

a. Nasal tip and lateral defect within one aesthetic unit.
b. Conchal bowl defects.
c. Scalp.
d. Septodermoplasty.

82.3 Level 3-Pedicled Skin Flaps

Pedicled skin flaps These are skin flaps that remain attached at their base to provide a blood supply and lymphatic drainage. They can be classified into random, axial and myocutaneous.

Random/local flaps Skin gets its blood supply either from direct cutaneous vessels which run superficial to the deep fascia or from indirect vessels which pass from feeding vessels through muscle or fascia to reach the skin. A random flap is one where there is an indirect or an unknown direct blood supply to the skin. When planning such a flap, the length of the flap should not exceed the width of the base otherwise the distal portion of the flap may become ischaemic.

Examples of random skin flaps are advancement (V–Y), rotational or transpositional (Z-plasty, bilobed and rhomboid) skin flaps. Although these flaps may be raised anywhere and run in any direction, careful planning is necessary to obtain optimal cosmesis. Where possible, the use of relaxed skin tension lines should be used.

Intraorally, the buccal fat pad advancement is quite commonly used to close small defects in the retromolar, buccal mucosa and lateral palate. The fat has to be carefully mobilised in order to maintain its blood supply, and tacking sutures placed to the adjacent mucosa to limit excess movement. A disadvantage of this flap can be trismus due to fibrosis.

Tongue flaps harvested from the dorsum have their place and can be used to close persistent oronasal/oroantral fistulae. This is a two-stage procedure, with division of the pedicle base at about 3 weeks so can only be used on cooperative patients due to the period of restricted oral function.

Axial flaps Fasciocutaneous axial flaps include submental, temporoparietal, paramedian forehead, supraclavicular artery island (SCAI) flap, internal mammary flap, deltopectoral flap and nasolabial flaps.

These are flaps with a named blood supply running superficial to the deep fascia supplying the overlying skin. The length of the flap corresponds to the area supplied by these vessels. The pectoralis major myocutaneous flap has replaced many of the indications for the deltopectoral flap, which would now only rarely be used. The paramedian forehead flap is a popular choice for reconstruction of the nose. There are various flaps that can be employed to close defects of the lip. Common examples include advancement flaps such as Gillies fan flap, the Karapandzic flap and bilateral advancement flap. Also, axial flaps such as the Abbe–Estlander flap composed of skin, muscle and mucosa with the pedicle containing labial vessels.

The main disadvantage of all these flaps is that the patient must submit to a two-stage procedure,

R

the second to return the pedicle to its original site after the distal portion has gained an adequate blood supply at its new site; this normally takes 3 to 4 weeks. Between stages, the patient must endure moist dressings to an unsightly granulating bed from which the flap has been lifted.

Musculocutaneous flaps There are an assortment of musculocutaneous flaps such as the pectoralis major, submental artery perforator, facial artery musculomucosal (FAMM), temporalis, sternoclei-domastoid, trapezius, latissimus dorsi, platysma, infrahyoid and masseter flaps.

Although a large number of head and neck musculocutaneous flaps have been described, the pectoralis major flap is now by far the most popular. This is a flap of skin, deep fascia and muscle based on the acromiothoracic artery, a branch of the first part of the axillary artery. It runs in a layer between the deep aspect of the muscle and its underlying fascia. The vessels perforate the muscle to supply the overlying skin. Its advantages are that it is straightforward to raise, provides good bulk and is reliable. Its main disadvantage is that its bulk may compromise function, and for this reason the radial forearm fasciocutaneous free flap has taken over much of its previous work. Two important points in technique in raising the flap are as follows:

1. Suture the muscle edge to the subcutaneous edge as the flap is raised to prevent shearing of the perforating vessels.
2. After measuring the flap, allow an extra 1 to 2 cm of pedicle length as the flap retracts on raising; it is important that the pedicle is not under tension when suturing the flap into position.

82.4 Level 4-Free Tissue Transfer

For the larger complex defects, these flaps provide the gold standard in terms of cosmesis and preservation of function. Good results require sound microvascular training and meticulous attention to detail. Raising the flap and preparing both the donor and recipient vessels and their subsequent anastomosis are critical areas in which small errors may cause the graft to fail. Good results come from expert training in a centre with an interest in such reconstructive surgery and also from microvascular courses. The success rate of free tissue transfer should be in the region of 95

to 98% depending on the complexity. Success rates will tend to be slightly less when pedicle length is an issue, such as reconstruction of the maxilla, or where the quality of the neck vessels are compromised, for example, in cases of osteoradionecrosis. The common free tissue transfer flaps in head and neck reconstruction with their main indications are as follows.

82.4.1 Soft Tissue Only

Radial forearm fasciocutaneous free flap The subcutaneous fat and skin are supplied by the perforating vessels that pierce the antebrachial from the radial artery. Allen's test is a useful pre-operative assessment before considering harvesting the flap. The veins are the two vena commitants and these usually join with the cephalic vein if traced high enough into the antecubital fossa. This is a commonly used flap with many advantages. However, the skin defect donor site and numbness over the distribution of the terminal superficial radial nerve are its main disadvantages. When thin pliable skin of relatively small surface area typically 5 by 6 cm, with a long pedicle, is required, then the radial forearm flap is an obvious choice. It is commonly used for reconstruction of the floor of mouth, tongue, lateral oropharyngeal wall, soft palate and the repair as a patch graft of a pharyngocutaneous fistula.

Anterolateral thigh flap The anterolateral thigh (ALT) flap is based on the lateral circumflex femoral artery perforators. It has become a popular flap for head and neck reconstruction, as it has relatively little donor site morbidity, and although takes more time to harvest than the radial, it can be raised at the same time as other procedures with twin operating. Sometimes the perforators are very small and the flap has to be abandoned. In this case, the incision can be used to provide the full-thickness graft to cover the radial flap if that is the next option of choice intraoperatively. Sometimes the ALT is very thick with adipose tissue. In these circumstances, it might be better to choose a different less bulky flap. However, if it is used, careful debulking can be performed so as not to damage the skin perforator(s). The ALT is ideal when larger skin area is required, and bulk following subtotal glossectomy and reconstructing the lateral skull base after petrosectomy. The area allows it to be tubed such as reconstruction of a neopharynx after pharyngolaryngectomy.

Rectus abdominis myocutaneous free flap This flap is based on the deep inferior epigastric artery and venae originating on the external iliac vessels just above the inguinal ligament. Generally, the flap has low morbidity except the abdominal scar. This is a bulky skin and muscle flap, and although its use has been surpassed by the ALT, it still has a role in microvascular reconstruction of the head and neck when thickness is needed. It could be considered in thinner patients for reconstruction following glossectomy or lateral skull base after petrosectomy.

Jejunal free flap This is a segment of small bowel with vascular supply from the superior mesenteric artery and accompanying vein within a root of mesentery. The flap is very reliable but necessitates an intra-abdominal procedure with all the attendant morbidity and delayed recover. Also, the length of pedicle can be short if the flap is not raised by a confident surgeon familiar with the small bowel anatomy. Its main problem is the need for open abdominal surgery often in patients who already have nutritional deficits and comorbidity. Its main use is as a tube reconstruction of a neopharynx after pharyngolaryngectomy.

82.5 Bone and Soft Tissue (Composite) Transfer

Composite osteocutaneous radial forearm free flap Like the soft tissue flap it is based on perforating vessels that pierce the antebrachial from the radial artery in congruity with a portion of flexor pollicis longus muscle. It is unicortical, from the outer surface of the radius bone and its length is limited by the insertions of pronator teres and pronator quadratus to about 8 cm. No more than 40% of the height of the radius should be harvested, and the donor site plated, in order to reduce the risk of a subsequent radial fracture. Fracture is associated with very poor functional outcome. This flap can be considered when the amount of bone volume required is small.

Iliac crest/deep circumflex iliac artery (DCIA) This flap is based on the DCIA from the external iliac system. Skin is not required as the internal oblique muscle can be used to line the oral cavity or orbit. Although it is possible to incorporate skin utilising the perforator over the bony crest, the skin is bulky and is relatively fixed so is limited in its positioning in the defect. The height of bone makes it suitable for a large maxillectomy defect and the concave shape ideal to restore the mandible.

Fibula The fibula bone and overlying skin is supplied by the peroneal artery. It is considered the workhorse of bone and composite reconstruction in the head and neck region. It allows two team operating. Perforating vessels to the skin are identified during the harvesting of the flap. Care must be taken to ensure a sufficient cuff of soleus and gastrocnemius muscle in order not to comprise the perforators at the final part of harvesting the skin paddle. Where length of cortical bone is required and the soft tissue defect is close to the resected bone, then the fibula has its place in reconstruction of both the mandible and maxilla.

Scapula The flap is based on the transverse branch of the circumflex scapular artery. The incorporation of the angular branch of the thoracodorsal artery (scapular tip) allows for more pedicle length and this can be very useful in the maxillary defect. The scapular flap provides a large area of skin which moves freely over the bone. The relatively large pedicle is usually undamaged by the effects of age, lifestyle and comorbidity. The drawback to the flap is the need to change the position of the patient intraoperatively and the inability to perform twin site surgery. This limits the choice of a scapula as a soft tissue only flap as the radial and ALT better fulfil this role. The flap is ideal for complex mandibular or maxillary defects.

Further Reading

Brennan P, Schliephake H, Ghali GE, Cascarini L. Maxillofacial Surgery. 3rd ed. St. Louis, MO: Elsevier; 2017

Hanasono MM. Reconstructive Surgery for Head and Neck Cancer Patients. Advances in Medicine. 2014;795483

Scott-Browns Otolaryngology, Head and Neck Surgery, 8th Edition, Volume 2. Editors-in-Chief - Watkinson JC & Clarke R. Published by CRC Press, Taylor & Francis group, Boca Raton, London, New York, 2018

Watkinson J, Gilbert RW. Stell and Maran's Textbook of Head and Neck Surgery and Oncology. 5th ed. Boca Raton, FL: CRC Press; 2012

Urken ML, Buchbinder D, Genden EM. Reconstruction of the Mandible and Maxilla. In: Cummings CC, ed. Otolaryngology Head and Neck Surgery. 4th ed. St. Louis, MO: Mosby Year Book Inc.; 2004:1618–1635

Related Topics of Interest

Hypopharyngeal carcinoma
Oral cavity carcinoma
Oropharyngeal carcinoma

83 Rhinitis—Allergic

Rhinitis is defined as at least two symptoms from a list comprising of rhinorrhoea, blockage, sneezing and nasal itching. Rhinitis is divided into infectious and noninfectious and the latter further subdivided into allergic (AR) and non-allergic rhinitis (NAR).

Allergic rhinitis (AR) is an immunoglobulin E (IgE)-mediated, type 1 hypersensitivity reaction in the mucous membranes of the nasal airways to an allergen or allergens. AR significantly reduces quality of life and interferes with school and work attendance and performance. Although it is very common, it is underdiagnosed and often undertreated. It is therefore not possible to give a confident incidence or prevalence, but it has been estimated to affect 10 to 30% of the United Kingdom population. It can be either seasonal (e.g., hay fever) or perennial (sometimes with seasonal exacerbations). Such a clinical classification is useful in United Kingdom practice for diagnosis and treatment and can be used to complement the allergic rhinitis and its impact on asthma (ARIA) classification. Some patients are atopic. Atopic means that they have a genetic susceptibility to form an immune (allergic) response to a range of commonly found allergens. An allergen that causes AR may also cause allergic asthma, atopic eczema (allergic dermatitis) and allergic conjunctivitis. It is a risk factor for asthma and control of AR is associated with better asthma control. These associations are more likely in atopic individuals. Those with a family history of atopy and firstborn children have a higher risk of developing AR.

83.1 Pathophysiology

Sensitisation to an allergen occurs in genetically predisposed people who are, to a variable degree, atopic. Allergens are captured by dendritic allergen-presenting cells. This activates T-helper (Th) cells and these activated Th cells, called Th2 cells, release cytokines, the most important of which is interleukin 4 (IL-4). IL-4 drives B cells to produce allergen-specific IgE. This IgE binds through its high-affinity receptor, to effector cells such as mast cells and basophils. Subsequent contact of a nasal allergen with two molecules of allergen-specific IgE on the surface of a mast cell triggers the immediate release of inflammatory mediators such as histamine, tryptase and prostaglandin causing an immediate inflammatory response. Cytokines, most importantly IL-4 again, are also released which permit the migration of leucocytes, particularly eosinophils, to the sensitised mucosa. These leucocytes in turn release their own cytokines leading to a late-phase inflammatory response.

83.2 Classification

The 2008 ARIA guidelines recommend the following classification:

a. Intermittent. Symptoms are present fewer than 4 days a week *or* for fewer than 4 consecutive weeks.
b. Persistent. Symptoms present for 4 or more days a week *or* for 4 or more consecutive weeks.

Intermittent and persistent can each be subdivided into mild or severe.

a. Mild. Symptoms are not troublesome and in particular do not cause sleep disturbance, impair daily leisure, do not impair sport activities and do not impair school or work.
b. Moderate to severe. Symptoms are troublesome and in particular disturb sleep, impair daily activities and impair attendance/performance at school or work.

In the United Kingdom, AR may also be classified as seasonal and perennial and used alongside the ARIA classification. Some patients may therefore have intermittent, mild, seasonal allergic rhinitis, etc.

83.3 Clinical Features

Seasonal rhinitis occurs at a time when the patient is most exposed to the allergen. For example, the following:

Grass pollen—late spring to early summer.

Tree pollen—early spring to late spring.

House dust mite—perennial but usually more severe in autumn, winter and early spring.

Work allergens—symptoms less marked at the end of the weekend or when on holiday.

The patient suffers from rhinorrhoea, nasal irritation and sneezing, nasal obstruction and nasal congestion (nasal breathing is fine, but patients have midfacial pressure and feel blocked). The

R

throat may be itchy or irritable and there may be associated itchy, red, watering eyes and urticarial upper and/or lower lid oedema that collectively can be mistaken for early periorbital cellulitis. This allergic conjunctivitis occurs in about 60% of those with AR and is the symptom that most reliably differentiates AR from other types of rhinitis.

On examination, the nasal mucosa usually appears moist, pale and swollen, and the turbinates hypertrophied. Sometimes the mucosa is injected, and the turbinates may have a blue hue. Signs of chronic rhinosinusitis may be present with or without nasal polyps. Nasal polyps, however, are more often seen in intrinsic rhinitis.

83.4 Investigations

1. *Skin tests* The epidermal prick test and the intradermal injection test use an allergen placed on the skin of the flexor aspect of the forearm. If the patient has an allergy to this, then a wheal and flare will come up within 20 minutes. A negative control (carrier substance) and a histamine-containing solution (positive control) are used to ensure that the patient is not allergic to the carrier substance and does react in the normal fashion to histamine. A battery of common allergens (e.g., pollens, moulds, feathers, house dust mite, animal epithelia, etc.) is compared with the controls by the wheal they produce. Specific substances can be used depending on the history. If the patient is highly sensitive, a widespread or even an anaphylactic reaction may result. Resuscitation equipment should be available although the epidermal prick test is safe if properly performed. If an adverse reaction occurs, a tourniquet should be placed proximally to contain the allergen and the patient given intravenous hydrocortisone, an antihistamine and adrenaline. Oral antihistamines, topical and oral steroids and tricyclic antidepressants may suppress the results.

2. *Blood tests* Total plasma IgE levels may be measured in the plasma radioimmunosorbent test (PRIST) and IgE to specific allergens in the radioallergosorbent test (RAST). These tests are more convenient, do not expose the patient to the risks of the skin tests, and do not rely on the use of a specific allergen. They are more expensive, less sensitive and less specific than skin tests. An eosinophilia may occur in an acute allergic reaction but is unusual in chronic AR.

3. *Nasal smears* An increase in eosinophils in a nasal smear may occur in allergic rhinitis but is not specific.

4. *Nasal challenge* A drop of the suspected allergen squeezed into the nose may cause rhinitis symptoms. The obstructive effect can be measured objectively by rhinomanometry pre- and post-challenge.

83.5 Management

NICE's clinical knowledge summary in management of AR provides an excellent detailed plan for treating patients according to their severity of symptoms and includes step-up advice for patients who respond poorly to initial treatment.

1. *Avoidance* or reduced exposure to the precipitating allergen is perhaps the most important and the least emphasised aspect of treatment.

2. *Selective oral antihistamines* selectively block histamine receptors and cause minimal or no drowsiness and can be given once daily (e.g., cetirizine, fexofenadine and loratadine). They are effective for congestion, rhinorrhoea and sneezing but less so for nasal blockage. They will also reduce associated throat and eye symptoms. Azelastine hydrochloride nasal spray is effective too, but the benefit of no systemic side effects must be weighed against the spray's unpleasant taste and occasional irritative effect on the nasal lining.

3. *Topical steroid sprays* and drops are now considered to be the cornerstone in the treatment of rhinitis. They are safe and effective for nasal blockage, nasal itchiness, watery rhinorrhoea and sneezing. Crusting and bleeding are the main side effects. Systemic absorption is less than 2% for the prescribable nasal steroids and they are therefore safe to use long term in most patients. Examples include fluticasone, mometasone and triamcinolone sprays.

4. *Oral steroids* for 7 to 10 days are very effective in rapidly reducing symptoms and, by reducing mucosal oedema, they allow nasal sprays to be more widely distributed within the nasal cavity. They may be used in poor responders to nasal steroids/antihistamine sprays.

R

5. *Topical anticholinergic drugs* (e.g., ipratropium bromide) may be effective if watery rhinorrhoea is the predominant symptom.

6. *Sodium cromoglycate* stabilises mast cell membranes and therefore prevents the release of the allergic response mediators. It has few side effects but needs to be used five to six times per day for adequate prophylaxis. It may be effective in children and can be used for allergic conjunctivitis.

7. *Desensitisation* immunotherapy involves exposure to regular small but increasing doses of an allergen to produce tolerance to the allergen by producing blocking IgG antibodies. It will only produce tolerance to the allergen presented. The presentation of allergen may be by subcutaneous injection (injection immunotherapy) or as a drop, spray or tablet of allergen sublingually (sublingual immunotherapy [SLIT]). Its main use is for those with life-threatening sensitivity to wasp and bee stings, peanuts and severe grass pollen allergy that has not responded to antihistamines/nasal steroids. The main complication of treatment is anaphylaxis and for this reason resuscitation equipment must be available.

8. *Leukotriene receptor antagonists* appear to have an additive effect to intranasal corticosteroids in controlling seasonal AR, particularly in patients with asthma.

9. *Surgical treatment* Turbinate reduction surgery is effective in increasing the calibre of the nasal airway. This may either significantly improve nasal obstruction or, in those who are still stuffy after surgery, it will allow nasal sprays to be more widely distributed throughout the nasal airway and therefore be more effective in controlling residual rhinitis symptoms. It does not help post-nasal drip and of course is not a cure for AR.

83.6 Follow-Up and Aftercare

Allergic rhinitis is usually managed by the patient's general practitioner. Referral to a specialist may be because of medical undertreatment. If such a patient is referred, then once symptoms are controlled, the GP should be given clear management instructions and perhaps guided to NICE's clinical knowledge summary.

Further Reading

Bousquet J, Khaltaev N, Cruz AA, et al; World Health Organization. GA(2)LEN. AllerGen. Allergic rhinitis and its impact on asthma (ARIA) 2008 update (in collaboration with the World Health Organization, GA(2)LEN and AllerGen). Allergy. 2008; 63(Suppl 86):8–160

Chhabra N, Houser SM. The surgical management of allergic rhinitis. Otolaryngol Clin North Am. 2011; 44(3):779–795, xi

NICE clinical knowledge summary on allergic rhinitis management, October 2015. Available at www.nice.org.uk

Seidman MD, Gurgel RK, Lin SY, et al; Guideline Otolaryngology Development Group. AAO-HNSF. Clinical practice guideline: allergic rhinitis. Otolaryngol Head Neck Surg. 2015; 152(1, Suppl):S1–S43

Related Topics of Interest

Rhinosinusitis—chronic (with nasal polyps)
Rhinosinusitis—chronic without nasal polyps
Rhinitis—non-allergic

84 Rhinitis—Non-Allergic

Rhinitis (nasal mucosal inflammation) may be classified as being either infective or non-infective and the latter further sub-divided into allergic and non-allergic rhinitis. Non-allergic rhinitis (NAR) is a diagnosis of exclusion. In a 2007 Danish study, it was found to affect a quarter of the population, of which half sought medical advice.

NAR accounts for about half of perennial rhinitis cases. It becomes more common with increasing age. Although NAR is common and significantly impacts on quality of life, it is surprisingly often under-treated. It has a multifactorial aetiology and is a risk factor for the development of asthma. For patients who do not have adequate symptom relief from medication, turbinate reduction surgery is effective in reducing nasal blockage.

84.1 Pathology

NAR has been divided into two types:

1. NAR associated with an identifiable cause.
2. Idiopathic rhinitis (previously called vasomotor or intrinsic rhinitis).

Eosinophilic rhinitis is usually placed in the idiopathic group because although such patients have a high number of eosinophils in their nasal mucous, the cause of this is unknown. Some patients demonstrate an intrinsic mucosal disorder of prostaglandin metabolism and there is an association of this type of rhinitis with aspirin hyper-sensitivity, asthma and aggressive nasal polyposis.

Regardless of the underlying aetiology, most patients demonstrate glandular hyperplasia and sub-mucosal vascular dilation. The nasal mucosa, particularly turbinate mucosa, becomes hyperaemic and hypertrophic. Eosinophil-laden polyps are more common in NAR than in allergic rhinitis (AR).

84.2 Predisposing Factors

- Familial tendency.
- A preceding nasal infection (nasal mucosal hyper-reactivity following viral or bacterial rhinitis).
- Occupational, such as irritation from hairsprays in hairdressers or chlorine in swimming instructors.
- Psychological and emotional factors.
- Endocrine (puberty, menstruation and pregnancy).
- Drugs (angiotensin-converting enzyme [ACE] inhibitors, β-blockers, methyldopa, aspirin and oral contraceptives).
- Pollution (atmospheric pollution, fumes, dust, industrial detergents and cigarette smoke).
- Climate changes in humidity and temperature.
- Alcohol.
- Smoking.

84.3 Clinical Features

- Anterior and posterior rhinorrhoea.
  A common misconception, even amongst chest physicians, is that post-nasal drip can cause chest symptoms. Most patients with NAR, who have a persistent sensation of post-nasal drip, do not have a visible post-nasal rhinorrhoea. If a higher volume of mucous is produced, there is nearly always a concomitant increase in muco-ciliary flow so that only the usual sheen of moist mucosa is seen when examining the posterior nares and nasopharynx. Moreover, many patients who complain bitterly of a post-nasal discharge do not have symptoms or signs of an anterior watery rhinorrhoea and conversely many patients with a marked anterior watery rhinorrhoea do not complain of a post-nasal drip. How does one explain this paradox? Probably the answer is simply that many patients with non-infective rhinitis (i.e. who have NAR or AR) have a hyper-reactive/hyper-sensitive posterior nasal and nasopharyngeal mucosa giving rise to a heightened awareness of normal mucociliary flow. This explains why various nasal applications may not help this symptom—because they may not reduce nasal sensitivity. It is likely that many patients who have non-infective rhinitis and who have a persistent cough simply have the chest equivalent of posterior nasal hyper-sensitivity, that is, bronchial hyper-reactivity or cough-variant asthma. In other words, they have an inflammatory process that affects both the lungs and the nose; it is not that one causes the other. Interestingly, controlling the inflammatory process in one system seems to reduce (but not resolve) symptoms in the other system too.

- Nasal obstruction.
For some patients with NAR, nasal obstruction is their main symptom, for others it is watery rhinorrhoea. Some patients have only mild daytime nasal obstruction, but they complain of marked blockage when lying flat trying to sleep. Nasal steroids and antihistamines are often not effective for such patients, but they do well from turbinate reduction surgery.
- Itching and sneezing are less common than with allergic rhinitis.
- Hyposmia, often mild, unless there are coexistent nasal polyps when more marked hyposmia or anosmia may occur.
- Coexistent sinus pathology may be present in up to 50% of cases. This may be primary, causing a secondary rhinitis, or secondary due to the compromise of sinus aeration and drainage. Examination generally reveals a red mucosa, often with copious secretions and hypertrophy of both middle and inferior turbinates, causing a consequent reduction in the airway size.

84.4 Investigations

NAR is a diagnosis of exclusion, and the aim of investigations is to identify other causes of rhinitis. Immunoglobulin E (IgE) estimation by PRIST and RAST and skin testing can be used to indicate allergy. If a systemic inflammatory process is suspected, an anti-neutrophil cytoplasmic antibody (ANCA) and ACE assay may be indicated as may be a nasal mucosal biopsy. A sinus computed tomography (CT) scan may help diagnose structural abnormalities and any coexistent sinus infection. A sinus magnetic resonance imaging (MRI) may be indicated, in addition to a CT, if inverted papilloma or sinus malignancy is suspected.

84.5 Medical Management

a. Antibiotics may be used to treat coexistent infection.
b. A short course of oral steroids may be indicated when there is marked nasal mucosal oedema and obstruction. This may allow control of mucosal oedema before the introduction of nasal steroids.
c. Nasal steroid sprays are more widely distributed within the nose when started at the end of a course of oral steroids. Oral and nasal steroids are not as effective in NAR, compared to AR, in controlling nasal obstruction.

d. Non-sedating antihistamines.
e. Topical ipratropium bromide has an anticholinergic effect and may reduce watery rhinorrhoea. Patients are probably best advised to self-titrate the dose, starting at one spray to each nostril twice daily building the dose up to a maximum of two sprays to each nostril three times daily. Patients should be advised to try to get a balance of obtaining symptom improvement while not over-drying the nasopharynx and oropharynx. Excessive throat drying on initial use may lead the patient to abandon the spray without a proper trial.
f. Systemic sympathomimetics can be helpful (e.g. pseudoephedrine), though they may produce unpleasant side effects such as dry mouth, constipation and excitability. They should not be used long term or in children.
g. Local nasal decongestants. Self-medication with topical vasoconstrictors (e.g. xylometazoline, ephedrine) is common and initially successful in bringing relief to the patient with enlarged turbinates by reducing turbinate blood flow. Unfortunately, when the effect wears off, there is a reflex vasodilation causing increased blood flow and turbinate engorgement (the so-called rebound phenomenon). Prolonged excessive use leads to an aggravation of symptoms, which eventually become unresponsive to the decongestant, and rhinitis medicamentosa may supervene. The treatment is to then stop the decongestant and prescribe a trial of topical nasal steroids. If the latter is not effective, then turbinate reduction surgery is indicated. Elderly patients who only have nocturnal nasal blockage may benefit from the controlled use of these decongestants, using one or two sprays to each nostril at night. Such usage is usually not associated with the rebound phenomenon, particularly if patients are advised to avoid use of the decongestant for a fortnight if they start to develop a degree of daytime blockage (indicating early rebound symptoms).

84.6 Surgical Management

Surgical treatment is useful for the control of symptoms, particularly nasal obstruction, when medical treatment is ineffective.

1. *Turbinate reduction surgery* Submucosal diathermy, linear diathermy, laser cautery, cryosurgery, coblation reduction and multiple

out fractures may be successful in the short term, but obstruction recurs in most cases because the remaining turbinate mucosa continues to be hyperplastic over the remaining inferior turbinate bone. The key to long-term benefit from nasal obstruction is to remove inferior turbinate bone so that the support for the hyperplastic mucosa is removed. Some surgeons favour turbinoplasty when much of the mucosa remains but the volume of the nasal airway increases by removing the supporting inferior turbinate bone. This has the advantage of a reduced risk of a severe epistaxis post-operatively compared to inferior turbinectomy. Inferior turbinectomy, where both the turbinate bone and the hyperplastic mucosa are excised, is associated with higher morbidity. An intra-nasal dressing is required post-operatively to tamponade the lateral nasal wall and there is a risk of a significant post-operative epistaxis once the intra-nasal dressing is removed. However, it remains the most effective procedure in relieving nasal obstruction long term.

2. *Vidian neurectomy* This operation was proposed for the relief of watery rhinorrhoea when there is no nasal obstruction. The vidian nerve (otherwise known as the nerve of the pterygoid canal) is formed by the union of the greater petrosal nerve and the deep petrosal nerve within the pterygoid canal. The deep petrosal nerve contains pre-ganglionic parasympathetic fibres from the facial nerve which synapse in the pterygopalatine ganglion. The post-ganglionic parasympathetic fibres of the greater petrosal nerve, upon synapsing in the pterygopalatine ganglion, distribute to the nose, palate and lacrimal gland through nerves leaving the pterygopalatine fossa. The deep petrosal nerve contains post-ganglionic sympathetic fibres which do not synapse in the pterygopalatine ganglion and supply the lacrimal gland and mucous glands and mucosa within the nasal cavity. The vidian nerve is divided or cauterised where it enters the pterygopalatine fossa. Half of the patients who have an initial benefit will have a recurrence of their symptoms with time.

3. *Endoscopic sinus surgery* to address concomitant sinus disease.

Further Reading

Scadding GK, Durham SR, Mirakian R, Jones NS. BSACI guidelines for the management of allergic and non-allergic rhinitis. Clin Exp Allergy. 2008; 38:19–42

Settipane RA, Kaliner MA. Nonallergic rhinitis. Am J Rhinol Allergy. 2013; 27(Suppl 1):S48–S51

Related Topics of Interest

Rhinitis—allergic
Examination of the nose
Rhinosinusitis—chronic (with nasal polyps)
Rhinosinusitis—chronic without nasal polyps
Functional endoscopic sinus surgery

85 Rhinoplasty

85.1 Introduction

Rhinoplasty is defined as an operation to change the structure of the nose and is one of the more commonly performed facial plastic surgery procedures. The aim of the surgery is to improve the shape of the nose, the nasal airway or frequently both. A key concept in rhinoplasty surgery is that form and function are inter-related.

Surgery involving the external structure of the nose is generally referred to as a rhinoplasty, and surgery to the external structure and the nasal septum classified as a septorhinoplasty. In reality, almost all rhinoplasty procedures affect the septum to some degree and many surgeons refer to all these cases as a septorhinoplasty.

This chapter will focus on surgery to the external structure of the nose, where the aim is to improve the cosmetic appearance while maintaining the nasal airway.

85.2 Pre-Operative Management

85.2.1 Should the Patient Have a Rhinoplasty?

For the majority of patients, a rhinoplasty is a positive experience. However, this is not always the case, and a key decision is whether a surgery should be offered. Patients must have a realistic expectation about what can be achieved with surgery and be willing to accept the limitations of what is possible. In reality, a rhinoplasty can generally produce a good improvement, but certainly not perfection. To justify a rhinoplasty on cosmetic grounds, there must be a noticeable abnormality which can be improved with surgery, and where the benefits outweigh the risks.

A significant minority of patients should not be offered a rhinoplasty, and it is only possible to reach a correct decision by taking sufficient time to discuss surgery. For this reason, most surgeons will see patients on two occasions.

It is mandatory to take clinical photographs prior to a rhinoplasty. It is particularly helpful to review the images with the patient to ensure that both surgeon and patient have a clear understanding of what is intended, and indeed possible.

85.3 Body Dysmorphic Disorder

On occasion, patients exhibit excessive, disproportionate anxiety about the appearance of their nose. This is a recognised psychological disorder known as body dysmorphic disorder. These patients often describe minor abnormalities in dramatic terms, and their concerns have a very negative impact on their quality of life. Although they are often desperate to undergo surgery, this is almost invariably counter-productive and leads to more unhappiness. Referral to a clinical psychologist or psychiatrist with an interest in this field is the way forward, although in reality many of these patients reject this option and continue to seek surgery.

85.4 Clinical Examination

Clinical examination initially involves inspection of the external shape of the nose. Palpation is helpful to assess deviation, cartilaginous and bony prominences and support of the nasal skeleton. The patient's skin type is particularly important in rhinoplasty, because thin skin tends to show irregularities, and thicker skin reduces the definition and contouring that can be achieved.

Anterior rhinoscopy is performed to examine the nasal septum and turbinates. The dynamic function of the nose should be examined, particularly any collapse of the nasal valves on quiet inspiration. Examination of the nasal cavity and post-nasal space with an endoscope is recommended, and is essential if the patient has airway obstruction or other rhinological symptoms.

85.5 Aesthetic Assessment

A rhinoplasty surgeon must be able to diagnose the anatomical abnormality causing the aesthetic concerns, and then plan a suitable operation to address these.

It is essential to have a structured method of examining nasal aesthetics. A helpful method is to assess the nose in thirds (nasal bridge, mid-third and tip) and then each half from the front view.

- Key features to be examined on front view include the width and any deviation of the nasal bones.

- The upper lateral cartilages and septum make up the mid-third of other nose and any deviation or asymmetry should also be identified.
- Finally, the symmetry and definition of the nasal tip is studied. It is also useful to trace the dorsal aesthetic line, which should curve gently from the eyebrow, down the sidewall of the nose to the nasal tip.

The nasal dorsal profile is examined, including the upper starting point of the nose which should be at the level of the upper eyelid fold. The ideal aesthetic profile will of course differ between men and women, and the presence of a dorsal hump or need for augmentation is assessed accordingly.

An important feature of the nose is the projection of the nasal tip which is the distance that the nasal tip projects forward from the face. The tip should be the high point of the nasal dorsum, and over- or under-projection of the tip should be recognised.

The rotation of the nasal tip is the angle between the nasal columella and the lip. Again, this differs between the male and female nose with an ideal angle of approximately 90 degrees in men and an increase in rotation in women to 100 to 110 degrees. The definition and contouring of the nasal tip, together with columellar and alar aesthetics should be assessed.

A comprehensive review of nasal assessment is beyond the scope of this chapter and this is available in texts recommended under further reading.

85.6 Informed Consent for Rhinoplasty

In an era of increasing medicolegal action taken against cosmetic surgeons, obtaining and documenting informed consent about a proposed rhinoplasty procedure is essential. The preoperative discussion should include the sequalae of surgery and possible complications including bleeding, possibility of packs, bruising, infection, numbness and septal perforation. It is recommended that other possible problems such as a loss of smell, skin changes and nasal obstruction are also discussed. Even in the most experienced hands, revision surgery may be required and this must be discussed with the patient.

It is important that these potential complications and the possibility of revision surgery are not only discussed but recorded in the case notes and consent form. The aims of the surgery should be clearly documented, together with the type of rhinoplasty recommended and the reason for this.

Written information should also be given and this action recorded in the case notes and on the consent form.

85.7 Surgical Approach

85.7.1 Endonasal versus Open Rhinoplasty

There are two approaches used in rhinoplasty, firstly, the endonasal or closed approach and secondly, the external or open approach. In endonasal rhinoplasty, incisions are made inside the nose to enable the skin to be elevated in situ, whereas in the open approach, incisions inside the nose are joined to a small external incision across the columella. This allows the skin and soft tissue envelope to be elevated and rotated exposing the underlying cartilages and bone.

There are advantages and disadvantages to each approach, and the type of surgery performed will depend on both the complexity of the surgery required and the experience and training of the surgeon. Traditionally, more complex cases such as revision or cleft nose surgery were performed via an open approach, and more straight forward primary cases performed using an endonasal approach. There is, however, now a great variation among those who specialise in this area of surgery, with many rhinoplasty surgeons performing almost all cases open and others the majority via an endonasal approach.

85.8 Surgical Techniques in Rhinoplasty

A detailed description of the many and varied surgical techniques used in rhinoplasty is beyond the scope of this chapter, and an overview is given.

A common request in rhinoplasty surgery is to reduce a dorsal nasal hump. Dorsal humps invariably involve bone and cartilage which is reduced. Medial and lateral osteotomies are then often required to in-fracture the nasal bones and narrow the bridge. Osteotomies may also be required to straighten deviated nasal bones.

During hump reduction, the upper lateral cartilages and septum are often reduced in height.

R

In recent years, the importance of preserving the upper lateral cartilages and reconstructing the mid-third of the nose to prevent collapse has been recognised. Various techniques are used to maintain the width of the mid-third of the nose. These include cartilage spreader grafts placed between the septum and the upper lateral cartilages or folding down the excess height of each upper lateral cartilage, so-called auto-spreader grafts.

The lower lateral cartilages can be reduced in size and the shape modified to improve the contour of the nasal tip. In recent years, there has been a move towards far more conservative resection of cartilage from the nose including the lower lateral cartilages. Modern techniques focus on cartilage preservation where possible, with re-contouring the cartilages using various sutures and grafts.

Cartilage grafts to augment, support or straighten the nose are frequently placed during a rhinoplasty. These grafts may be harvested from the nasal septum, or from the pinna if there is insufficient cartilage in the septum due to injury, infection or previous surgery. Grafts from the conchal bowl of the pinna can be harvested with limited morbidity and are widely used. They are, however, rather soft and generally not suitable for structural grafting in rhinoplasty.

On occasion, autogenous rib cartilage is used when large or strong structural grafting is required, although this does carry a significantly increased morbidity and stay in hospital. Irradiated cadaveric donor rib is commercially available in some countries and is used by many surgeons. Synthetic grafts may be used, although these are not favoured by most specialist rhinoplasty surgeons due to an increased risk of extrusion and infection.

85.9 Post-Operative Management

The nose is protected with an external splint for a week or so, and the patient is reviewed in the early post-operative period to ensure healing is proceeding without complication.

It is important to make patients aware that it takes many months for the swelling of the nose to settle before the final result can be judged. Rhinoplasty patients often need considerable support from their surgeon during the post-operative period.

Further Reading

Sclafani AP. Rhinoplasty: The Experts' Reference. Stuttgart: Thieme Medical Publishers; 2015

Nolst Trinite GJ, ed. Rhinoplasty: A Practical Guide to Functional and Aesthetic Surgery of the Nose. The Hague, The Netherlands: Kugler Publications; 2005

Rollin K. Mastering Rhinoplasty: A Comprehensive Atlas of Surgical Techniques. 2nd ed. New York, NY: Daniel, Springer Science & Business Media;, 2010

Tardy ME. Rhinoplasty: The Art and the Science. Vol 1. Philadelphia, PA: WB Saunders; 1997:2–125

86 Rhinosinusitis—Appropriate Terminology

Rhinosinusitis is defined differently in children and adults according to the most recent EPOS 2012 conference summary.

86.1 Adult Definition

1. Inflammation of the nose and the paranasal sinuses characterized by at least two nasal *symptoms*. At least one nasal symptom should be from the group—nasal blockage, nasal obstruction, nasal congestion and nasal discharge (anterior or posterior rhinorrhea). The second group of symptoms, which are not essential, and of which, at most, only one counts towards the two symptoms required for formal diagnosis, are: facial pain, facial pressure, a reduction or loss of olfaction.
2. There should also be either (a) endoscopic *signs* of nasal polyps and/or mucopurulent nasal discharge primarily from the middle meatus and/or mucosal oedema/mucosal obstruction primarily in the middle meatus and/or (b) computed tomography (CT) mucosal changes within the ostiomeatal complex and/or sinuses.

86.2 Paediatric Definition

Similar to the adult definition except that in the second group of symptoms a reduction or loss of olfaction is replaced by the presence of a cough.

86.3 Chronic Rhinosinusitis

This is defined as rhinosinusitis symptoms that have been present for 12 weeks or longer. It is sub-divided into chronic rhinosinusitis (CRS) with nasal polyps (CRSwNP) and CRS without nasal polyps (CRSsNP).

CRSwNP is a CRS as defined earlier with bilateral endoscopically visualized polyps present in the middle meatus.

CRSsNP is a CRS as defined earlier with no polyps visible within the middle meatus, if necessary following application of nasal decongestant.

The definitions emphasize there is a wide range of disease in CRS that includes polypoidal changes within the sinuses or middle meatus. To avoid overlap it excludes polypoidal disease present in the nasal cavity.

86.4 Acute Rhinosinusitis

Acute rhinosinusitis (ARS) is defined as rhinosinusitis symptoms that have been present for less than 12 weeks.

ARS is most commonly caused by common cold viruses. EPOS 2012 thus sub-divided ARS into viral ARS or post-viral ARS, the latter replacing non-viral ARS from the 2007 definition.

Viral ARS is defined as rhinosinusitis symptoms lasting less than 10 days with complete resolution.

Post-viral ARS is defined as an increase of rhinosinusitis symptoms after 5 days or persistent symptoms after 10 days but with less than 12 weeks duration.

Post-viral ARS is meant to encompass non-viral ARS causes and true post-viral ARS.

Please remember that only a small percentage of patients with post-viral ARS have a bacterial aetiology, which is then called acute bacterial rhinosinusitis (ABRS). ABRS is therefore a sub-set of post-viral ARS. Bacteria may be the initial causative agent (primary ABRS) or secondary to an initial viral ARS (secondary ABRS).

86.5 Acute Bacterial Rhinosinusitis

ABRS is suggested by the presence of at least three of the following symptoms/signs:

- Discoloured discharge (with unilateral predominance) and purulent secretion in the nasal cavity.
- Severe local pain (with unilateral predominance).
- Fever > 38°C
- Elevated ESR/CRP (erythrocyte sedimentation rate/C-reactive protein).
- Double sickening (deterioration after an initial milder phase of illness).

Further Reading

Fokkens WJ, Lund VJ, Mullol J, Bachert C. et al. The European Position Paper on rhinosinusitis and nasal polyps 2012. Rhinology. 2012; 23:1–299

Related Topics of Interest

Rhinosinusitis—chronic (with nasal polyps)
Rhinosinusitis—chronic without nasal polyps

R

87 Rhinosinusitis—Acute

Both the maxillary and frontal sinuses drain through narrow spaces, clefts and gaps between the ethmoid cells, into the middle meatus. The anterior ethmoid cells also drain into the middle meatus, but the posterior ethmoids drain into the superior meatus. Any condition narrowing or blocking these channels may lead to secretion retention and poor ventilation, thus predisposing to consequent infection. The commonest cause (98% according to the National Institute of Clinical Excellence) is viral acute rhinosinusitis (ARS) from common cold viruses. Viral ARS usually resolves of its own accord after 2 to 3 weeks but occasionally may progress to post-viral ARS. Post-viral ARS requires antibiotics and if inadequately treated may progress to chronic rhinosinusitis (CRS). There are specific definitions for the different types of rhinosinusitis and these are covered in Chapter 86, Rhinosinusitis—Appropriate Terminology. It should be appreciated that most patients with acute facial pain have a non-sinogenic cause.

87.1 Predisposing Factors

1. Local
   a. Acute viral upper respiratory tract infection from common cold viruses or influenza.
   b. Tonsillitis.
   c. Pre-existing rhinitis (allergic, vasomotor, rhinitis medicamentosa, etc.).
   d. Nasal polyps.
   e. Nasal foreign body.
   f. Nasal anatomical variations (septal deviation, abnormal uncinate process, middle turbinate or ethmoid bulla) narrow the infundibulum and may predispose to its occlusion when there is intercurrent disease.
   g. Nasal tumour.
   h. Dental extraction or infection (diseases of the upper premolars and upper first molar in particular, as these dental roots are particularly close to the maxillary sinus floor).
   i. Swimming and diving.
   j. Fractures involving the sinuses.

2. General
   a. Debilitation.
   b. Immunocompromise.
   c. Mucociliary disorders (e.g. Kartagener's syndrome, cystic fibrosis).

   d. Atmospheric irritants (dust, fumes and tobacco smoke).

Acute inflammation of one or all the sinuses may occur (pansinusitis). The ethmoid and maxillary sinuses are clinically the most commonly affected, followed by the frontal and sphenoid sinuses in that order.

87.2 Pathology

Most cases follow a viral upper respiratory tract infection which involves all the respiratory epithelium including the paranasal sinuses. Such infections cause hyperaemia and oedema of the mucosa, which then block the ostia. There will be cellular infiltration and an increase in mucus production. The infections will also paralyse the cilia, leading to stasis of secretions predisposing to a secondary bacterial infection. The usual causative bacterial organisms are *Streptococcus pneumoniae*, *Haemophilus influenzae* (accounting for 70% of cases in adults), *Streptococcus pyogenes*, *Moraxella catarrhalis* and *Staphylococcus aureus*. *Klebsiella pneumoniae*, *Escherichia coli* and *Streptococcus milleri* may spread from a dental source. Acute fungal infections (e.g. mucormycosis and aspergillosis) are rare but may develop in immunocompromised or elderly diabetic patients.

87.3 Clinical Features

The symptoms usually occur several days after developing an upper respiratory tract infection. The patient will have pain over the infected sinus, nasal congestion, fullness in the face, malaise and possibly a pyrexia. The fullness in the face and pain may be exacerbated by bending forward or stooping down.

Specific features may indicate the sinus that is infected. Pain developing in the cheek or upper teeth indicates maxillary sinus involvement. Frontal sinusitis produces pain in the forehead and tenderness below the eyebrows. Ethmoid sinusitis may cause pain between the eyes accompanied by frontal headache. Sphenoid infection may produce retro-orbital pain, or pain anywhere across the vault.

Anterior rhinoscopy may show red oedematous nasal mucosa and turbinates. Flexible or rigid endoscopy may reveal pus in the middle meatus or sphenoethmoidal recess. It may also be possible to elicit tenderness over the infected sinus. Percussion over the upper teeth may elicit tenderness. This suggests either a dental cause or that the inflamed floor of the maxillary sinus lies very close to the dental roots (in particular, U4/5/6) so that the vibration transmitted by percussion irritates the inflamed maxillary sinus mucosa.

87.4 Differential Diagnosis

Reading Chapter 35, Headache and Facial Pain, will be a reminder of the plethora of causes of non-sinogenic acute facial pain which includes the following:

1. Migraine.
2. Cluster headaches.
3. Atypical facial pain.
4. Dental pain.
5. Trigeminal neuralgia.
6. Paroxysmal hemicrania.
7. Temporal arteritis.
8. Herpes zoster and post-herpetic neuralgia.
9. Erysipelas.
10. Sinonasal tumour.

87.5 Investigations

- An elevated white cell count and C-reactive protein (CRP) will confirm an acute infection. The erythrocyte sedimentation rate (ESR) may also be raised possibly indicating the presence of infection for some time.
- Pus from the nose should be cultured and blood cultures should be taken if there is significant systemic upset.
- A high-definition coronal computed tomography (CT) scan of the sinuses may be indicated in the deteriorating patient or if a complication of rhinosinusitis is suspected (see Chapter 90, Rhinosinusitis – Complications). Modern rapid-sequence multi-slice CT scanning allows the viewer to control the window setting so that both soft tissue and bone window images and coronal, axial and sagittal planes are viewed.

87.6 Management

The aims of treatment are to resolve and limit the course of the acute infection, to prevent complications and to correct any precipitating factors. In October 2017, the National Institute for Clinical Excellence (NICE) produced an updated Clinical Knowledge Summary (CKS) and recommended treatment summary for acute sinusitis. NICE points out that 98% of ARS is of viral aetiology and will settle in 2 to 3 weeks without antibiotics. In such patients, antibiotics should only be prescribed immediately if the patient has a comorbidity which puts him or her at a high risk of a complication. For all other patients, only if symptoms suggest acute bacterial rhinosinusitis (ABRS) should antibiotics be prescribed. NICE recommends phenoxymethylpenicillin 500 mg qds for 5 days as a first-line treatment unless the patient is systemically unwell or at high risk of a complication of ABRS, when co-amoxiclav 625 mg three times daily for 5 days is recommended as a first-line treatment. For those patients allergic to penicillin, doxycycline or erythromycin is recommended as a first-line treatment for 5 days. A second-line antibiotic is recommended if no improvement with first-line treatment occurs after 2 to 3 days. Co-amoxiclav is recommended for those initially prescribed phenoxymethylpenicillin. For those initially prescribed co-amoxiclav, a discussion with microbiology is recommended. If the patient has symptoms or signs suggesting sepsis at any stage or is felt to be developing a complication of ABRS, then referral to hospital is indicated.

87.6.1 Medical Treatment

In the acute stages the patient should have the following treatment:

- Bed rest and adequate simple analgesia (e.g. paracetamol and non-steroidal anti-inflammatory drugs [NSAIDs]).
- A decongestant (e.g. pseudoephedrine or xylometazoline) in viral ARS or a nasal steroid in ABRS (both level 1a evidence).

An antibiotic may be required if symptoms suggest ABRS rather than viral ARS (see NICE guidelines above).

The condition can also be helped by the use of ipratropium bromide nasal spray in viral ARS (level 1a evidence) and saline nasal irrigation (level 1a evidence). Decongestants may reduce nasal oedema thereby facilitating ventilation of the sinuses. Oral antihistamines are only recommended by NICE if the patient has a coexistent nasal allergy.

R

87.6.2 Surgical Treatment

Most patients with ARS are treated in primary care. Those admitted to hospital have either developed a complication of ABRS such as periorbital cellulitis or they have become septic despite being on oral antibiotics or symptoms, such as facial pain, have increased. Such ABRS patients may just need intravenous antibiotics, but some who fail to respond may require surgery, for example, an endoscopic middle meatal antrostomy and anterior ethmoidectomy for those with severe localised maxillary pain. This will not only allow ventilation and drainage of infection in the maxillary sinus but will also promote drainage from the other sinuses as oedema in the middle meatus settles. Any pus obtained should be cultured.

87.7 Follow-Up

After resolution, the patient should have an outpatient follow-up to determine if further treatment is required such as long-term nasal steroids or any (further) surgery. Correction of precipitating factors (e.g. septoplasty for septal deviation) may be necessary. It may be that symptoms persist beyond 12 weeks when the patient is said to have CRS. This may require treatment as advised in the Chapter 88.

Further Reading

Banigo A, Watson D, Ram B, Ah-See K. Orofacial pain. BMJ. 2018; 361:k1517

Chow AW, Benninger MS, Brook I, et al; Infectious Diseases Society of America. IDSA clinical practice guideline for acute bacterial rhinosinusitis in children and adults. Clin Infect Dis. 2012; 54(8):e72–e112

NICE CKS: Acute sinusitis. Last updated October 2017. Available at www.nice.org.uk

NICE prescribing guidelines for acute sinusitis (NG79). Last updated October 2017. Available at www.nice.org.uk

Rosenfeld RM, Piccirillo JF, Chandrasekhar SS, et al. Clinical practice guideline (update): adult sinusitis. Otolaryngol Head Neck Surg. 2015; 152(2, Suppl):S1–S39

Related Topics of Interest

Rhinosinusitis—appropriate terminology
Rhinitis—allergic
Rhinitis—non-allergic
Rhinosinusitis—chronic without nasal polyps
Rhinosinusitis—fungal
Rhinosinusitis—complications
Functional endoscopic sinus surgery
Headache and facial pain

R

88 Rhinosinusitis—Chronic without Nasal Polyps

Rhinosinusitis is defined differently in children and in adults. Please see Chapter 86, Rhinosinusitis-Appropriate Terminology for the correct definitions and classification. Chronic rhinosinusitis without nasal polyps (CRSsNP) is diagnosed when rhinosinusitis symptoms and signs have been present for more than 12 weeks, but there are no polyps visible within the middle meatus. The causes of CRSsNP are the same as those causing acute rhinosinusitis (ARS) but with CRSsNP mucosal oedema and infected secretions persist, causing chronic inflammation. Saline nasal douching, intra-nasal steroids and a long course of antibiotics may be indicated before considering surgery.

88.1 Pathology

There is an increase in vascularity and vascular permeability. This leads to oedema and hypertrophy of the mucosa which may become polypoidal. Goblet cell hyperplasia and a chronic cellular infiltrate occur. Ulceration of the epithelium results in the formation of granulation tissue. Multiple small abscesses occur in the thickened mucosa and fibrosis of the sub-mucosal stroma supervenes. The changes in the mucosa over this time may be irreversible, and when the original cause of infection has been treated, the lining may then not revert to normal.

88.2 Symptoms

Nasal obstruction, nasal congestion, anterior or posterior nasal discharge, facial pressure or pain and a reduction or loss of olfaction are the presenting symptoms.

Cacosmia (unpleasant smell) may occur in infections of dental origin when a dental root infection discharges into the maxillary sinus. This occurs when the maxillary bone capping the roots of the premolars and first molar is thin so that dental root infection can erode and break through the bone to discharge into the maxillary sinus. The patient is therefore usually free of facial pain because there is no pus being retained under pressure. If the bone capping the dental roots is thick, then the abscess will be contained within the maxilla

and the patient will develop localised maxillary swelling and severe pain.

88.3 Signs

Chronic irritation of the nasal airway and repeated rubbing of the nose may lead to vestibulitis and epistaxis. Chronic pharyngitis may occur and often lead to throat irritability and throat clearing. Throat clearing can cause secondary laryngeal irritability and signs of chronic laryngitis. If the patient has a chronic cough, it may be due to laryngeal irritability, but it may be due to a primary chest condition coexisting with chronic rhinosinusitis (CRS). Such chest conditions might include emphysema, bronchial hyper-reactivity, cough-variant asthma, allergic asthma and late-onset asthma. Coexisting chest symptoms are common because there is an association of CRS with chest conditions. To be clear, it is not that the chest condition is caused by CRS, or vice versa, but that the two conditions coexist with the same aetiological trigger. Clinical examination will show mucosal oedema and mucopurulent discharge primarily from the middle meatus, but no nasal polyps.

88.4 Differential Diagnosis

It is not uncommon to mistakenly ascribe chronic facial pain and headaches to sinus disease. Most facial pain is non-sinogenic. The definition of CRS becomes important in comparing studies on the disease, because different patient inclusion criteria may affect study results.

After a thorough history, examination and, if necessary, further investigations (including computed tomography [CT] and/or magnetic resonance imaging [MRI] scanning), patients with chronic facial pain broadly fall into one of three groups:

1. Patients with facial pain/headaches due to a primary sinogenic cause.
2. Those with facial pain/headaches due to a non-sinogenic cause.
3. Those where it is not certain whether the symptom is sinogenic or not. In this group, there may be no endoscopic signs of CRSsNP, for example, but a sinus CT shows frontal recess

opacity or infundibulum opacity with maxillary sinus mucosal thickening. In these cases, an assessment as to whether the CT findings match a patient's symptoms is made (e.g. left frontal headaches and CT shows left frontal recess opacity) to determine the way forward.

88.5 Radiology

A multi-slice CT scan of the sinuses on bone setting windows may be indicated if maximum medical treatment does not resolve symptoms and signs of CRSsNP. Extra fine cuts of 0.5 mm are indicated if frontal recess disease is suspected, otherwise 1-mm slices are usually sufficient. An MRI scan of the sinuses with gadolinium may be indicated to complement the CT and allow secretions to be differentiated from solid tissue if neoplasia is suspected (e.g. inverted papilloma and malignant disease).

88.6 Treatment

The principal aims of treatment are to correct the predisposing cause, to ventilate the sinus and to restore normal mucosal lining in the sinus.

88.6.1 Medical

Macrolide antibiotics have been clearly demonstrated to benefit patients with lower airway disease because of an antibacterial and an anti-inflammatory effect. The benefit for patients with CRSsNP is less clear. Two double-blind, placebo-controlled studies have provided contradictory results, but the dose of azithromycin in one of these studies may have been too low. Patients with normal levels of IgE seem to do better when treated with long-term (> 3 months) macrolide antibiotics (erythromycin, clarithromycin or azithromycin) compared to those with elevated levels of IgE. Saline nasal douching and nasal steroids will also improve symptom control and together with a long-term course of a macrolide antibiotic are recommended as a first-line treatment.

88.6.2 Surgical

a. Endoscopic sinus surgery
   Endoscopic sinus surgery (ESS) is indicated for those patients who have not adequately benefited from medical treatment. Occasionally,

surgery may be indicated as a first-line treatment for those with severe disease. EPOS 2012 recommended that symptoms are scored by a visual analogue scale (VAS) and those who score an average of less than 3 should have initial medical therapy. Those with a higher score may be considered for primary surgery according to the signs and CT findings. In the United Kingdom, most rhinologists still do not use a VAS to assess patients' symptoms and most would recommend a trial of maximum medical therapy initially before proceeding with further investigations and considering surgery. The extent of surgery depends on which sinuses are diseased. The progression of endoscopic sinus surgery means more extensive ESS procedures are now routinely performed, such as an endoscopic fronto-ethmoidectomy, to ensure all diseased sinus groups are opened and wide ventilation created. The increased availability of image guidance allows more extended applications of ESS surgery, such as Draf frontal sinus procedures.

b. Open sinus surgery procedures
   Open procedures are rare because in nearly all cases inflammatory disease can be accessed endoscopically. The main indication for open surgery now is for malignant disease. Even with malignancy, surgery is usually a combination of open and endoscopic surgery. Rhinologists not involved in managing malignancy will not perform sufficient number of cases to gain or maintain a reasonable expertise. Historical open operations on the sinuses may still be asked about in the examinations. They are listed below, but details of each procedure and its complications should be sought from an operative textbook.
   - Chronic maxillary sinusitis:
     Caldwell–Luc procedure (this is the one open operation that all rhinologists should be able to confidently perform).
   - Chronic ethmoid sinusitis: Intra-nasal ethmoidectomy. External ethmoidectomy (Patterson's operation).
     Transantral ethmoidectomy (Horgan's operation).
   - Chronic frontal sinusitis:
     External fronto-ethmoidectomy (Howarth's operation).
     Osteoplastic flap procedure (MacBeth's operation).

- Chronic sphenoiditis:
  Transantral ethmoidectomy or an external fronto-ethmoidectomy is performed to gain access to the face of the sphenoid.

Further Reading

Chong LY, Head K, Hopkins C, et al. Saline irrigation for chronic rhinosinusitis. Cochrane Database Syst Rev. 2016; 4:CD011995

Chong LY, Head K, Hopkins C, Philpott C, Schilder AG, Burton MJ. Intranasal steroids versus placebo or no intervention for chronic rhinosinusitis. Cochrane Database Syst Rev. 2016; 4:CD011996

Rosenfeld RM, Piccirillo JF, Chandrasekhar SS, et al. Clinical practice guideline (update): adult sinusitis. Otolaryngol Head Neck Surg. 2015; 152(2, Suppl):S1–S39

Related Topics of Interest

Rhinitis—allergic
Functional endoscopic sinus surgery
Rhinitis—non-allergic
Rhinosinusitis—chronic (with nasal polyps)
Rhinosinusitis—complications

R

89 Rhinosinusitis—Chronic (with Nasal Polyps)

Rhinosinusitis is defined differently in children and adults according to the most recent EPOS 2012 conference summary. Please see Chapter 87, Rhinosinusitis-Appropriate Terminology for the correct definitions and classification. Chronic rhinosinusitis (CRS) with nasal polyps is common and is caused by an inflammatory response to a trigger in predisposed individuals. In many instances, the trigger is not identified. Saline nasal douching, nasal and oral steroids and antibiotics are all used to control nasal polyps. Surgery is reserved for those with significant symptoms after maximum medical therapy and should be regarded as just one part of a package of ongoing care for such patients.

89.1 Chronic Rhinosinusitis

This is defined as rhinosinusitis symptoms that have been present for longer than 12 weeks. It is sub-divided into CRS with nasal polyps (CRSwNP) and CRS without nasal polyps (CRSsNP). CRS is common, with an overall worldwide prevalence of 11%, and with a geographic variation of 7 to 27%. There is a strong association of rhinitis and rhinosinusitis with asthma across all ages. This association is strongest in CRS and allergic rhinitis. CRS in the absence of nasal allergies is positively associated with late-onset asthma.

89.2 Chronic Rhinosinusitis with Nasal Polyps

In certain predisposed individuals, an inflammatory nasal condition (such as chronic infection, non-allergic rhinitis, a viral URTI or, in some cases, an unknown trigger) can lead to marked swelling of the sinus and nasal mucosa. This seems particularly to affect the mucosa in the region of the middle turbinate and middle meatus. Polyp formation results when this swelling becomes sufficiently pronounced. Anomalies in the synthesis of prostaglandin and related compounds, collectively known as eicosanoids (these function in diverse physiological and pathological systems including triggering or inhibiting inflammation, allergy and other immune responses) may play a role in polyp formation. In Samter's triad, for example it has been shown there is an overproduction of eicosanoids. There are a wide range of such compounds and so it may be that there are other prostaglandins over-produced in other inflammatory conditions, triggering polyp formation.

89.3 Pathology

Polyps demonstrate marked oedema of connective tissue stroma. The stroma contains a variety of inflammatory mediators such as histamine, prostaglandins and leukotrienes. There is a marked eosinophilic and histiocytic infiltrate and the epithelium displays goblet cell hyperplasia and, in some areas, squamous cell metaplasia. A polyp forms when the oedematous stroma ruptures and herniates through the basement membrane. Nasal polyps are rare in childhood, and if they occur one should suspect cystic fibrosis or immune deficiency.

89.4 Clinical Features

Nasal polyps may be asymptomatic and found incidentally but, even when they are small, patients may complain of a feeling of congestion or pressure high in the nose and may have hyponasal speech. As the polyps enlarge there is increased nasal obstruction and usually anterior or posterior rhinorrhoea. Airflow over the olfactory cleft and sphenoethmoidal recess is increasingly impeded causing hyposmia and often anosmia with concomitant hypoageusia. Headaches, pressure sensation in the face and secondary infective sinusitis may occur. In severe cases the polyps may be visible at the external nares and widening of the intercanthal distance may occur (telecanthus). The polyps are insensate. A history of epistaxis or contact bleeding should raise suspicion of neoplastic polyp. Clinical examination of the nose is not complete without an endoscopic examination (rigid or flexible) to visualize the polyps and any associated signs such as rhinitis, rhinorrhea, suppuration and deviated septum. Patients can then be appropriately categorized.

89.5 Investigations

There are few essential investigations. Skin tests or a radioallergosorbent test may identify a co-existent allergic rhinitis though most patients with nasal polyps are not allergic. Those to be treated by endoscopic sinus surgery (ESS) should have a multi-slice computed tomography (CT) scans of the sinuses when fine cuts (0.5 mm) in coronal, axial and sagittal planes should be available. Such scans provide an indication of disease extent, a map of the paranasal sinuses and may identify anatomical variations associated with an increased risk of ESS complications. It may also show signs suggesting fungal infection (fungal ball—single sinus involvement, hyperintense calcified deposits within a hypodense mass; allergic fungal sinusitis—opaque sinuses with central hyperdense opacification; chronic invasive sinusitis—mottled hyperintense lucency, irregular bone destruction, bone sclerosis and extra-sinus extension localized to the area of bone erosion). Remember a CT scan will not distinguish between retained mucous, mucopus or polyps. Following surgical removal, the polyps should always be sent for histological analysis, especially unilateral polyps or unusual looking polyps. Microbiology for both bacteria and fungi may also be indicated depending on the nature of the secretions.

89.6 Management

89.6.1 Medical

The EPOS 2012 conference summary recommended patients be categorized into mild, moderate or severe disease according to the severity of symptoms and signs. A visual analogue score (VAS) for symptoms is suggested with 0 to 3 being mild; 4 to 7 being moderate and 8 to 10 being severe. Routine UK practice, presently, does not involve using a VAS. There is no formal grading system for clinical signs but a reasonable approach may be to grade polyps as mild if they are limited to the middle meatus, moderate if polyps extend below the middle turbinate but not to the nasal floor and severe if polyps extend to the floor. Interestingly, despite the recommended grading, the initial treatment and escalation of treatment are similar. Probably the main point of categorization is to record patient response to a treatment. For all grades of polyps, a low bioavailability nasal steroid spray and a saline nasal wash are recommended. Saline irrigation will help to thin and wash away the inspissated mucous that CRSwNP patients produce, allowing nasal steroids to then coat nasal polyps more reliably. Steroid drops, an increased dose of nasal steroid spray or a short course of oral steroids, are

suggested for poor responders. A long (at least 12 weeks) course of doxycycline may reduce polyp size and sensation of blockage as well as reducing post nasal drip (level 3 evidence), particularly when immunoglobulin E is not elevated. It is possible other antibiotics such as azithromycin may have the same effect. For patients who continue to have poor symptom control, a CT scan of the sinuses and surgical removal are recommended. Post-operatively long-term saline nasal irrigation is recommended and nasal steroids as required.

89.6.2 Surgical

Good symptom control can be obtained with an endoscopic polypectomy under either local or general anaesthetic. A more radical clearance by means of an endoscopic fronto-ethmoidectomy leads to better longer-term disease control probably because there are fewer contact areas remaining and topical treatments can work more effectively. Surgery is best performed with a combination of powered micro-debriders and through-cutting instruments to avoid mucosal stripping. Computer-aided navigation systems for ESS may increase safety in difficult regions, such as the frontal recess, but surgical expertise and sensible decision making is paramount. Initially, in North America, these systems did not reduce complications because they gave relatively inexperienced surgeons confidence to attempt more radical surgery.

89.7 Follow-Up and Aftercare

Long-term saline nasal douching is recommended. This treatment alone reduces rhinitis activity, probably by washing away the sticky mucous that CRSwNP patients produce. Intranasal steroids reduce recurrence in the first year and may make a difference to the recurrence rate long term. In aggressive CRSwNP, regular follow-up to catch and treat recurrent polyps is a reasonable strategy. Such patients may require an increased frequency of saline douching, long-term nasal steroid drops and occasional courses of oral steroids to maintain disease control following surgery.

89.8 Antro-Choanal Polyp

An antro-choanal polyp is uncommon. Maxillary sinus mucous cysts however are common incidental CT findings that cause no symptoms. Occasionally, such cysts will expand to fill the sinus and then mushroom out of the sinus through the natural ostium or an accessory fontanelle to form a polyp within the middle meatus which then extends backwards, sometimes through the choana (note choana means posterior opening so calling the choana the posterior choana is incorrect). Therefore, the maxillary component of these polyps is often cystic and the nasal portion solid and similar to a simple nasal polyp.

The patient, commonly a young adult, presents with unilateral nasal obstruction, which may be worse on expiration owing to the ball valve-like effect of the polyp in the choana. If sufficiently large, it may produce bilateral obstruction and cause otological symptoms because of blockage of the Eustachian tube orifice. Anterior rhinoscopy may look normal as only a thin stalk extending posteriorly may be present in the middle meatus nose. Endoscopic examination reveals the polyp.

A CT scan is the best investigation, providing a map of the maxillary and anterior ethmoid sinuses.

Treatment is by ESS. After removal of the solid nasal portion of the polyp, an uncinectomy and middle meatal antrostomy (if the polyp has not already dilated the natural ostium) are performed to improve access to the maxillary sinus. The polyp stalk is then grasped and with a very gentle rocking movement, sometimes over the course of several minutes, the attachments of the antral portion of the polyp are released and the antral portion removed. Failure to completely remove the antral component may result in a recurrence of the polyp. Repeated recurrences may mean a Caldwell–Luc procedure is required.

Further Reading

Lind H, Joergensen G, Lange B, Svendstrup F, Kjeldsen AD. Efficacy of ESS in chronic rhinosinusitis with and without nasal polyposis: a Danish cohort study. Eur Arch Otorhinolaryngol. 2016; 273(4):911–919

Andrews PJ, Poirrier AL, Lund VJ, Choi D. Outcomes in endoscopic sinus surgery: olfaction, nose scale and quality of life in a prospective cohort study. Clin Otolaryngol. 2016; 41(6):798–803

Related Topics of Interest

Rhinosinusitis—acute
Rhinosinusitis—chronic without nasal polyps
Functional endoscopic sinus surgery
Rhinitis—non-allergic

90 Rhinosinusitis—Complications

In rhinosinusitis, spread of infection beyond the walls of the sinus is uncommon, but complications can be life changing and life threatening. Complications are most commonly caused by acute rhinosinusitis but may also be seen with an acute exacerbation of chronic rhinosinusitis.

90.1 Classification

- Periorbital and orbital complications.
- Osteomyelitis (maxilla or frontal bone).
- Intracranial complications (meningitis, intracranial abscess and cavernous sinus thrombosis).
- Mucocele.
- Locoregional complications (pharyngitis, laryngitis and otitis media).

90.2 Periorbital and Orbital Complications

These can occur at any age, but are more common in children, particularly under the age of 6 years. There is usually a history of a viral upper respiratory tract infection (URTI) preceding a periorbital/orbital complication. A secondary suppurative acute rhinosinusitis occurs, which then rapidly involves the orbit and periorbital tissues. In adults, there may be pre-existing chronic rhinosinusitis. The usual bacteria causing such a complication are therefore the bacteria that cause acute and chronic rhinosinusitis without polyps (CRSsNP), particularly *Streptococcus pneumoniae* and *Haemophilus influenzae*.

Periorbital cellulitis and orbital abscess may occur from direct spread of suppurative organisms from the ethmoid sinuses, particularly in children. It can also spread from thrombophlebitis of mucosal vessels in the ethmoid and rarely the frontal sinuses. In teenagers and adults, it is occasionally secondary to frontal sinusitis. In children, areas of lamina papyracea are variably deficient and here, only a thin fibrous layer fills the deficiency to separate the orbit from the ethmoid sinuses. By early teens, the lamina papyracea is fully developed, and there is then a complete bony barrier between the ethmoid sinuses and orbit.

Complications are still classified according to Chandler et al. This classification provides a reminder of the usual order of disease progression as well as providing a treatment plan. The orbital septum forms a natural barrier. This is a fibrous framework of the eyelids which is thickened towards the lid margin to form the tarsal plates. Infection may localise in front of the septum as a pre-septal (or periorbital) cellulitis or posterior to the septum as orbital or intracranial infection.

90.2.1 Chandler's Classification of Orbital Complications of Sinusitis

Stage 1 Pre-septal or periorbital cellulitis. There is lid oedema, which can be marked and usually lid erythema. There is no proptosis, usually no conjunctival chemosis, normal and painless eye movements and normal colour vision. The C-reactive protein (CRP) is raised, but often not markedly in the first 24 hours, and there is usually only a low-grade pyrexia (< 38°C) in the early stages. An urticarial reaction can mimic pre-septal cellulitis. In this situation, there may be conjunctival chemosis, but there is no pyrexia, the white cell count (WCC) is normal and the CRP is normal.

Stage 2 Post-septal or orbital cellulitis. There is orbital inflammation but no abscess formation. The eye is proptosed, conjunctival chemosis is usually present, and there is pain with ocular movements. Colour vision is usually normal. There is usually no diplopia. The WCC is raised and there is a neutrophil leukocytosis. The CRP is significantly raised. It may only be possible to distinguish stage 2 from stage 3 by performing a sinus and orbit computed tomography (CT) scan with gadolinium.

Stage 3 Sub-periosteal abscess. Symptoms and signs may be similar to stage 2, but there is more marked proptosis, greater pain on ocular movement, and there may be diplopia and a progressive deterioration of colour vision, particularly red and green.

Stage 4 Orbital abscess. Severe and often rapidly progressive proptosis, ophthalmoplegia, chemosis and diplopia. Vision may be rapidly lost.

Stage 5 Intracranial involvement, particularly cavernous sinus thrombosis. Cavernous sinus thrombosis may follow an initial stage 1 to 4 orbital complication or facial cellulitis. It may initially affect just one side before usually becoming bilateral. It occurs due to thrombophlebitis of the superior ophthalmic vein which passes from the posterior orbit through the superior orbital fissure to the anterior end of the cavernous sinus. There is severe proptosis, meningism (severe headache and photophobia), a swinging pyrexia, ophthalmoplegia due to the involvement of cranial nerves (CNs) III, IV, V1 and V2 and papilloedema.

90.2.2 Management

Immediate liaison with an ophthalmologist is recommended due to the risk of blindness. This occurs because of raised intra-orbital pressure causing ischaemia and septic necrosis of the optic nerve. Visual acuity, red–green colour vision, visual fields, pupillary reflexes, and the optic disc should be examined at least once a day for stage 1 and at least twice daily for other stages. Red–green colour blindness is an early sign of the optic nerve's function being impaired. Absence of the ipsilateral (optic nerve impairment) and contralateral (oculomotor nerve impairment) light reflex will occur with visual impairment. In the latter, the contralateral eye is stimulated with light and the affected eye is observed for a reduction or a loss of pupillary constriction compared to the stimulated eye.

All patients who are graded Chandler's stage 2 or greater either at presentation or after disease progression, should have a contrast-enhanced, high-resolution CT scan of the sinuses and orbits. Therefore, significant proptosis, pain on ocular movement, reduced ocular movement, ophthalmoplegia and colour vision impairment are all symptoms that immediately warrant a CT scan to determine if there is a sub-periosteal or an orbital abscess.

If the CT shows stage 3 or 4 disease, then drainage of the intra-orbital collection is recommended as an emergency. For stage 3 disease, and particularly if the abscess is greater than 4 mm at its largest width, the abscess should be drained. Some surgeons feel an abscess less than 4 mm in a patient without visual symptoms and signs can be managed with intravenous antibiotic and frequent reassessment.

For drainage, an external approach using the lower half of a Lynch–Howarth incision is recommended. Elevation of the orbital periosteum allows one to reach sub-periosteal pus under pressure. An external ethmoidectomy is performed which allows continuous drainage of the abscess cavity from the orbit through the ethmoid sinus and middle meatus into the nasal cavity. Even for a rhinologist, who is an expert endoscopic sinus surgeon, an endoscopic approach to find and drain the abscess is very difficult, not only because of middle meatal oedema and friable mucosa, but because the lamina at the site of an abscess is usually more posterior and superior than the surgeon thinks. Also, the orbital periosteum anterior to the abscess is inflamed and more adherent to the lamina than usual. If the lamina here is removed in error, the orbital periosteum may easily tear exposing orbital fat and increasing the chances of infection spreading to the orbital contents. Coexisting maxillary sinusitis may require an endoscopic middle meatal antrostomy. For stage 4 disease, the expertise of an ophthalmologist is required.

90.3 Osteomyelitis

This only occurs in diploic bone and thus only in the maxilla of children and the frontal sinus of adolescents and adults. The common organism is *Staphylococcus aureus*.

Osteomyelitis of the maxilla is rare and usually only seen in third world countries. It presents as a painful swelling of the cheek and lower eyelid. Treatment comprises intravenous antibiotics and debridement when necessary.

Osteomyelitis of the frontal bone is also rare, but it may be extensive and dangerous. There is a buildup of dull local pain with oedema of the forehead and the upper eyelids. This is potentially a life-threatening condition because usually the inner table of the frontal sinus lining the meninges is thinner than the outer wall and if there is necrosis of the inner table or there is thrombophlebitis spread, there is a risk of intracranial complications, particularly an extradural or a frontal lobe abscess. Thrombophlebitis of the frontal sinus may spread to involve the superior sagittal sinus, a life-threatening complication. A contrast-enhanced, high-resolution CT scan/venogram or a magnetic resonance imaging (MRI)/magnetic resonance angiography (MRA)/magnetic resonance venography (MRV) will illustrate the extent of the problem. A sub-periosteal abscess of the forehead may form (Pott's puffy tumour) if the thicker outer table of the frontal sinus necroses. Prompt treatment with high-dose intravenous antibiotics, surgical drainage of the frontal sinus and debridement may be necessary.

90.4 Intracranial Complications

The cavities of the frontal, ethmoidal and sphenoid sinuses are closely related to and separated by a thin wall of bone from the anterior cranial fossa.

Infection may involve the brain and meninges from either direct spread or retrograde thrombophlebitis. Meningitis is the commonest complication, but encephalitis, intracranial abscess (extradural, subdural or intracerebral) and venous sinus thrombosis may complicate sinus infections. The clinical features of meningitis are well known. A lumbar puncture may identify the causative organism, but it is essential to exclude raised intracranial pressure before this is done by examining for papilloedema.

Venous sinus thrombosis from thrombophlebitis is life threatening. Cavernous sinus thrombosis will cause a high spiking fever, and a reduced and varying conscious level from cerebritis, cerebral infarction and cerebral oedema. The eyes will proptose and an ophthalmoplegia of the cranial nerves which travel in the cavernous sinus will occur (III, IV, VI and ophthalmic and maxillary branches of V). The central retinal vein drains into the superior ophthalmic vein and then into the cavernous sinus. The facial vein drains into the inferior ophthalmic vein which also drains into the cavernous sinus. Efferent veins of the cavernous sinus on each side are the inferior petrosal sinus, which passes through the jugular foramen to enter the internal jugular vein just below the skull base and the superior petrosal sinus, which passes to the sigmoid sinus. Therefore, retrograde spread of thrombophlebitis from the cavernous sinus may spread to the lateral sinus (the collective term for transverse and sigmoid sinuses) and the internal jugular vein.

The ear, nose and throat (ENT) surgeon should maintain a high index of suspicion of an intracranial complication in sinusitis patients who become drowsy or show neurological symptoms or signs. A CT or preferably an MRI scan with enhancement may assist in diagnosis. Intracranial complications should all be treated with high-dose intravenous antibiotics. An extradural or subdural abscess will require drainage by a neurosurgeon, together with drainage of the offending sinuses by an ENT surgeon. The mortality and morbidity after intracranial complications is considerable. Up to 25% of patients may die and nearly a third of surviving patients will suffer with epilepsy.

90.5 Mucocele

A mucocele may develop when the outlet from a sinus becomes permanently blocked. It occurs most commonly in the frontal sinus, but also in the ethmoid, maxillary and sphenoid sinuses. There is an accumulation of sterile mucus which becomes increasingly viscous. The mucocele exerts pressure on the sinus walls causing bone erosion and therefore bone thinning. The continued high intra-mucocele pressure allows the thin bone to expand. This leads to displacement of adjacent structures, especially the orbit when diplopia and proptosis may result. The main complaints are headache and swelling. These features can be dramatic if infection supervenes (pyocele). A high-resolution CT scan of the sinuses and orbit will define disease extent.

Treatment is surgical drainage and marsupialisation of the sinus, usually endoscopically. An external fronto-ethmoidectomy (Howarth's operation) and the osteoplastic flap procedure (Macbeth's operation) for an occluded frontal sinus are now much less common with the advent of image guidance. Image guidance allows a Draf II a/b or even Draf III to be safely performed to create wide frontal drainage.

90.6 Locoregional Complications

Regional complications occur because of infection and inflammation spreading through the rest of the upper aerodigestive tract mucosa. Mucopus from sinusitis is carried back through the nasal airway into the pharynx and may cause a pharyngitis. Invasion of the sub-epithelial lymphoid tissue will produce a granular pharyngitis and visible lymphoid nodules due to lymphoid hyperplasia. Further downward spread may lead to irritation of the vocal cords causing a laryngitis. Sinusitis is also implicated as a cause and complication of tonsillitis and otitis media.

Further Reading

Carr TF. Complications of sinusitis. Am J Rhinol Allergy. 2016; 30(4):241–245

Chandler JR, Langenbrunner DJ, Stevens ER. The pathogenesis of orbital complications in acute sinusitis. Laryngoscope. 1970; 80(9):1414–1428

Hakim HE, Malik AC, Aronyk K, Ledi E, Bhargava R. The prevalence of intracranial complications in pediatric frontal sinusitis. Int J Pediatr Otorhinolaryngol. 2006; 70(8):1383–1387

Related Topics of Interest

Rhinosinusitis—acute
Rhinosinusitis—chronic without nasal polyps
Rhinosinusitis—chronic (with nasal polyps)
Functional endoscopic sinus surgery

91 Rhinosinusitis—Fungal

Fungal sinusitis is now being recognised more frequently because of advances in diagnostic techniques (nasendoscopy, computed tomography [CT] and magnetic resonance imaging [MRI] sinus scanning) and the awareness of different subtypes of the disease in both immunocompetent and immunocompromised patients. Awareness of the entity of acute invasive fungal sinusitis when managing immunocompromised patients may allow an early diagnosis and can be lifesaving.

Steroids, antifungals, antibiotics (for secondary bacterial infection) and saline nasal douching are the mainstay of medical treatment. Endoscopic sinus surgery is indicated for mycetoma and to debride and ventilate sinuses, when indicated, in other subtypes of fungal sinusitis.

91.1 Classification

Fungal sinusitis may be divided into invasive, non-invasive and granulomatous groups. The non-invasive and granulomatous groups are immunocompetent (have normal immunity), but the invasive groups are immunocompromised.

91.1.1 Non-Invasive Fungal Sinusitis

Mycetoma

These are masses of fungal debris that usually occur in the maxillary or sphenoid sinuses.

Patients are usually immunocompetent and non-atopic. *Aspergillus fumigatus* is the most common organism isolated. Treatment is by endoscopic removal of the debris and ventilation of the sinus. There is usually no requirement for antifungal or any other systemic therapy.

Allergic Fungal Sinusitis

This is an eosinophilic form of recurrent chronic allergic hypertrophic rhinosinusitis that is clinically, histopathologically and prognostically distinct from other forms of rhinosinusitis. It occurs in atopic immunocompetent adults and is usually associated with nasal polyps and asthma. The commonest organisms are those from the dematiaceous family which include *Alternaria*,

Bipolaris, and *Curvularia*s Patients have a type 1 hypersensitivity reaction that often presents after a seemingly innocent upper respiratory tract infection (URTI). Patients usually have a positive *Bipolaris* skin test result and high serum levels of allergen-specific immunoglobulin E (IgE). Acute-onset nasal obstruction and rhinorrhea are the main symptoms. Nasendoscopy reveals inspissated mucous, impressive mucosal oedema and middle meatal polyps. Endoscopic sinus surgery to clear the sinuses of polyps, ventilate the sinuses and remove collected mucous is indicated with a post-operative course of oral steroids, itraconazole and life-long saline nasal douching. Recurrences are common and are treated with steroids and itraconazole. A prolonged course of itraconazole does not seem to reduce recurrences. There may be a role for immunotherapy in the future for this condition, but it is not yet available. Working with an allergist may be helpful to optimise patient symptom control.

91.1.2 Invasive Fungal Rhinosinusitis

Acute Invasive Fungal Sinusitis

This is a rare, highly aggressive and life-threatening form of fungal sinusitis affecting severely immunocompromised patients. These include patients with leukaemia, aplastic anaemia, uncontrolled insulin-dependent diabetes, those having chemotherapy or who are immunosuppressed due to transplantation. *Aspergillus*, *Mucor*, and *Rhizopus* are the commonest causative organisms. The fungus rapidly spreads through sinus mucosa and bone to involve the brain and eye. Sinoscopy shows ulcerated and black necrotic issue. Microscopically, blood vessels are invaded by fungus, causing ischaemia and gangrene. Treatment is a combination of aggressive surgical debridement, high doses of antifungal medication and adequate hydration. Mortality is high.

Chronic Invasive Sinusitis

This is also called chronic indolent sinusitis. Over several months, it produces a slowly progressive, destructive sinusitis which rarely invades blood vessels and causes minimal inflammatory reaction. It occurs in mildly immunosuppressed patients such as those with diabetes, AIDS patients on treatment, those on long-term corticosteroids or immunosuppressives such as methotrexate for conditions such as severe rheumatoid arthritis. It may erode the bony sinus wall allowing the sinus to expand. It most commonly affects the ethmoid and sphenoid sinuses and therefore expansion of these sinuses can cause involvement of the eye and hypertelorism. *Aspergillus fumigatus* is the most commonly found fungus on culture. Treatment is to widely ventilate the affected sinuses and suction/excise all debris and inspissated mucous. Antifungal treatment is then instituted, ideally itraconazole for 4 to 6 months, and, if possible, measures taken to improve the patient's immunity.

Granulomatous Invasive Fungal Sinusitis

This is rare in the West and North America and is usually seen in patients from India, Pakistan, Saudi Arabia, UAE and Sudan in immunocompetent patients. Over the course of typically 2 to 4 months, patients present with an enlarging mass in the nose, sinuses, orbit or cheek. Treatment is by surgical debridement of the mass, removal of all debris from the sinuses and wide ventilation of the affected sinuses. All removed tissue and secretions are sent for histopathology and microbiology. This shows granulomas and usually *Aspergillus flavus* is cultured. Itraconazole, the drug of choice, should be given post-operatively for 4 to 6 months and saline nasal douching performed two or three times daily long term.

Further Reading

Middlebrooks EH, Frost CJ, De Jesus RO, Massini TC, Schmalfuss IM, Mancuso AA. Acute invasive fungal rhinosinusitis: a comprehensive update of CT findings and design of an effective diagnostic imaging model. AJNR Am J Neuroradiol. 2015; 36(8):1529–1535

Payne SJ, Mitzner R, Kunchala S, Roland L, McGinn JD. Acute invasive fungal rhinosinusitis: a 15-year experience with 41 patients. Otolaryngol Head Neck Surg. 2016; 154(4):759–764

Related Topics of Interest

Rhinitis—allergic
Rhinitis—non-allergic
Functional endoscopic sinus surgery
Rhinosinusitis—complications

R

92 Robots in ENT/Head and Neck Surgery

92.1 Introduction

Transoral robotic surgery (TORS) was initially conceived for oropharyngeal cancer. The traditional treatment for this primary site, until the turn of the millennium, had been open surgery. The emergence of transoral laser microsurgery (TLM) offered the prospect of a surgical procedure with less morbidity. Publication of several reports of good oncological control with TLM combined with low morbidity led to interest in primary surgery for this site being rejuvenated. While TLM has shown undoubted oncological efficacy in this setting, most of work on TLM primarily pertained to tumours of the tonsil. Because of difficulties with resecting cancers of the tongue base via an endoscope, a microscope and coaxially mounted laser, the tongue base continued to be an orphan site with very few reports presenting data on TLM outcomes for this sub-site. Even for tonsil cancers, surgeons and multi-disciplinary teams were slow to adopt TLM for several reasons. The technique is difficult to teach which resulted in a shallow learning curve. TLM involves cutting through the tumour to identify its depth, with further sampling of the defect to confirm clear margins; thus, pathological margin assessment of the transected specimen was beset with controversies and frequently resulted in patients receiving double or triple modality treatment.

The manoeuvrability and optics of robotic systems, the prospect of en bloc resection and rapid adoption of robotic technology at other primary sites were attractive to head and neck surgeons. TORS offered the optimal balance of transoral access with limited morbidity, en bloc resection and a more rapid learning curve.

This chapter will address the rationale and evidence base supporting TORS for primary and recurrent cancers of the head and neck, and the emerging role of TORS in the investigation of the unknown primary tumour. This chapter will also briefly discuss the trials that are ongoing currently in this field.

92.2 Rationale for Incorporating TORS into the Treatment of Oropharyngeal Malignancies

92.2.1 HPV-Related Squamous Cell Cancers

The rising incidence of human papillomavirus (HPV)-related squamous cell carcinoma (SCC) at this primary site has been a key driving force in transoral surgery for oropharyngeal cancer. Affecting a relatively younger patient group, HPV-related SCC responds well to treatment; thus, survivorship issues become important. It is well recognised that radical doses of chemoradiotherapy (CRT) used to treat head and neck cancer (with the aim of organ preservation) cause significant morbidity for patients in the short and long term. In patients receiving CRT, top complaints at various time points are consistently xerostomia and dysphagia, both seen after CRT. In a meta-analysis of 230 patients included in three large trials (RTOG 91–11, RTOG 97–03 and RTOG 99–14), 43% of patients were found to still be experiencing grade 3 or higher toxicity in the long term. Prospective observational studies suggest that both the above side effects can be reduced or avoided with a primary TORS approach. In a systematic review involving 20 case series, including eight intensity-modulated radiotherapy (IMRT) studies (1,287 patients) and 12 TORS studies (772 patients), while the oncological outcomes were comparable, the adverse events profile was different: oesophageal stenosis (4.8%) and osteoradionecrosis (2.6%) for IMRT, haemorrhage (2.4%) and fistula (2.5%) for TORS. Incorporation of TORS into the treatment strategy allows clinicians to tailor adjuvant therapy in patients who would otherwise receive standard CRT.

92.2.2 Non–HPV-Related Squamous Cell Cancers

These cancers typically have a worse prognosis than HPV-positive SCC. All available level 1 evidence for this group of patients supports non-surgical treatment. The French 94–01 phase III multi-centre randomised trial recruited 226 patients, comparing radiotherapy alone with radiotherapy and concomitant chemotherapy. Although explicit HPV testing was not done, the patient cohort with large primary sites and small nodal disease is indicative of HPV-negative tumours. They posted 5-year overall survival (22.4 vs. 15.8% [$p = 0.05$]) and locoregional control (47.6 vs. 24.7% [$p = 0.002$]) favouring the latter arm. Several prospective datasets where HPV-negative cancers have been treated by TORS and adjuvant radiation indicate high control rates, from 80 to 94%. However, selection bias in these studies is inevitable. As discussed above, the morbidity and mortality rates attributed to open surgery do not apply to surgical practices in the current day, and especially to transoral surgery; data on 30-day mortality from the U.K. national head and neck database indicate a mortality of less than 1%. For these reasons, more multi-disciplinary teams (MDTs) are in favour of incorporating a transoral resection for these tumours where feasible.

92.3 Non-Squamous Cancers

Minor salivary gland tumours are the most common non-squamous cancers seen in this anatomical site. The primary management is surgery. Following careful assessment, if access is found to be optimal, as is often the case with these tumours, transoral resection with or without adjuvant radiation offers equivalent control rates with less disruption of anatomy, and thus quicker recovery.

92.4 Robotic Technology

Although several robotic systems are currently available, the most commonly used system is the da Vinci, marketed by Intuitive, and will be described in this chapter. TORS represents a stepwise evolution in transoral surgery, the foundations for which have been laid by TLM. However, unlike TLM, tumours need not be in the 'line of sight' of the surgeon, a desirable attribute when resecting tumours of the base of tongue, supraglottis or hypopharynx. The hardware in the da Vinci system allows telescopes to achieve excellent three-dimensional visualisation of patient and tumour anatomy, and operating instruments to be controlled remotely within this visual field with excellent manoeuvrability. Robotic surgery with the Intuitive system is performed via a patient side cart comprising of the telescope and two (of the three available) robotic arms mounted on a mobile platform, which are docked into the patient's mouth. The operator remotely controls these three instruments from a surgeon console across the operating room (▶ Fig. 92.1); the robot eliminates tremor and allows hand movements in 7 degrees of freedom which would be impossible with the human wrist.

92.5 Theatre Setup for TORS

An examination under anaesthetic is performed at a separate sitting to assess the size, extent and resectability of the primary tumour. For the robotic resection, patients are positioned supine and mouth opening is maintained with an appropriate retractor, the choice depending on the site of tumour. Two commonly used retractors include the Boyle Davis or Feyh–Kastenbauer retractor; the latter has been extensively modified to incorporate a range of concave tongue blades that increase the intra-oral space and it possesses a larger frame that allows easier intra-oral docking of the robotic arms with less instrument clashes. The patients' face and eyes are appropriately protected to avoid accidental injury. The operating telescope is inserted into the patients' mouth and two instruments (at least one of which is an energy device to cut tissues and the other a grasper to retract tissues) are positioned either side of this (▶ Fig. 92.2).

An assistant at the head of the patient helps with smoke evacuation, suction, application of ligatures and retraction. This allows four independently controlled instruments to be used simultaneously in the intra-oral environment, providing unparalleled manoeuvrability.

92.6 TORS for Oropharynx and Supraglottic Cancers

Tonsil cancer The principle of TORS surgery is en bloc resection with a clear margin. The foundations for en bloc resection of tonsil cancers via a transoral route had been laid back in the 1950s when

R

R

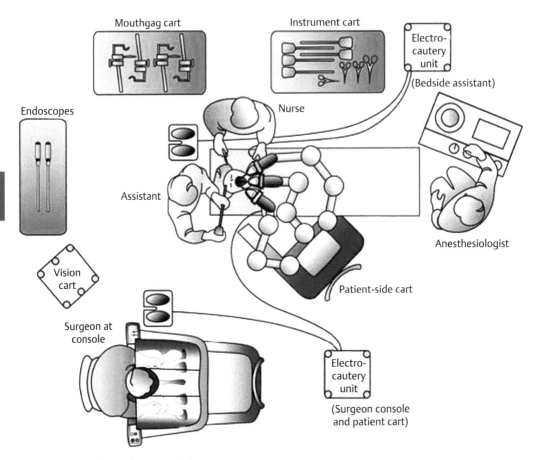

Fig. 92.1 Theatre layout for transoral robotic surgery.

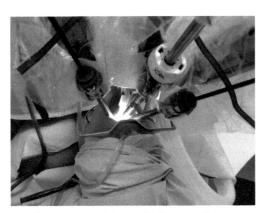

Fig. 92.2 Close-up picture of the three robotic arms docked in the mouth. The middle arm is the telescope, with the other two arms being a choice of instruments based on the operator's preference.

P. C. Huet described this procedure. This involved transoral resection of the tonsil and the superior constrictor muscle deep to the parapharyngeal space. TORS radical tonsillectomy is one of the first procedures that is undertaken by surgeons in the early stages of their TORS practice. The first report of TORS radical tonsillectomy was published in 2007 in a cohort of 27 adult patients with tonsil tumours staged T1 to T3, with a negative margin of 93%, 0% mortality and an acceptable complication rate of 4% gastrostomy-dependent at 6 months. A global multi-institutional study that collated outcomes for 410 patients from 11 centres demonstrated 2-year locoregional control rates of 91.8% and disease-free survival of 91%. TORS is currently used and approved by the Food and Drug Administration (FDA) for T1 and T2 cancers in the United States.

The aim of resecting tonsil tumours with TORS is to ensure compartmental resection of the tonsil, the constrictor bed it sits on along with a cuff of soft palate and the tongue base to ensure histologically negative margins. A detailed description is outside the scope of this work, but in brief, the steps are incision through the pterygomandibular raphe to identify the parapharyngeal space with the help of the medial pterygoid tendon, separating the constrictor muscles from the parapharyngeal fat, mobilising the superior pole of the tonsil with an adequate cuff of tissue from the soft palate, progressive dissection in the parapharyngeal space to free the stylopharyngeus and pharyngeal constrictors down to the pre-vertebral fascia, resecting a cuff of tongue base between the anterior and posterior tonsillar pillars to ensure a good inferior margin, resecting at least a centimetre segment of styloglossus to ensure histologically negative margin and progressive transection of the constrictor muscle along with the stylopharyngeal musculature to achieve an en bloc resection. Post-operatively, the tonsil defect is left to heal on its own and complete mucosalisation normally takes place within 6 weeks, however, patients commence oral feeds before that and usually are free of nasogastric feeds within days.

Tongue base cancers TORS is used for T1 and T2 tongue base cancers, but given the relative rarity of these tumours, the bulk of published data includes this site along with tonsil tumours. The principles of the operation are similar to tonsil tumours where an en bloc resection is performed. Careful assessment of the scans will need to be performed to assess the location and lateralisation of the tumour. Tumours crossing the midline are not good candidates for TORS. The operation commences with an incision along the posterior one-third of the tongue. This is deepened followed by a midline cut towards the vallecula. The vallecula identifies the depth of the resection needed and lateral margin is established.

Supraglottic cancers TORS is an excellent tool for supraglottic laryngectomy and allows en bloc resection with good clearance of the pre-epiglottic space in early-stage (T1 and T2) cancers.

92.7 Management of the Neck

In the setting of squamous cancers of the above sites, the neck nodes will invariably require attention. There remains some debate as to whether the tonsil and neck dissection should be performed at the same time or be staged. There are advantages and disadvantages to both approaches. Performing the tonsil resection and neck dissection at the same time allows for a single operative procedure, but with a small risk of creating a fistula into the neck. A staged operation, where the neck dissection is performed first reduces the risk of a fistula into the neck, and allows for full use of the allocated robotic time that is available for surgical teams on specified days. This approach does necessitate that the two procedures are separated by days. The risk of a fistula into the neck is also influenced by the levels of the neck that are dissected. No consensus exists, but many surgical teams will perform a level II to IV neck dissection for N1 and N2a necks, while others dissect level I to IV. It is generally agreed that at the time of the neck dissection, individual branches of the external carotid artery (lingual, facial and ascending pharyngeal) are identified and individually ligated to reduce the risk of post-operative haemorrhage after transoral surgery.

92.8 Post-Operative Adjuvant Treatment

It is essential and mandatory that prior to setting up a transoral robotic surgical practice, institutional agreement and protocols should be in place for surgical and radiation oncology treatment for these patients. It is especially relevant in the setting of HPV-positive oropharyngeal cancer, where significant controversy exists about the role of the surgery given the high oncological efficacy of radiation therapy or chemoradiation therapy. It is strongly recommended that where ongoing trials are available, patients be recruited into these trials.

Adjuvant radiation is based on the results of pathological examination, patient factors and institutional practice. In general, adjuvant radiation is delivered in the presence of positive margins and adverse features in the primary cancer or the neck dissection specimen. However, several prospective datasets have questioned the value of concurrent chemoradiation therapy in the adjuvant setting for HPV-positive tumours and deintensification regimes are being tested in ongoing trials.

R

92.9 Transoral Robotic Surgery for the Unknown Primary

It is entirely conceivable that HPV-positive micro-cancers originate from the palatine and lingual tonsils. Random biopsies will have a low probability of primary site detection given the large area of the tongue base. Tongue base mucosectomy involves removal of full thickness of the tongue base mucosa up to the muscle layer, from the level of the circumvallate papillae to the vallecula, in patients who have had full radiological work-up and no primary is evident. It can be combined with tonsillectomy, at the same time or performed when the tonsils have been removed and shown no tumour. This technique can identify the primary site in over 50% of patients who have no radiological evidence of a primary site.

92.10 Recurrent Cancer

The standard of care for recurrent oropharyngeal cancers is open resection. In selected cases, TORS has shown good oncological outcomes for this patient group, very comparable to open resections. However, significant expertise with TORS is needed prior to embarking on these procedures. Free flap reconstruction is not needed in most cases as the defect will heal by secondary intention. In cases where the resection is through into the neck or where the tissue is felt to be unhealthy, TORS-assisted free flap inset is needed and can be performed.

92.11 Rehabilitation

Patients planned for robotic resections, especially with recurrent cancer, will need pre-surgical speech and swallow assessment, and a multidisciplinary approach is mandatory for these patients. Appropriate feeding routes are decided based on this assessment. Post-operative swallowing rehabilitation can then be provided according to the individual patient's needs.

92.12 Other Uses of Robots in ENT/Head and Neck Surgery

Robotics has been used to deal with benign tumours of the parapharyngeal and retropharyngeal spaces. Several reports confirm the applicability and benefit of robotics in surgery for obstructive sleep apnoea and skull base surgery via the transoral route. Although this chapter has focused on transoral robotic surgery, significant progress has been made in applying robotic technology for minimal access thyroid surgery, neck dissection and cochlear implantation. With the emergence of more robotic systems at reduced costs, and given the significant advantages of the robotic interface, robotic surgery is here to stay. The ENT surgeon of the future will see robotic surgery integrated into clinical care in several spheres of practice.

Further Reading

Chang EHE, Kim HY, Koh YW, Chung WY. Overview of robotic thyroidectomy. Gland Surg. 2017; 6(3):218–228

Gil Z, Amit M, Kupferman ME, eds. Atlas of Head and Neck Robotic Surgery. Switzerland: Springer International Publishing; 2017

Hachem RA, Rangarajan S, Beer-Furlan A, Prevedello D, Ozer E, Carrau RL. The role of robotic surgery in sinonasal and ventral skull base malignancy. Otolaryngol Clin North Am. 2017; 50(2):385–395

Hamilton D, Paleri V. Role of transoral robotic surgery in current head & neck practice. Surgeon. 2017; 15(3):147–154

Toh ST, Hsu PP. Robotic obstructive sleep apnea surgery. Adv Otorhinolaryngol. 2017; 80:125–135

Weinstein G, Malley B. Transoral Robotic Surgery (TORS). San Diego, CA: Plural Publishing Inc; 2010

George Garas, Neil Tolley. Robotics in otorhinolaryngology–head and neck surgery. Ann Roy Coll Surg. 2018;100(Suppl 7):34–41

Related Topic of Interest

Oropharyngeal carcinoma

93 Salivary Gland Diseases

There are four major salivary glands—two parotids and two submandibular glands—and multiple minor salivary glands which occur throughout the upper respiratory tract, notably in the oral cavity and oropharynx. Most patients with salivary gland disease will present with a complaint of swelling, pain, alteration in taste (foul taste), dryness of the mouth (xerostomia) or drooling (sialorrhoea). Patients with enlargement of their salivary glands (sialomegaly) pose a particularly interesting diagnostic dilemma and are often used as examination cases.

93.1 Pathology

1. Infection
   a. Viral: mumps virus, coxsackie virus, echovirus and human immunodeficiency virus (HIV).
   b. Bacterial: staphylococcal, actinomycosis, tuberculosis and leprosy.
2. Neoplasm
   a. Benign: pleomorphic adenoma, Warthin's tumour and oncocytoma.
   b. Malignant: mucoepidermoid carcinoma, acinic cell carcinoma, adenoid cystic carcinoma, adenocarcinoma, squamous cell carcinoma and lymphoma.
   c. Non-epithelial: haemangioma, lymphangioma and neurofibroma.
3. Inflammatory
   a. Sjögren's syndrome
   b. IgG4-related disease
4. Metabolic
   Hypothyroidism, diabetes, Cushing's disease, cirrhosis, gout, bulimia and alcoholism.
5. Drug induced
   Coproxamol (dextropropoxyphene and paracetamol), oral contraceptive pill, thiouracil, phenylbutazone and isoprenaline.
6. Sialectasis
   Progressive destruction of the alveoli and parenchyma of the gland accompanied by duct stenosis and cyst formation. Many cases are thought to be congenital. Epithelial debris or calculi may be found in the main ducts.
7. Pseudoparotomegaly
   These disorders should be kept in mind as they may mimic sialomegaly: hypertrophic masseter, winged mandible, mandible tumours, dental cyst, branchial cyst, pre-auricular lymph node, sebaceous cyst, lipoma and neuroma of the facial nerve.

Salivary neoplasms will be covered in Chapter 94. Sjögren's syndrome and IgG4 related disease merit special mention as they are regularly asked about in examinations.

93.2 Sjögren's Syndrome

This is an autoimmune disease which is characterised by periductal lymphocytes in multiple organs. It is diagnosed usually in middle-aged women (9:1). The salivary glands are affected in approximately 40% of all cases. In 4.3% of patients, the disease will progress to a non-Hodgkin's lymphoma. Sjögren's syndrome originally described dry mouth (xerostomia), dry eyes (keratoconjunctivitis sicca) and rheumatoid arthritis, with no mention of salivary gland swelling.

93.2.1 Classification

The American–European Consensus Group's (AECG) criteria, proposed in 2002, are still the most commonly used criteria for the diagnosis of Sjögren's syndrome although a new set of criteria has been proposed by the Sjögren's International Collaborative Clinical Alliance (SICCA) and accepted by the American College of Rheumatology (ACR) in 2012.

AECG Criteria

Four of the six listed criteria must be present for a diagnosis which must include either the fifth or sixth criterion. Alternatively, if three out of the four objective criteria are present, then this is adequate for a diagnosis.

1. Ocular symptoms—dry eyes for more than 3 months, foreign body sensation and use of tear substitutes more than three times daily.
2. Oral symptoms—dry mouth, frequent use of liquids to aid swallowing and recurrent salivary gland swelling.
3. Ocular signs—positive Schirmer's test performed without anaesthetic.
4. Oral signs—abnormal parotid sialography or salivary scintigraphy findings, abnormal sialometry finding (< 1.5 mL of unstimulated saliva flow in 15 minutes).
5. Positive minor salivary gland biopsy (biopsy showing focal lymphocytic lymphadenitis).
6. Positive anti-SSA or anti-SSB antibodies.

S

ACR Criteria

These were developed to improve specificity of criteria for entry into clinical trials and use of objective tests. The diagnosis of Sjögren's syndrome requires at least two of the following three criteria:

1. Positive serum anti-SSA and/or anti-SSB antibodies *or* positive rheumatoid factor and anti-nuclear antibody titre of at least 1:320.
2. Ocular staining score of at least 3.
3. Focal lymphocytic sialadenitis with at least one focus every 4 mm² in a labial minor salivary gland biopsy.

The disease can be further classified into the following:

a. Primary Sjögren's syndrome (or sicca complex) consisting of the above but with no connective tissue component.
b. Secondary Sjögren's syndrome, which consists of xerostomia, xerophthalmia, a positive minor salivary gland biopsy and a connective tissue disorder, usually rheumatoid arthritis (occasionally systemic lupus erythematosus).

93.3 IgG4-Related Disease

This is a chronic inflammatory autoimmune condition characterised by tissue infiltration with lymphocytes and immunoglobulin G4 (IgG4) secreting plasma cells and fibrosis. Several different diseases are now considered to be manifestations of IgG4-related disease. These include type 1 autoimmune pancreatitis, Riedel's thyroiditis, Mikulicz's disease, Küttner's tumour (now known as IgG4-related sialadenitis), inflammatory pseudotumours (in various sites of the body), mediastinal fibrosis and some cases of retroperitoneal fibrosis.

93.4 Sarcoid

This can cause parotid enlargement in about 5 to 10% of sufferers. Bilateral involvement is the rule, and the gland is usually not tender but firm and smooth. Heerfordt's syndrome, also referred to as uveoparotid fever, is a rare manifestation of sarcoidosis. The symptoms include inflammation of the eye (uveitis), swelling of the parotid gland, chronic fever and, in some cases, facial nerve palsy.

93.5 History

The diagnosis is often obvious from the clinical findings. A focused history should include the age of the patient (think of mumps or congenital sialectasis), the number of glands affected (tumours are unilateral apart from Warthin's which is bilateral in 5–14%), whether the swelling is exacerbated by eating (sialolithiasis [calculi] and ductal stenosis), duration of symptoms (benign tumours grow slowly and malignant ones rapidly) and any related pain (infection, calculus or malignancy—particularly adenoid cystic carcinoma). Lymphoma may present as a localised or diffuse swelling and should always be considered, but especially in elderly patients. There should be a thorough review of systemic symptoms (metabolic causes). A patient with sialomegaly, dry mouth and rheumatoid arthritis or another connective tissue disorder may have Sjögren's syndrome. Any medication the patient is taking should be noted. A dry mouth can be caused by anti-depressants, anxiolytic agents, anti-hypertensive medication, diuretics and antihistamines. Drooling (sialorrhea) is sometimes seen in patients with cerebral palsy, Parkinson's disease or following a cerebrovascular accident. The social history including alcohol intake and risk of HIV infection (patient may present with a lymphoepithelial cyst or parotid node) may be relevant in some cases.

93.6 Examination

Inspect the enlarged gland and then all the other salivary glands. Inflamed skin over the swelling should make one consider an infection or skin involvement from a malignant lesion. The facial nerve should be tested as facial weakness also raises the suspicion of malignancy. Before palpating the lesion be sure to ask if it is tender; this is kind to the patient and a good habit in clinical medicine—it is essential in an examination! Palpation should determine whether the lesion is local or diffuse, solid or cystic, mobile or fixed and whether other glands are affected. Inspect the oral cavity and palpate all the glands bi-manually. In the floor of the mouth, a submandibular calculus may be felt or pressure on a parotid gland may express pus from the parotid duct. Then examine the pharynx to look for a parapharyngeal lesion (in particular one arising from the deep lobe of the parotid), which may push the tonsil medially. Complete the ENT examination and perform a general examination if systemic or disseminated neoplastic disease is suspected.

93.7 Investigations

1. *Blood tests* Rheumatoid factor, anti-nuclear factor and abnormal electrophoresis are sometimes found in Sjögren's syndrome. Specific Sjögren's antibodies may also be present (anti-SSA and/or anti-SSB at a titre of at least 1:320). Tests for relevant endocrine disorders may be appropriate. The serum IgG4 levels may be elevated in IgG4 disease. An elevated angiotensin-converting enzyme (ACE) may assist in diagnosing sarcoid.

2. *Radiography* A plain film can be useful as it may reveal a radiopaque submandibular calculus. Most submandibular gland calculi are radiopaque, but most parotid calculi are radiolucent. Ultrasound scan will reveal most calculi (acoustic shadowing), possible duct dilation, will delineate a space-occupying lesion or generalised gland enlargement and is usually the investigation of choice. A plain or magnetic resonance (MR) sialogram (the latter if there is a radiologist with an interest in salivary gland disease) is also a useful investigation for benign salivary gland disease. Duct stenosis, calculi and sialectasis can all be diagnosed if sialography is possible and it can also be therapeutic in clearing the duct of debris. Magnetic resonance imaging (MRI) scanning is usually the preferred investigation in neoplastic disease to delineate any potential deep lobe involvement and to assess the tumour's relationship to the facial nerve.

3. *Biopsy* Incisional biopsy should not be performed as there is a risk of seeding neoplastic disease. Fine-needle aspiration biopsy or fine-needle core biopsy are safe, often useful, but the results should be interpreted in conjunction with clinical suspicion as incorrect reports are not uncommon, especially with cystic lesions. A parapharyngeal mass should never be biopsied through the pharynx because there may be uncontrollable bleeding if the patient has a vascular lesion. Sublabial biopsy is the definitive investigation to confirm the diagnosis in Sjögren's syndrome (periductal lymphocytic infiltration should be found).

93.8 Management

The management and specific treatment of the patient depend on the cause.

- The acute phase of infection will require analgesia, hydration, antiseptic mouthwash and antibiotics if considered to be bacterial.

- Obstructive sialadenitis (sialolithiasis) accounts for more than 50% of major salivary gland disease and usually occurs in the submandibular gland. Calculi, ductal stenosis and mucous plugs are the usual pathology. Small calculi (3–4 mm maximum) can be removed endoscopically (sialendoscopy) from the submandibular (Wharton's) or parotid (Stenson's) duct with the use of micro-instruments such as baskets and balloons. Patients with calculi larger than 4 mm may be treated with Holmium:YAG laser lithotripsy. Stenosis or debris in the ducts can also be treated with dilation and irrigation.

- Occasionally, the size of a stone or its position in the duct, and a patient with recurrent symptoms, may necessitate surgical excision of the gland. The morbidity of these interventions should be borne in mind. Submandibular gland excision carries specific risks of haematoma, wound infection and nerve damage (marginal mandibular branch of facial nerve, lingual nerve and hypoglossal nerve). Parotid gland excision caries specific risks of haematoma, seroma, wound infection, facial nerve weakness, numbness of the ear (greater auricular nerve damage), salivary fistula and gustatory sweating on the cheek (Frey's syndrome).

Management of Sjögren's syndrome is in supporting the patient's symptoms (reduction of dry mouth with hydration and artificial saliva preparations, prevention of corneal complications and minimising the risk of fungal infection) and monitoring for risk of lymphoma (high risk of non-Hodgkin's lymphoma).

IgG4 disease and sarcoid are both usually treated with steroids. Steroid-sparing immunosuppressive agents might be considered including rituximab, azathioprine, methotrexate and cyclophosphamide.

Further Reading

Bradley PJ, Guntinas-Lichius O. Salivary gland Disorders and Diseases: Diagnosis and Management. Stuttgart: Thieme publications; 2011

Gallo A, Capaccio P, Benazzo M, et al. Outcomes of interventional sialendoscopy for obstructive salivary gland disorders: an Italian multicentre study. Acta Otorhinolaryngol Ital. 2016; 36(6):479–485

Related Topic of Interest

Salivary gland neoplasms

94 Salivary Gland Neoplasms

Neoplastic tumours may be benign or malignant, and malignant tumours can be primary or metastatic. In addition, if one can remember the epithelial and the non-epithelial histology of the affected organ, an excellent working framework is easily established. Salivary gland tumours are no exception in this respect, except that some salivary neoplasms are characterised by diverse histological appearance and variable biological behaviour. The distinction between tumour types can be difficult, particularly based on material from fine-needle aspiration. There are several other aspects of salivary gland tumours that make them interesting; the commonest benign tumour (pleomorphic adenoma) has malignant transformation potential and, although considered benign, there is a propensity of recurrence after treatment. It is not surprising that with such a wealth of pathology, clinical features, investigation issues and contentious treatment options that salivary gland neoplasms are a regular examination subject.

94.1 Pathology

Salivary glands are a common source of benign pathology; malignant tumours are rare. Approximately 300 cases/year of primary salivary gland malignancy are registered in the United Kingdom, of which fewer than 10 occur in children. The worldwide incidence is estimated at 0.5 to 3 per 100,000 per year, accounting for about 2 to 5% of all head and neck malignancies.

The World Health Organization (WHO) histological classification of salivary tumours now includes over 40 variants and includes tumour-like lesions (e.g. salivary gland cysts). A simplified classification is presented below:

1. *Benign* Pleomorphic adenoma, Warthin's tumour (adenolymphoma), myoepithelioma, basal cell adenoma, oncocytoma and cystadenoma.
2. *Malignant* Mucoepidermoid carcinoma, adenoid cystic carcinoma, acinic cell carcinoma, adenocarcinoma, squamous cell carcinoma (SCC), undifferentiated carcinoma, carcinoma ex-pleomorphic adenoma and polymorphous low-grade carcinoma.
3. *Haematolymphoid* Hodgkin's lymphoma, diffuse large B-cell lymphoma and extra-nodal marginal zone B-cell lymphoma.

4. *Non-epithelial* Haemangioma, lymphangioma and neurofibromas.

Carcinomas are often further classified as high grade, low grade or mixed, the latter inferring a variable behaviour depending on the histological picture. It should be recognised that the clinical behaviour rather than the histology of a tumour can provide a better treatment guide, and it is recommended that clinical factors in addition to histology and grade are considered when planning treatment. Salivary gland tumours are uncommon in children, but a greater proportion of them (30%) are malignant (usually low-grade mucoepidermoid carcinoma).

A good approximation to remember is that 80% of all salivary tumours are in the parotid, 80% of parotid tumours are benign, and 80% of the benign tumours that arise in the parotid are pleomorphic adenoma. Warthin's tumour is the second most common benign lesion. The most common malignant tumour is mucoepidermoid carcinoma, followed by acinic cell carcinoma and adenoid cystic carcinoma. It is also important to remember that the parotid gland is a common site for metastases from SCCs arising in the skin of the head and neck.

Approximately, half of the tumours arising in the submandibular gland are benign (pleomorphic adenomas) with the remainder being malignant (adenoid cystic carcinoma is the most common, followed by mucoepidermoid carcinomas and carcinoma ex-pleomorphic adenoma).

Most minor salivary gland tumours arise on the soft palate (35%), followed by the upper lip (25%) and buccal mucosa. Half the tumours are benign (usually pleomorphic adenoma) and the remainder are malignant (mucoepidermoid carcinoma, adenoid cystic carcinoma and polymorphous low-grade adenocarcinoma).

94.2 Benign Tumours

Pleomorphic adenoma is the commonest benign salivary tumour. The sex distribution is equal and the peak age incidence is in the fifth decade. It has a pseudocapsule of compressed salivary tissue into which the tumour usually has many protuberances. It arises from intercalated duct cells and myoepithelial cells. Microscopically, it comprises epithelial and mesodermal elements

S

with a mucopolysaccharide stroma giving rise to a characteristic mixed staining pattern. If the capsule is ruptured during removal, then tumour may implant, causing recurrence. They usually present as slow-growing painless tumours. Pleomorphic adenoma has an estimated rate of malignant transformation of 1% per year, so excision is recommended in most cases if there are no surgical contraindications.

Warthin's tumour (adenolymphoma) is a benign tumour, usually seen in the tail of the parotid gland in elderly men. The peak incidence is the seventh decade and the male–female ratio is 7:1. It is reported to be more common in smokers. They are soft and cystic tumours which are thought to arise from heterotopic parotid tissue in the lymph nodes within the parotid gland. Ten percent are bilateral, but rarely synchronously. Treatment can be by excision and, unlike pleomorphic adenoma, recurrence almost never occurs. As these tumours have no malignant potential, and if there is a confident diagnosis, observation only is a management option.

Oncocytoma is a benign eosinophilic tumour (also called oxyphil adenoma) that arises from intra-lobular ducts or acini. It is usually found in the superficial lobe of the parotid. It can undergo malignant change and treatment is also by excision with a cuff of tissue.

94.3 Malignant Tumours

Mucoepidermoid carcinoma is the commonest malignant major salivary gland tumour and arises in any salivary tissue, but predominantly the parotid gland. It is the commonest salivary neoplasm in children. Low-grade or well-differentiated tumours usually behave in a benign fashion, intermediate ones are more aggressive and high-grade or undifferentiated tumours metastasise early to regional lymph nodes and carry a poor prognosis. However, the behaviour is not always accurately predicted by the histological appearance. Five-year survival varies between 86% for low-grade and 22% for high-grade tumours.

Adenoid cystic carcinoma is overall (for all glands) the commonest malignant salivary gland tumour and may arise from any salivary tissue, but is more common in minor than in major salivary glands. The sex incidence is equal and they are seen most often in patients in their sixth decade.

The tumour usually presents as a slow-growing mass and tends to spread along nerve sheaths. The patients often complain of facial pain and may present with a facial paresis. The incidence of lymph node metastases is low. Local recurrences are common and distant metastases occur in 30 to 40% patients, usually in the lungs, many years later. Stage I and II cancers can be cured although the survival curve never flattens even after 20 years. Patient with stage III and IV diseases have a poor prognosis with low survival rates at 10 years. Patients with lung metastases may live up to 5 years before succumbing to the disease.

Acinic cell carcinoma is the third most common cancer of the parotid gland. They grow slowly and usually do not spread to local nodes. However, they do recur or present with distant metastases many years after apparent disease-free survival. This is reflected in excellent survival rates of 90% at 5 years, which drops to 55% at 20 years.

Polymorphous low-grade adenocarcinoma is increasingly recognised, particularly as a tumour of the minor salivary glands on the soft palate. It is rare in the parotid. It is easily confused with pleomorphic adenoma and adenoid cystic carcinoma histologically. It generally behaves in an indolent, low-grade fashion, but can be unpredictable with perineural invasion and lymph node metastases.

Squamous cell carcinoma Most cases of SCC are metastases to the parotid from skin cancers. Associated neck nodes are common, so that these cases should also have an elective selective neck dissection, even in an N0 neck. SCC has a propensity for early extracapsular extension and in the parotid, this threatens local structures and prompt surgical intervention should be the rule. A few weeks' delay can make a significant difference with tumours readily invading the skin and increasing the complexity of any planned surgery.

Lymphomas may develop in intraparotid lymph nodes. The risk of lymphoma is increased in patients with Sjögren's syndrome. They can be confused with Warthin's tumour on cytology and larger tissue samples are usually requested and immunohistochemistry required.

94.4 Clinical Features

The usual presentation is a slow-growing painless mass. Rapid growth, pain, tethering of the skin, ulceration of the skin, cervical lymphadenopathy and facial nerve paralysis are all suggestive of malignancy. Tumours low in the tail of the parotid gland can easily be confused with an upper cervical lymph node. Bilateral parotid tumours are most common in Warthin's tumours and HIV-related lymphoepithelial cysts.

All patients with a mass in a salivary gland should have an inspection and palpation of the mass itself. Oral examination should be with inspection of the relevant salivary gland duct. The submandibular duct (Wharton's duct) orifice found in the floor of the mouth and the parotid (Stenson's duct) situated opposite the upper second molar. Peroral palpation can be useful to assess extent of tumours, particularly with submandibular gland tumours. Inspection of the oropharynx for parapharyngeal extension should be performed, which will usually manifest as medialisation of the tonsil. Facial nerve assessment is mandatory, as is neck node palpation. The head and neck skin should be checked for cancers.

94.5 Investigations

Fine-needle aspiration biopsy (FNAB) This is now established as the primary diagnostic tool for salivary gland lesions, but the role of FNA in the diagnosis of benign and malignant salivary gland disease still carries some controversy. It is a relatively painless procedure, has few complications (seeding of the tumour does not appear to occur) and may prevent an ill-advised and often ill-fated incisional or excisional biopsy of a parotid mass. However, it is far from straightforward with issues regarding aspiration technique, adequacy of specimen, cytological expertise and limitations of interpretation. If the result of FNA is at variance with other findings, then clinical judgement should prevail.

Imaging Ultrasound scan (USS) provides invaluable information about the site, size and nature of salivary gland tumours and the presence of any significant cervical lymphadenopathy. The position of a tumour in the superficial or deep aspect of the parotid gland is established by identification of its relation to the retromandibular vein. It is usually combined with FNA (USS-guided FNAB [USSgFNAB]) which improves the adequacy rate. In experienced hands, this can distinguish malignant from benign disease in 80 to 90% of cases. Cross-sectional imaging is not essential in straightforward benign tumours, but magnetic resonance imaging (MRI) scanning of a parotid tumour is useful in the assessment and delineation of anatomical structures, extension to the deep lobe and relation to the facial nerve.

94.6 Staging

The classification applies only to carcinomas of the major salivary glands. Tumours arising in minor salivary glands are not included. The staging of metastatic neck nodes for salivary gland cancer is similar to that for other metastatic disease. T stage according to the eighth edition of the UICC/AJCC staging manual is as follows:

T1 Tumour 2 cm or less in greatest dimesion without extraparenchymal extension.*

T2 Tumour more than 2 cm but not more than 4 cm in greatest dimension without extraparenchymal extension.*

T3 Tumour more than 4 cm and/or tumour with extraparenchymal extension.*

T4a Tumour invades skin, mandible, ear canal and/or facial nerve.

T4b Tumour invades base of skull, and/or pterygoid plates, and/or encases carotid artery.

*Extraparenchymal extension is clinical or macroscopic evidence of invasion of soft tissues or nerve, except those listed under T4a and 4b. Microscopic evidence alone does not constitute extraparenchymal extension for classification purposes.

The UICC are cognisant of the other factors which are relevant to the prognosis of salivary gland tumours and present a prognostic factors grid. This includes tumour-related factors (histological grade, tumour size, local invasion, perineural invasion and neck metastases), host factors (patient age, facial palsy and pain) and management related (resection margins, residual disease and adjuvant radiotherapy [RT]).

94.7 Management

94.7.1 Submandibular Gland Tumours

Benign tumours are excised in a supra-capsular plane, but malignant tumours require a wide excision (> 2 cm margin in aggressive tumours). There is a high risk of metastases in high-grade

S

mucoepidermoid carcinoma, (SCC, anaplastic tumours and carcinoma ex-pleomorphic adenoma), so N0 patients should also have an elective selective neck dissection (levels I–III). Tumours greater than 4 cm diameter have a significantly worse prognosis and should have adjuvant RT. Post-operative RT is also advised for high-grade tumours, extracapsular spread (ECS) in neck nodes, recurrent disease treatment, and for adenoid cystic carcinomas.

94.7.2 Parotid Gland Tumours

Benign Superficial parotidectomy with identification and exposure of the facial nerve (found 1 cm inferior and 1 cm deep to the tragal pointer and bisecting the angle of the insertion of the digastric muscle into the digastric ridge) was traditionally the preferred procedure. It is now generally accepted that an adequate margin in benign tumours is a cuff of 1 to 2 mm. There is thus an increasing recognition that lesser operations that remove less tissue are acceptable. Partial parotidectomy or hemi-superficial parotidectomy have become commonplace. Extracapsular dissection is an option and even endoscopically assisted parotidectomy is as effective, in selected patients. It is preferable that these procedures should be performed by expert surgeons in appropriately selected cases, such as small tumours confined to the superficial lobe. A 'lumpectomy' procedure should not be done due to high recurrence rates. Recurrence will occur if there has been incomplete excision and may occur if there has been tumour spillage.

Tumour spillage carries an increase in the rate of recurrence over a prolonged period and therefore long-term follow-up is recommended in such cases. Adjuvant RT for such cases should be discussed in a multi-disciplinary team (MDT) setting, but the use of RT in these cases is controversial and is generally not recommended especially in younger patients due to the risk of radiation-induced tumours.

Management of recurrent tumour is difficult. It can be multi-focal and as the facial nerve may be involved, its sheath may need to be stripped. The facial nerve should, if at all feasible, not be sacrificed; rarely, radical surgery is needed with resection of the facial nerve. The facial nerve may be encased in scar tissue so the traditional method of finding it may have to be augmented by exposing it in the mastoid bone or more hazardously a peripheral branch traced back. There is a high rate of transient facial nerve paresis in this group of patients. The patient should be discussed in the MDT for the suitability of post-operative RT to reduce recurrence.

Malignant For small, low-grade superficial tumours, a partial parotidectomy with a margin of at least 1.5 cm may suffice, but otherwise a total conservative parotidectomy is advocated with resection of adjacent structures if necessary to achieve an en bloc resection. A functioning facial nerve should be preserved unless found to be infiltrated with tumour at the time of resection. If the nerve is sacrificed because of involvement, then primary nerve grafting should be performed. The greater auricular nerve as a donor is an option, but it may be involved, so the sural nerve may be preferred.

Neck dissection should be performed in patients with clinical or radiological evidence of nodal disease. A prophylactic selective neck dissection (levels I–III) should be performed for patients with high-stage (T3/T4) and/or clinically high-grade tumours (i.e. adenocarcinoma, squamous and undifferentiated carcinomas, high-grade mucoepidermoid carcinoma and carcinoma ex-pleomorphic adenoma).

Adjuvant RT is recommended for large tumours (> 4 cm), recurrent disease, patients with incomplete or close margins, perineural invasion, extension beyond the gland, nodal disease, in metastatic disease and is usually indicated for adenoid cystic carcinomas and high-grade tumours.

94.7.3 Minor Salivary Gland Tumours

Benign tumours of the palate can be safely resected sub-periosteally without removing palatal bone. Proven benign tumours in soft tissue can be removed by careful local dissection. Most malignant cases are treated in a similar way to SCC, with en bloc resection with depth of excision compatible with treatment of SCC to ensure adequate resection margins. Therapeutic neck dissection is indicated for lymph node involvement. Elective neck dissection is indicated for high-stage and clinically high-grade disease such as high-grade adenocarcinoma, invasive carcinoma ex-pleomorphic adenoma, SCC, high-grade mucoepidermoid and undifferentiated carcinoma. Post-operative RT is indicated for microscopic residual disease, large tumours

(> 4 cm), aggressive undifferentiated tumours and adenoid cystic tumours.

Further Reading

Foresta E, Torroni A, Di Nardo F, et al. Pleomorphic adenoma and benign parotid tumors: extracapsular dissection vs superficial parotidectomy—review of literature and meta-analysis. Oral Surg Oral Med Oral Pathol Oral Radiol. 2014; 117(6):663–676

Medina JE. Salivary gland tumours. Curr Opin Otolaryngol Head Neck Surg. 1993; 1:91–96

Roland NJ, Caslin AW, Smith PA, Turnbull LS, Panarese A, Jones AS. Fine needle aspiration cytology of salivary gland lesions reported immediately in a head and neck clinic. J Laryngol Otol. 1993; 107(11):1025–1028

Sood S, McGurk M, Vaz F. Management of salivary gland tumours: United Kingdom National Multidisciplinary Guidelines. J Laryngol Otol. 2016; 130(S2):S142–S149

Witt RL. The significance of the margin in parotid surgery for pleomorphic adenoma. Laryngoscope. 2002; 112 (12):2141–2154

Related Topics of Interest

Salivary gland diseases
Examination of the head and neck

S

95 Septal Perforation

A septal perforation is most commonly located in the anterior, cartilaginous septum except for that caused by syphilis, which normally occurs more posteriorly in the bony septum. Most perforations are either due to trauma, most commonly from nose picking, or iatrogenic, usually as a complication of septal surgery, particularly when the Killian incision is used. Septal perforations are usually preceded by ulceration except when following a septal haematoma or abscess when an area of ischaemia occurs. Patients with a septal perforation are commonly used in the rhinology section of examinations.

95.1 Aetiology

1. *Trauma*
   a. Iatrogenic.
      - Septal surgery. A perforation may arise from torn, opposing mucoperichondrial flaps where cartilage has been removed, from a septal haematoma or septal abscess.
      - Nasal packing that has been traumatically placed or from epistaxis balloons left in situ for a prolonged period or at too high a pressure.
      - Nasal cautery. There are two important points to mention. First, the mucosa over Little's area is quite thick inferiorly but thin at midheight. Therefore, if the latter area has bilateral nasal cautery, this can result in bilateral opposing septal burn ulceration, predisposing to a septal perforation. Secondly, nasal cautery to Little's area is contraindicated in the presence of Little's nasal vestibulitis. This is because the vestibulitis may be the cause of the epistaxis, so the vestibulitis should be treated medically and this may obviate the need to perform nasal cautery. Finally, cauterising infected tissue causes more necrosis and may allow infection to spread to cartilage, increasing the risk of a septal perforation from the vestibulitis.
      - Nasal cannulas are used for patients with chronic obstructive pulmonary disease (COPD) requiring long-term oxygen delivery or intensive therapy unit (ITU)/coronary care unit (CCU) patients requiring short-term oxygen delivery. They can cause trauma to the anterior nasal septum.
   b. Self-inflicted nasal trauma (nose picking). Trauma from nose picking may cause ulceration to mucosa over Little's area, which then becomes infected with *Staphylococcus aureus*. This causes infected crusts and may lead to cartilage necrosis and a perforation.
   c. Injury (assault, road accident and sport injury). Trauma may cause a septal haematoma. Haematoma in contact with septal cartilage causes cartilage resorption and mucosal ischaemia. The haematoma may become infected and the resulting septal abscess causes septal cartilage necrosis and mucosal infection. These scenarios may cause a septal perforation and a dorsal nasal saddle if the cartilage necrosis extends to the superior margin of the quadrangular cartilage.

2. *Infection* Syphilis, tuberculosis, *Mycobacterium kansasii* and invasive fungal sinusitis.

3. *Neoplasm* Squamous cell carcinoma, adenocarcinoma, basal cell carcinoma, T-cell lymphoma (midline nasal granuloma) and malignant melanoma.

4. *Inflammatory* Wegener's granulomatosis, sarcoidosis, polyarteritis nodosa, systemic lupus erythematosus, chronic relapsing polychondritis and cryoglobulinaemia.

5. *Chemicals* Cocaine (see Chapter 20, Epistaxis), button batteries (see Chapter 31, Foreign Bodies in ENT), chromium, nickel, alkaline dusts, bevacizumab (a monoclonal antibody that inhibits vascular endothelial growth factor and has been associated with ischaemic or inflammatory septal ulceration/perforation) and snuff.

6. *Idiopathic.*

95.2 Clinical Features

Posterior septal perforations involving the bony septum (perpendicular plate of the ethmoid and the vomer), or quadrangular cartilage where the anterior margin lies posterior to the nasal valve, are usually asymptomatic. Anterior perforations are often asymptomatic too, but may present with recurrent epistaxis, crusting and nasal obstruction. The severity of the symptoms depends on the position and the size of the perforation. Usually, the larger the perforation and more anterior its position, the more symptomatic is the patient. A small perforation (< 7 mm) may cause whistling from turbulence on nasal breathing.

95.3 Investigations

Patients who have an active perforation margin, that is an angry, friable margin, should be investigated further. Such patients may also have mucosa on the lateral nasal wall with a similar appearance. The following tests should be performed:

- Full blood count (FBC), erythrocyte sedimentation rate (ESR), C-reactive protein (CRP), angiotensin-converting enzyme (ACE) assay, fluorescent treponema antibody (FTA) for syphilis and anti-neutrophil cytoplasmic antibody (ANCA) for Wegener's granulomatosis.
- Chest radiograph may show lesions in tuberculosis, Wegener's granulomatosis or sarcoid.
- Urinalysis (haematuria or proteinuria may result from nephritis in Wegener's granulomatosis or polyarteritis).
- Biopsy from the edge of the perforation. Biopsy from an inactive edge is not indicated.

95.4 Treatment

The first objective is to treat the causative disease process before specific treatment of the perforation.

Swabs from symptomatic patients nearly always grow *S. aureus* and resolving such an infection may be very tricky because the infection often involves infected and exposed septal cartilage, particularly the posterior margin. Such patients may have seen several clinicians previously and have been prescribed an anti-*Staphylococcus* application for a week or two without follow-up. Such an approach will hardly ever resolve the problem. What is needed is a clinician who is committed to their patient and a patient who trusts the clinician and so is more likely to comply with advice given. This means that time is taken at the first consultation to explain to the patient the treatment plan and to reassure the patient that compliance with the plan will probably, eventually, provide a clean dry nose.

1. Medical therapy:
   A recommended treatment plan is as follows:
   - Soften the nasal crusts with a cotton wool ball soaked in warm water and placed in each nostril until the crusts soften (about 10 minutes), then gently remove the crusts with a finger.
   - Apply mupirocin 2% nasal ointment to both nares in sufficient quantity to cover the whole perforation circumference. The nostrils are then gently externally massaged to adequately distribute the ointment. The nozzle of the tube is quite fine, so it is best that the patient places the nozzle into both nares and squeezes to apply the ointment. Using a cotton ear bud to apply the ointment is not recommended because the ointment simply sticks to the cotton bud and little gets into the nose.
   - The ointment is applied four times daily and initially the crust removal should be done prior to each application. Within just a few days the crust production dramatically reduces so that after a week crust softening/ removal is usually necessary only twice daily (but the mupirocin continues to be applied four times daily). After a fortnight, the mupirocin is swapped to Naseptin cream qds for a further fortnight, provided the patient is not allergic to peanuts (the Naseptin contains peanut oil). The patient is reviewed after the first week of treatment to ensure compliance and that sufficient ointment is being applied. It is important to reinforce the need for compliance because the nose at this early stage of treatment feels much improved and it is tempting for patients to reduce their commitment. The patient is further reviewed after completion of the first 4-week cycle of treatment and a decision whether to proceed with a second 4-week cycle made.

Usually, if the nose is not pristine after a second cycle, it is because of exposed cartilage at the posterior margin. The exposed cartilage can be excised by mobilising mucosal flaps around the circumference, excising a rim of the exposed cartilage while preserving mucosa and replacing the mucosal flaps which will then heal. It is important that after finishing the anti-*Staphylococcus* treatment Vaseline is applied to both nares qds for several months. This is because the mucosa around the perforation has usually undergone metaplastic change, due to chronic infection, to a squamous, non–mucous-producing lining that will crust. It is usual that after several months the metaplastic mucosa, if prevented from drying, will revert to a normal mucous-producing nasal mucosa. With this management plan, most symptomatic perforations become and remain asymptomatic.

2. Surgical intervention:
   If an inactive perforation continues to be symptomatic, usually causing problematic whistling, then some surgeons advocate occluding the perforation with a Silastic septal button. Paradoxically, anterior perforations that cause a whistle, but no other symptom may be enlarged to about 7 to 8 mm. However, although this usually stops the whistling, it does increase the chance of the patient developing problems from drying and crusting of the perforation edge in the future.

An alternative strategy is to close or repair the perforation. One review found an extensive range of surgical treatment techniques, but reported results were rarely statistically significant. It is difficult to be categorical about the effectiveness of a surgical treatment method; nonetheless, each technique has its own advantages and drawbacks. Successful surgical closure of a septal perforation is related to the size of the perforation and the activity of the perforation edge. In perforations with an inactive edge and less than 35-mm diameter, a 95% success rate is possible in experienced hands using bilateral local flaps with an interposition graft. Unilateral local flaps are almost never successful and are not advised. The interposition graft is usually tragal cartilage, which has much less tendency to curl than conchal cartilage, or porcine collagen sheet. The local flap involves rotating a long nasal mucosal flap that starts on the lateral nasal wall beneath the inferior turbinate and is then elevated and mobilised on a broad front of the nasal floor and septum. Large perforations may require a superior septal flap too, to cover the superior third of the perforation.

Further Reading

Goh AY, Hussain SS. Different surgical treatments for nasal septal perforation and their outcomes. J Laryngol Otol. 2007; 121(5):419–426

Hulterström AK, Sellin M, Monsen T, Widerström M, Gurram BK, Berggren D. Bacterial flora and the epidemiology of staphylococcus aureus in the nose among patients with symptomatic nasal septal perforations. Acta Otolaryngol. 2016; 136(6):620–625

Watson D, Barkdull G. Surgical management of the septal perforation. Otolaryngol Clin North Am. 2009; 42(3):483–493

S

Related Topics of Interest

Nasal trauma
Non-healing nasal granulomata

96 Sinonasal Tumours

Tumours of the nasal cavity and sinuses are rare and may be benign or malignant. Because of the hidden nature of the nasal cavities and sinuses, a high index of suspicion is required to avoid delay in diagnosis. This chapter addresses the key issues of sinonasal tumours and highlights their characteristics, management and outcomes.

96.1 Clinical Presentation

96.1.1 Benign Nasal Tumours

Benign nasal tumours often present as a unilateral nasal polyp. The usual symptoms are as follows:

- Nasal obstruction. This is generally unilateral unless a tumour fills the area of the nasopharynx.
- Epistaxis. Spontaneous bleeding is not usual but is usually induced by forceful nose blowing.
- Anosmia. Loss of the sense of smell may be associated with obstruction to airflow reaching the olfactory cleft.

Occasionally, a benign tumour may obstruct the sinus ostium and lead to a complication such as a mucocele, a mucopyocele and orbital swelling.

96.1.2 Malignant Nasal Tumours

Malignant tumours similarly cause a mass effect and obstruct the nasal airway. They can therefore also present with nasal obstruction. Loss of sense of smell may also arise from obstruction of airflow to the olfactory clefts but can also be due to direct involvement of olfactory mucosa by the tumour.

The cardinal symptoms of a malignant sinonasal tumour are a unilateral bloodstained nasal mucus discharge and facial pain.

Malignant tumours can also invade local tissues and induce secondary problems according to the direction of spread (▶Table 96.1). Metastasis to regional cervical lymph nodes and distant spread may also cause symptoms and signs and should always be considered.

96.2 Initial Clinical Management

Any patient presenting with unusual sinonasal symptoms and signs or a unilateral polyp or mass within the nose should undergo a thorough

▶ **Table 96.1** Local effects of sinonasal tumours

Relative to nasal cavity	Susceptible structure	Clinical effects
Anterior	Facial skin	Fungating tumour
Lateral	Orbit	Proptosis
	Infraorbital nerve	Diplopia/impaired vision
	Pterygomaxillary fossa	Facial numbness Trismus
Posterior	Eustachian tube	Otitis media with effusion
Medial	Nasal septum	Spread across midline
Superior	Anterior skull base	Invasion into intracranial cavity Loss of sense of smell
Inferior	Teeth/gingiva/ palate	Spread to oral cavity Local pain Palatal fistula

endoscopic assessment of the nasal cavities after suitable vasoconstriction.

A multi-planar computed tomography (CT) scan of the sinuses should be considered and obtained. Should there be any possibility of the tumour mass being malignant, an urgent enhanced magnetic resonance imaging (MRI) scan should be arranged.

It is difficult to predict the histological nature of a nasal polyp/mass on clinical grounds alone, and attention should be given to histological confirmation. A biopsy should be deferred until after any imaging While it may be possible to obtain a biopsy in clinic, the risk of inducing significant bleeding should be considered. Ideally, the patient should be admitted urgently for assessment under general anaesthesia. The surgeon can then either simply take a diagnostic biopsy or choose to debulk and possibly resect the mass, as long as this does not induce severe haemorrhage or compromise further treatment.

Once the histology is known, all patients with malignant tumours should then be presented for discussion at the local head and neck or skull base multi-disciplinary team (MDT) meeting.

Further scans may be required, according to the agreed MDT protocol. These are likely to include MRI of the neck and CT of the chest, abdomen and pelvis.

S

96.3 Specific Benign Sinonasal Tumours

96.3.1 Sinonasal Papilloma

Sinonasal papillomas are the commonest sinonasal tumour, (0.5–4% of all sinonasal tumours) and the estimated incidence is 1/1,000,000/year. They are more common in men and the peak age at presentation is the fifth to sixth decade.

The term sinonasal papilloma encompasses exophytic, inverted and oncocytic papillomas.

a. Exophytic papilloma

These present as warty-looking growths in the anterior nasal cavity, particularly on the nasal septum. The lesions may be multiple and may spread to other regions within the nasal cavity. They are virally related and have a propensity for recurrence, even if completely excised. They do not carry any risk of malignant transformation. However, it should be noted that the histology can be confused with well-differentiated squamous cell carcinoma.

b. Inverted papilloma

The inverted papilloma derives its name from the pattern of cell growth as seen histologically. In practice, there may be areas of exophytic growth as well.

The endoscopic appearance can be variable and range from a smooth, pale and lobulated polypoid lesion to a dusky red, irregular tumour. Generally, they are quite large at the time of diagnosis unless they have been found as an incidental finding in patients presenting with chronic rhinosinusitis.

About half of these tumours arise from the maxillary sinus. The rest arise from the ethmoid/nasal cavity and a smaller number occur in the frontal sinus and sphenoid. Tumours that affect the frontal sinus have nearly always originated in the anterior ethmoid and encroached into the frontal sinus through the natural ostium.

The tumour characteristically causes focal hyperostosis that is evident on the CT scan (▶ Fig. 96.1). The preferred staging system is that described by Krouse (▶ Table. 96.2).

Most tumours can be completely removed endoscopically, even if this includes extended endoscopic techniques into the maxillary, frontal and sphenoid sinuses. External surgery is now limited to extensive tumours affecting the extremes of the frontal sinus and maxillary sinus.

The tumour may sometimes behave aggressively and cause bone erosion. There is a small but significant risk of malignant transformation, estimated to be less than 2%. There is a significant risk of local recurrence of approximately 20%. The risk of recurrence is decreased by cleaning the bone adjacent to the tumour origin with a diamond drill, endoscopic-targeted tumour base surgery and taking frozen sections of the tumour margins.

Following tumour removal, the patient should be reviewed and assessed for tumour recurrence regularly for up to 5 years.

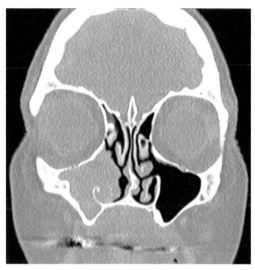

Fig. 96.1 Coronal CT scan showing hyperostosis in the lateral wall of the right maxillary sinus secondary to inverted papilloma.

S

▶ **Table 96.2** The melanoma seven-point checklist lesion system

T1	Tumour confined to the nasal cavity
T2	Tumour confined to the ethmoid sinus and medial/superior portion of the maxillary sinus
T3	Tumour involving the lateral or inferior portions of the maxillary sinus/or frontal sinus/or sphenoid sinus
T4	Tumour extending beyond the nose and paranasal sinus boundaries or malignant disease

Source: Krouse JH; Laryngoscope, 2000; 110(6): 965–968

c. Oncocytic papilloma

The oncocytic papilloma is the least common variety of sinonasal papilloma and behaves very similarly to inverted papilloma. The name is derived from the histological features of cylindrical oncocytic cells within the tumour.

96.3.2 Benign Bony Sinus Tumours: Fibro-Osseous Lesions

Fibro-osseous lesions are unusual and include fibrous dysplasia, ossifying fibroma and sinus osteoma.

Fibrous dysplasia presents as a diffuse slow-growing lesion in one or more sites that may affect the sphenoid, orbital apex, maxilla and frontal bone. It normally presents with facial asymmetry. When active, the bone can be very vascular, and surgery is best deferred until the condition becomes quiescent.

Ossifying fibroma is a rare tumour that can be locally aggressive.

Sinus osteoma is the most common of these bony lesions, but the incidence is unknown. They tend to occur in the ethmoid and frontal sinuses. They may present as an incidental finding on a CT scan, either as a very small tumour or a large bony mass.

Large osteomas are more likely to be symptomatic and expand into the orbit causing proptosis. If the frontal os is obstructed, a frontal mucocele may form. The latter can develop into a mucopyocele and cause intracranial or periorbital infection. Asymptomatic osteomas do not necessarily need operative intervention, as long as a sinus complication is not imminent. Interval scans are a perfectly reasonable way of monitoring tumour activity.

While endoscopic resection may be possible, careful consideration should be given to conventional external approaches, such as creating an osteoplastic flap or performing a craniofacial resection.

96.4 Juvenile Nasopharyngeal Angiofibroma

The juvenile nasopharyngeal angiofibroma (JNA) is an encapsulated slow-growing hormonally related vascular tumour with a fibrous stroma that normally presents in adolescent and young adult males.

The tumour derives a blood supply from feeding vessels of both the external and internal carotid arterial systems, but intracranial arterial connections often connect with the internal carotid artery. It is a slow-growing tumour that is locally invasive. It originates in the region of the sphenopalatine foramen and expands medially into the nasopharynx and nasal cavities, where it causes nasal obstruction and recurrent nosebleeds. The tumour can also expand into the infratemporal fossa, orbit, sphenoid sinus, skull base and intracranial cavity in the region of the cavernous sinus.

Biopsy should be avoided because of the risk of catastrophic haemorrhage. Treatment is surgical and many of these tumours are now successfully removed endonasally. Surgery is not without risk, given the vascularity of the tumour. Pre-operative tumour embolisation within a couple of days of surgery will help to minimise this risk. In young children, the use of a cell saver and autotransfusion during surgery should be considered.

There is a significant risk of tumour recurrence following surgery due to invasion of the vidian canal in the region of the basisphenoid. It is therefore important to completely clear this, and ideally, drill the basisphenoid to limit the likelihood of recurrence.

96.5 Miscellaneous Rare Tumours

Unilateral nasal masses can sometimes arise due to very unusual pathology, such as meningioma, pleomorphic adenoma and haemangiopericytoma.

96.6 Malignant Sinonasal Tumours

Malignant tumours of the nose and sinuses are very uncommon. The problem with growing in a relatively hidden site is that they are often large and quite advanced at the time of presentation. Most tumours arise from the epithelium (80%), but the diversity of other cell types explains the range of alternative tumour types, which include the following:

- Squamous cell carcinoma.
- Adenocarcinoma.
- Olfactory neuroblastoma.
- Salivary gland tumours (e.g. adenoid cystic carcinoma).

- Mucosal malignant melanoma.
- Lymphoma.
- Sarcoma.
- Metastasis.

96.6.1 Squamous Cell Carcinoma

Squamous cell carcinoma is rare, but the most common malignant sinonasal tumour, with a general incidence of 1:100, 000. The peak age is 55 to 65 years and it is slightly more common in men (men: women 1.5:1). Clinically, the most common site is the maxillary sinus (60–70%), followed by the nasal cavity/ethmoid (10–25%).

Unusual variants include verrucous carcinoma, spindle cell, basaloid, papillary, acantholytic and adenosquamous carcinoma. Non-keratinising squamous cell carcinoma (NKSCC) is now an accepted term that used to be known as schneiderian, cylindrical, or transitional cell carcinoma. A sinonasal undifferentiated carcinoma (SNUC) is another very unusual cancer that is locally very aggressive and typically extensive and inoperable at the time of presentation.

96.6.2 Adenocarcinoma

Adenocarcinoma accounts for 10 to 20% of all sinonasal malignancies. The association between this tumour and exposure to hardwood dust is well established. Pathologically, the tumour is categorised into a non-intestinal type of high and low grade and the more common intestinal-type adenocarcinoma (ITAC), associated with wood dust. The rare possibility of metastasis from a distant tumour site should always be excluded.

The tumour occurs more commonly in the ethmoid (40%), but it can affect with other areas within the nose and sinuses. The endoscopic appearance is variable, and it can be a smooth polypoid mass or friable and irregular. The tumour should be resected if possible as the role of radiotherapy is unproven. Wide excision is recommended because of the possibility of widespread field change.

96.6.3 Staging of Sinus Carcinoma

Carcinoma of the nasal cavity and sinuses should be staged with the up-to-date UICC/AJCC staging system (currently the 8th edition). A summary of which is as follows.

96.7 Maxillary Sinus

T1 Tumour limited to the mucosa with no erosion or destruction of bone.
T2 Tumour causing bone erosion or destruction, including extension into the hard palate and/or middle nasal meatus, except extension to posterior wall of maxillary sinus and pterygoid plates.
T3 Tumour invades any of the following: bone of posterior wall of maxillary sinus, subcutaneous tissues, floor or medial wall of orbit, pterygoid fossa or ethmoid sinuses.
T4a Tumour invades any of the following: anterior orbital contents, skin of cheek, pterygoid plates, infratemporal fossa, cribriform plate and sphenoid or frontal sinuses.
T4b Tumour invades any of the following: orbital apex, dura, brain, middle cranial fossa, cranial nerves other than maxillary division of trigeminal nerve (V2), nasopharynx or clivus.

96.8 Nasal Cavity and Ethmoid Sinus

T1 Tumour restricted to one sub-site of nasal cavity or ethmoid sinus, with or without bony invasion.
T2 Tumour involves two sub-sites in a single site or extends to involve an adjacent site within the nasoethmoidal complex, with or without bony invasion.
T3 Tumour extends to invade the medial wall or floor of the orbit, maxillary sinus, palate or cribriform plate.
T4a Tumour invades any of the following: anterior orbital contents, skin of nose or cheek, minimal extension to anterior cranial fossa, pterygoid plates and sphenoid or frontal sinuses.
T4b Tumour invades any of the following: orbital apex, dura, brain, middle cranial fossa, cranial nerves other than V2, nasopharynx or clivus.

96.8.1 Olfactory Neuroblastoma (Esthesioblastoma)

Olfactory neuroblastoma arises from cells in the olfactory mucosa within the olfactory cleft. It is locally invasive and typically erodes the anterior skull base, expanding superiorly into the anterior

S

cranial fossa. The prognosis depends on the stage of the disease and the histopathological features. The Kadish system describes three groups:

Group A—tumour limited to the nasal cavity.

Group B—tumour localised to the nasal cavity and paranasal sinuses.

Group C—tumour extension into adjacent areas, for example, orbit and anterior cranial fossa.

Other systems such as that described by Dulgerov are based on the UICC/AJCC system. The key determinants in prognosis have been shown to be orbital invasion, cranial fossa invasion and the presence of metastases. Metastatic spread to regional cervical lymph nodes occurs in up to 25% of cases, sometimes affecting nodes on both sides of the neck. Regional metastasis to the neck can take several years to present, with a median time of 5 years.

96.8.2 Adenoid Cystic Carcinoma

The adenoid cystic carcinoma is a salivary gland malignancy that arises mainly in the maxillary sinus (60% of cases). It presents with unilateral nasal obstruction and nosebleeds. However, it can also cause facial pain, paraesthesia or numbness due to its characteristic behaviour of spreading along nerves. Occasionally, the tumour is hidden in the pterygopalatine fossa, and will not be visible within the nose. The CT and MRI images need careful evaluation and typically show expansion of the pterygomaxillary fissure. Such tumours can be accessed endoscopically via the posterior wall of the maxillary sinus, facilitating biopsy and access for reducing tumour bulk.

Complete excision is often not possible because of neural spread into the skull base and intracranial cavity. Post-operative radiation is nearly always necessary.

Long-term survival is poor (7% at 10 years) and death is typically due to local recurrence, although pulmonary metastases are always a long-term risk.

96.8.3 Lymphoma

Occasionally, lymphomas may originate within the ethmoid and maxillary sinus and present with unilateral nasal obstruction and bleeding. Once the diagnosis has been confirmed by endoscopic biopsy, the patient should be referred to haematology, where tumour staging can be undertaken according to the specialist protocol. Treatment is determined by the specific histology and tumour stage, and normally consists of a combination of radiotherapy and chemotherapy. These tumours are often very responsive, and the tumour mass disappears with treatment. Long-term follow-up is necessary; sinonasal endoscopy is important in detecting recurrence.

96.8.4 Mucosal Melanoma

Mucosal malignant melanoma is an uncommon condition that typically presents late with progressive nasal obstruction. It is invasive and aggressive, and tumours can be extremely vascular and prone to significant bleeding during surgery. There has recently been a trend to resect these tumours endoscopically rather than by conventional open techniques. The endoscope may facilitate good local clearance, and outcome results have been encouraging. Ideally, surgery should be followed by radiotherapy, although there is no evidence to support locoregional control or survival.

96.9 Management of Malignant Tumours

Modern day health care ensures that all patients with these rare malignant tumours of the nose and sinuses are presented at a centralized MDT meeting.

The management of sinonasal tumours should be on an individual basis, taking account of the local extent, regional spread and distant metastases. The MDT should define whether the proposed treatment is curative or palliative, and consider whether specific treatment is required for the orbit, anterior skull base and neck. The introduction of positron emission tomography CT (PET-CT) has had an impact on the management of this patient group and helps with the early detection and identification of distant tumour spread and recurrence.

Generally, cervical lymph node involvement at the time of diagnosis of the sinonasal malignancy is low. Ethmoid sinus tumours have low rates of lymph node involvement and subsequent nodal recurrence. The situation, however, changes if the T stage is high and the tumour is squamous and undifferentiated.

MDT assessment and discussion often results in patients being referred for further consideration by other MDT groups. Examples include the lung cancer, melanoma and sarcoma MDT groups. Similarly, patients with lymphoma are referred to the specialist lymphoma group. Collaborative work with other specialty groups is now positively encouraged. This has enabled significant improvements in planning reconstruction following tumour resection.

When deciding on surgical management of a tumour, it is most important to take into consideration the tumour biology and behaviour, as this will affect the overall outcome. The established concepts of en bloc tumour resection and specific tumour margins are controversial and have been challenged in the management of sinus tumours. The long-term outcome results following endoscopic piecemeal tumour removal have been encouraging and seem to be equally as good as open resection.

96.10 Surgery for Malignant Sinonasal Tumours

96.10.1 Endoscopic Tumour Resection

There has been a paradigm shift in the surgical approach to these tumours.

There is now a definite place for endoscopic resection, sometimes combined with open approach surgery.

Endoscopic resection of tumours has been shown to have outcomes that are equal to conventional open surgery. However, the endoscopic technique allows for lower morbidity and shorter hospital stays. Frozen section can be used to confirm that margins are clear. Image-guided surgery can be used to aid endoscopic tumour resection and future developments include preoperative tumour mapping and colour coding of resection areas.

Tumour assessment should consider the feasibility of endoscopic reception and the risks that it entails. Tumours that invade the facial soft tissues are already beyond endoscopic resection. However, some contraindications are relative. Vascular tumours would also pose a problem; embolisation within a couple of days of surgery should be considered. Extensions into the ptergomaxillary and infratemporal fossae are relative contraindications that may be overcome. Similarly, invasion into the intracranial cavity would be difficult to clear.

The tumour pathology also has to be taken into account. Endoscopic resection of an olfactory neuroblastoma has been shown to result in good local control. Endoscopic resection of adenocarcinoma has been shown to give a 92% survival with a median follow-up of 30 months. Disease control and survival following endoscopic resection of squamous cell carcinoma is, however, significantly worse.

96.10.2 Open Surgery and Reconstruction

The two main open conventional surgical approaches that enable resection of sinonasal malignant tumours are maxillectomy and craniofacial resection.

Approaches to the maxilla include a transcutaneous incision (Weber–Ferguson) or a transoral route utilising a midfacial degloving procedure. Various extensions can facilitate additional exposure to the ethmoid sinuses, lateral and posterior maxilla. Consideration should be given to the palatal defect and whether or not to close this with an obturator or to repair the defect with a vascularised flap.

Craniofacial resection (CFR) facilitates good exposure of the anterior skill base to enable clearance of tumours of the ethmoid and olfactory cleft. Three types of craniofacial resection are described:

Type I CFR: This is done via an extended lateral rhinotomy incision. This facilitates resection of orbital contents during tumour resection.

Type II CFR: A shield-shaped midline window frontal craniotomy facilitates excellent exposure of the cribriform plates from above. Tumours can be resected en bloc and the dura repaired with fascia lata or pericranium.

Type III CFR: This technique is utilised only for large tumours with significant intracranial involvement and includes a large frontal craniotomy combined with a lateral rhinotomy incision.

96.11 Non-Surgical Oncological Therapy

96.11.1 Radiotherapy

Radiation therapy is used as an adjunct to surgery with an 'intent to cure' or for palliation in incurable oncological disease. Typically, post-operative radiotherapy is used within a few weeks of surgery. Occasionally, it may be used before surgery if it will facilitate less aggressive surgery that may, for example, lead to preservation of an eye.

S

Conventional radiotherapy utilises megavolt photons produced by a linear accelerator, typically in doses of 60 to 70 Gy fractionated over 30 to 35 sessions over 6 to 7 weeks. Intensity-modulated radiotherapy (IMRT) is well suited to sinus tumours enabling enhanced therapeutic doses to the tumour bed while limiting doses to sensitive nearby tissues. It avoids low-dose radiation therapy to areas of the tumour bed that would lead to inadequate treatment and an increased risk of local recurrence. Proton beam radiation is a new form of therapy that not yet in general use, but, has the advantage of a rapid dose falloff that could be highly advantageous to treating tumours that are adjacent to vital intracranial structures.

The response and effectiveness of radiotherapy treatment will depend on the individual tumour type and biology: tumours such as squamous sinus carcinoma, adenocarcinoma and olfactory neuroblastoma are all radiosensitive. However, the damage to nearby anatomical structures, such as the eye, lacrimal gland, optic nerve, pituitary gland and brain, all need to be considered and doses should be managed accordingly.

Radiotherapy of sinus tumours inevitably leads to a dry crusty nose, often associated with anosmia. Once the acute inflammatory effects of radiotherapy have abated, the nasal crusts should be cleared endoscopically and the patient started on frequent saline rinses.

Regional lymph node disease is uncommon with sinonasal malignancy, but neck imaging is essential in the staging process. If neck disease is present, it should be treated with an appropriate neck dissection and possibly adjuvant radiotherapy depending on the pathological stage of the neck.

96.11.2 Chemotherapy

Chemotherapeutic regimes are well established for the treatment of lymphoma and lymphoproliferative disease, but evidence to support its routine use in other sinonasal malignancy is limited. It may be a helpful adjunct in the palliative treatment of advanced disease, such as poorly differentiated/undifferentiated carcinoma with metastatic disease or in neuroendocrine tumours.

Chemotherapeutic agents may be given at the induction of radiotherapy with the intention of reducing tumour size, or during the course of radiotherapy as a radiation sensitiser.

Patients receiving this combination must be relatively fit and able to withstand the toxic effects that typically accompany this particular treatment regime.

Further Reading

Brierley JD, Gospodarowicz MK, Wittekind C. TNM Classification of Malignant Tumours. 8th ed. Wiley Blackwell Publishers; 2017

Lund VJ, Clarke PM, Swift AC, McGarry GW, Kerawala C, Carnell D. Nose and paranasal sinus tumours: United Kingdom National Multidisciplinary Guidelines. J Laryngol Otol. 2016; 130(S2):S111–S118

Lund VJ, Stammberger H, Nicolai P, et al; European Rhinologic Society Advisory Board on Endoscopic Techniques in the Management of Nose, Paranasal Sinus and Skull Base Tumours. European position paper on endoscopic management of tumours of the nose, paranasal sinuses and skull base. Rhinol Suppl. 2010; 22:1–143

97 Skin Cancer—Melanoma

This chapter deals with the diagnosis and principles of management of cutaneous and mucosal melanoma of the head and neck.

97.1 Cutaneous Melanoma of the Head and Neck

Cutaneous melanoma is a malignant tumour of neural crest–derived cutaneous melanocytes. The incidence of melanoma is increasing rapidly and has done for the last few decades. It is caused by ultraviolet radiation (UVR) in susceptible individuals, especially if exposure occurs at a young age. Fair-skinned individuals, who burn easily in the sun, have fair or red hair and have a tendency to freckles are particularly vulnerable. The presence of atypical or dysplastic naevi and a family history (2%) are also relevant. A history of intense burning sun exposure of young unacclimatised white skin is the major risk factor for melanoma. This contrasts with the chronic sun damage which causes non-melanoma skin cancers.

Despite the increased incidence, the prognosis has improved. This improvement is mostly attributable to a higher proportion of thinner tumours because of earlier diagnosis and reflects the considerable effort expended in raising public and professional awareness of melanoma. Although melanoma is the major cause of skin cancer mortality, it is usually curable if treated at an early stage. In contrast, melanoma in its advanced stages is incurable.

Cutaneous melanoma is divided into sub-types based on clinical features and pathology:

- Superficial spreading melanoma.
- Nodular melanoma.
- Lentigo maligna melanoma (LMM).
- Acral lentiginous melanoma.
- Desmoplastic neurotropic melanoma.

97.1.1 Superficial Spreading Melanoma

This is the most frequently encountered type of melanoma. It is usually an asymmetrical pigmented lesion with irregular borders, pigmentation and outline. Patients may have noted growth, a change in sensation, colour, crusting, bleeding or inflammation of the lesion.

97.1.2 Nodular Melanoma

This usually has a shorter length of presentation and a greater tendency to bleeding and ulceration. It may occur both in sun-exposed and non-exposed areas of the skin. Clinically, it appears as a well-circumscribed blue/black lesion with areas of nodularity and involution within.

97.1.3 Lentigo Maligna Melanoma

This occurs most often in sun-damaged skin on the head and neck of older patients. It may be preceded by a pre-invasive (in situ) lesion called lentigo maligna (LM) before progressing in some instances to an invasive melanoma (LMM).

97.1.4 Acral Lentiginous Melanoma

The least common type of melanoma is the acral lentiginous melanoma. This may occur on the palms, soles and beneath the nails. It is more common in Afro-Caribbeans and Asians.

97.1.5 Desmoplastic Neurotropic Melanoma

This lesion is predominantly found in the head and neck. It has a greater propensity to local recurrence than other forms of melanoma, probably due to its tendency for perineural spread.

97.1.6 Clinical History

Do not concentrate on the lesion and forget it is attached to a patient. A history of sun exposure and involvement of any other risk factors should be documented. Avoidance advice should be supplemented with leaflets whenever possible. Document intercurrent diseases and the use of anticoagulant medication which will have implications for operative bleeding. Appropriate and safe arrangements for stopping these medications should be made (and the advice given in writing to the patients as they otherwise may forget).

97.1.7 Clinical Examination

The clinical diagnosis of melanoma can be difficult and various methods relating to the clinical history and examination findings have been suggested. Even then, the accuracy of diagnosis varies according to a clinician's experience. Suspicious pigmented lesions are best examined in a good light with or without magnification and should be assessed using the seven-point checklist or ABCDE systems as given in ▶ Table 97.1 and ▶ Table 97.2.

Dermatoscopy is useful for diagnosis when used by those trained and experienced in the technique. Dermatoscopy refers to the examination of the skin using a handheld skin surface microscope. It is mainly used to evaluate pigmented lesions in order to distinguish melanoma and pigmented basal cell carcinoma, from benign melanocytic naevi and seborrhoeic keratoses. A high-quality lens giving 10 to 14 times magnification and a lighting system enables visualisation of sub-surface structures and patterns. With dermatoscopy, there is considerable improvement in the sensitivity (detection of melanomas) as well as specificity (percentage of non-melanomas correctly diagnosed as benign), compared with naked eye examination.

Examination of the cervical nodes is essential. It should be remembered that the nodes most often affected are those in the parotid gland, superficial jugular, upper deep cervical and occipital nodes. Lymphatic drainage is not always predictable and sentinel node biopsy using lymphoscintigraphy is a popular investigation for melanoma. Patients presenting with regional metastatic melanoma of unknown primary origin should be seen by a dermatologist for a skin examination, an ophthalmologist for examination of the eye and a head and neck surgeon for visualisation of the upper aerodigestive tract.

97.1.8 Investigations

Despite widely used checklists, the clinical diagnosis of melanoma can be difficult and a biopsy is needed for diagnosis. The thickness of the lesion influences both its treatment and its prognosis. It is essential, therefore, to obtain a full-thickness biopsy of suspected lesions. Excisional biopsy is the preferred technique and is aimed at excising the lesion with a 2 to 5-mm peripheral margin, including a cuff of subdermal fat. Excisional biopsy may not be practical when the lesion is large or located near structures such as an eyelid or lip and punch biopsy is an alternative.

Clinically palpable lymph nodes should undergo fine-needle aspiration, ideally under ultrasound control, for a cytological diagnosis. MRI and CT can help to stage the disease particularly if there is concern that it may involve underlying structures. The use of scans to detect distant metastases is indicated in patients with high-risk melanoma. In this instance, a chest, abdominal and pelvic CT scan are used. Imaging of the brain is recommended in patients with stage IV disease. Positron emission tomography CT (PET-CT) is also increasingly used to investigate for distant metastases in melanoma.

Occult nodes may be diagnosed by sentinel lymph node biopsy (SLNB). SLNB involves the administration of a radio-colloid into the site of the excision biopsy. Pre-operative lymphoscintigraphy identifies the approximate location of the sentinel nodes and intra-operative use of blue dye and a gamma-probe aid in location of the sentinel node. Regional lymph node metastases identified should be treated by a neck dissection. SLNB has replaced elective lymph node dissection in melanoma, but there is controversy as to whether it improves disease-specific survival and its routine use has been questioned. It is currently recommended in stage IB disease and above.

97.1.9 Staging Systems

The extent of the primary tumour (T-stage) for melanoma is classified after excision. For

▶ Table 97.1 The melanoma seven-point checklist lesion system

Major features	Minor features
Change in size of lesion	Inflammation
Irregular pigmentation	Itch/altered sensation
Irregular border	Lesion larger than others Oozing/crusting of lesion

▶ Table 97.2 The ABCDE lesion system

A	Geometrical **A**symmetry in two axes
B	Irregular **B**order
C	At least two different **C**olours in lesion
D	Maximum **D**iameter > 6 mm
E	**E**levation of lesion

S

malignant melanoma (MM), the regional lymph nodes (N stage) have a specialised system reflecting the concept and presence of micro-scopic (clinically occult), macroscopic (clinically apparent) and satellite (tumour nests or nodules within 2 cm of the primary) or in-transit (involves skin or subcutaneous tissue > 2 cm from the primary) metastases.

TNM Staging System 8th Edition for Melanoma

pTX	Primary tumour cannot be assessed.
pT0	No evidence of primary tumour.
pTis	In situ melanoma (Clark's level I).
pT1	Tumour 1 mm or less in thickness.
pT1a	Less than 0.8 mm without ulceration.
pT1b	Less than 0.8 mm with ulceration or 0.8 mm to 1 mm in thickness.
pT2	Tumour more than 1 mm but less than 2 mm in thickness.
pT2a	Without ulceration.
pT2b	With ulceration.
pT3	Tumour more than 2 mm but less than 4 mm in thickness.
pT3a	No ulceration.
pT3b	With ulceration
pT4	Tumour more than 4 mm in thickness.
pT4a	No ulceration.
pT4b	With ulceration.

97.1.10 Treatment

Patients with melanoma must have their care managed by a hospital-based multi-disciplinary team (MDT) with specialist skills.

97.1.11 Surgical Excision

Wide local excision is the most effective treatment for cutaneous melanoma. The optimal width of excision margins has been contentious. The current recommended excision margins for cutaneous melanoma are shown below. It should be noted that these recommendations are for cutaneous melanomas in all body sites. In the head and neck region, anatomical restrictions and cosmetic considerations sometimes prohibit such generous margins. Even in these circumstances, however, the width of excision should remain as uniform as possible around the lesion.

MM Recommended Excision Margins

- In situ melanoma (lentigo maligna): 5 mm peripheral margins.
- Lesions less than 1 mm thick: 1 cm excision margins.
- Lesions 1 to 2 mm thick: 1 to 2 cm excision margins.
- Lesions 2.1 to 4 mm thick: 2 to 3 cm margins (2 cm preferred).
- Lesions thicker than 4 mm: 2 to 3 cm margins.

The surgical defect after wide local excision should be closed primarily whenever possible. If primary closure is not possible, reconstruction by local flaps or skin grafts will be required. Local flaps are the preferred option when the surgical defect is on the face, because of a superior aesthetic outcome. It should be noted that grafts and flaps may interfere with the accuracy of later performed SLNB. If there is any doubt as to the adequacy of diagnosis or surgical clearance, definitive recon-struction should be delayed pending histological confirmation.

Neck nodes should be investigated by ultrasound (US)-guided fine-needle aspiration biopsy or core biopsy. Immunohistochemistry may be required to distinguish melanoma from high-grade lym-phoma. If diagnostic doubt remains, then an open biopsy may be necessary, but it should be done with a wound that can be excised if the diagnosis is confirmed, when a neck dissection is necessary. Usually, a superficial parotidectomy and neck dis-section should be performed unless the parotid gland is clear on scans and the natural lymphatic drainage of the primary site is not through the gland, whereupon the parotid can be spared.

97.1.12 Chemoradiotherapy

Primary radiotherapy is not advocated in the management of early-stage malignant melanoma other than in elderly patients with extensive facial lentigo maligna melanoma. There is no consensus that radiotherapy is beneficial following surgery, but for patients with cervical lymph node disease it is frequently used. Similarly, there is no cur-rently defined role for chemoradiation in nodal disease. Recent adjuvant trials in metastatic malig-nant melanoma have included immunotherapy (interferon, IL-2) and anti-angiogenic agents, such

S

as bevacizumab. About 50% of melanomas show a mutation in the *BRAF* gene. If this mutation is present, then patients with distant metastatic disease will have a 60 to 70% chance of responding to a BRAF inhibitor drug such as vemurafenib or dabrafenib.

97.1.13 Follow-Up

All patients should be given information and written instruction about self-surveillance. Patients who have a confirmed diagnosis should have a whole-body examination undertaken by a dermatologist.

97.2 Mucosal Melanoma of the Upper Aerodigestive Tract

Mucosal melanoma of the upper aerodigestive tract is rare and has a poor prognosis. Most patients present in the sixth decade and the most common sites of head and neck mucosal melanoma are the nasal and oral cavities. No risk factors for the development of this disease have been identified, but it is thought that there is a preceding atypical melanocytic hyperplasia.

97.2.1 Clinical Presentation

Sinonasal melanoma presents with nasal obstruction, discharge and bleeding. The commonest site is the anterior portion of the nasal septum. Oral mucosal melanoma most often presents as a painless mass on the alveolar gingiva and palate. They may or may not be pigmented and cause ulceration and bleeding.

97.2.2 Management

Imaging and endoscopic assessment should be performed for staging. Localised disease is best treated by excision with clear surgical margins. However, the outcome for extensive disease is poor. There are high rates of local recurrence and distant metastases and a median survival rate of less than 2 years. This should be remembered before radical procedures are recommended with significant morbidity inflicted on an already ill patient. Mucosal melanoma is acknowledged as a radioresistant tumour, but some authorities recommend RT to help with local control in short courses using hypofractionated schedules.

Further Reading

Ahmed OA, Kelly C. Head and neck melanoma (excluding ocular melanoma): United Kingdom National Multidisciplinary Guidelines. J Laryngol Otol. 2016; 130(S2):S133–S141

National Collaborating Centre for Cancer. Melanoma: Assessment and Management. London: National Institute for Health and Care Excellence; 2015

Kyrgidis A, Tzellos T, Mocellin S, et al. Sentinel lymph node biopsy followed by lymph node dissection for localised primary cutaneous melanoma. Cochrane Database Syst Rev. 2015(5):CD010307

Thomas JM. Where is the evidence base for benefits of sentinel node biopsy in melanoma? BMJ. 2013; 346:f675

Brierley J, Gospodarowicz M, Wittekind C. UICC TNM Classification of Malignant Tumours. 8th ed. Oxford, UK: Wiley-Blackwell; 2017

Related Topic of Interest

Skin cancer—non-melanoma

98 Skin Cancer—Non-Melanoma

This chapter deals with the diagnosis and principles of management of skin cancer. Skin cancer is the most common malignancy in the world, and its incidence is increasing. Cutaneous malignancy is divided into melanoma and non-melanoma skin cancer (NMSC).

98.1 Types of NMSC

There are several types of NMSC, but by far the most common types are basal cell carcinoma and squamous cell carcinoma.

- Basal cell carcinoma (BCC).
- Squamous cell carcinoma (SCC).
- Merkel's cell carcinoma (MCC).
- Skin appendage carcinoma (e.g. sebaceous carcinoma, micro-adnexal carcinoma).
- Sarcoma (e.g. dermatofibrosarcoma, angiosarcoma and Kaposi's sarcoma).

98.2 Aetiology

The main risk factor is sun exposure and consequently the head and neck, the hands and the forearms are the sites most commonly affected. The risk factors can be related to the individual or the environment.

98.2.1 Individual Risk Factors

- Inherent factors
  Male gender, pale complexion, fair hair, skin freckles, blue eyes and increasing age.
- Genetic syndromes
  Xeroderma pigmentosa increases the risk of developing SCC, BCC and malignant melanoma (MM). It is caused by a defect in DNA repair and synthesis. Gorlin's syndrome is characterised by multiple BCCs. Patients with albinism, epidermolysis bullosa and porokeratosis are predisposed to skin cancer.
- Immunosuppression
  Patients who have had an organ transplant are at high risk of developing all types of skin cancers because of their long-term immune suppression from medications like cyclosporin. The risk increases with time following the transplant and is higher in older patients and white-skinned people who have had

excessive sun exposure. These patients often have multiple and fast-growing tumours, which may pose difficulties in their management. Their compromised immune status is also strongly correlated to poor prognosis after treatment. Skin cancers comprise 40 to 50% of post-transplant malignancies. The place of retinoids as a prophylactic agent is promising. Individuals with AIDS are more prone to develop SCC at a younger age.
- Chronic inflammatory disorders
  Chronic scarring and inflammation are the most important risk factors in black skin. SCC may arise in the scars of skin burns or chronic ulcers (Marjolin's ulcer). Actinic keratosis can also be a precursor of cutaneous SCC and these tend to be less aggressive.

98.2.2 Environmental

- Ultraviolet (UV) radiation
  Ultraviolet exposure is the main risk factor. Individuals working outside for extended periods of time were historically most at risk, but recently recreational sun exposure has become an important predisposing cause. UVB is more carcinogenic than UVA.
- Ionising radiation
  Miners, airline pilots and patients with a past history of radiotherapy are at increased risk.
- Chemical carcinogens
  Occupational exposure to arsenic and polycyclic hydrocarbons has been implicated, as have tobacco and psoralens.

98.3 Basal Cell Carcinoma

This is the most common malignancy in humans. There are five histological subtypes which are important to identify because of their distinct clinical behaviour.

- Nodular.
- Superficial.
- Basosquamous.
- Pigmented.
- Morphoeic.

Nodular BCC is the most common and has the distinctive features of a raised rolled edge nodule, with a pearly appearance and local telangiectasia. They can be locally invasive. Central ulceration may occur and this has led to the term 'rodent ulcer'.

Superficial BCC is the least aggressive type and is characterised by dry, scaly and erythematous plaques. Basosquamous BCC is a more aggressive lesion, having histological features of BCC and SCC. It also has some metastatic potential. Pigmented BCCs tend to occur in darker-skinned individuals and may be confused with melanoma. Morphoeic BCCs are pale, indurated lesions, which have indistinct borders. As such there is a propensity to incomplete excision as they may be more extensive than they initially appear.

98.4 Squamous Cell Carcinoma of the Skin

SCC usually affects elderly males with the highest incidence in those aged 85 years or older. The lesions may arise in areas of actinic (solar) keratosis with transformation rates of 5 to 20%, or in areas of SCC in situ (Bowen's disease) where the transformation rates are only around 5%.

SCC typically presents as an enlarging firm papule or plaque that may be rough or smooth. As the tumour enlarges, it often ulcerates. It is often asymptomatic, but it can cause tenderness, itching or bleeding. Squamous cell carcinoma of the nasal vestibule is frequently misdiagnosed, feigning vestibulitis or local trauma. SCC of the ear canal is often diagnosed late as it can look like many other more common conditions of the ear canal. The lip, ear and nose are more prone to metastasise than other sun-exposed sites.

Regional metastases are uncommon, occurring in about 5%, but increases to 20 to 25% in larger and poorly differentiated tumours, recurrent tumours and those which are incompletely excised. The nodes within the parotid gland, superficial jugular nodes and upper deep cervical nodes are the usual sites.

98.4.1 Keratoacanthoma

Keratoacanthoma (KA) is classically a symmetrical, rapidly growing skin tumour, with a shoulder of stretched normal skin and a central keratin plug. These tumours reach their maximum size in 3 months and then begin to resolve spontaneously. They are now considered to be a well-differentiated SCC.

98.5 Merkel's Cell Carcinoma

This is a rare neuroendocrine tumour of the skin, so called because it is thought to arise from mechanoreceptor (Merkel) cells. It occurs most commonly in the elderly Caucasian population. Its aetiology is unknown, but ultraviolet radiation is thought to be an important factor. Merkel's cell polyomavirus has recently been linked to MCC although there is no developed clinical use for this at present. MCC is difficult to identify clinically and is often misdiagnosed as a benign lesion. It usually presents as a papule or subcutaneous nodule. These are highly aggressive tumours with a propensity to local recurrence and metastatic spread. Its nature is more often likened to MM than SCC. Patients have a poor prognosis and management should be in a specialist centre and by multi-disciplinary team (MDT). Smaller lesions may be treated by surgery, but they are also radiosensitive and adjuvant radiotherapy and chemoradiotherapy may be used for larger lesions and more extensive disease.

98.6 Investigations

The vast majority of NMSC will be suitable for immediate excision biopsy and repair without any other investigation. However, a punch biopsy for histology can be very useful before embarking on potentially disfiguring surgery of the face if the lesion is large and there is diagnostic doubt.

Clinically palpable lymph nodes should undergo fine-needle aspiration, ideally under ultrasound control, for cytological diagnosis. In NMSC cases, magnetic resonance imaging (MRI) and computed tomography (CT) can help to stage the disease particularly if there is concern that it may involve underlying structures (e.g. scalp lesions invading the skull or the maxillary spine in SCC of the columella). Scans are not needed in the N0 neck but can help define the presence of metastatic nodal disease in high-risk cases and palpable disease. A CT scan of the chest may be important in high-risk cases to exclude lung metastases.

98.7 Staging Systems

The TNM staging system for NMSC has been problematic, but continues to evolve with available data. Many other systems have been advocated (e.g. the O'Brien P/N system or the Wang system) and have their uses, but are not universally accepted. The current TNM staging for NMSC is described below for T-stage. N staging follows that of mucosal head and neck cancers.

98.7.1 TNM Staging System 8th Edition for NMSC

TX Primary tumour cannot be assessed.

T0 No evidence of primary tumour.

Tis Carcinoma in situ.

T1 Tumour 2 cm or less in greatest dimension.

T2 Tumour is greater than 2 cm but less than 4 cm.

T3 Tumour is greater than 4 cm in greatest dimension or minor bone erosion or peri neural invasion or deep invasion (invasion beyond the subcutaneous fat or > 6 mm).

T4a Tumour with gross cortical bone/marrow invasion.

T4b Tumour with skull base or axial skeleton invasion (i.e. foramen of skull base or verte bral invasion).

98.8 Treatment

Surgical excision of head and neck skin cancer is the mainstay of treatment. Many patients with pre-cancerous, small, and low-risk lesions will have their procedures performed in the community and non-specialist units. Patients with SCC, high-risk BCC and melanoma must have their care managed by a hospital-based MDT with specialist skills. The following patients should be discussed in a skin cancer MDT:

- All patents with SCC.
- High-risk BCCs (larger tumours, involved margins and recurrent lesions).
- Patients with suspected melanoma.
- Patients with an unusual or rare skin cancer.
- Patients considered for Mohs' surgery.
- High-risk patients (immunocompromised, genetically predisposed conditions).
- Metastatic disease.
- Patients considered for radiotherapy.
- Patients for clinical trials.

98.8.1 Surgical Excision

Local, complete and primary excision with a pre-determined margin is the aim. The recommended margins for NMSC differ in the available guidelines, but acceptable ranges for the *minimum* margin are below. The deep margin should include fat. Histological confirmation of clearance can be confirmed by utilising Mohs' micrographic surgery, frozen section or waiting for results from paraffin section. It is always good practice to mark resected specimens with an ori-entation suture, so that further excision can target the close or involved margin if necessary.

98.8.2 NMSC Recommended Excision Margins

- BCC more than 2 cm should be excised with a 4- to 5-mm margin.
- Low-risk SCC should be excised with a margin of 4 to 5 mm. High-risk SCC should be excised with greater than 6-mm margin.
- SCCs that are larger than 2 cm should have at least a 6- to 10-mm margin.
- Lesions with high risk of recurrence should be treated with delayed reconstruction or Mohs' micrographic surgery.

Ideally, the surgical defect after excision should be closed primarily. If primary closure is not possible, reconstruction by a local flap or skin graft will be required. Local flaps are the preferred option when the surgical defect is on the face, because of better skin match and so a superior aesthetic outcome. Rarely, distant flaps will be required for complex or very large surgical defects. If there is any doubt as to the adequacy of surgical clearance, definitive reconstruction should be delayed pending histological confirmation. Incompletely excised lesions should be discussed at the MDT. Re-excision would be recommended for all incompletely excised SCCs and high-risk BCCs or where there is deep margin involvement.

Elective neck dissection is not done routinely for NMSC as there is no evidence to show that it improves mortality, and it adds to the patient's morbidity. If parotid lymphadenopathy is present, then a neck dissection (levels I–III) should also be performed as a high proportion of patients with parotid lymph node involvement will have occult cervical metastases. Patients with parotid and neck nodes need a parotidectomy and levels I to V selective neck dissection.

98.8.3 Mohs' Micrographic Surgery

Mohs' micrographic surgery is a precise technique in which excision of the skin is carried out in stages and each stage checked histologically. It is advocated for use in cases where it is critical to obtain a clear margin while preserving the maximum amount of normal surrounding tissue. Its use is encouraged for recurrent and high-risk aggressive growth pattern BCCs such as morphoeic type BCCs and SCCs. Mohs' surgery may have a role in the primary treatment of cutaneous melanoma of the head and neck, especially that of the face. The main problems with this technique include the length of the procedure, the need for special equipment and training and the relatively high cost. However, there is good evidence that both local recurrence and metastases are lower after Mohs' micrographic surgery and because tissue removal is minimised, there are better cosmetic outcomes.

98.8.4 Radiotherapy

The cure rates for radiotherapy are over 90% for most NMSC lesions, but the long-term cosmesis, particularly for young patients, is often inferior to that following other treatments and there is an increased risk of secondary malignancies. However, radiotherapy is a useful treatment for a sub-set of patients with NMSC who cannot, or prefer not to, be treated by surgery. Radiotherapy still has an important role in the treatment of elderly patients, and as an alternative to mutilating surgery in the treatment of advanced disease. It has a role in the palliative treatment of patients with large, inoperable and recurrent SCC, or if there are inoperable metastases in lymph nodes or elsewhere. Post-operative radiotherapy can be used in cases when the margins of excision appear to be incomplete on histopathological examination, although this is not desirable. It also has a role in adjuvant treatment of extracapsular nodal disease following neck dissection.

98.8.5 Destructive Techniques

1. Curettage and cautery
   This technique is performed using a curette to remove the tumour and the base of the tumour destroyed using either hyfrecation or cautery. It should only be used by experienced practitioners and may be used to treat small well-defined BCCs (< 4 mm) and in situ SCCs (< 1 cm). It is safe and well tolerated, and usually produces a good cosmetic outcome. It is suitable for patients with multiple lesions. However, the histology may be difficult to interpret as the lesion may be incompletely removed and margins of excision cannot be assessed.

2. Cryotherapy/cryosurgery
   Cryotherapy is the destruction of skin lesions using liquid nitrogen. It is a cost-effective treatment and may be used in specialised centres for low-risk superficial BCC and in situ SCC. It is, however, inadvisable to use cryotherapy if SCC is suspected unless an incisional biopsy is taken first to confirm the diagnosis of an in situ SCC.

3. Photodynamic therapy
   Photodynamic therapy (PDT) involves the use of light therapy in combination with a topical photosensitising agent to destroy cancer cells. Its use has been well described in the treatment of KA, in situ SCC and superficial BCC. The advantages claimed of PDT include a low rate of adverse effects and good cosmesis. The disadvantages are that the patient must be available for a period of at least 3 to 4 hours for treatment, and that the photosensitiser and equipment are relatively expensive. It is not recommended for invasive SCC.

4. Topical drug therapies
   There are number of topical drug therapies including the immune response modifier imiquimod and 5-fluorouracil cream. These are effective treatments for small primary superficial BCCs and in situ SCC.

98.9 Follow-Up

All patients should be given information and written instruction about self-surveillance. Patients who have a confirmed diagnosis of SCC should have a whole-body examination undertaken by a dermatologist. Patients with completely excised BCC or low-risk SCCs do not need long-term surveillance and should be discharged from formal follow-up when they have fully recovered from the treatment. Those patients with a recurrent or multiple BCCs and those with a high-risk SCC should be reviewed for 2 to 5 years.

S

Further Reading

Brierley J, Gospodarowicz M, Wittekind C. UICC TNM Classification of Malignant Tumours. 8th ed. Oxford, UK: Wiley-
Blackwell; 2017

Martin RCW, Clark J. Non-melanoma and melanoma skin cancer.
Stell and Maran's Textbook of Head and Neck Surgery and Oncology. 5th ed. Arnold, London: Hodder; 2012:734–753

Newlands C, Currie R, Memon A, Whitaker S, Woolford T.
Non-melanoma skin cancer: United Kingdom National Multidisciplinary Guidelines. J Laryngol Otol. 2016;
130(S2):S125–S132

Telfer NR, Colver GB, Morton CA; British Association of Derma-
tologists. Guidelines for the management of basal cell carcinoma. Br J Dermatol. 2008; 159(1):35–48

Related Topics of Interest

Cervical lymphadenopathy
Reconstructive surgery
Skin cancer—melanoma

S

99 Smell and Taste Disorders

The sense of smell and taste are phylogenetically our oldest sensory modalities. Smell and taste disorders are under-reported and increase with age. It is important to appreciate that these disorders have a significant impact on quality of life. In the elderly, they may be one of the first signs of cognitive impairment that leads to Alzheimer's disease. The patient's mental state may be affected by smell and taste disorders, there being an increased incidence of depression, seasonal affective disorder and anorexia.

99.1 Epidemiology

Studies have found that on objective testing, about 25% of adults over 50 years and 60% over the age of 80 have olfactory impairment. Of those tested, only 10% had self-reported a reduction to their GP suggesting that symptoms are significantly under-reported.

99.2 Terminology

Anosmia—an inability to detect an odour.
Hyposmia—a reduced sense of olfaction.
Dysosmia—distorted or inappropriate sense of olfaction which can be sub-classified into the following:

a. Parosmia—an altered perception of an odour. If this altered perception is an unpleasant odour, then it is called cacosmia.
b. Phantosmia—the perception of an odour when none is present.
c. Agnosia—an ability to detect but not differentiate/interpret different odours.

Ageusia—an inability to detect taste.
Hypogeusia—a reduced sense of taste.
Dysgeusia—a distorted sense of taste which can be sub-classified into the following:

a. Parageusia—an altered perception of taste. If this altered perception is unpleasant, then it is called cacogeusia.
b. Phantogeusia—the perception of a taste when none is present.
c. Agnosia—the ability to detect but not differentiate/interpret different tastes.

There are three chemosensory contributions to smell and taste:

1. Olfaction.
2. Gustation.
3. Common chemical sensation.

99.3 Physiology

Olfaction is provided by an area of specialised pseudostratified neuroepithelium in the vault of the nasal cavity. It extends from the cribriform plate onto the nasal septum medially and onto the medial aspects of the superior and middle turbinates laterally, as far as the anterior margin of the vertical attachment of the middle turbinate to the lateral lamina of the lamina cribrosa. Odorant molecules (those molecules with the ability to bind and stimulate olfactory receptors) are carried into the nasal cavity with inspiratory and expiratory airflow. They may then dissolve in, and diffuse through, the overlying mucus, or they may combine with specific odorant-binding proteins and be transported through the overlying mucus layer. The free molecules or odorant/protein complexes then attach to receptor proteins, resulting in the production of an intracellular secondary messenger (usually cyclic adenosine monophosphate [AMP]), with subsequent cell depolarisation and a neural action potential. The olfactory neurons pass through the cribriform plate and sensory information passes to the olfactory bulb and then onto the thalamus, hypothalamus and olfactory cortex. The different odorants have different rates and degrees of solubility in the overlying mucus. Neither do all olfactory receptors respond identically to a particular odorant, nor are the olfactory receptors equally distributed in the nasal cavity. It is likely that all these factors have a bearing on smell recognition.

Gustation is served by the taste buds, which are modified epithelial cells found throughout the oral cavity, although there are regional differences in their concentration and distribution. There are concentrations of taste buds in three types of papillae on the tongue.

E

1. Fungiform papillae. Located on the anterior two-thirds of the tongue, there are about 30 papillae each with about 100 taste buds supplied by the chorda tympani.
2. Circumvallate papillae. Located at the junction of the middle third and posterior third of the tongue, there are about 12 papillae each with about 250 taste buds supplied by the glossopharyngeal nerve.
3. Foliate papillae. Located in the folds of the lateral border of the tongue and housing 1,000 to 1,500 taste buds supplied by the glossopharyngeal nerve.

Note that the filiform papillae, which coat the anterior two-thirds of the tongue (and which are absent in patches in geographic tongue), do not have taste buds.

Bitter tastes are better perceived on the posterior tongue, sweet and salt on the anterior tongue and sour on the lateral border. A fifth taste sense, umami, is a savoury sense due to its recognising glutamate and is the reason why monosodium glutamate may be added to certain foods. Neural stimulation occurs after dissolution of the tastant in a similar fashion to olfaction although the neural pathways are more complex. Several different cranial nerves are involved, with their primary afferents synapsing in the tractus solitarius in the medulla, before sensation passes onto the thalamus and cortex.

Common chemical sensation (irritation, heat and textural quality) and pain are served by free nerve endings from branches of the trigeminal nerve in the oral cavity and nose with a contribution from the glossopharyngeal and vagus nerves in the oropharynx. These fibres are stimulated by (unpleasant) mechanical, thermal or chemical stimuli. Information is ultimately passed to the cortex via the thalamus.

99.4 Aetiology of Olfactory Disturbance

It is uncommon for common chemical sensation or taste to be lost; there is much redundancy in the neural supply and the sensory distribution is relatively wide. It is more likely that olfaction may be lost or impaired. Most patients who have lost or had a reduction in the sense of olfaction will complain of a reduction in their taste sense

when there is none because olfaction enhances taste sense. Olfaction and taste sense reduce with increasing age. The aetiology can be compared with the classification of hearing loss and fall into three main groups: conductive or impaired transport, sensory and neural.

The main causes of disorders of olfaction are as follows:

1. Sinonasal disease (20–30%) causes a conductive and occasionally a sensory reduction or loss of olfaction. In most cases, this is due to a mechanical obstruction (polyps, mucosal swelling in rhinitis, etc.) preventing odorants from reaching the olfactory epithelium in the narrow nasal vault, although in some cases the local inflammatory response may alter the overlying mucus or injure the receptor cells.
2. Upper respiratory tract infection (15–20%) can cause a sensory loss due to an injury to the peripheral olfactory receptors by a neurotrophic virus.
3. Head injury (20%) may cause a neural injury from shearing of the olfactory filaments as they pass through the cribriform plate or direct contusion of the olfactory bulb or cortex.
4. Idiopathic (20%). Probably many are due to an injury of the sensory receptors from a sub-clinical neurotrophic upper respiratory tract (URT) viral infection.
5. Others (15–20%). Systemic disease, causing nasal granulomatosis such as sarcoidosis or Wegener's granulomatosis with polyangiitis, endocrine dysfunction (diabetes mellitus, hypothyroidism), metabolic and connective tissue disorders, drug therapy (aminoglycosides and some chemotherapy agents), neurological and degenerative brain conditions (Parkinson's disease, Alzheimer's disease, motor neuron disease [MND] and multiple sclerosis), toxin exposure (intranasal zinc products and formaldehyde), iatrogenic from septoplasty or sinus/anterior skull base surgery, sinonasal malignancy, radiotherapy or as an age effect.

99.5 Aetiology of Gustatory Disturbance

Loss of olfaction without injury to the taste buds may reduce gustation because olfaction enhances the perception of taste. The causes of gustatory loss include many of the causes of olfactory loss and include a URT infection (URTI), head injury, drugs, neurological or degenerative brain conditions, endocrine disorders, poor oral hygiene, malignancy of the oral cavity and surgery to treat malignancy, radiotherapy to the oral cavity, nutritional deficiency (decreased zinc, copper and nickel levels from anorexia or malabsorption), HIV, systemic disease (Sjögren's syndrome as part of calcinosis, Raynaud's phenomenon, oesophageal dysmotility, sclerodactyly and telangiectasia [CREST] or other autoimmune disease, cirrhosis and renal failure with uraemia).

99.6 Investigations

A thorough history must be taken and a note made of upper respiratory infection or head injury. A full upper aerodigestive tract examination, including nasopharyngoscopy, should be undertaken to establish a local cause. Computed tomography (CT) and/or magnetic resonance imaging (MRI) of the sinuses may be required. Further general investigations will be dictated by the clinical features and may include an objective measurement of olfaction. Commercial 'scratch and sniff' kits are available using a forced choice technique which greatly increase their sensitivity, for example, the University of Pennsylvania Smell Identification Test (UPSIT). Evaluation of taste is not as well developed but taste strips with varying concentrations of four taste senses (sweet, sour, salt and bitter) are available. They can be useful for deciding if a patient is suffering from a smell or taste disorder or suggest they may be malingering.

99.7 Management

Sinonasal disease should be managed as appropriate to the condition. It has the best prognosis in terms of response to treatment. Reassurance regarding the absence of serious pathology should be stressed to the post-URTI and head injury groups. A small proportion in both groups (10–20%) will improve with the passage of time. A nasal steroid spray is a reasonable treatment in the rhinitis, post-URTI or idiopathic group of patients. The steroid is an anti-inflammatory and may create an environment advantageous to recovery of olfaction. Zinc and magnesium supplements have been reported as helpful.

Systemic causes are treated as for that condition and drug-induced problems may require a change of medication. Interestingly, loss of sense of smell seems to provoke a disproportionate degree of emotional upset and even depression which may require specific treatment.

Further Reading

Allis TJ, Leopold DA. Smell and taste disorders. Facial Plast Surg Clin North Am. 2012; 20(1):93–111
Hüttenbrink KB, Hummel T, Berg D, Gasser T, Hähner A. Olfactory dysfunction: common in later life and early warning of neurodegenerative disease. Dtsch Arztebl Int. 2013; 110 (1–2): 1–7, e1

Related Topics of Interest

Rhinitis–allergic
Halitosis
Rhinitis—non-allergic
Rhinosinusitis–chronic (with nasal polyps)

100 Snoring and Sleep-Related Breathing Disorder

Sleep-related breathing disorder is a spectrum of breathing disorders occurring during sleep and comprises simple snoring, upper airway resistance syndrome and obstructive sleep apnoea.

100.1 Definitions

- Snoring: A noise generated from turbulence due to partial upper airway obstruction during sleep.
- Apnoea: A period of no airflow at the nose or mouth for at least 10 seconds.
- Hypopnoea: Breathing where there is a 30% or greater reduction in normal tidal volume.
- Apnoea–hypopnoea index (AHI): The number of periods of apnoea and hypopnoea per hour.

Sleep apnoea can be obstructive, central or mixed. In obstructive sleep apnoea, there is partial (hypopnoea) or complete (apnoea) upper airway obstruction yet the patient continues to make respiratory efforts to overcome this. In central apnoea, respiratory effort and consequently airflow, ceases for a while. Central apnoea is due to a defect of autonomic control of respiration in the medulla or in the peripheral chemoreceptors resulting in a failure of respiratory drive. It is a symptom of serious neurological disease and is not considered further here.

Obstructive sleep apnoea (OSA) is diagnosed if the AHI is more than 5. Obstructive sleep apnoea is classified as mild (AHI = 5–15), moderate (AHI = 15–30) or severe (AHI > 30).

Upper airway resistance syndrome (UARS) is diagnosed if the AHI is less than 5 but patients have some of the symptoms and signs of OSA. Patients with UARS may progress to OSA if factors that are contributing to UARS are not addressed.

100.2 Pathophysiology

The noise of snoring is produced by vibration of the soft palate and pharyngeal walls caused by turbulent airflow and the Bernoulli effect from a partial obstruction. The obstruction occurs when the negative intra-luminal pharyngeal pressure exceeds the ability of the dilators to hold the pharynx open. Any cause of airway narrowing from nares to glottis can contribute to increased airway resistance. Neuromuscular incoordination interfering with the reflex activity of the pharyngeal dilators associated with inspiration, increased compliance and bulk of pharyngeal tissues, the Venturi effect and the decreased muscle tone associated with sleep can all predispose to upper airway collapse. This obstruction has three effects:

1. Hypoxia, which may cause cardiac dysrhythmias, and if severe and prolonged may lead to pulmonary and systemic hypertension and cor pulmonale.
2. Increased negative intrathoracic pressure and increased cardiovascular strain.
3. Arousal, which is an attempt to overcome the obstruction and caused by increased serum levels of carbon dioxide. Frequent arousal results in poor sleep quality.

Patients with severe OSA have an increased mortality due to cardiovascular disease.

100.2.1 Clinical Features

Snoring and OSA in adults are more common with increasing age, in men (2:1 M/F ratio), in the obese (body mass index [BMI] > 30), in those with a neck size of more than 17 inches and in those with a high alcohol intake. Snoring occurs in 10% of men under 30 years and 40% of men over 60 years, while OSA can be found in approximately 6% of men. In children, it most commonly occurs around the age of 5 when lymphoid hyperplasia is at its greatest. Snoring can be immensely socially disruptive and may lead to marital difficulties. OSA often leads to excessive daytime somnolence, morning headaches, personality change including depression, intellectual deterioration (inattention, memory loss and poor work performance), reduced libido and impotence and an increased risk of causing a road traffic accident. The DVLA should be informed of a diagnosis of OSA; it is the doctor's responsibility to alert the patient of this need, and it is the patient's responsibility to carry this out.

It is important to establish whether the patient has simple snoring, UARS or OSA and to identify exacerbating factors, for example, medication causing drowsiness, endocrine disorders such as hypothyroidism or diabetes. One should try to identify the site and level of obstruction including anatomical factors such as retrognathia or benign tonsillar hyperplasia. A thorough history and examination is needed. When taking the history, it is preferable to have the bed partner present.

100.2.2 Investigations

1. *Body mass index* This measurement helps define the degree of obesity. It is calculated by dividing the weight in kilograms by the square of the height in metres (kg/m^2). A normal BMI is 19 to 25, overweight 26 to 30, obese 30 to 40 and very obese greater than 40. Palatal surgery is less effective in patients with a body mass index of greater than 30. This is probably because these patients are more likely to have OSA caused by multi-segmental or tongue base level collapse.

2. *General investigations* Full blood count (FBC), thyroid function tests (TFTs), chest radiograph and electrocardiogram (ECG).

3. *Epworth sleepiness scale* This is a self-scoring questionnaire to identify those who may have OSA and therefore should have a sleep study. Eight situations are described and for each situation the patients must score themselves according to their chance of dozing.
The situations are described below:

   a. Sitting reading a book.
   b. Watching television.
   c. Sitting inactive in a public place, for example, a meeting or theatre.
   d. Lying down to rest in the afternoon when circumstances permit.
   e. Sitting talking to someone.
   f. Sitting quietly after lunch without alcohol.
   g. In a car, stopped in traffic or at traffic lights.
   h. In a car, as a passenger for an hour.

   The situations are scored as below:
   0   Would never doze.
   1   Slight chance of dozing.
   2   Moderate chance of dozing.
   3   High chance of dozing.

Interpretation of total score/24 is as follows:
0–5   Low normal daytime sleepiness.
6–10   High normal daytime sleepiness.
11–12   Mild excessive daytime sleepiness.
13–15   Moderate excessive daytime sleepiness.
16–24   Severe excessive daytime sleepiness.

Those with a score of 11 or higher should be referred for a sleep study to determine if the patient has UARS or OSA.

4. *To identify sleep apnoea* An overnight sleep study. Polysomnography is the gold standard and involves recording an electroencephalogram (EEG), electromyogram (EMG) (to detect periodic limb movements), ECG, airflow, abdominal and chest movements, oxygen saturation, body position monitor and microphone recording of the snoring. This is expensive in terms of time and equipment but is an ideal research tool. Effective screening sleep studies may be performed. Overnight pulse oximetry alone will detect all those with severe OSA but may provide some false-positive results if the oximeter is not secured and may miss some patients with moderate OSA. It does not detect arousals, which are triggered by high negative intrathoracic pressure and low serum CO_2 rather than hypoxia and may not distinguish between UARS and mild OSA.

5. *Site of obstruction* To differentiate between palatal and tongue base or multi-segmental obstruction, a variety of tests have been developed to assess the dynamic airway including sleep nasopharyngoscopy, drug-induced sedation endoscopy and, the most widely used test, the Muller manoeuvre. This involves positioning, per nasally, a flexible fibre-optic endoscope to the level of the tongue base with the patient in the sitting position and with the mouth closed. The patient inhales vigorously while the nares and mouth are occluded (akin to sucking through a straw) and the degree of hypopharyngeal collapse noted. The manoeuvre is then repeated with the endoscope positioned just above the soft palate (velopharyngeal level). This allows the level and degree of obstruction to be identified in up to 85% of cases.

100.2.3 Treatment

Snoring and OSA are often multi-factorial conditions with a variety of primary causative factors, hence there will never be a single treatment to cure snoring. Accurate assessment is essential and will guide treatment. Weight loss to reduce BMI to the normal weight range (< 25) may reduce neck size and tongue base bulk. Exercise helps to increase palatal and pharyngeal muscle tone which in turn helps to prevent airway collapse in the presence of negative pharyngeal pressure. In the early evening, exercise promotes restfulness too.

Good sleep hygiene All patients with sleep-related breathing disorder will benefit from practising good sleep hygiene. This means getting into good habits and practices and creating the correct environment for a better-quality sleep.

Personal habits

- Establish a regular bedtime routine, getting to bed and rising at similar times each day.
- Regular exercise helps to reduce stress, anxiety and depression. Exercise, particularly late afternoon exercise, can cause somnolence a few hours later when the body has recovered and cooled, allowing sleep to come more readily. Avoid vigorous exercise too close to bedtime.
- Eating healthily and not too close to bedtime.
- Avoid caffeine, nicotine and alcohol close to bedtime (within 4 hours ideally) as these may act as stimulants.
- Our circadian rhythm is triggered by light and darkness, so try to be outdoors for periods during the day and evening and have minimal light when sleeping.
- Some find relaxation techniques such as yoga or meditating help to relax the mind and promote restfulness.

Sleep environment

- Associate the bedroom with sleep. Do not watch television or look at electronic devices.
- Keep the bedroom dark so as not to disrupt one's circadian rhythm, quiet and cool.
- Have a comfortable bed.

100.3 Nasal Obstruction

Medical treatment of rhinitis, the use of the 'Nozovent' nasal splint or Breathe Right nasal strips to open the nasal valve or surgical correction of a septal deviation, turbinate hypertrophy or nasal polyps may all help snoring by overcoming nasal obstruction. If nasal continuous positive airway pressure (CPAP) or pharyngeal surgery are

contemplated, nasal obstruction should be corrected first.

Oropharyngeal obstruction causing simple snoring and OSA.

1. Uvulopalatopharyngoplasty (UPPP) involves tonsillectomy and excision of the uvula. Laser palatoplasty involves excision of the uvula and scarring of the soft palate with the laser in a variety of ways to induce palatal stiffness. This surgery can be very painful and complications include nasopharyngeal reflux, pharyngeal stenosis and a dry mouth.
2. Laser-assisted uvulopalatoplasty (LAUP) is a technique in which the uvula is vapourised by the laser and troughs created through the soft palate to each side of the uvula base to form a neo-uvula. LAUP is sometimes performed under a local anaesthetic.
3. Somnoplasty. Low-temperature radiofrequency energy (coblation) is delivered via a needle placed into the soft palate. This results in an area of scarring and hence stiffening of the soft palate. It is recommended for certain individuals with simple snoring.
4. In 2011, a polar bear–shaped pillow fitted with a robotic arm and called Jukusui-Kun, which gently brushes the snorer's cheek when loud snoring or reduced oxygen saturations are detected, was described in Japan. No trial of Jukusui-Kun has yet been published.

All these procedures, except Jukusui-Kun, have an initial 75 to 85% success rate in significantly reducing snoring. This success rate reduces with time because patients continue to suffer reducing pharyngeal muscle tone with age and may also gain weight. Further palatal stiffening with a laser or coblation may be required.

5. Adenotonsillectomy. In children, OSA is in most cases adequately dealt with by adenotonsillectomy as this is the usual site of obstruction. With a history of OSA sedative premed should be avoided.

100.4 Continuous Positive Airway Obstruction

In moderate-to-severe OSA due to tongue base and multi-segmental airway collapse, surgery is not particularly effective and anaesthetic risk

S

is significant. Nasal CPAP is the gold standard treatment. Air under pressure is delivered via a tight-fitting nasal mask. The air acts as a pneumatic splint holding the upper airway open and thus preventing snoring and obstructive episodes. It can be extremely effective, but compliance is often a problem, even with the newer, smaller masks. The latest AutoSet devices are more expensive but much better tolerated. They have sensors that detect obstructive episodes and they can then intermittently deliver positive pressure respiration.

100.5 Maxillofacial

1. Mandibular positioning devices. This appliance is worn in the mouth overnight. It is like an upper and lower gum shield attached in such a way as to bring the lower jaw forward. This in turn draws the tongue base forward enlarging the oropharyngeal airway. Long-term tolerance of these devices can be poor. The long-term effects on the temporomandibular joints are not known.
2. Hyoid suspension techniques to advance the hyoid and hence move the tongue base forward have been tried with some success. In retrognathia, mandibular osteotomies may be required. In patients with morbid obesity and life-threatening obstructive sleep apnoea,

bi-maxillary and bi-mandibular advancement osteotomies have been performed together with significant success rates reported.

100.6 Tracheostomy

In severe OSA, when all other forms of treatment have failed, a tracheostomy can be lifesaving and, in such patients, significantly improve their quality of life.

Further Reading

Lazard DS, Blumen M, Lévy P, et al. The tongue-retaining device: efficacy and side effects in obstructive sleep apnea syndrome. J Clin Sleep Med. 2009; 5(5):431–438

Marin JM, Carrizo SJ, Vicente E, Agusti AG. Long-term cardiovascular outcomes in men with obstructive sleep apnoea-hypopnoea with or without treatment with continuous positive airway pressure: an observational study. Lancet. 2005; 365(9464):1046–1053

Smith I, Nadig V, Lasserson TJ. Educational, supportive and behavioural interventions to improve usage of continuous positive airway pressure machines for adults with obstructive sleep apnoea. Cochrane Database Syst Rev. 2009(2):CD007736

Related Topics of Interest

Adenoids
Tonsillectomy
Tracheostomy

101 Speech and Swallow Rehabilitation Following Head and Neck Surgery

Swallow and communication rehabilitation are required following head and neck cancer surgery as a result of alteration to the anatomy and physiology. The speech and language therapist (SLT) provides assessment, diagnosis and treatment of speech, language, voice and swallowing problems from the point of diagnosis throughout and beyond surgical and non-surgical treatment. The therapy provided by the SLT focuses on either rehabilitating the individual's swallow or communication compromise or providing compensatory strategies to optimise function. There are physical, emotional and psychosocial components to this therapeutic intervention.

101.1 Background

The nature of the therapeutic intervention provided by the SLT is dependent on the aetiology of the dysfunction, the degree of compromise the individual presents with, the rehabilitation potential and the patient's engagement with the therapeutic process. In order to provide appropriate rehabilitation, it is fundamental that the normal swallow process is first understood.

101.1.1 Normal Swallow Function

Swallow function is dependent on the sequencing and timing of oral, pharyngeal and laryngeal musculature to broadly facilitate the following tasks:

- Achieve adequate closure of the lips.
- Mastication.
- Creation of intraoral pressure.
- Propulsion of the food or fluid bolus from the anterior to the posterior oral cavity.
- Lift and closure of the soft palate against the pharynx.
- Approximation of the tongue base against the posterior pharyngeal wall.
- Closure of the laryngeal inlet.
- Raise and anterior tilt of the larynx and hyoid, facilitating epiglottic retroflexion and opening of the cricopharyngeus.
- Pharyngeal stripping and tightening of the superior, medial and inferior constrictors.
- Oesophageal motility.

Head and neck surgery may alter this normal sequence in a variety of ways, at any phase of the swallow. Patients with dysphagia may present in the following ways: coughing before, during or after swallow, describing pain on swallow, reporting recurrent chest infections or describing a sensation of food sticking; this list is not exhaustive. Rehabilitation interventions from the SLT must be based on careful and comprehensive assessment to ensure the correct therapy is provided to treat the presenting issue.

101.1.2 Compensatory and Rehabilitation Strategies

Strategies to improve swallow function may include the following:

- Postural changes to alter the direction and speed of bolus flow.
- Manoeuvres to augment the timing and physiological components of swallow.
- Exercise regimens to maintain and improve targeted muscle strength.
- Heat or flavour stimulation to improve sensory awareness.
- Alteration to the viscosity of food or drinks to facilitate safe transit through the pharynx reducing the risk of penetration or aspiration.

These interventions are prescribed with the aim of either rehabilitating swallow to recover function or compensating with strategies to optimise function. Rehabilitation following salvage surgery may be challenging as a result of delayed healing, wound breakdown and the potential for fistula formation. These parameters should be described to patients, so they are counselled appropriately for the potential for a prolonged recovery.

101.2 Oral Cavity Surgery

Oral cavity reconstruction may alter the function of the articulators and muscle groups including the tongue, floor of mouth, buccal cavity and palate, all fundamental for effective speech and swallow. In broad terms, the tumour size, the number of swallow structures involved and the degree of swallow dysfunction at the point of diagnosis are useful indicators regarding expected function following surgery.

101.2.1 Pre-Operative Assessment

Rehabilitation for dysphagia following oral cavity reconstruction can begin at the 'pre-treatment' assessment. An assessment of swallow using various fluid and food types may be undertaken, where the SLT will advise on particular strategies to improve swallow competence. This intervention is provided to optimise swallow pre-operatively, to reduce the potential impact of dysphagia, and to attempt to facilitate early understanding of what rehabilitation entails. It also provides the individual with the opportunity to meet the clinical team, ask questions and consider the impact of the surgery, with the support of their carers and/or family.

Compensatory strategies at the pre-operative phase may involve postural changes, dietary modifications and/or swallow manoeuvres. At presentation, people with oral cavity cancer frequently report pain on mastication, and weight loss. In this circumstance, the SLT may suggest the patients to tilt their head during swallow to the side of their mouth unaffected by the tumour to utilise the most effective musculature. Conversely, if a patient presents with a vocal cord palsy, and laryngeal phase dysphagia, the SLT may advise that the patients turn their head to the side of the palsy, to reduce the impact of the laryngeal incompetence and the vocal cord palsy. Manoeuvres such as an effortful swallow may also be added to this intervention to improve the efficiency of swallow.

101.2.2 Post-Operative Assessment

Communication and swallow may be optimised by assessing the patients from the first or second post-operative day, during their stay in the intensive care unit. In this circumstance, therapy may be provided to enable the patient to communicate when they have a tracheostomy in place, which compromises their ability to make their needs known following surgery. The SLT may provide information on ways the patient may mouth words and use non-verbal means of communication. The SLT can also facilitate timely decannulation of the tracheostomy by enabling the individual to either swallow and/or expectorate excess saliva effectively and safely.

101.2.3 Dysphagia Rehabilitation

Swallow assessment following oral cavity surgery usually happens from day 3 to 7 post-operatively, dependent on surgeon preference, institutional norms, type of reconstruction and whether the patient has received previous chemo- and or radiotherapy. Swallow assessment may begin with clear fluids only to assess for any presence of fistula. Once the teams are convinced the surgical site is patent, the patient is likely to progress to free fluids and diet. This usually begins with single texture or pureed consistencies and builds up to mixed textures and soft foods as the post-operative oedema reduces.

Swallow rehabilitation may be provided for some time beyond discharge from the inpatient ward. However, an aim of the early post-operative intervention from the SLT is to improve function to a point that the patient can manage enough oral intake and return to activities of daily living outside of the acute hospital in a meaningful way. Patients may leave hospital swallowing various consistencies of fluid or diet in order that they may return home safely without the requirement for alternative means of feeding such as a nasogastric (NG) tube. It is unrealistic to expect the swallow will have returned to 'normal' at the point of discharge.

101.2.4 Speech Rehabilitation

Speech rehabilitation tends to focus on placement and approximation of the articulators within the surgically altered oral cavity, so that consonant and vowel sounds may be achieved effectively. This may include the provision of specific exercises, as well as demonstrating and enabling the individual to create voice and sounds in appropriate ways. The person who has undergone oral cavity surgery requires encouragement and support to manage the difficulties associated with altered speech function. This includes supporting the individual to cope with the embarrassment and isolation which may accompany altered speech and swallow function. The relationship between depression and disfigurement has been identified, which highlights the value of acknowledging both the

S

psychosocial and physical compromises patients may experience.

101.3 Laryngeal Surgery

Laryngeal surgery alters the protection of the airway pre-, intra- and post swallow. The specific impact of partial laryngeal surgery, either supracricoid or vertical partial hemi-laryngectomy, is different to total laryngectomy, and therefore requires specific rehabilitation strategy and preparation.

101.3.1 Pre-Operative Assessment

At the pre-operative phase, the individual undergoing any type of laryngeal surgery requires specific information from the MDT about the planned surgical intervention. This includes accessible and appropriate information about not only what the operation involves and the structures and function it will alter, but also the expected long-term outcomes and rehabilitative aims. It is only with this information that patients may engage most effectively and have the opportunity to best understand their forthcoming surgery.

It is fundamental that people who undergo laryngectomy have the opportunity to meet a person who has undergone this surgery previously, so that they may observe the stoma, understand the concept of surgical voice restoration and the reality of life beyond laryngectomy. In rare cases, meeting someone who uses oesophageal speech or an electrolarynx may be most appropriate, although this is the exception rather than the rule. Primary puncture at the point of surgery is the usual practice in the United Kingdom.

People who undergo partial laryngeal surgery should be seen by the SLT and the surgeon in joint consultations, so that information on surgery and function may be tailored accordingly. This group of patients also benefit from meeting a person who has undergone similar surgery. Explanation of the practical impact of the surgical procedure on voice and swallow is required to inform the patient's expectations. The selection of appropriate individuals to undergo this type of surgery is important and the following parameters should inform the process: the chronological versus biological age, comorbidity and pulmonary function, cognition, motivation and engagement in the challenging rehabilitation process.

Pre-operative exercises may also be provided by the SLT including the Masako manoeuvre (to improve base of tongue to posterior pharyngeal wall function), Mendelsohn manoeuvre (to improve laryngeal elevation and duration of upper oesophageal opening) or the supraglottic swallow (to close the vocal cords pre-swallow and protect laryngeal inlet). This helps to prepare the patient for the nature of the post-operative rehabilitation, and to practice the techniques before surgery.

Advice, support and counselling should also be provided by the SLT to address the psychosocial and emotional impact of the diagnosis and planned treatment. The administration and collection of quality of life and functional outcomes should not be overlooked, as these tools enable the clinician and the individual to quantify, determine and track both the degree of presenting dysfunction and its impact on day-to-day life.

101.3.2 Post-Operative Assessment

Following laryngectomy, there is a nil by mouth phase to facilitate optimal healing. The duration of this tends to last from 3 to 10 days depending on the nature of the reconstruction, whether the patient has undergone previous chemo-and/or radiotherapy and the preference of the surgical team. The SLT will support the patient to communicate effectively, will advise on the placement of a soft laryngectomy tube, if appropriate, and along with nursing staff will monitor for any adverse signs such as wound breakdown, infection or fistula formation. Voicing via the tracheo-oesophageal puncture should be avoided until anastomotic leak has been ruled out; however, the patient will be taught management and cleaning of the puncture during this post-operative phase.

101.3.3 Dysphagia Rehabilitation

After partial laryngeal surgery, the SLT will provide intensive swallow rehabilitation. This may involve the following:

- Providing techniques such as postures, manoeuvres, and exercise.
- Advising on secretion management using swallow techniques rather than medical management of saliva.

- Providing reassurance regarding pain/discomfort/sensation changes/anxiety/control.
- Advising on appropriate time for cuff deflation.
- Ensuring collaborative decision making regarding decannulation.
- Assessing for appropriate time for commencing fluid/oral intake/NG removal.
- Providing instrumental assessment.
- Assessing voice quality—introducing voice exercises.

It is also important to note that this type of surgery frequently results in laryngeal penetration and/or aspiration. This should not cause the SLT to stop or reduce the intensity of therapy, rather the tolerance of controlled aspiration is likely to be part of the normal rehabilitation trajectory.

Like oral cavity surgery, the rehabilitation process for both voice and swallow following total and partial laryngeal surgery goes on beyond the post-operative phase in hospital, where the SLT will provide ongoing physical, emotional and psychosocial support for the individual and their family or carers.

101.4 Conclusion

There is a complex interface which exists between the physical symptoms an individual who undergoes head and neck surgery may present with, and the impact and effect of these symptoms on his or her quality of life, emotional and psychosocial well-being. With this in mind, the therapy provided by the SLT should be evidence based, tailored to meet the needs of the individual, and recognised as a fundamental component of the surgical intervention.

Further Reading

Clarke P, Radford K, Coffey M, Stewart M. Speech and swallow rehabilitation in head and neck cancer: United Kingdom National Multidisciplinary Guidelines. J Laryngol Otol. 2016; 130(S2):S176–S180

Groher ME. Laryngectomy. In: Edels Y, ed. Dysphagia—Diagnosis and Management. London: Butterworths; 1984

Langmore SE, Schatz K, Olsen N. Fiberoptic endoscopic examination of swallowing safety: a new procedure. Dysphagia. 1988; 2(4):216–219

Logeman J. The Evaluation and Treatment of Swallowing Disorders. San Diego, CA: College Hill press; 1983

Logeman J. Manual for the Videofluoroscopic Study of Swallowing (Ltd Ed.). Austin, TX: Pro-Ed; 1993

Taub S, Bergner LH. Air bypass voice prosthesis for vocal rehabilitation of laryngectomees. Am J Surg. 1973; 125(6): 748–756

Related Topics of Interest

Laryngeal carcinoma
Laryngectomy
Reconstructive surgery
Speech and language therapy for benign voice disorders

S

102 Speech Audiometry

In many animals the sense of hearing is adapted for a specific purpose. In the human, the ear is specifically tuned to the speech frequencies (500–4,000 Hz). One of the main functions of the human ear is therefore the perception of speech. Indeed, most of the handicap of hearing loss is due to loss of the ability to perceive the spoken word. Speech audiometry provides a measure of this ability and any corresponding deficit. Voice tests can be considered as a very basic form of speech audiometry. However, in general, speech audiometry implies the formal qualitative assessment of a subject's perception of speech. It serves as a measure of disability produced by any hearing impairment, but it is not without its limitations, for example, usually tested in a soundproof room and often through earphones delivering the stimulus to each ear separately, which is different to a real-world situation. It is, however, useful in a variety of contexts including the following:

a. Assessment and diagnosis of peripheral and central hearing disorders.
b. Prediction of the usefulness of a hearing aid and as a counselling tool.
c. Evaluation of the benefits of certain surgery (pre- and post-operative assessment), such as stapedectomy and cochlear implantation.
d. Medicolegal assessment and as a means to cross-check the validity of pure-tone audiometry.

102.1 Materials

1. *Instruments* Testing is performed in a sound-proof room, with the volume controlled from the audiometer, which presents speech material to the subject via loudspeakers or headphones. Live speech material presented by a tester using a microphone is prone to variation in both intensity and accent. Standardised, prepared speech material presented by CD or computer and controlled by the audiometer is much more desirable. The use of headphones, as opposed to the free-field situation with loudspeakers, allows each ear to be tested individually and allows the non-test ear to be masked.

2. *Speech material* Phonemes are the building blocks of speech and represent the smallest unit of recognisable speech sound (e.g. ay, aw, ah, etc.). There are 49 phonemes in the English language. Speech material is chosen to provide a representative balance of phonemes and can be presented as words, sentences or synthetic sentences which have no meaning. A great number of lists of appropriate speech material have been developed by various agencies, for example, Medical Research Council, Institute of Hearing Research, Fry, Boothroyd and Manchester junior word lists, and Bench, Koval and Bamford (BKB) sentences (University of Manchester). There are also international word lists and ideally word lists in the patient's first language will provide optimum results.

102.2 Procedure

The subject is seated in a soundproof room and instructed in the test procedure. The recorded word lists are presented to the patient monaurally over headphones at various sound intensities. As speech audiometry is a suprathreshold test, masking of the non-test ear is usually required. Masking sounds in speech audiometry are chosen to try and recreate an appropriate noise background such as speech, cocktail party and babble noise. Pink noise and wide band noise (equal energy for each octave over the hearing range) are usually used when these are unavailable.

The first presentation is usually at 20 to 30 dB greater than the pure-tone average for the frequencies 500, 1,000 and 2,000 Hz. Subsequent presentations are usually made at +10, +20, –10 and –20 dB from this level, although more may be required. The patient is asked to repeat the words as accurately as possible and the percentage of words or phonemes, which are correctly repeated at each sound intensity (dB) is calculated and plotted on a graph.

The graphical display is compared with the calibration graph for that particular machine, which will have been obtained by testing otologically normal individuals on that machine, using the same tapes and test environment. The recorded data can then be used to formulate certain scores, and the shape of the graph used to give information regarding the type of deafness.

S

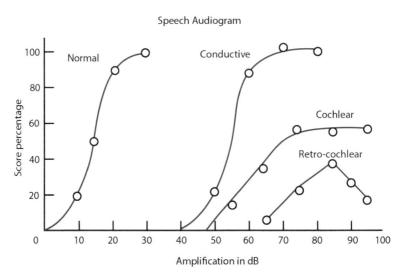

Fig. 102.1 Some typical speech audiometry curves.

102.3 Scoring

a. The maximum speech recognition score (SRS) is the subject's maximum score, no matter how loud the volume is turned up. It is a measure of optimal performance and should be 100% when normal.

b. The speech recognition threshold (SRT) is the sound intensity (dB) at which the subject can correctly repeat 50% of the presented words.

c. The optimum speech level is the level at which the maximum SRS is obtained.

d. The half optimum hearing threshold level of speech (HOHTLS) is the level corresponding to 50% of the maximum SRS. If the patient has a speech impediment or his or her first language is not English, then difficulties in scoring may occur.

102.4 Shape of the Graph

If the hearing is normal, all the words will be understood if they are played loudly enough. The result is a sigmoid-shaped curve with a steep, near-vertical portion in the middle.

In patients with a conductive hearing loss, all the words will be understood, but they must be played louder than for a normal subject. The curve is parallel to the normal but is shifted to the right (i.e. greater half peak level elevation [HPL]) in proportion to the degree of hearing loss. The maximum SRS is still 100% as discrimination is preserved. In patients with a sensorineural hearing loss, there is usually a loss of ability to discriminate speech, and consequently the maximum SRS is often less than 100%. The gradient of the middle portion of the curve is often less and a plateau may be reached in which further increases in sound intensity do not improve discrimination. In severe cases 'rollover' may occur: beyond a certain point any further increase in sound intensity causes a reduction in the discrimination score. This type of curve is typical of a retrocochlear lesion (▶ Fig. 102.1).

102.5 Specific Uses

102.5.1 Non-Organic Hearing Loss

Speech audiometry can be used in the investigation of non-organic or feigned hearing loss. Two tests exist as below:

1. Delayed speech feedback (DSF). The subject is asked to read text aloud. The speech is relayed to the test ear with a delay of 1 to 200 ms. If there is normal hearing in the test ear, stammering and a raised voice are almost inevitable.

2. Competition tests. The patient is asked to repeat speech material delivered to the good ear while competing speech material is introduced to the test ear. If the hearing is normal, stuttering is likely when the competing material is 40 dB louder than the test material.

102.6 Central Function

Speech audiometry can also be used as a test of central auditory function. This can be done using a variety of techniques, including speech messages in competing noise, competing messages and overlapping messages in each ear, accelerated, interrupted and filtered speech. For further details on this, the reader is referred to Keith and Pensak (1991).

Further Reading

Marriage JE, Salario-Corbetto M. Psychoacoustic audiometry, Chapter 51 in Scott-Browns Otolaryngology, Head and Neck Surgery, 8th Edition, Volume 2. Editors-in-Chief–Watkinson JC & Clarke R. Published by CRC Press, Taylor & Francis group, Boca Raton, London, New York, 2018

Katx J. Handbook of Clinical Audiology. 7th ed. Philadelphia, Baltimore, New York: Wolters Kluwer; 2015

Keith RW, Pensak ML. Central auditory function. Otolaryngol Clin North Am. 1991; 24(2):371–379

Related Topics of Interest

Non-organic hearing loss
Clinical assessment of hearing
Pure-tone audiometry
Vestibular schwannoma

S

103 Speech and Language Therapy for Benign Voice Disorders

103.1 Introduction

Speech and language therapists (SLT) with specialist training and experience have a unique role in working alongside the ear, nose and throat (ENT) physician to reach an accurate diagnosis of a voice disorder and to identify an effective treatment plan.

Many classification systems exist to categorise voice disorders, the scope of which is beyond this chapter. Changes in the voice may result from structural, neuromuscular or inflammatory processes, or from inappropriate patterns of muscle tension in and around the larynx. Muscle tension disorders are often further subdivided to include psychogenic voice disorders, where unresolved emotional conflict is converted into significant muscle tension in the larynx that impedes normal voice production.

Recently, there has been an increase in the awareness and understanding of upper airway disorders, such as inducible laryngeal obstruction (ILO, formerly known as vocal cord dysfunction) and laryngospasm. The majority of upper airway patients report episodic changes to their breathing and are referred to respiratory clinics. However, some patients highlight significant throat tightness and voice changes that may lead them to be referred to ENT. Symptoms are usually episodic and result from paradoxical narrowing of the vocal folds on inspiration, but this may not be apparent on laryngeal examination. It is essential to refer patients with a history and presentation suggestive of ILO to a specialist upper airway team for multi-disciplinary assessment and treatment. Other patient groups presenting to ENT clinics and who may require voice therapy are professional voice users, including singers, and transgender clients.

103.2 Referral to SLT

All patients with a voice disorder must be evaluated by an ENT physician prior to commencing voice therapy. This allows identification of relevant medical factors affecting the voice and visualisation of any structural or functional changes in the larynx that underpin the voice disorder. It is impossible to form an effective therapy plan without knowing the status of the larynx. Reduction of laryngeal irritation through early management of nasal symptoms and/or acid reflux also aids voice recovery.

Assessment may be carried out in regular ENT clinics, but there are now many specialist voice clinics run jointly by ENT and SLTs across the United Kingdom and abroad. They have the benefit of combined expertise of the ENT physician and SLT, bringing together medical and surgical knowledge with finely tuned perceptual voice skills, understanding of the physiology of voice production, and an ability to determine suitability for voice therapy. Joint voice clinics are often furnished with more advanced, high-resolution imaging systems, including stroboscopy, that allow detailed analysis of the mucosal wave and areas of tension and stiffness in the vocal cords. Images should be recorded and viewed, with the patients, to enhance understanding of their symptoms and increase compliance with the proposed treatment plan. Recording of images also allows for pre- and post-surgical/post-therapeutic comparison.

Some voice disorders, such as those related to papilloma, severe Reinke's oedema and occult cysts, are unlikely to resolve without surgical intervention. However, there is still a valuable and effective role for voice therapy, dovetailing with ENT input, in reducing compensatory behaviours that may have magnified the change in voice quality and in providing pre- and post-operative advice, especially in preventing recurrence.

Specific referral processes vary according to setting, but referrals to the voice SLT should include, as a minimum, any medical factor affecting the voice, a summary of laryngeal appearance and function, any proposed surgical intervention or onward referrals and a brief statement of voice quality on the day of assessment.

103.3 SLT Assessment

A typical initial voice assessment consists of a detailed case history, perceptual assessment by the SLT, rating scales completed by the patient, voice recording +/− instrumental analysis and, where appropriate, palpation of the larynx.

The case history provides an opportunity for the patients to summarise their symptoms and the background to the voice difficulties, focusing on factors that they believe to be relevant, and to express the current impact of the voice changes on their life. The therapist will carefully insert additional questions as necessary to yield information on general health, sense of well-being, lifestyle and work considerations, voice use and any past or current emotional stress that may have resulted in laryngeal tension or disrupted healthy breathing patterns.

Throughout the case history, the skilled SLT will tune into the sound of the voice, including pitch and resonance, and make observations on voice technique, posture, breathing pattern and muscle tension. Voice quality may fluctuate as the patient is talking and the SLT will note any potential connections between voice changes and subject matter.

Use of rating scales and instrumental analysis varies greatly across voice services. Hirano's GRBAS scale is commonly used, despite its limitations, for rating overall severity of voice change and specific parameters of roughness, breathiness, asthenia and strain, with therapists making additional comments on pitch, loudness and resonance. The Voice Handicap Index provides a good measure of the impact of the voice disorder on the patient. Instrumental analysis previously rested on the use of computer-based systems, such as the Laryngograph and Computerised Speech Lab (CSL), and yielded many acoustic and aerodynamic measurements, highly applicable for research purposes. There are now many mobile apps available to both patient and therapist, clinical governance issues notwithstanding, that allow immediate analysis of pitch, loudness and voice quality. These are useful for pre-and post-therapy measures as well as for biofeedback during therapy sessions.

By the end of the initial session, the therapist aims to co-ordinate the findings from all assessment sources and provide a coherent and meaningful explanation of the voice problem to the patient. It is essential to have an agreed understanding of the cause of the current voice difficulty and of the onward treatment plan. The goals of therapy should be clear with an estimate of the number and timing of therapy sessions.

103.4 SLT Management

Voice therapy is typically delivered on a 1:1 basis, although group work can be highly effective for voice education and preventative work. Goals of therapy vary according to assessment and diagnosis and may be curative, preventative, facilitative, rehabilitative or supportive.

Explanation of the voice symptoms, vocal tract care and voice conservation is appropriate for most patients with voice difficulties. It is crucial that the patients understand the specific factors responsible for the change in their voice, in order to know what needs to change. Education and understanding are fundamental to securing a patient's willingness to engage in therapy.

Additional therapy approaches are determined by individual goals and assessment findings and may be direct (physiological) and/or indirect (psychosocial).

A direct, physiological approach aims to modify features of voice production to achieve the most appropriate and acceptable voice quality for the patient with the least possible effort. The skilled voice therapist has at his or her disposal a wide variety of techniques and will be led intuitively by each patient and his or her voice to select the most effective. Techniques may focus on improving breathing pattern, adjusting vocal fold contact, reducing excessive muscular effort (often in the false vocal folds, but throughout the entire vocal tract as necessary), modifying pitch and intonation patterns and the use of pacing and phrasing to reduce talking on residual air. Specific treatment programmes, such as Estill Voice Training and the Accent Method, may be employed, as well as specific exercises that have stood the test of time in the world of voice, such as chant talk and yawn-sigh, and more recent frameworks, such as resonant voice and flow phonation. Therapeutic nasendoscopy is a highly effective therapy tool to allow a patient to modify voice use with visual biofeedback, and laryngeal massage is invaluable in breaking engrained patterns of muscle tension in some cases.

Indirect treatment approaches may be used with patients whose voices are affected by emotional or psychological factors. Some voice therapists have undertaken training in psychological techniques, in order to integrate direct and indirect approaches seamlessly during therapy, but in some cases, onward referral to a psychologist or counsellor may be helpful. Indirect approaches include Cognitive Behaviour Therapy, Acceptance and Commitment Therapy, and Solution-Focused Therapy. In addition, many patients benefit from their own practices of yoga, mindfulness and Alexander Technique, for example.

S

Ideally, patients will make steady progress towards their goals once therapy is underway and a block of up to six therapy sessions is usually sufficient to achieve the agreed aims. Where progress is slower than expected or absent, it is wise to refer the patient back for ENT or joint voice clinic review and adapt the management plan, if necessary.

Further Reading

Behrman A. Speech and Voice Science. 3rd ed. San Diego, CA: Plural Publishing; 2017

Boone D, McFarlane S, Von Berg S. The Voice and Voice Therapy. 7th ed. Boston, MA: Allen & Bacon; 2005

Carding P, Bos-Clark M, Fu S, Gillivan-Murphy P, Jones SM, Walton C. Evaluating the efficacy of voice therapy for functional, organic and neurological voice disorders. Clin Otolaryngol. 2017; 42(2):201–217

Royal College of Speech and Language Therapists. (2009). Resource manual for the commissioning and planning services for SLCN: Voice. https://www.rcslt.org/speech_and_language_therapy/commissioning/voice_plus_intro. Accessed 23 July 2018

Shewell C. Voice Work: Art and Science in Changing Voices. Chichester, NH: Wiley-Blackwell; 2009

Related Topics of Interest

Speech and swallow rehabilitation following head and neck surgery

Voice disorders

Vocal fold paralysis

104 Stertor and Stridor

104.1 Definitions

Stertor is noisy breathing caused by turbulence due to partial obstruction of the upper respiratory tract (URT) above the larynx.

Stridor is noisy breathing caused by turbulence due to partial obstruction of the URT at the laryngeal or tracheal level.

Stertor and stridor may co-exist. Obstruction below the trachea, for example, due to a foreign body or consolidation from infection, will typically cause an expiratory wheeze. This can sometimes be confused with stridor in the clinical setting.

104.2 Stertor

Stertor may present at any age and may be caused by single or multiple levels of obstruction to the airway above the larynx.

104.2.1 Congenital (present at birth) Stertor

Nose

Neonates are obligate nasal breathers and complete nasal obstruction will cause a respiratory arrest. Partial nasal obstruction at birth may progress to total nasal blockage with development, depending on the cause and its extent.

Choanal stenosis or atresia.

External nasal deformity due to a craniofacial abnormality or nasal trauma.

Deviated nasal septum from birth trauma or congenital nasal mass.

Congenital nasal mass such as the following:

1. Dermoid, nasoalveolar, dentigerous and mucous cysts deforming or projecting into the nasal airway.
2. Masses arising from the anterior skull base such as a meningocele, encephalocele, meningoencephalocele or glioma.

Nasopharynx

Craniofacial abnormality, especially Apert's and Crouzon's syndromes. Congenital cystic or solid mass such as a dermoid or haemangioma.

Oral cavity and oropharynx

Micrognathia to a craniofacial abnormality, especially Treacher Collins and Pierre Robin syndromes. In these, a small mandible and hypotonia allows the normal-sized tongue to fill the mouth and, by falling backward (glossoptosis), obstruct the oropharynx.

True macroglossia, either from congenital masses such as a haemangioma or lymphangioma or as part of a syndrome such as Beckwith–Wiedemann syndrome, obstructs both the oral cavity and oropharynx.

Relative macroglossia due to a small mouth without micrognathia, but normal tongue, most frequently in children with Down's syndrome.

Lingual thyroid and thyroglossal cyst.

Congenital neurological conditions causing hypotonia.

Congenital neck masses, such as a cystic hygroma, causing extrinsic compression of the upper airway.

104.2.2 Acquired Stertor

Nose

Trauma causing external nasal and septal deviation, septal haematoma or a secondary septal abscess.

Rhinitis, rhinosinusitis and nasal polyps.

Iatrogenic, from nasal stenosis or intra-nasal adhesions following nasal surgery including septorhinoplasty.

Acquired nasal masses, which may be benign such as meningocele or malignant such as an olfactory neuroblastoma, lymphoma or sinus carcinoma.

Systemic diseases causing nasal obstruction, such as Wegener's granulomatosis or sarcoidosis.

Foreign body.

Nasopharynx

Adenoid hyperplasia.

Juvenile angiofibroma.

Nasopharyngeal carcinoma or lymphoma.

Iatrogenic such as nasopharyngeal stenosis from palatal surgery.

Acute tonsillitis, especially to infectious mononucleosis.

Parapharyngeal and retropharyngeal abscess.

S

Oral cavity and oropharynx

Acquired macroglossia from (a) benign causes such as a haemangioma or as part of an anaphylactic reaction, or (b) malignant causes such as an exophytic tongue carcinoma.

Oral cavity/oropharyngeal carcinoma, including tonsillar and tongue base cancer.

Mandibular trauma causing poor mouth opening or trismus.

Benign tonsillar hyperplasia.

Infection of the oral cavity (a) acute tonsillitis, particularly glandular fever tonsillitis causing significant tonsillar hyperplasia, (b) Ludwig's angina. Epiglottitis.

Foreign body.

Extrinsic compression

Infection (such as a parapharyngeal abscess or infected branchial cyst), benign neck lumps such as a deep lobe parotid pleomorphic adenoma or malignant neck disease (e.g. high-grade lymphoma or large metastatic lymph nodes).

104.2.3 Clinical Features

Stertor is usually inspiratory and harsh/gruff sounding. A full history should ascertain length of onset, symptom progression, aggravating and relieving factors, whether there is sleep apnoea, an intercurrent URT infection (URTI) or if trauma has occurred. Examination should include the patient's weight, body mass index, collar size and craniofacial assessment. Careful neck, external nose and oral cavity examination is necessary as is endoscopic examination of the nose and laryngopharynx (contraindicated in acute epiglottitis). The pulse, temperature, respiratory rate and blood pressure should be monitored.

104.2.4 Investigations

These depend on the patient's clinical features. A full blood count, erythrocyte sedimentation rate (ESR) and C-reactive protein (CRP) are required when an infective cause is suspected. Oxygen saturation should be monitored. A lateral soft tissue neck radiograph or a magnetic resonance imaging (MRI) scan may be indicated to show the site of airway obstruction. In a child, it is important to extend the neck to prevent the retropharyngeal soft tissue causing a pseudomass.

104.2.5 Treatment

This depends on the cause, progression and severity of the stertor and on whether it is causing complications (see cross references).

Complications are directly related to the airway obstruction when there may be acute or chronic hypoxia and hypercapnia, include pulmonary hypertension and right ventricular failure (cor pulmonale), failure to thrive and impaired neurocognitive development in children, central respiratory arrest (in the first 3 months of life neonates are obligatory nasal breathers) and acute total airway obstruction.

104.3 Stridor

104.3.1 Congenital Stridor

Larynx

- Supraglottis: Laryngomalacia, web, saccular cyst and cystic hygroma.
- Glottis: Web, vocal cord paralysis.
- Subglottis: Web, stenosis and haemangioma.

Trachea and bronchi: Web, stenosis, tracheomalacia, tracheo- and bronchogenic cyst and compression from vascular and other mediastinal tumours.

104.3.2 Acquired Stridor

- Trauma: Thermal and chemical, iatrogenic (intubation and surgical) and blunt and sharp external.
- Inflammatory: Acute laryngitis, acute laryngotracheobronchitis and diphtheria.
- Foreign body: Laryngeal, tracheal, bronchial and external compression from an oesophageal foreign body.
- Allergy: Angioneurotic oedema of the larynx or trachea.
  Extrinsic allergic alveolitis.
- Neoplasia:
  - Benign, for example, laryngeal papillomatosis.
  - Malignant, for example, laryngeal carcinoma.

104.3.3 Clinical Features

Classically, supraglottic stridor is inspiratory because the negative inspiratory intra-laryngeal pressure draws in the supraglottic soft tissues on inspiration and passive opening occurs on expiration. Glottic and subglottic airway obstruction is associated with inspiratory or biphasic stridor. Upper tracheal obstruction causes stridor because of turbulence of air flowing through a narrow but rigid airway that doesn't collapse. It too may be inspiratory but is usually biphasic. Lower tracheal obstruction is also usually biphasic, but in the smaller bronchi and bronchioles obstruction accentuates the physiological constriction occurring in expiration to cause an expiratory wheeze.

A full history is particularly important. It should cover time of onset (acute or chronic) and progression, presence of a respiratory tract infection, the possibility of a foreign body, previous surgery and recovery thereafter (particularly thyroid/parathyroid surgery). Time spent intubated in a paediatric high dependency unit (HDU)/intensive treatment unit (ITU) or adult ITU should be determined. Previous episodes of cyanosis and their trigger should be noted. The voice and cry should be assessed and exacerbating factors noted (e.g. feeding or exercise). Relieving factors such as medication (steroids or β_2-agonists), neck position or lying erect or supine should be determined as should the smoking and alcohol history, patient weight, general health and reflux history.

Examination of the nose, throat and neck is indicated if circumstances permit. It is vital to be aware of the risk of causing a rapid and life-threatening deterioration of the patients' airway in certain instances if they become distressed by the examination. This is especially but not exclusively so in children. Before a decision to examine the airway is made, the clinician needs to have assessed the vital signs (pulse, temperature, respiratory rate and blood pressure), obtained oxygen saturations with oximetry and observed the effort of breathing (looking for intercostal recession, subcostal recession and tracheal tug) and listened to the chest. This may allow a working diagnosis to be made. Flexible nasopharyngolaryngoscopy may then be appropriate, but this usually only allows accurate assessment of the airway to the level of the vocal cords. Investigations should not delay the management of the airway.

104.3.4 Investigations

A lateral soft tissue neck and chest radiograph, or a computed tomography (CT) scan of the larynx and lungs may be appropriate. For certain conditions, including foreign body aspiration and innominate artery compression, chest radiographs may suggest the correct diagnosis. It must be emphasised radiographs may be normal in children with a bronchial foreign body. Therefore, if the history is suggestive, bronchoscopy may still be indicated even with a normal chest radiograph. Rigid endoscopy with spontaneous ventilation is still the gold standard of investigation as it allows the most complete examination of the upper aerodigestive tract. Depending on circumstances a ventilating bronchoscope may be used to examine the airways and extract a tracheal or main bronchus foreign body.

104.3.5 Treatment

Treatment depends on the diagnosis and the severity of symptoms.

Further Reading

Denoyelle F, Garabédian EN. Propranolol may become first-line treatment in obstructive subglottic infantile hemangiomas. Otolaryngol Head Neck Surg. 2010; 142(3):463–464

Digoy GP, Burge SD. Laryngomalacia in the older child: clinical presentations and management. Curr Opin Otolaryngol Head Neck Surg. 2014; 22(6):501–505

Thompson DM. Laryngomalacia: factors that influence disease severity and outcomes of management. Curr Opin Otolaryngol Head Neck Surg. 2010; 18(6):564–570

Related Topics of Interest

Paediatric airway problems
Laryngeal carcinoma
Oropharyngeal carcinoma
Nasopharyngeal tumours
Adenoids
Nasal trauma
Nasal swellings
Foreign bodies in ENT

S

105 Sudden Hearing Loss

Sudden hearing loss is a significant subjective decline in the hearing acuity occurring over a relatively short time period. Usually, only one ear is affected and the aetiology is frequently not identified. It can be classified into conductive and sensorineural causes. The following list covers many causes but is not exhaustive.

105.1 Conductive Causes

- External ear canal occlusion, for example, from wax or a foreign body.
- Infection, for example, otitis externa, acute otitis media or chronic otitis media.
- Acute serous otitis media.
- Ear trauma, from a direct blow, acoustic or barotrauma (see Related Topics of Interest).
- Iatrogenic—post-surgical.

105.2 Sensorineural

- Idiopathic.
- Iatrogenic—post-surgical.
- Serous and purulent labyrinthitis.
- Viral, for example, measles and mumps virus.
- Cerebellopontine angle tumours, for example, vestibular schwannoma, cholesterol granuloma, congenital dermoid and meningioma.
- Temporal bone fractures, particularly transverse fractures.
- Causes of perilymph fistula including round window rupture, for example, from blast trauma or barotrauma.
- Ménière's *disease* (primary endolymphatic hydrops) and secondary endolymphatic hydrops (which may cause Ménière's *syndrome*).
- Ototoxic drugs, particularly aminoglycoside antibiotics and chemotherapeutic drugs.
- Central causes, for example, following a brainstem cerebrovascular accident.
- Autoimmune inner ear disease.

The most common causes of sudden hearing loss, in the absence of any other significant otological symptoms, are impacted wax, where water exposure may cause swelling and subsequent hearing loss, acute serous otitis media, normally following an air flight with a concurrent upper respiratory tract infection or idiopathic sensorineural hearing loss (SNHL). The first two of these conditions are usually easily recognised on examination and should be treated on their merits.

The hearing loss that accompanies ear infection, trauma, Ménière's disease, cerebrovascular event or other recognised aetiological cause, is usually very obviously secondary to the more troublesome primary symptoms of each condition. The reader is therefore directed to the relevant chapters for a more thorough coverage of these conditions.

The rest of this chapter will therefore focus on the condition of idiopathic sudden sensorineural hearing loss (ISSHL).

105.3 Definition

There are many definitions of ISSHL, but probably the one in most widespread use, and certainly in use in the United Kingdom is the presence of at least 30-dB hearing loss in at least three audiometric frequencies, occurring over a 72-hour (3 day) period (all the 3s!). As prior audiometry may not be available then, this often means comparing the affected with the unaffected ear.

105.4 Clinical Features

It is a relatively uncommon condition with an estimated incidence of 8:100,000 cases per year. In most cases of ISSHL, there is the presumption of some form of inflammation of the inner ear or cochlear nerve, possibly due to viral infection, vascular disturbance or immunological dysfunction. These suggestions come from previous temporal bone studies (and are not mutually exclusive), but a definitive aetiology is still awaited.

The patient will typically present with a relatively recent onset of a sensation of blockage, pressure and altered hearing. Tinnitus is a frequent accompanying symptom. Occasionally, there may be initial vertigo or unsteadiness. A thorough history and examination will not reveal any obvious identifiable cause. Subsequently, and with appropriate special investigations, a cause may be identified but this will be in less than 10%. The remainder will be labeled as idiopathic of which approximately two-thirds will recover spontaneously.

Anecdotally, mild and low-tone hearing losses are thought to have a better prognosis than more severe or high-tone hearing loss. Co-existent tinnitus does not influence prognosis, but the presence of vertigo is felt to be a poor prognostic sign, presumably reflecting more widespread labyrinthine involvement. The prognosis for recovery is also felt to be better with earlier treatment; significant benefit is unlikely beyond 6 weeks from the onset of symptoms.

Many ISSHL patients who present to primary health care are told they have a middle ear effusion as the cause of their symptoms, and reassured that it will recover when the effusion clears (in the absence of any actual effusion). Most are then treated with only symptomatic medicines or perhaps antibiotics and an opportunity for early treatment is missed. Given that many GPs will ring on-call ear, nose and throat (ENT) doctors for advice, this will be discussed further under management.

105.5 Management

The first and most important investigation is to qualify and quantify the hearing loss. Confirmation of a SNHL requires access to tuning forks, a microscope and an audiologist to obtain an impedance audiogram and an air and bone conduction pure-tone audiogram. Subsequent investigations are likely to include magnetic resonance imaging (MRI) scanning if the asymmetrical hearing persists, and blood tests including full blood count (FBC), urea and electrolytes (U&Es), thyroid function tests (TFTs), lipids, syphilis serology and an autoimmune screen.

Having established the presence of a SNHL, treatment may be offered. There are many treatments that have been suggested for this condition, but good-quality evidence of benefit is lacking. Most patients do not require admission into hospital unless the aetiology (e.g. trauma, purulent labyrinthitis) dictates and they can usually be investigated and managed as an outpatient.

Suggested treatments include steroids—both oral and intratympanic, hyperbaric oxygen therapy (HBOT), antivirals, rheologic agents (e.g. dextrans), vasodilators (including Ginkgo biloba and carbogen) and vitamin supplements among many others!

There have been several meta-analyses looking at this subject and the current Cochrane review findings for ISSHL are summarised as follows:

1. The value of steroids in the treatment of ISSHL remains unclear because the evidence obtained from randomised controlled trials is contradictory in nature. There is no consensus therefore on whether they should be prescribed. The last review was April 2013.
2. The effectiveness of vasodilators in the treatment of ISSHL remains unproven. Last review was September 2008.
3. HBOT significantly improved hearing in patients with ISSHL. Patient numbers reported are small and because of methodological shortcomings and poor reporting, this result should be interpreted cautiously, but an appropriately powered trial was thought appropriate. Last Cochrane review was in 2009. It may be reasonable to offer HBOT if such facilities exist locally, for acute but not long-standing ISSHL.

There is no evidence that any other medication makes any difference to outcome (most such treatments report a response rate of 60%, about the same as those who spontaneously recover with no treatment), and so in both U.K. and U.S. guidance there are no other recommended treatments.

In the context of a request for advice from a GP, it would seem reasonable to see the patient and a 7- to 14-day course of steroids would not be unreasonable in an otherwise fit patient and in the absence of any contraindications. This would have the benefit of an early treatment and avoid the risk of a complaint of delayed or missed treatment (which medicolegally, evidence shows, is not a reasonable complaint).

Subsequent monitoring of the hearing by pure-tone and/or speech audiometry is desirable to determine whether the hearing is stable, improving or declining. This will enable the patient's disability and handicap to be assessed, and to allow provision of supportive treatment in the form of counselling, hearing aids and tinnitus management as required.

Further Reading

Burton MJ, Harvey RJ. Idiopathic sudden sensori-neural hearing loss. In: Gleeson M, ed. Scott-Brown's Otolaryngology, Head and Neck Surgery. 7th ed. London: Hodder Arnold; 2008;3:3577–3593

Jarvis SJ, Giangrande V, John G, Thornton AR. Management of acute idiopathic sensorineural hearing loss: a survey of UK ENT consultants. Acta Otorhinolaryngol Ital. 2011; 31(2):85–89

O'Connell BP, Hunter JB, Haynes DS. Current concepts in the management of idiopathic sudden sensorineural hearing loss. Curr Opin Otolaryngol Head Neck Surg. 2016; 24(5):413–419

Stachler RJ, Chandrasekhar SS, Archer SM, et al; American Academy of Otolaryngology-Head and Neck Surgery. Clinical practice guideline: sudden hearing loss. Otolaryngol Head Neck Surg. 2012; 146(3, Suppl):S1–S35

Related Topics of Interest

Barotrauma
Labyrinthitis
Ménière's disease
Ototoxicity
Otitis media—chronic
Vestibular schwannoma
Otitis media—acute

E

106 Suppurative Otitis Media—Acute

106.1 Definition

Otitis media is an inflammation of the mucosa of the middle ear cleft, the collective term for the eustachian tube, tympanic cavity, attic, aditus, antrum and mastoid air cells. The prefix, acute, sub-acute or chronic, relates to the duration of the condition with acute taken to imply a time period of up to 3 weeks, sub-acute as 3 weeks to 3 months, whereas chronic implies 3 months or more. Acute suppurative otitis media (ASOM) is an acute, pus-producing, usually bacterial, inflammatory process affecting the whole of the middle ear cleft.

106.2 Epidemiology

ASOM is common and is most prevalent between the ages of 6 and 24 months with some series reporting at least one episode by the age of 2 years, in up to 80% of children. Boys are more prone than girls and the incidence falls steeply after the age of 5. There is evidence from the United States of a significant drop in incidence since the introduction of the polyvalent *Streptococcus pneumoniae* vaccine. Similar benefits have been found from the Hib vaccine (see Chapter 19, Epiglottis).

106.3 Associated Risk Factors

- Young age—often related to teething, which may increase saliva production and the risk of eustachian tube salivary reflux.
- Family history—more likely if one or both parents suffered similarly in childhood.
- Day care/nursery—the greater the number of children in the care facility, the greater the risk (if > 4 children).
- Breast-feeding—a minimum of 3 months of post-natal breast-feeding seems to provide some protection.
- Cigarette smoke exposure.
- Pacifier/dummy use—associated with a very slight increased risk—however, parenting benefits may outweigh the very slight risk of ASOM.
- Socioeconomic—correlation with deprivation, poverty and crowded housing.
- Race and ethnicity—some races seem to exhibit a particularly high risk of the condition—Native Americans, Canadian Inuits and Australian Aborigines.

106.4 Microbiology

Respiratory viruses and bacteria have been cultured from middle ear aspirations. The commonest bacteria are *S. pneumoniae* (40–50%), *Haemophilus influenzae* (30%) and *Moraxella catarrhalis* (10%). Group A streptococci are also found (2–10%). The commonest viruses are respiratory syncytial virus (RSV), adenovirus and influenza type A virus.

ASOM may occur as a primary infection, but more typically it will occur as a secondary infection after a viral upper respiratory tract infection (URTI). The URTI will lead to swelling and dysfunction of the eustachian tube. Infants have a short, wider and a more horizontally placed eustachian tube, which is more prone to dysfunction in the presence of nasopharyngeal inflammation. An effusion will follow and subsequent viral or bacterial infection can then arise. Pathogenic bacteria have been isolated from the nasopharynx in up to 97% of children with ASOM.

Bacteria can also enter the middle ear cleft via a perforated tympanic membrane or more rarely be blood-borne.

106.5 Clinical Features

The cardinal symptom of this condition is earache. This often starts and is worse at night, probably due to reduced eustachian tube opening during sleep and increased mucosal oedema when prone or dependent. It may occur as a solitary symptom or may follow symptoms of URTI. The pain may rapidly increase as inflammation progresses and may cease to respond to simple analgesics. The child may start to become systemically unwell. Although associated with reduced hearing, this is rarely volunteered as a symptom during an acute episode. These symptoms may rapidly improve if rupture of the tympanic membrane occurs, due to inflammatory and pressure necrosis. This may produce a mucopurulent and sometimes blood-stained otorrhoea. Perforation may also occur in the absence of significant pain, especially if there is a pre-existing atelectatic segment.

Initial examination may reveal a dull tympanic membrane, although wax may obscure the view. Hyperaemia rapidly follows and leashes of vessels may be seen running along or parallel to the malleus handle. Soon radial vessels are visible on the drumhead and a middle ear effusion occurs. The drumhead takes on a full (i.e. opposite to retraction), red and angry appearance, and pus may be seen bulging posteroinferiorly. Pressure necrosis of this region may cause the drumhead to rupture allowing mucopus to drain into the external ear canal. Children are usually fretful, look unwell and often have a high-grade fever (> 39°C) and, rarely, there may be signs of complications of ASOM.

106.6 Treatment

1. Explanation and advice. This is a condition that is usually self-limiting.
2. Simple supportive treatment for the inevitable accompanying symptoms including fluids, topical or systemic decongestants and simple analgesia such as ibuprofen (anti-inflammatory) and paracetamol (antipyretic).
3. Antibiotics in appropriate dosage may be required. A Cochrane review is underway to address this point but a recent 'state of the art' panel review (see Further Reading) suggests a 7- to 14-day course of amoxycillin as first choice (or possibly co-amoxiclav), which will cover the most common pathogens provided the patient is not allergic to penicillin (erythromycin or clarithromycin are suitable alternatives) and the organisms are not resistant. In these circumstances, gleaned from bacterial sensitivity studies or lack of clinical response, a suitable alternative should be chosen. Microbiological advice may be helpful. Oral medication is usually adequate in the absence of complications. There is some evidence that a longer course of antibiotics is more likely to result in clearing of middle ear effusion. Some authors advocate a prolonged (6 weeks) course of antibiotics in children with frequent, recurrent episodes.
4. Grommet insertion may be helpful for those children suffering repeated and frequent episodes.
5. Conditions predisposing to ASOM should be treated on their own merit after resolution. These include adenoidal enlargement and adenoiditis, and those with an immune disorder.

106.7 Complications of Acute Otitis Media

These complications are fundamentally a result of spread of the infective process beyond the confines of the middle ear cleft, and can occur in both acute and chronic otitis media:

- Acute mastoiditis (osteomyelitis of the mastoid bone and air cells).
- Acute petrositis should the petrous apex become involved, which may progress to cause Gradenigo's syndrome.

Gradenigo's syndrome comprises the following:

- Acute otitis media.
- An ipsilateral abducent nerve palsy causing paralysis of the external rectus muscle of the eye.
- Pain in the distribution of the ipsilateral trigeminal nerve.

The respective cranial nerves are only separated by a layer of dura from the petrous apex, so that inflammation from an aerated petrous apex can extend to involve these adjacent nerves. An extradural abscess or pachymeningitis (meningitis extending to the dural layer) of this region from a generalised meningitis may also cause the combined cranial nerve signs, without an accompanying otitis media.

- Meningitis.
- Citelli's abscess is a sub-periosteal abscess which has spread through the medial aspect of the mastoid, into the digastric fossa.
- Bezold's abscess is an abscess which has tracked inferiorly within the sheath of sternomastoid to form a fluctuant mass along its anterior border.
- Extradural and subdural abscess.
- Cerebellar, temporal lobe and perisinus abscess.
- Lateral sinus thrombosis, rarely extending in an antegrade direction to thrombose the internal jugular vein and in a retrograde direction causing a cavernous sinus thrombosis.
- Otitic hydrocephalus.
- Lower motor neuron facial nerve paralysis. The at-risk population is that group of patients with a congenital dehiscence of the horizontal portion of the facial nerve. This arises in 6% of the population.
- Serous and suppurative labyrinthitis.

106.8 Otological Sequelae of ASOM

- Non-suppurative middle ear effusion (otitis media with effusion). This persists for over 30 days in 40% of children and for over 3 months

in 10%. This can predispose to atelectasis of the tympanic membrane and cholesteatoma.
- High-tone sensorineural hearing loss, perhaps secondary to bacterial toxins migrating across the round window.
- Tympanic membrane perforation.
- Adhesions between the tympanic membrane, ossicles and the medial wall of the middle ear.
- Tympanosclerosis which may spread from the tympanic membrane to the ossicular chain, fixing the latter.
- Erosion of the ossicular chain, in particular, the long process of the incus, especially following recurrent episodes of ASOM.

Further Reading

Atkinson H, Wallis S, Coatesworth AP. Acute otitis media. Postgrad Med. 2015; 127(4):386–390

Montague M-L, Hussain SS. A child with recurrent acute otitis media. Clin Otolaryngol. 2007; 32(3):190–192

Schilder AGM, Marom T, Bhutta MF, et al. Panel 7: otitis media: treatment and complications. Otolaryngol Head Neck Surg. 2017; 156(4_suppl, 4S):S88–S105

Venekamp RP, Sanders SL, Glasziou PP, Mar CBD, Rovers MM. Antibiotics for acute otitis media in children. The Cochrane Library Published Online; 2015:23

Related Topics of Interest

Tympanosclerosis
Tympanoplasty
Cholesteatoma
Suppurative otitis media—chronic
Suppurative otitis media—complications

S

107 Suppurative Otitis Media—Chronic

Chronic otitis media (COM) refers to an abnormality of the pars tensa or pars flaccida. It may be classified into four distinct entities:

1. Inactive mucosal (dry perforation).
2. Active mucosal (wet perforation).
3. Inactive squamous (retraction pocket and atelectasis).
4. Active squamous (cholesteatoma).

The previous classification of tubotympanic (safe) and tympanomastoid (atticoantral/unsafe) disease is little used now and probably misleading. This chapter describes COM entities without cholesteatoma.

107.1 Inactive Mucosal Chronic Otitis Media (Dry Perforation)

This describes a permanent perforation of the pars tensa without middle ear inflammation. This usually occurs after an episode of acute otitis media (AOM), where the drum has ruptured and failed to heal. Recurrent episodes of ruptured AOM will further increase this risk. Ventilation tube placement in the drum has a 2% chance of leaving a permanent perforation. Longer-term ventilation tubes such as T tubes are associated with much higher permanent drum perforation rates, around 20%. Perforations may occasionally result from other trauma or when an atelectatic drum or localised retraction perforates. The combined pathology may be evident on careful micro-otoscopic examination and the surgeon must always be mindful of epithelium that may be displaced within the middle ear. In perforations, the epithelium and mucosa usually meet at the perforation edge. However, the epithelium may migrate medially on the undersurface of the drum towards the annulus and manubrium technically forming a cholesteatoma. The surgeon must be careful to see and remove this at surgery to avoid a residual middle ear cholesteatoma.

107.2 Active Mucosal Chronic Otitis Media (Wet Perforation)

A dry (inactive) perforation may become infected (active) when pathogens gain entry to the middle ear cleft either via the eustachian tube, often triggered by an upper respiratory tract infection (URTI), or via the ear canal where contaminated bath, swimming pool or sea water are the most common sources. The mucosa becomes oedematous and fibrotic with hypervascularity and influx of inflammatory cells. Blood vessel proliferation and fibroblast activity form granulation tissue. This tissue may coalesce forming a polyp which may protrude through the perforation which tends to bleed easily on instrumentation. The inflammatory process promotes osteoclast activity initiating a resorptive osteitis of the ossicles. This may result in ossicular erosion, particularly the long process of incus, and also the stapes crura or manubrium.

107.3 Inactive Squamous Chronic Otitis Media (Retraction and Atelectasis)

This is medial retraction of the pars tensa or pars flaccida that has potential to become active with keratinous debris (cholesteatoma). Negative middle ear pressure is thought to initiate the retraction, but other factors may perpetuate or contribute to it. Retraction is a dynamic state and may reverse in the early stages. As retraction advances, changes occur in the membrane leading to further likely irreversible weakness. Episodic mesotympanic inflammation may cause contractile adhesions between the middle ear wall and the retracted drum exacerbating the problem. In the pars tensa, retractions may be localised or more generalised. Atelectasis refers to a drum that has lost some of its elastic features and becomes hyper-compliant. Numerous classifications exist for grading the extent of retraction, the most commonly used being those of Sade and Tos.

107.4 Sade (1979)—Pars Tensa

Stage 1—Mild retraction of tympanic membrane.
Stage 2—Retraction onto incudostapedial joint.
Stage 3—Retraction onto promontory.
Stage 4—Adhesion of pars tensa to medial wall (of middle ear).

107.5 Tos and Poulsen (1980)—Pars Flaccida

Type 1—Retraction towards (but not onto) neck of malleus, airspace visible behind.

Type 2—Retraction onto neck of malleus with no visible airspace between membrane and malleus.
Type 3—Retraction of membrane extends beyond osseous malleus but full extent seen.
Type 4—Erosion of outer attic wall (scutum).

107.6 Active Squamous Chronic Otitis Media (Cholesteatoma)

This is the presence of keratinous debris within a matrix of epithelium in the middle ear cleft. Infection may co-exist causing a wet malodorous discharge and inflammatory changes similar to that found in active mucosal COM. Cholesteatoma is described further in another chapter (see Chapter 10).

107.7 Clinical Features

COM can be readily detected using otoscopy. Micro-otoscopic examination, when possible, is preferable. Considerably better detail is appreciated and binocular vision aids depth perception of any drum retraction and extent of any disease. Otoendoscopic examination of the ear is becoming increasingly popular in the outpatient setting and as an adjunct in surgery for COM. This has the advantage of angulated view of the drum or middle ear to detect the depth of disease. Photographic documentation of findings greatly enhances clinician–patient explanation of their disease and is very helpful in monitoring activity/progression of COM.

With pars tensa perforations, deafness is roughly proportional to the size of a perforation. An air–bone gap of more than 30 dB is unusual and suggests an ossicular discontinuity. The patient may notice the hearing improves when the ear discharges indicating there is an ossicular discontinuity which has been bridged by mucopus or a polyp. This sometimes occurs with cholesteatoma or in retraction where the drum remains in contact with an eroded incus or stapes. Tinnitus, typically high pitched, and vertigo, typically momentary and initiated by sudden head movement, are usually associated with a high-tone sensorineural hearing loss secondary to toxins reaching the perilymph through the oval or round window. With cholesteatoma, erosion of the labyrinth (labyrinthine fistula) may cause acute vertigo or a more generalised intermittent disequilibrium. Intracranial and severe cochleovestibular symptoms are unusual as is a lower motor neuron facial palsy.

107.8 Management

1. Dry perforations
   Management options are surgical repair of the perforation, a hearing aid to manage any hearing impairment or no treatment. 'No treatment' includes advice on how to prevent the perforation becoming infected. This includes water precautions where pre-made or custom-moulded ear plugs can be helpful. No treatment is a suitable option for a dry perforation where there are no or very infrequent infections and where any hearing impairment is minimal or otherwise being well managed with a hearing aid.

   Hearing aids offer a safe method of overcoming any hearing impairment. Moulded aids, however, may cause water trapping in the ear canal (from moist air via the perforation) which may increase the risk of infection. Open fit, ventilated or bone conducting devices may overcome this if it becomes problematic for any individual patient.

   Tympanoplasty surgery in expert hands has a perforation closure rate of around 95%. Larger perforations, anterior perforations, surgeon inexperience and revision surgery are associated with lower success rates. The prime goal achieved will be a waterproof ear with reduced chance of infections. Any air–bone gap caused by the perforation is usually improved and ossiculoplasty may be needed to correct any ossicular chain abnormalities. Consideration must be given to the overall hearing impairment and hearing status of the other ear. If closure of the air–bone gap will not improve the overall hearing disability, then tympanoplasty for hearing gain alone may not be worthwhile. Patient factors such as desire to swim, occupation, lifestyle, age and general health will all influence the decision to proceed with surgery or not (see Chapter 117, Tympanoplasty).

2. Wet perforations
   Active infection is treated with regular aural toilet to remove infected debris or granulation and topical medication. Aural toilet is best achieved with microsuction. Topical aminoglycoside, usually with steroid, is highly effective at treating active mucosal COM. Several studies have demonstrated topical treatment is more effective than aural toilet alone, or systemic (oral or parenteral) antibiotics. Aminoglycosides

S

are potentially ototoxic, although the significance of this in active COM is not entirely clear. The Safety of Medicines Regulatory Authority in the United Kingdom continues to consider topical aminoglycosides contraindicated in the presence of a drum perforation. ENT UK has published guidance and recommendations for their use in the presence of a wet perforation. Topical fluoroquinolones have no proven ototoxicity and are as effective at treating infection. Most available are licenced for ophthalmic use and are thus used in the ear 'off license'. However, the MHRA has recently approved a combination topical ciprofloxacin and dexamethasone preparation for use in an open middle ear. Therefore this, or other fluoroquinolones, should be used where possible.

Tympanoplasty surgery to seal the perforation and prevent infection is very effective. Attempts to dry the ear up before surgery will facilitate surgery, but probably does not materially affect surgical success. Adjuvant cortical mastoidectomy is sometimes performed to help remove active disease, but the evidence points to this adding little to success rates overall (see Chapter 117, Tympanoplasty)

3. Retraction pockets and atelectasis
   Retraction may resolve, remain static or progress to cholesteatoma. When identified, a retraction should at least be monitored for potential progression. In those over the age of 12 years, eustachian tube function is more likely to be normal. Thus, in the over 12-year group, retractions should be stable. Periodic monitoring in the clinic over time (2–5 years) will help determine this. If the pocket remains stable, then further observation is less likely to be of benefit. For those under the age of 12 years, there is a greater chance a retraction will be unstable. Children should be kept under review. Children with otitis media with effusion (OME) and retraction have a high chance of resolution when the OME resolves (70%). Retraction without complication rarely requires any treatment. Where there is impending ossicular erosion or the pocket starts to become active, the options are to excise the retraction with no graft or, more

commonly performed, to excise and reconstruct the defect (with fascia or perichondrium or cartilage, etc.). A frank discussion must be undertaken with the patient or parents about the pros and cons of intervention and the likely outcomes of treatment versus no treatment. Placement of a ventilation tube, may on the face of it, seems like a reasonable treatment, to help ventilate the middle ear and prevent further retraction. The main evidence base comes from studies of retraction in OME, where ventilation tube placement greatly increases the rates of retraction. However, whether this principle translates to eardrums with retractions but without OME is uncertain.

4. Cholesteatoma
   Untreated cholesteatoma will continue to expand and locally erode anatomy within the temporal bone. The only effective treatment is surgical eradication, although regular aural toilet and topical treatment of concurrent infection is an option for those who are not surgically fit. The principal aims of surgery are to eradicate disease and preserve function of the middle ear. This is discussed in detail in the cholesteatoma chapter, Chapter 10.

Further Reading

Phillips JS, Yung MW, Burton MJ, Swan IR. Evidence review and ENT-UK consensus report for the use of aminoglycoside-containing ear drops in the presence of an open middle ear. Clin Otolaryngol. 2007; 32(5):330–336

Sade J. The atelectatic ear. In: Sade J, ed. Monograms in Clinical Otolaryngology, Secretory Otitis Media and Its Sequelae. New York, NY: Churchill Livingstone; 1979:64–88

Tos M, Poulsen G. Attic retractions following secretory otitis. Acta Otolaryngol. 1980; 89(5–6):479–486

Tos M, Stangerup SE, Larsen P. Dynamics of eardrum changes following secretory otitis. A prospective study. Arch Otolaryngol Head Neck Surg. 1987; 113(4):380–385

Related Topics of Interest

Suppurative otitis media—acute
Suppurative otitis media—complications
Tympanoplasty
Cholesteatoma
Mastoid surgery

108 Suppurative Otitis Media—Complications

The complications of otitis media (OM) are associated with a high morbidity and may be life threatening with an 8% mortality risk from intracranial complications. Complications can arise from all forms of active otitis media including cholesteatoma, middle ear mucosal disease and acute otitis media. The complications occur by spread of infection:

- *Directly* via the oval or round window to reach the labyrinth, through osteomyelitic bone to reach the dura and lateral sinus, or to affect a congenitally dehiscent facial nerve.
- *By retrograde propagation* of small foci of thrombophlebitis, of emissary veins, which may extend through the temporal bone and dura to the major venous sinuses to cause a lateral sinus thrombosis and by further extension a cerebellar or temporal lobe abscess.
- *Along the periarteriolar spaces* to cause a temporal or cerebellar lobe abscess.

Browning, in a retrospective study, has calculated that the annual risk of a patient with chronic otitis media developing an otogenic intracerebral abscess is approximately 1 in 10,000, and 1:3,500 for developing meningitis.

The complications may be classified as extracranial or intracranial.

108.1 Extracranial Complications (~ 40%)

- Mastoiditis/post-aural abscess—75% of extracranial complications.
- Chronic otitis externa and meatal stenosis.
- Ossicular discontinuity from ossicular erosion.
- Middle ear adhesions.
- Tympanosclerosis which may spread from the tympanic membrane over the ossicular chain causing ossicular chain fixation.
- Lower motor neuron facial nerve palsy.
- Serous or purulent labyrinthitis.
- Labyrinthine fistula.
- Petrositis and Gradenigo's syndrome (signs of acute suppurative otitis media [ASOM], an ipsilateral abducent nerve palsy and pain in the distribution of the ipsilateral trigeminal nerve).

- Bezold's and Citelli's abscess—also complications of acute otitis media.
- Luc's abscess—secondary to acute OM is invariably a rare abscess beneath temporalis muscle caused not by a breach through the mastoid bone but by pus tracking from the middle ear along the external auditory meatus beneath meatal skin and then tracking deeply and superiorly at the bony/cartilaginous meatal junction.
- Squamous cell carcinoma of the middle ear.

108.2 Intracranial Complications (~ 60%)

- Extradural, subdural, intracerebral (cerebellar and temporal lobe) abscess—70%.
- Lateral (transverse and sigmoid) sinus thrombosis. This may extend to involve the superior and inferior petrosal sinus, the cavernous sinus, the sinus confluence, the superior sagittal sinus and the internal jugular vein. There is often a concomitant extradural or subdural abscess which may have precipitated the formation of the thrombus.
- Meningitis.
- Otitic hydrocephalus.

108.3 Clinical Features

Patients with acute intracranial complications usually present to the neurosurgeons and are most likely to be seen by an ENT surgeon after recovery from the acute episode. Patients with OM who present with unilateral or occipital headaches, visual disturbance, vomiting, clumsiness, forgetfulness or drowsiness should have a full neurological examination looking in particular for signs of raised intracranial pressure, meningitis and localising cerebellar and temporoparietal lobe signs. A deep throbbing otalgia and serosanguinous discharge may herald malignant change.

108.4 Investigations

A high-definition CT scan of the petrous temporal bone will show the extent of mastoid disease although it may not distinguish cholesteatoma from mucosal disease. A gadolinium-enhanced MR scan can make the diagnosis of an intracranial venous thrombosis (simple thrombus shows an intermediate signal, vascularised thrombus, granulation tissue and slow-flowing blood a high signal and fast-flowing blood no signal) and intracranial abscess (shows a centre of low attenuation with an outer rim of high signal). A CT venogram or MR venogram will confirm the diagnosis if the enhanced MR is suspicious for but not diagnostic of a lateral sinus thrombosis.

108.5 Treatment

Principles:

1. High-dose intravenous antibiotics to commence after taking a culture swab of the aural discharge.
2. Early liaison with the neurosurgeons to manage intracerebral abscess.
3. Treatment of initiating otological disorder.

Subdural and extradural abscesses require a cortical mastoidectomy to provide adequate exposure before drainage. A lateral sinus thrombosis should have as a minimum a cortical mastoidectomy and removal of the lateral sinus plate to expose the lateral sinus. The diagnosis should be confirmed by needling the sinus. After confirmation, some authorities propose doing no more and treating the patient with high-dose intravenous antibiotics. Others advocate opening the sinus and evacuating clot, trying to obtain free bleeding from each end. This might mean then having to pack the cortical cavity with a temporalis muscle flap reinforced if necessary with bismuth iodoform paraffin paste (BIPP) to control bleeding. Tying the internal jugular vein high up in the neck to prevent infective embolisation during evacuation of infected clot is no longer thought necessary because of the risk of retrograde propagation of the thrombosis to involve the sagittal sinuses.

A facial palsy secondary to acute OM is invariably a neuropraxia. The nerve does not require decompressing and should recover rapidly with aggressive treatment of the infection. The facial palsy in chronic OM is usually secondary to compression from cholesteatoma or granulation tissue. Most otologists advocate an urgent mastoidectomy and decompression of the vertical segment of the facial nerve though this has recently been challenged. If there is an actively discharging ear, others would observe for at least 48 hours with the patient on intravenous antibiotics. In this instance, the palsy may be a neuropraxia of a dehiscent horizontal segment of the nerve, found in 6% of ears.

Labyrinthine fistulae may be caused by erosion of bone by cholesteatoma and by osteitis with the formation of granulation tissue. In cholesteatoma, the matrix usually becomes apposed to the endosteum within the fistula and a protective walling off does not arise. If a fistula is suspected from clinical signs and operative findings then either (1) the matrix can be left over the affected portion of the labyrinth and a canal wall down procedure performed leaving an open cavity, or alternatively, (2) the matrix can be peeled off under constant irrigation and the fistula immediately sealed with fascia or muscle as the final manoeuvre in surgery.

Further Reading

Browning GG, Merchant SN, et al. Chronic otitis media. In: Michael Gleeson, ed. Otorhinolaryngology and Head and Neck Surgery. 7th ed. London: Hodder Arnold; 2008:3395–3445

Herzog JA, Smith PG, Kletzker GR, Maxwell KS. Management of labyrinthine fistulae secondary to cholesteatoma. Am J Otol. 1996; 17(3):410–415

Related Topics of Interest

Cholesteatoma
Suppurative otitis media—acute
Suppurative otitis media—chronic

109 Temporal Bone Cancer

Cancer of the external auditory canal and middle ear is rare. Severe otalgia, bloody otorrhoea and visible irregularity are suspicious clinical features. The mainstay of treatment is surgery, usually with post-operative radiotherapy. The minimal operation is a lateral temporal bone resection. The morbidity of surgery with very advanced cancers is high and the chance of cure is generally poor.

109.1 Epidemiology and Pathology

Primary cancers of the temporal bone are comparatively rare, with an incidence of less than 1 per million per year. Mostly, they are squamous cell carcinomas (SCCs) arising in the external auditory meatus (EAM). Middle ear SCC is even less common. The only aetiological factor relevant in some cases is chronic inflammation, in the form of otitis externa or suppurative otitis media, or an unstable, chronically infected post-surgical mastoid cavity.

These cancers arise from the epithelial surface and spread along that surface and deeply into the underlying bone. Further local spread depends on the anatomical location of the primary cancer, but can extend superiorly through the tegmen into the middle cranial fossa; anteriorly into the temporomandibular joint (TMJ) or parotid gland; posteriorly into the mastoid air cells; or medially into the middle ear and labyrinth. The facial nerve can be involved medially and posteriorly. Extensive spread along the lateral skull base can involve other cranial nerves (IX, X and XII). Lymph node metastasis can be to intraparotid lymph nodes, and/or to cervical lymph nodes (most commonly to level 2).

Other tumour types include basal cell carcinoma (generally conchal bowl/lateral EAM), skin adnexal cancers and melanoma. Parotid cancers can invade into the temporal bone and EAM and can be confused with a primary temporal bone cancer. Any age group can be affected, although the incidence generally increases with age.

109.2 Clinical Features

While rare, cancer should be considered in any patients with more than one of chronic otalgia, bloody otorrhoea, bleeding, mass in the ear (often granulation tissue/ulceration), facial swelling or facial palsy. Some patients may have a long history of chronic middle or external ear infection. The diagnosis should also be considered in any patient with chronic suppurative otitis media (CSOM) or a mastoid cavity who develops increasing pain. Late diagnosis of patients with cancers of the EAM and middle ear (ME) is not uncommon. Different pathologies can present in a similar way. These include pseudotumoural skull base osteomyelitis of the temporal bone (also called necrotising or malignant otitis externa), and inflammatory diseases such as granulomatosis with polyangiitis.

109.3 Investigations

Diagnosis is achieved by biopsy of the EAM or ME, achievable in many cases in clinic. In some cases, examination and biopsy under anaesthesia may be required.

Both computed tomography (CT) and magnetic resonance imaging (MRI) are required (temporal bone and neck). CT (fine cut, high resolution) is essential for assessing EAM erosion, extent of middle ear and mastoid involvement, spread into jugular bulb, carotid canal, tegmen, TMJ, parotid and beyond. MR differentiates mucosal swelling or mastoid fluid from tumour, is superior at ascertaining dural or brain involvement and gives more detail of parapharyngeal space and infratemporal fossa involvement. Both can also stage the neck. In addition, a CT of thorax should be done to exclude distant metastasis, as with other head and neck cancers.

A pure-tone audiogram should be performed. It informs the patient and clinicians about the level of hearing and will help to inform its subsequent management.

109.4 Staging

There is no Union for International Cancer Control (UICC) or American Joint Committee on Cancer (AJCC) staging system for cancers of the temporal bone or lateral skull base. However, many use the revised Pittsburgh staging system (▶ Table 109.1). Standard UICC staging is used for neck and distant metastases.

▶ **Table 109.1** Modified Pittsburg staging system

T1	Tumour limited to the EAC without bony erosion or evidence of soft tissue extension.
T2	Tumour with limited EAC erosion (not full thickness) or radiological findings consistent with limited (< 0.5 cm) soft tissue involvement.
T3	Tumour eroding the osseous EAC (full thickness) with limited (< 0.5 cm) soft tissue involvement of middle ear and/or mastoid, or causing facial paralysis at presentation.
T4	Tumour eroding the cochlear, petrous apex, medial wall of middle ear, carotid canal, jugular foramen or dura or with extensive (> 0.5 cm) soft tissue involvement.

Abbreviation: EAC, external auditory canal.

109.5 Treatment and Prognosis

As with all head and neck cancers, all cases should be discussed in the setting of a head and neck cancer multi-disciplinary team (MDT), with expertise in lateral skull base surgery.

Treatment for cure is through primary surgery with an en bloc temporal bone resection and, usually, post-operative radiotherapy. The influence of middle ear involvement on prognosis is critical. T1 and T2 lesions (lateral to the tympanic membrane) have cure rates between 80 and 100% with true en bloc resections without breach of the tumour. T3 and T4 5-year survival results vary from dismal to as high as 50% in some series. If the modified Pittsburg staging is applied to middle ear carcinomas, they are all at least T3.

109.6 Surgery

A lateral temporal bone resection (LTBR) should be regarded as the minimum oncological operation for T1 and T2 lesions.

The essential elements of LTBR are (1) excision lateral to the facial nerve; (2) conchal bowl resection; (3) bony cuts: mastoid to middle fossa dura (or leaving a thin layer of bone), anteriorly into zygomatic aircells and TMJ, inferiorly to stylomastoid foramen, hypotympanum to TMJ.

This can be modified with additional steps, which include resection of the entire pinna and periauricular skin; condyle/mandible, parotid,

extension of resection into parapharyngeal space and infratemporal fossa, neck dissection, facial nerve sacrifice and cable graft.

Extended temporal bone resection (ETBR) is required for more extensive tumours involving the middle ear. The essential elements of ETBR are (1) facial nerve sacrifice; (2) posterior and middle craniotomy; (3) labyrinthectomy; (4) transection of internal auditory canal; (5) resection of petrous tip; (6) exposure of intrapetrous portion of the carotid; (7) total parotidectomy.

This can be modified with additional steps including craniectomy (squamous temporal bone; sphenoid wing, posterior fossa); mandibulectomy; parapharyngeal/infratemporal fossa resection; extension to jugular foramen; lower cranial nerve sacrifice; dural resection.

For very advanced cancers, careful consideration needs to be given as to whether the risks and consequences of aggressive resection are justified given the small chance of cure. Dural involvement is a highly adverse prognostic indicator. A small proportion of these patients might be curable, but dural spread along the middle fossa is often quite wide (and therefore not totally resectable), and, if there is cerebral involvement, the chance of cure is tiny.

Resection of the intrapetrous carotid is possible. If this is the case, or anticipated as a possibility, patients can benefit from pre-operative radiological permanent occlusion of the carotid artery, subject to successful balloon occlusion. However, the cancer mortality in this group of patients with petrous apex involvement is high, due to, among other factors, difficulties achieving full microscopic resection around this area. The post-operative morbidity is also extremely high due to, among other things, multiple cranial nerve deficits from a resection of this extent. Thus, for this group of patient, surgery is not a particularly attractive option in the main.

109.6.1 Parotidectomy

The parotid gland may be either involved directly by tumour, or be harbouring intraparotid lymph node metastases (it may contain the primary echelon lymph node). Therefore, for all resections, at least a superficial parotidectomy should be carried out. For advanced T3/T4 temporal bone SCCs, total parotidectomy should be carried out, which also facilitates access to the parapharyngeal space, infratemporal fossa and masticator space. For basal

T

cell carcinoma (BCC) without evidence of direct invasion into or near the parotid gland, parotidectomy can be omitted.

109.6.2 Facial Nerve

Pre-operative facial nerve dysfunction due to facial nerve involvement by tumour requires sacrifice of the nerve as part of the resection. For some patients with normal function pre-operatively, it may be technically impossible to resect a tumour, with curative intent, without nerve sacrifice. When the facial nerve is sacrificed, the proximal stump at the limit of the sacrifice should be sent for frozen section pathology.

When facial nerve sacrifice is necessary, steps to bring about dynamic re-animation or static facial elevation should be considered. It should be borne in mind that, with the exception of oculoplastic interventions, the best time to perform these interventions is at the time of tumour resection, as virtually every patient in this group will go on to have post-operative radiotherapy.

- Dynamic re-animation: A cable graft from middle ear facial nerve to intra- or extra-parotid branches can be performed if there is enough proven tumour-free proximal facial nerve. Otherwise a facial–hypoglossal anastomosis can be considered. Useful donor nerves include greater auricular nerve, sural nerve or lateral cutaneous nerve of thigh (easily available if harvesting an anterolateral thigh free flap).
- Static facial elevation: Static procedures can be employed, using temporalis myoplasty (Labbé) or sling/fascia lata for oral commissure/cheek suspension.

109.6.3 Reconstruction

Dural defects are normally repaired with non-vascularised tissue such as autologous fascia lata grafts or synthetic materials.

Reconstruction of the skin defect should be considered in parallel with the volume defect created, this being determined by the extent of temporal bone resection, parotidectomy and mandibulectomy in particular.

For smaller skin defects without much volume loss, options include radial forearm free flap, cervicofacial rotation flap and temporalis flap.

These can be used to reconstruct small skin/auricle defects with modest volume loss.

For most defects after temporal bone resection, the anterolateral thigh free flap offers optimal reconstruction, providing bulk/contouring, and enough skin for most defects (which can be reduced by de-epithelisation if the auricule is not resected). It also allows vascularised fascia lata to be used for static facial re-suspension and/or the lateral cutaneous nerve of the thigh for an interpositional facial nerve graft.

The use of pectoralis major flap is sub-optimal as the lateral skull base is at or beyond the limits of rotation in many cases.

109.6.4 Neck Dissection

In the setting of cN0 neck, selective neck dissection should be performed for all temporal bone SCC. The levels dissected will vary according to the extent and location of tumour but will generally comprise of 1b, 2 and 3. However, the apex of level 5 may also need to be included.

As for any head and neck cancer, N+ necks require comprehensive neck dissection, although level 1a (sub-mental) can be spared.

109.6.5 Post-Operative Care Issues

In addition to facial nerve issues, all lower cranial nerves essential for swallowing and voice (IX, X and XII) are at risk of injury or sacrifice in surgery for advanced tumours. Care of the patient in this situation must include close involvement of speech and language therapy. Interventions include either pre- or post-operative percutaneous gastrostomy, nasogastric tube and tracheostomy if aspirating on saliva. Later interventions include vocal cord medialisation and cricopharyngeal myotomy.

Ipsilateral total (sensorineural) or total conductive hearing deficit is an inevitable outcome of temporal bone resection. Pre-operative audiological assessment of the contralateral ear will identify patients with a pre-existing deficit. This may be corrected or improved with appropriate aiding. Total conductive hearing loss can be rehabilitated through an osseointegrated bone anchored hearing aid (BAHA). Total hearing loss can be rehabilitated through either BAHA or a BICROS aid.

Post-operative vertigo is expected if there is resection of a functioning labyrinth. If vestibular compensation is protracted and incomplete, referral for vestibular rehabilitation services should be considered.

109.7 Radiotherapy

109.7.1 Post-Operative Radiotherapy

The decision regarding post-operative radiotherapy is based on an individualised MDT discussion with interaction between surgeon, pathologist and clinical oncologist.

In general, T1 and T2 SCCs without adverse histological features (particularly perineural infiltration) and with proven clear margins may not require adjuvant therapy. However, all other cases (the majority) will require post-operative radiotherapy.

109.7.2 Primary Radiotherapy

When primary surgery is not considered possible, or too morbid, definitive radiotherapy may be used. While surgery is the preferred primary treatment, radiotherapy does offer effective short–medium-term survival/local tumour control and, sometimes, cure.

Synchronous treatment with cisplatin can be considered; however, ototoxicity is enhanced compared with radiotherapy alone and brain toxicity is also likely to be increased.

Further Reading

Homer JJ, Lesser T, Moffat D, Slevin N, Price R, Blackburn T. Management of lateral skull base cancer: United Kingdom National Multidisciplinary Guidelines. J Laryngol Otol. 2016; 130(S2):S119–S124

Masterson L, Rouhani M, Donnelly NP, et al. Squamous cell carcinoma of the temporal bone: clinical outcomes from radical surgery and postoperative radiotherapy. Otol Neurotol. 2014; 35(3):501–508

Moody SA, Hirsch BE, Myers EN. Squamous cell carcinoma of the external auditory canal: an evaluation of a staging system. Am J Otol. 2000; 21(4):582–588

Rosenthal EL, King T, McGrew BM, Carroll W, Magnuson JS, Wax MK. Evolution of a paradigm for free tissue transfer reconstruction of lateral temporal bone defects. Head Neck. 2008; 30(5):589–594

Shinomiya H, Hasegawa S, Yamashita D, et al. Concomitant chemoradiotherapy for advanced squamous cell carcinoma of the temporal bone. Head Neck. 2016; 38(Suppl 1):E949–E953

Related Topics of Interest

Cervical lymphadenopathy
External ear conditions
Facial nerve palsy
Vocal fold paralysis

110 Temporal Bone Fractures

110.1 Background

Temporal bone fractures (TBFs) occur as a result of severe head injury, from either blunt or penetrating trauma. The main issues relevant to the otolaryngologist are damage to the facial nerve, inner ear, ossicles, tympanic membrane, external auditory canal, persistent cerebrospinal fluid (CSF) leak either from the ear or nose or temporal bone meningoencephalocele formation. Severe penetrating injury could also cause vascular injury to the internal carotid artery (ICA), jugular bulb or sigmoid sinus or the lower cranial nerves as they exit the jugular foramen. Considerable force is usually required with consequent loss of consciousness and the potential for serious associated injuries that require neurosurgical management. These will take priority over managing the issues relevant to the otolaryngologist, which may not become apparent for several days or even weeks. Sometimes the patients may not have other injuries and only require overnight observation in terms of their overall head injury. These patients will present earlier. Rarely a TBF may occur secondary to mandibular trauma, with a localised fracture of the external ear canal posterior to the temporomandibular joint.

110.2 Pathogenesis/ Classification

TBFs are traditionally classified (Ulrich) according to the direction of the fracture compared with the line of the petrous temporal bone.

- Longitudinal fractures (80% of fractures), usually caused by blunt trauma to the side of the head, travel medially from the squamous temporal bone into the middle ear or mastoid and then towards the petrous bone. They often cross the facial nerve at the geniculate ganglion, causing a temporary palsy that will resolve, and passing anterior to the otic capsule. They are more commonly associated with ossicular chain disruption, middle ear fluid, haemotympanum and tympanic membrane (TM) perforation all contributing to a conductive hearing loss.
- Transverse fractures (20% of fractures), typically caused by trauma to the back of the head, pass from the occipital bone anterolaterally, crossing either the mastoid and middle ear or through the otic capsule or the internal auditory canal (IAC), with a higher incidence of severe facial nerve injury and damage to the cochlea giving a sensorineural hearing loss. In reality, many fractures do not follow this presentation and are known as mixed fractures.

More recently, TBFs have been classified according to whether they spare the otic capsule or not as this appears to be a better predictor of whether severe facial nerve injury or CSF leak will occur.

An understanding of the pathophysiology of facial nerve injury is essential in understanding its management. When the facial nerve is injured in TBF, it may be subjected to blunt force causing either neuropraxia or axonotmesis, depending on severity, or sharp trauma (e.g. from bone fragments) causing neurotmesis. There may be a combination of all three types of injury, with the pre-dominant one determining the prognosis. A neuropraxia results in a conduction block which will resolve in a few weeks. Both axonotmesis and neurotmesis result in distal wallerian degeneration, which usually occurs over a period of 3 to 14 days. There will also be significant oedema that may result in further injury, because the nerve is confined within a bony canal, converting neuropraxia to axonotmesis. Following wallerian degeneration, the nerve fibres have to regrow from the point of injury into the distal nerve sheath, at approximately 1 mm per day. A complete transection, a bone fragment or fibrosis may prevent some nerve fibres finding the distal sheath, resulting in loss of neurons to the distal muscles. The nerve fibres grow up the nerve sheath in an uncontrolled fashion, inevitably resulting in some aberrant regeneration and subsequent synkinesis.

A patient with an initial incomplete palsy must have had a substantial proportion of nerve fibres that were initially uninjured. Subsequent deterioration is likely to be caused by conversion to neuropraxia secondary to oedema. These patients are likely to return to normal function without the need for surgical treatment.

It should also be noted that a patient with a complete palsy will often be able to close his or her eyelid initially because there will still be resting tone within the facial muscles and the lid closes by relaxation of levator palpebrae superioris, which is innervated by the oculomotor nerve.

T

110.3 Acute Management

Resuscitation should be carried out using the standard ABC formula. Any suggestion of vascular injury should be managed as per zone III of the neck, with an angiogram performed and embolisation, balloon occlusion or stenting to the intratemporal ICA performed if necessary. Pre-dominantly, acute management will be performed by the trauma team alongside the neurosurgeons with the otolaryngologist mainly involved with managing trauma to the neck.

110.4 History

Once the patient is stable and conscious, the history should focus on his or her facial function, inner and middle ear status and whether there is any evidence of CSF leak.

Ideally, the time course of facial palsy should be elicited, determining whether the palsy was of delayed onset or initially incomplete. In reality, this is often not possible as other features of the head injury will have taken precedence. Eye witness accounts are likely to be unreliable as the eye will still have closed as described above. It should be noted whether the patient has any eye discomfort currently that may require acute treatment.

Further history should note whether there has been discharge from the ear (blood or serous), hearing loss, tinnitus, vertigo or imbalance or any clear, watery and ipsilateral rhinorrhoea.

110.5 Examination

Facial function needs to be carefully assessed. Attention needs to be paid to any movement at the forehead, orbicularis oculi, orbicularis oris and in the midface in order to grade the palsy. Eyelid closure should not be used in the early days after injury. The eye should be assessed for any corneal or conjunctival inflammation.

The ear is assessed with otoscopy, noting blood or clear fluid within the canal, lacerations to the canal indicative of a fracture, injury to the tympanic membrane or a haemotympanum. Clinical hearing tests and tuning fork tests will help determine the nature of any hearing loss.

Features of a vestibular injury may include horizontal paralytic nystagmus (fast phase away from the injured ear), a positive head impulse test ipsilateral to the injury or a positive Unterberger's

test depending on the severity of the injury and time delay since the injury occurred.

CSF rhinorrhoea may be assessed by noting the presence of clear fluid arising from the ipsilateral eustachian tube on nasendoscopy.

110.6 Investigations

Imaging If there is suspicion of a TBF, then a high-resolution computed tomography (HRCT) scan of the temporal bone is required. The patient may have had a CT head as part of his or her initial assessment that may demonstrate the fracture, but the higher resolution of the temporal bone scan is more helpful to determine the precise course of the fracture line and to look for bone fragments that may be compressing the facial nerve. A pneumolabyrinth is a sign that the otic capsule has been involved in the fracture. A large fracture may also cause meningoencephalocele formation. While a CT will provide an indication of this, magnetic resonance imaging (MRI) may be required for certainty.

Hearing tests Once the patient is well enough, then a pure-tone audiogram should be carried out to determine the nature of any sensorineural or conductive hearing loss.

Electrophysiology If the patient has a complete facial palsy and there is no reliable history of delayed onset, then electrophysiology should be considered to assess facial function, again once the patient is well enough. Electroneuronography (ENoG) is carried out initially to assess wallerian degeneration. This test consists of applying monitoring needle electrodes into the distal facial muscles bilaterally and then a stimulating electrode just in front of both mastoid processes, such that the main facial nerve trunk is stimulated as it arises through the stylomastoid foramen. The amplitude of the action potential on the electro-myogram (EMG) is then compared between both sides. A loss of greater than 90% is indicative of a severe injury and correlates well with a poorer outcome. These patients benefit from surgical exploration with nerve decompression and repair if necessary. Because of the time course of wallerian degeneration with the potential for further deterioration due to oedema, the test should not be performed before 3 days and will need to be repeated up to 14 days after the injury. Some authors recommend daily testing (assuming the initial test demonstrates reasonable function),

T

but, as this is an uncomfortable test involving significant resources, a more pragmatic view may be to carry the test out at 7 and 14 days post-injury. By 6 to 8 weeks, neuropraxia should have resolved and an EMG may start to show action potentials indicative of a recovering nerve.

110.7 Consequences and Management

110.7.1 Facial Palsy

In patients who develop a facial palsy hours or days after injury or in whom the palsy is partial, the injury is likely to be secondary to a neuropraxia and a conservative policy should be adopted. Steroids may be considered if they are not otherwise contraindicated because of other features of the head injury. ENoG and EMG will provide an indication of the severity of the injury and the prognosis in those patients where the history is not clear. If the summating potential is more than 10% of normal after 14 days, the prognosis is good, with about 90% recovery to House–Brackmann grade I or II. If it is less than 10% after 14 days, then the consensus view is to explore the nerve. If the fracture line appears close to the labyrinthine segment or internal auditory meatus (IAM), then these areas may need to be decompressed and an opinion should be sought from a skull base surgeon. If the hearing has been lost following a fracture through the otic capsule, then a translabyrinthine approach may be used; otherwise a combined middle fossa/transmastoid approach will be required. The surgeon must be prepared to mobilise and/or graft the nerve should a significant transection have occurred, depending on the length of nerve involved.

110.7.2 CSF Leak and Meningoencephalocele Formation

CSF otorrhoea or rhinorrhoea is confirmed by the presence of β_2-transferrin (also known as tau protein). Conservative management with bed rest, head elevation and stool softeners will usually allow the leak to settle within 10 days. A lumbar drain may be considered if the leak does not appear to be settling. The use of prophylactic antibiotic cover is controversial. Should the leak persist greater than 10 days, then surgical exploration will be required by a skull base surgeon.

If the leak requires surgical repair or there is formation of a meningoencephalocele, then, depending on the size and site of the defect, it is usually possible to repair directly with a trans-mastoid and/or middle fossa approach or a translabyrinthine approach if there is already a profound sensorineural hearing loss. Large defects may require eustachian tube obliteration, blind sac closure of the external ear canal with removal of the tympanic membrane and a fat graft (usually harvested from the abdomen or the thigh) to the middle ear and mastoid cavities. If obliteration is required in the presence of good hearing, then this can be rehabilitated with a bone conduction hearing aid (BCHA) as it will not be possible to use a conventional hearing aid.

110.7.3 Inner Ear Trauma

Vestibular injury should be managed in the same way as labyrinthitis, with acute vestibular suppressants and then longer-term vestibular rehabilitation to facilitate central compensation if necessary.

The patient's sensorineural hearing loss will be managed with an ipsilateral conventional hearing aid for mild-to-severe loss and contralateral routing of signal (CROS) hearing aids or a BCHA for profound hearing loss as per any cause of single-sided deafness. Bilateral profound hearing loss can occasionally occur in the presence of bilateral TBF and will require rehabilitation with cochlear implantation. Extremely rarely, there have been reports of bilateral cochlear nerve avulsion and then the only option for auditory rehabilitation is with an auditory brainstem implant.

Fluctuating vertigo and hearing loss might suggest an ongoing perilymph fistula which may need surgical exploration. This may be difficult to distinguish from secondary endolymphatic hydrops which may also occur. Benign paroxysmal positional vertigo is not uncommon after any head injury.

110.7.4 Tympanic Membrane Damage

Tympanic membrane perforations can occur as a result of direct penetrating trauma, barotrauma

T

or shearing forces from a fracture. They should be managed conservatively, initially with water precautions and antibiotics only if there is infection. Many will heal spontaneously, but if there is no evidence of healing after 6 to 8 weeks, then a tympanoplasty may be considered. As with any tympanic membrane perforation, some patients may elect to continue with conservative management.

Clinicians should also be mindful of the possibility of longer-term retraction and cholesteatoma formation if the tympanic membrane is damaged. These will be managed in the standard way.

110.7.5 Ossicular Damage

Conductive hearing loss (CDHL) may occur secondary to acute haemotympanum, effusion, tympanic membrane perforation and ossicular disruption or damage or in the longer term due to fibrosis or tympanosclerosis. Clinical examination, tympanometry and the high-resolution CT scan will help to delineate the cause although some defects, such as fractures of the crura of the stapes or footplate, will probably not be seen.

An initial conservative period is sensible to allow effusions to settle. Because of the limitations of ossicular reconstruction, mild CDHL of less than 20 dB will likely be treated conservatively. More severe CDHL may warrant surgical exploration via a tympanotomy for consideration of ossicular reconstruction. Careful attention should be paid to the stapes and footplate during surgery as well as incus and malleus mobility. Conservative management with audiological rehabilitation with a conventional hearing aid would also be appropriate for any CDHL.

110.7.6 External Auditory Canal

Fractures of the external auditory canal (EAC) may cause bony displacement. Many of these will require no further treatment, but canal stenosis and cholesteatoma formation may occur in the longer term and require surgical management.

Further Reading

Johnson F, Semaan MT, Megerian CA. Temporal bone fracture: evaluation and management in the modern era. Otolaryngol Clin North Am. 2008; 41(3):597–618, x

Schubl SD, Klein TR, Robitsek RJ, et al. Temporal bone fracture: evaluation in the era of modern computed tomography. Injury. 2016; 47(9):1893–1897

Related Topics of Interest

Facial nerve palsy
External ear conditions

111 Thyroid Disease—Benign

Benign thyroid disease can be analysed from three different aspects, which are often inter-related. These are non-toxic thyroid goitre (NTG), hypothyroidism and hyperthyroidism. Patients with NTG are the most important from a surgical standpoint as it is this group that is often referred to otorhinolaryngologists/head and neck surgeons by general practitioners for primary management. In the United Kingdom, it is estimated that up to 15% of the population have a goitre and that when using ultrasound up to 50% of women and 30% of men might have thyroid nodules. Although thyroid nodules are common, the incidence of thyroid cancer is relatively low (See Chapter 112). However, its incidence is increasing rapidly. It is therefore necessary that patients are adequately evaluated.

111.1 Classification of Goitre

1. *Non-toxic goitre* These may be both physiological and pathological. Physiological goitres include puberty, pregnancy and with the contraceptive pill. The causes of pathological goitres include iodine deficiency. Nodular goitre may be solitary or multi-nodular. The differential diagnosis of the solitary thyroid nodule (STN) includes colloid nodule, adenomatoid nodules, follicular adenoma, thyroid cyst or carcinoma. Multi-nodular goitre (MNG) is defined as an enlarged thyroid gland with multiple nodules of different size and consistency. It can be associated with iodine deficiency, which is endemic in patients living at high altitude such as the Alps or Himalayas. The majority of patients with MNG are euthyroid, and present with an asymptomatic enlargement of the thyroid gland or increasing symptoms of compression. Patients with hypothyroidism may or may not have a goitre. Hypothyroidism may be congenital or acquired. The former is usually due to congenital absence or atrophy of the thyroid and if untreated, it leads to cretinism. Rarely, it is associated with inherited dyshormonogenesis such as Pendred's syndrome (which is the association of congenital hypothyroidism with high tone deafness). Acquired hypothyroidism is usually idiopathic or due to surgical ablation of the gland, post-treatment of thyrotoxicosis with radioiodine or Hashimoto's (lymphocytic)

thyroiditis. Treatment is with thyroid hormone replacement. The starting dose is usually T4 100 to 125 µg/d. In the presence of sub-clinical hypothyroidism (high thyroid-stimulating hormone (TSH) > 10 mU/1, normal free T4), patients should be treated with T4 (100 µg/d) if antibodies are positive, if there are convincing symptoms or a past history of radioiodine treatment.

2. *Toxic goitre (hyperthyroidism)* Patients with thyrotoxicosis usually either have Graves' disease or a solitary toxic nodule. Graves' disease is caused by circulating thyroid-stimulating immunoglobulins (IgGs) which bind to TSH receptors to increase thyroid hormone production. These IGs are usually associated with thyroid eye disease (thyroid ophthalmopathy), which is caused by a specific antibody named exophthalmos-producing substance (EPS). EPS targets retro-orbital tissue to cause oedema of fat and muscle. Graves' disease may also be associated with signs of vitiligo, pre-tibial myxoedema, fatigue, atrial fibrillation, weight loss and other autoimmune disorders such as pernicious anaemia.

Hyperthyroidism is usually treated either medically using antithyroid drugs (carbimazole or propylthiouracil) or with radioiodine. About 50% of patients will relapse following medical treatment after 6 months. In these patients, together with those who have significant thyroid ophthalmopathy or those who request surgery, surgery either with a 'near-total' or 'total' thyroidectomy is an alternative option. Radioiodine can also be used to treat large toxic MNG in the elderly and infirm, when good shrinkage is achievable. Patients who have solitary toxic nodules are usually best dealt with surgically.

Some patients who have had a MNG for a long time can develop thyrotoxicosis (Plummer's disease). These patients are often elderly with co-existent morbidity such as ischaemic heart disease, and the rise in T4 is often associated with atrial fibrillation. Because of this, these patients usually have cardiac signs (and not eye signs) and are usually treated medically. Recurrent thyrotoxicosis is treated on its merits, but may require further treatment with either the same or another modality. Many patients (whatever their treatment)

T

will be hypothyroid post-treatment and will be on long-term thyroxine replacement therapy.

Surgical thyroidectomy indications in hyperthyroidism are as follows:

- Failure to medical or radioiodine treatment.
- Suspected malignancy.
- Compression symptoms.
- Dysthyroid eye disease or thyroid ophthalmopathy.
- Patient choice.
- Allergy to iodine and amiodarone.
- Children.

3. *Inflammatory goitre—thyroiditis*
   a. *Hashimoto's thyroiditis* This is an autoimmune disorder most common in middle-aged women. Antibodies are directed against thyroglobulin and/or microsomal peroxidase. They cause lymphocyte infiltration, atrophy and regeneration of the thyroid, and ultimately a goitre. The gland is usually firm, but rubbery. Initially, patients are hyperthyroid, but may become hypothyroid as the disease progresses. Once the diagnosis is made, patients should be treated with thyroxine suppression and have thyroid function tests once a year. Surgery may be required for an enlarged gland causing obstructive symptoms or when there is an indeterminate or suspicious fine-needle aspiration cytology (FNAC) result that necessitates definitive diagnosis. These patients are at a high risk of subsequently developing a thyroid lymphoma.
   b. *De Quervain's thyroiditis* This condition results as a consequence of acute viral infection. Etiological viruses include coxsackie virus, mumps and adenovirus. Some cases develop post-partum. This is a flu-like illness, and associated with diffuse swelling and tenderness of the gland. There is usually both a transient hyperthyroidism and production of autoantibodies. Treatment is with symptomatic non-steroidal anti-inflammatory drugs (NSAIDs), β-blockers and corticosteroids in severe cases.
   c. *Riedel's thyroiditis* This is a rare condition associated with a woody hard, sometimes tender, irregular thyroid gland which histologically shows marked fibrosis. This is thought by some to signify a fibrotic reaction to an underlying carcinoma or lymphoma.

4. *Neoplastic goitre* This can be a benign adenoma or malignant tumour. The overall risk of malignancy in a STN has been reported to be between 4 and 7% and in a MNG between 2 and 11%. This incidence can be even higher in endemic areas.

5. *Miscellaneous goitres* There are a number of other causes of an enlargement of the thyroid gland. These include tuberculosis, sarcoidosis, amyloid, HIV infection, drug-associated thyroiditis and radiation.

111.2 Clinical Assessment

Depending on the cause and duration of the goitre, patients may be euthyroid, hyperthyroid or hypothyroid. A drug history is important because some are goitrogens, for example, sulphonylureas. The goitre may produce discomfort on swallowing, dysphagia (implying oesophageal compression) or stridor (implying tracheal compression or involvement of the recurrent laryngeal nerve). It is important to confirm that the swelling moves with swallowing and to note its size, position and any intrathoracic or retrosternal involvement. The latter is suspected from dullness to percussion over the manubrium or the inability to find a plane between the goitre and the clavicle. The rest of the neck requires examination for the presence of lymph nodes, and the examination of the larynx with fibre-optic endoscopic nasolaryngoscopy is mandatory for the evaluation of vocal cord movement.

111.3 Investigations

All patients with a goitre should have their thyroid function and thyroid antibody status checked. In addition, all euthyroid patients should have an ultrasound (US) guided with or without FNAC performed and a vocal cord check is advised in those with any voice change, difficulty in swallowing and breathing, and in those patients undergoing surgery. A chest X-ray is not usually required and flow loops are not helpful unless the patient has an incidental intrathoracic goitre. Serum calcium and calcitonin may be indicated when there is clinical suspicion of multiple endocrine neoplasia or medullary thyroid carcinoma.

- US is now part of the baseline assessment in patients with nodular goitres. It provides information about size, number of nodules and the status of the other lobe and neck. It will provide evidence of the characteristics of the nodules for being solid, cystic or mixed. Cystic nodules are rarely neoplastic. Hypoechoic nodules, micro-calcification, irregular margins, high vascularity and evidence of associated lymphadenopathies are all features of malignancy. It also aids the FNAC by decreasing the sample error and by increasing its accuracy.

- Radionuclide scintigraphy using Tc_{99} or I^{123} can be used to identify whether a nodule is 'hot' (takes up isotope) and therefore is functioning, or is 'cold' (and therefore not functioning). More than 90% of lesions identified with scintigraphy will not concentrate the radio-nuclide and therefore will appear 'cold'. These clinically solitary non-functional nodules may represent an adenoma, carcinoma, a cyst or a dominant nodule in a non-palpable MNG. The likelihood of malignancy in a truly solitary cold nodule is between 10 and 20%. The rate of malignancy in truly functioning nodules (hot)

is less than 5%. Scintigraphy is only used in the evaluation of thyroid nodules if there is evidence of hyperthyroidism.

- FNAC is safe, cheap and reliable with a diagnostic accuracy of approximately 90% and is therefore together with the US the initial investigation of choice for a STN. The diagnostic strategy for evaluating the thyroid nodule is shown below.
- Anatomical imaging with computed tomography (CT) scan with contrast is useful to assess patients with compression symptoms, suspicion of intrathoracic extension or malignancy. It is an excellent modality to evaluate the neck for nodes, the visceral compartment of the neck, the mediastinum and the chest.

111.4 Management

Patients presenting with STN or non-toxic MNG should be managed by the following guidance from the British Thyroid Association (▶Fig. 111.1).

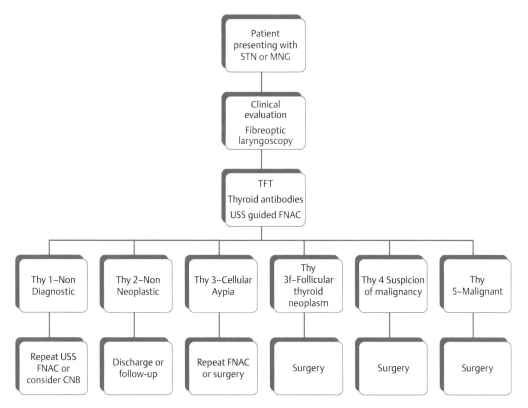

Fig. 111.1 British Thyroid Association guidelines for management of patients presenting with STN or non-toxic MNG.

111.4.1 Surgical Management

Surgery is the mainstay of many thyroid disorders. These include thyroid cancer, MNGs with compressive symptoms and thyrotoxicosis.

The current indications for surgery in thyroid disorders include the following:

1. Suspected or proven malignancy.
2. Cosmetic or quality-of-life reasons.
3. Compressive symptoms.
4. Thyrotoxicosis.
5. Failure to medical treatment.

111.4.2 Types of Surgery

The following operations can be performed on the thyroid gland:

1. Isthmusectomy.
2. Lobectomy.
3. Sub-total thyroidectomy.
4. Near-total thyroidectomy.
5. Total thyroidectomy.

A lumpectomy is removal of the nodule alone with minimal surrounding thyroid tissue. This is not recommended as it would cause significant fibrosis compromising any subsequent removal of the gland. A total lobectomy completely removes one thyroid lobe with the isthmus. A sub-total thyroidectomy is bilateral removal of more than one-half of the thyroid gland on each side plus the isthmus and is rarely performed. A 'near-total' thyroidectomy is a total lobectomy and the isthmusectomy with removal of more than 90% of the contralateral lobe and is often done to preserve blood supply to parathyroids on one side. A 'total' thyroidectomy is removal of both thyroid lobes and the isthmus with preservation of the parathyroids and a completion thyroidectomy is a subsequent procedure to convert a lesser operation into a near-total or total thyroidectomy. In general, the minimum operation that should be done on the thyroid gland is a total lobectomy or in the case that the nodule is in the isthmus an isthmusectomy.

111.5 Complications of Thyroidectomy

Along with the hazards of any surgical operation there are specific potential local and general complications of thyroidectomy.

1. Injury to related anatomical structures
   a. *Injury to the recurrent laryngeal nerve* The incidence of damage to the recurrent laryngeal nerve is approximately 2%. It is related to the experience of the surgeon and increased for operations involving malignancy and for revision surgery.
   b. *Injury to the external branch of the superior laryngeal nerve* The incidence is unknown but is increased in surgery for cancer, surgery for large goitres, and can be reduced when operations are performed by an experienced surgeon.
   c. *Injury to the trachea* This can occur in patients with large goitres or locally invasive thyroid cancer.
   d. *Pneumothorax* This can occur in surgery for retrosternal or intrathoracic goitres and often requires chest drainage.

2. Hormonal
   a. *Hypoparathyroidism which is secondary to parathyroid removal or ischaemic injury to the glands* This may recover and if so is covered with calcium replacements, but permanent damage is treated with replacement therapy using alphacalcidol.
   b. *Thyroid crisis or thyroid storm* This occurs in poorly control patients undergoing surgery for thyrotoxicosis.
   c. *Hypothyroidism* This is best considered a sequelae. Five to 10% of patients with positive antibodies undergoing hemithyroidectomy can develop hypothyroidism.
   d. Late recurrence of thyrotoxicosis (incomplete removal of the toxic gland to include the pyramidal lobe).

3. Complications of the wound site
   a. *Haemorrhage which can be immediate or delayed* This may cause laryngeal oedema and airway obstruction. Treatment will require wound exploration and drainage.
   b. *Tracheomalacia* This only occurs in less than 2% of elderly patients with large goitres.
   c. *Wound infection* This is less than 1% and often occurs after wound re-exploration of haematoma.
   d. *Poor scarring* This occurs due to poor surgical technique. Patients with darker skins have a higher incidence of hyperthrophic or keloid scars.

111.6 Follow-Up and Aftercare

In those patients who have had a hemi-thyroidectomy, thyroid function is checked at 6 weeks to check the contralateral lobe is functioning normally and if not, a further blood test is done at 3 months. If there is still evidence of sub-clinical hypothyroidism, patients may well require long-term thyroxine replacement therapy. This is particularly common in the elderly and in those who have positive thyroid antibodies. Patients who have had a near-total or total thyroidectomy usually require immediate thyroxine replacement therapy and all patients following thyroidectomy should have a vocal cord mobility checked so that the true incidence of cord paresis for one particular surgeon can be documented. Corrected serum calcium levels should be performed routinely 24 hours post-operatively to counteract iatrogenic hypoparathyroidism.

Further Reading

Bliss RD, Gauger PG, Delbridge LW. Surgeon's approach to the thyroid gland: surgical anatomy and the importance of technique. World J Surg. 2000; 24(8):891–897

Godballe C, Madsen AR, Pedersen HB, et al. Post-thyroidectomy hemorrhage: a national study of patients treated at the Danish departments of ENT Head and Neck Surgery. Eur Arch Otorhinolaryngol. 2009; 266(12):1945–1952

Lorente-Poch L, Sancho JJ, Ruiz S, Sitges-Serra A. Importance of in situ preservation of parathyroid glands during total thyroid-ectomy. Br J Surg. 2015; 102(4):359–367

Nixon IJ, Simo R. The neoplastic goitre. Curr Opin Otolaryngol Head Neck Surg. 2013; 21(2):143–149

Perros P, Boelaert K, Colley S, et al; British Thyroid Association. Guidelines for the management of thyroid cancer. Clin Endocrinol (Oxf). 2014; 81(Suppl 1):1–122

Related Topic of Interest

Thyroid disease—malignant

T

112 Thyroid Disease—Malignant

Thyroid carcinoma (TC) is the most common endocrine malignancy, but it is relatively rare. Current incidence in the United Kingdom is approximately 5 per 100,000 in women; however, incidence rates are projected to rise by 74% in the United Kingdom to 11 cases per 100,000 people by 2035. It is predicted that nearly 7,000 cases of TC will be diagnosed in the United Kingdom in 2035. Despite this increasing incidence the survival rates remain static.

112.1 Aetiology

The cause for most TC is unknown. However, several factors are now known to be important in its causation. These are as follows:

- Natural diet-deficient iodine.
- Increased secretion of thyroid-stimulating hormone (TSH).
- Benign thyroid disease. Adenomas, multi-nodular goitres and thyroiditis.
- A previous history of ionising radiation. Patients who had radiotherapy treatment or are survivors of atomic explosions or accidents are at higher risk especially children and adolescents.
- Family history. Familial adenomatous polyposis patients have an increased risk of TC.
- Previous history of cancer. Patients who have been treated for non-Hodgkin's lymphoma, breast cancer, oesophageal cancer and testicular cancer are at higher risk.
- Factors related to women and reproduction. Pregnancy, use of oral contraceptives, hormonal replacement therapy (HRT) and menopause have been implicated in some studies, but the evidence is not conclusive.

Other factors such as diabetes, acromegaly and obesity have also been implicated.

112.2 Classification

There are various types of thyroid tumours and these are shown in ▶ Table 112.1.

1. *Papillary adenocarcinoma or papillary thyroid carcinoma (PTC)* PTC (along with follicular adenocarcinoma) is a differentiated thyroid cancer (DTC) and accounts for 80% of thyroid malignancy. It occurs in all ages and is the

▶ **Table 112.1** Classification of thyroid tumours

Benign	Malignant
• Follicular cell adenoma	Primary
• Hurthle cell adenoma	• Papillary carcinoma (80%)
• Teratoma	– Pure papillary
	– Mixed papillary—follicular
	– Follicular variant
	• Follicular carcinoma (10%)
	• Hurthle cell carcinoma
	• Medullary carcinoma (5%)
	• Anaplastic carcinoma
	• Lymphoma
	• Sarcoma
	• Squamous cell carcinoma
	Secondary
	• Kidney, lung, colon and breast

commonest type of thyroid cancer in children. It usually presents as a solitary thyroid nodule (STN), but is often multicentric (up to 60% of cases). PTC either exists in a pure papillary form, as mixed papillary/follicular carcinoma, or as the follicular variant papillary carcinoma. It is associated with a high incidence of cervical lymphadenopathy which may, on occasion, be the only initial presenting feature. Less than 10% will have distant metastases, which are usually to the lungs.

2. *Follicular adenocarcinoma or follicular thyroid carcinoma (FTC)* FTC occurs in older age groups between 40 and 60 years and is seldom seen under the age of 30. It is less common than PTC (10% of all thyroid malignancy) and usually presents as a STN or occasionally with either distant bony metastases or cervical node involvement (about 10%). While PTC can be identified on fine-needle aspiration cytology (FNAC), it is not possible to diagnose a FTC using this technique, since it cannot distinguish an adenoma from a carcinoma. Therefore, a diagnostic/therapeutic thyroid lobectomy is usually required.

3. *Medullary thyroid carcinoma (MTC)* MTC accounts for about 5% of all cases of thyroid malignancy. MTC arise from the para-follicular or C cells which secrete calcitonin, and this can be a valuable tumour marker. It may occur as part of the multiple endocrine neoplasia (MEN)

syndrome, as familial non-MEN disease or in sporadic form. In patients with MEN, it is frequently bilateral (90%) and multi-focal, and cervical node metastases are common. The autosomal dominant MEN2A is associated with pheochromocytomas (10%) and parathyroid hyperplasia (60%). MEN2B is medullary carcinoma associated with mucosal neuromas, pheochromocytomas, and Marfan's syndrome. Genetic screening is now possible for familial disease using the RET proto-oncogene.

4. *Thyroid lymphoma (TL)* Primary TLs are uncommon and account for fewer than 5% of all lymphoma cases. They usually present as a rapidly increased swelling of the neck in an elderly woman and there is often a history of Hashimoto's thyroiditis. The clinical presentation can be identical to anaplastic carcinoma and both these conditions should be excluded from each other by core needle or open biopsy. Once the diagnosis is made, patients require formal staging and treatment is with radiotherapy plus or minus chemotherapy.

5. *Anaplastic thyroid carcinoma (ATC)* ATCs are common in elderly patients and many are superimposed on a long-standing multi-nodular goitre. They present with rapid thyroid enlargement, are aggressively malignant and rapidly invade surrounding structures. They have a poor prognosis. Its histology comprises of swarms of small cells and can be difficult to distinguish from lymphoma, which has a good prognosis. Therefore, immunohistochemical staining for cytokeratin squamous cell marker and CD4/CD8 lymphoid cell markers is required. Treatment of anaplastic carcinoma has changed over the past few years. For patients with localised ATC, good performance status, and no evidence of local invasion or distant metastases, surgery could be considered to achieve local control and minimise local invasion and progression. Radiotherapy is often ineffective, a tracheostomy may be required and most patients are dead within 1 year.

112.3 Clinical and Diagnostic Evaluation and Treatment Setting

- Clinical evaluation should include history, full head and neck examination including fibre-optic laryngoscopy to assess the airway and the status of the vocal cords.
- All patients should have thyroid function (TSH, fT4 and fT3) tests and thyroid antibodies. Patient with history of MEN or MTC should have calcitonin levels.
- All patients should be investigated with ultrasound (US)-guided FNAC. US and cytological features should be documented as per current validated scoring systems including The British Thyroid Association or American Thyroid Association (Bethesda).
- In patients with suspected lymphoma, poorly differentiated carcinomas, anaplastic carcinomas or metastatic carcinomas, a core needle biopsy or incisional biopsy can be considered to establish diagnosis.
- Patients with advanced disease should have cross-sectional imaging with computed tomography (CT) or magnetic resonance imaging (MRI). Whole body staging for lymphoma is done with positron emission tomography CT(PET-CT).
- All cases should be discussed pre-operatively at the thyroid cancer multi-disciplinary team meeting (TCMDT) or tumour board (TCTB).

112.4 Staging

All patients should be accurately staged. Staging should be done according to the latest UICC TNM staging (▶ Table 112.2).

112.5 Prognostic Factors and Risk Stratification

It is important to assess risk in patients with DTC using prognostic scoring systems. This enables a more accurate prognosis to be given and the appropriate treatment decisions to be made. There are several, risk assessment and staging tools and any of them can be used to assign patients to high-, intermediate-, or low-risk categories. TNM and MACIS probably yield the most useful prognostic information.

Factors contributing to high-risk categories are older age, male gender, poorly differentiated histological features, tumour size, extrathyroidal extension (ETE) and metastatic spread. Adequate management at a TCMDT treatment also influences prognosis.

There is, however, controversy as to how these different risk stratification tools influence outcomes.

▶ **Table 112.2** TNM classification of thyroid cancer

T stage
T1 ≤ 2 cm in greatest dimension limited to the thyroid.
T1a ≤ 1 cm, limited to the thyroid.
T1b > 1 cm but ≤ 2 cm in greatest dimension, limited to the thyroid.
T2 > 2 cm but ≤ 4 cm in greatest dimension, limited to the thyroid.
T3 > 4 cm in greatest dimension limited to the thyroid or any tumour with minimal ETE (e.g. extension to sternothyroid muscle or perithyroid soft tissues).
T4a Tumour of any size extending beyond the thyroid capsule to invade subcutaneous soft tissues, larynx, trachea, oesophagus or recurrent laryngeal nerve.
T4b Tumour invades pre-vertebral fascia or encases carotid artery or mediastinal vessels.
T4a Intrathyroidal anaplastic carcinoma.
T4b Anaplastic carcinoma with gross ETE.
N stage
N0 No regional lymph node metastasis.
N1 Regional lymph node metastasis.
N1a Metastases to level VI (pre-tracheal, para-tracheal, and pre-laryngeal/delphian lymph nodes).
N1b Metastases to unilateral, bilateral or contralateral cervical (levels I, II, III, IV or V) or retropharyngeal or superior mediastinal lymph nodes (level VII).
M stage
M0 No distant metastasis.
M1 Distant metastasis.
Group staging

	Under 45 years	45 years and older
Stage I	Any T, any N, M0	pT1, N0, M0
Stage II	Any T, any N, M0	pT2, N0, M0
		pT3, N0, M0
Stage III		pT4, N0, M0
		Any pT, N1, M0
Stage IVᵃ		Any pT, any N, M1

ᵃUndifferentiated or anaplastic carcinomas are all stage IV.
Note: From 2018, the group staging will be amended to adjust for better prognosis and risk stratification, so the cutoff for group staging will be 55 years of age.

Current management of DTC, using adequate evaluation, assessment and risk stratification tools should be able to provide improved local control, disease-specific and overall survival for these patients. The concept of dynamic risk stratification (DRS) has been introduced with the aim to predict which treatments should be used, the need for post-treatment adjuvant therapies and the intensity and length of follow-up.

112.6 Management

Surgery is the mainstay of the treatment of thyroid cancer. Surgeons performing operations for confirmed or suspected thyroid cancer should be core members of the TCMDT or TCTB. In the United Kingdom and Denmark, surgeons should be contributing to the Thyroid National Registry.

Complex and lymph node surgery should be undertaken by nominated surgeons, in cancer centres with specific training in and experience of thyroid oncology.

▶ Table 112.3 lists patients deemed to be *high risk* and these patients should be considered for level VI lymph node dissection (pre-tracheal and para-tracheal nodes from the hyoid bone superiorly to the level of the sternal notch inferiorly). Lobectomy should include the isthmus in all patients. Sub-total thyroidectomy is not an appropriate operation for thyroid cancer.

Frozen section histology may be of use in confirming suspected PTC (THY4) but is not recommended for use in cases of suspected FTC (THY3).

112.7 Surgical Treatment

112.7.1 Initial Surgery for Known PTC

A strategy for the surgical treatment of PTC is detailed in ▶ Table 112.4.

112.8 Initial Surgery for FTC

The majority of patients undergoing surgery for FTC will be undiagnosed at the time of the initial surgery (THY3 or Bethesda IV). Frozen section histology is not recommended. An operative strategy for surgical treatment of follicular cancer is outlined in ▶ Table 112.5.

Low-risk patients with a diagnosis of minimally invasive tumour less than 2 cm following lobectomy may be managed by lobectomy and TSH suppression alone in most cases. No clear recommendations currently exist for low-risk minimally invasive tumours of 2 to 4 cm and these cases should be discussed individually at MDT. In some cases, lobectomy and TSH suppression alone may be sufficient. Hurthle cell cancers (follicular oncocytic) tend to be more aggressive tumours and should be treated by total (completion) thyroidectomy (see ▶ Table 112.5).

▶ **Table 112.3** Differentiated thyroid cancer high-risk patients

High-risk DTC patients
Male
Age > 45 y
Tumour > 4 cm
Extracapsular spread (ECS)
Extrathyroidal extension (ETE)

Abbreviation: DTC, differentiated thyroid cancer.

▶ **Table 112.5** Initial surgery for follicular thyroid cancer

Recommendation	Clinical details	
	High-risk patient	Low-risk patient
	> 45 y Tumour < 4 cm Extracapsular invasion Extrathyroidal disease Hurthle cell tumours	Female < 45 y
Thyroid lobectomy	No	Yes
Total thyroidectomy	Yes	No
Level VI nodal dissection	Only where clinically involved nodes present	No

▶ **Table 112.4** Initial surgery for known papillary thyroid cancer

Recommendation	Tumour < 1 cm	Tumours > 1 cm	T3 and T4 tumours +N1 level VI nodes
	With no other clinical features such as extrathyroidal spread, nodal involvement, etc.	Papillary cancer diagnosed following thyroid lobectomy Multi-focal disease Thyroid radiation in childhood Familial disease (1st degree)	Treat all the above tumours as high risk
Thyroid lobectomy	Yes	No	No
Total thyroidectomy	Discuss at MDT	Completion or total	Yes
Prophylactic level VI nodal dissection	No	In high-risk patients	Yes
Therapeutic level VI nodal dissection (clinically involved)	Yes	Yes	Yes

Abbreviation: MDT, multi-disciplinary team.

112.9 Management of Lymph Nodes in DTC

Therapeutic level VI nodal dissection is recommended when the presence of lymph node metastasis is confirmed by FNA/core or open biopsy/frozen section. Prophylactic level VI lymph node dissection is advised in high-risk patients, but it is associated with a higher incidence of recurrent laryngeal nerve (RLN) injury and transient and permanent hypoparathyroidism. Prophylactic level VI nodal dissection is not recommended in low-risk, small papillary and most follicular cancers.

Clinically involved lateral cervical lymph nodes should be managed by selective neck dissection (levels II–V). Isolated lymph node excision 'berry picking' is not advocated as it leads to high rates of recurrence. Involvement of level I or level VII nodes is rare in DTC and should only be dissected if involved. Prophylactic lateral neck compartment dissection for node-negative (clinically/radiologically N0) patients is not recommended in DTC, however, it can be considered in patients with locally advanced neck disease or poorly differentiated tumours.

112.10 Completion Thyroidectomy

Completion thyroidectomy is not needed in low-risk, small (< 1 cm), unifocal, intrathyroidal and clinically node-negative tumours.

112.11 Locally Advanced Disease

Where possible, locally advanced disease should be resected. In an attempt to perform curative resection, unilateral RLN sacrifice may be necessary. Where both nerves are involved, then residual tumour may be left to protect the nerve/s and residual disease treated with external beam radiation and/or radioiodine.

Extensive resection of trachea, larynx and oesophagus should only be considered if potentially curative. Where disease is unresectable, radiotherapy and radioiodine should be considered.

112.12 Initial Surgery for MTC

Patients with proven MTC should be treated with total thyroidectomy and levels VI and VII neck dissection.

112.13 Management of Lymph Nodes in MTC

Patients with lateral neck metastases should be treated with a minimum of a selective neck dissection including levels II, III, IV and V as well as levels VI and VII. In patients with clinical and radiological N0 necks, the measurement of the calcitonin will determine the extent of the neck dissection. If the calcitonin level is less than 200 pg/mL, then only an ipsilateral neck dissection is required, but if the level is more than 200 pg/mL, then a bilateral neck dissection (levels II–Vb) is required.

112.14 Post-Operative Management

112.14.1 Radioactive Iodine Ablation

The role of radioactive iodine (RAI) in management of DTC is evolving. There is no place for RAI in MTC as C cells do not uptake iodine. The recognition that RAI has side effects and can be associated with second primary malignancies along with a recognition that outcome for many patients treated with surgery alone is excellent has led to refinement in the indications for RAI. While high-risk patients are still candidates for RAI, low-risk patients are not. Many patients will fall between these two groups and clinical decision making must be personalised. Comparison of low- and high-dose RAI shows no benefit to high doses in intermediate- and low-risk patients. Further work is ongoing to determine whether such patients can be managed without RAI at all.

- Definite indications for RAI: Tumour greater than 4 cm, distant metastases, ETE, more than 10 involved lymph nodes and more than 3 nodes with extranodal extension.
- Definite indications to omit RAI: Microcarcinoma, follicular carcinoma less than 2 cm with no or minimal vascular invasion.

T

- Consider RAI: Tumour 1 to 4 cm/microscopic ETE/aggressive histology/widely invasive/nodal metastasis greater than 6 mm/lymph node ratio greater than 0.7/extranodal extension/thyroglobulin level detectable post-operatively.
- The dose of RAI 1.1 GBq is as effective as 3.7 GBq for T1–T2 N0 lesions.

112.14.2 Recombinant TSH

Thyroid hormone withdrawal is the traditional preparation for RAI to achieve high TSH levels at the time of therapy. However, with the increasing availability of recombinant TSH (rTSH) patients can now safely be prepared for RAI without long periods of hypothyroidism. There are significant cost implications, however, which may limit the use of rTSH in some health care systems.

- Preferred preparation for RAI over thyroxine withdrawal.
- Improved patient quality of life and reduced radiation exposure to normal tissues.

112.14.3 External Beam Radiotherapy

Most DTC concentrates iodine and therefore external beam radiotherapy (EBRT) is not required. However, as thyroid cancer de-differentiates, iodine avidity is lost. In such cases, EBRT provides a means of improving locoregional control in selected patients. The side effects are more significant than RAI. The indications of EBRT in MTC are similar to those in DTC.

- Can be used in combination with RAI.
- Appropriate only in select cases:
  - Unresectable lesions.
  - Gross residual disease.
  - Gross ETE.
  - De-differentiating disease which does not concentrate iodine.

112.15 Post-Treatment Follow-Up

Most patients with DTC do well. These patients can be identified both pre- and post-operatively. Following surgery, assessment of the vocal cords should be performed for all patients and those who develop hypocalcaemia require close monitoring. Serial clinical examination, ultrasound and thyroglobulin (Tg) dependent on DRS. The follow-up intensity is based on assessment of risk. Patients with an excellent response will have an annual review (Tg and US).

112.16 Monitoring Thyroglobulin Levels

Tg is used as a tumour marker. Following total thyroidectomy and RAI, the aim is to render the Tg undetectable. However, for many patients (including those managed with lobectomy alone) Tg will be measurable and can be followed. Increases in Tg levels are normally associated with recurrent disease and should trigger imaging investigations. Tg trends can be used as a prognostic aid in managing patients with recurrent disease.

- Check at 6 and 12 months.
- Then, annually if undetectable.
- For patients with detectable Tg, consider 6 monthly monitoring.
- Imaging for rising or persistently elevated Tg (US/CT/MRI/bone scan/PET/I^{131} whole body scan).

112.17 TSH Management

A high TSH stimulates cells of thyroid origin to divide. For this reason, TSH suppression was once considered the standard of care for all thyroid cancer patients. However, it now appears that high-risk patients are likely to benefit most. Elderly patients, particularly those with cardiac risk factors, should be managed carefully as thyrotoxicosis may present a greater risk than the thyroid cancer for which they are treated.

- Balance of cardiac/skeletal risk versus risk of recurrence.
- 'Excellent' response 0.3 to 2 mU/L (normal).
- 'Indeterminate' response 0.1 to 0.5 mU/L (mild suppression).
- 'Incomplete' response less than 0.1 mU/L (suppression).
- 'Indeterminate or incomplete' response.
  - Appropriate imaging.
  - Individualised follow-up depending on patient needs.

T

112.18 Medullary Thyroid Cancer

Patients with MTC are followed up with serial calcitonin levels. Calcitonin levels may remain elevated. TSH suppression is not necessary. If recurrence is suspected, then patients should be investigated with US FNAC, CT, MRI or PET-CT as appropriate.

112.19 Specific Scenarios

112.19.1 Micropapillary Thyroid Cancer

As imaging improves and is applied more widely, an increasing number of microcarcinomas are diagnosed. They are extremely low risk and may even be considered normal. Ideally, clinical teams should avoid biopsy in sub-centimetre lesions. However, when diagnosed, clinicians must manage the patient appropriately. Some groups, particularly in Japan, are now recommending observation. In Europe, however, most clinicians recommend surgical resection with minimal morbidity.

- Extremely low risk.
- Lobectomy alone unless:
  - Multi-focal with risk factors.

112.19.2 Locally Advanced Thyroid Cancer

Around 5% of patients present with locally advanced (cT4a) disease. Invasion of the RLN, airway or oesophagus must be identified pre-operatively in order to plan surgery and provide informed consent. Decision making in such cases is complex and should be co-ordinated by an experience team. Both patient and tumour factors are critical in making the correct individualised choice.

- Balance of risk–benefit on individual case basis.
- Surgery to control central neck and achieve negative margin.
- Post-operative EBRT and RAI.
- TSH suppression and close follow-up.

112.19.3 Poorly Differentiated Thyroid Cancer

As DTC de-differentiates towards ATC, it becomes more aggressive. Poorly differentiated thyroid cancer (PDTC) is associated with large-volume disease, ETE, nodal metastases and poor outcome. Few large series exist; however, aggressive management for an aggressive malignancy is recommended.

- Intermediate outcome between differentiated and anaplastic.
- Aggressive surgery to resect all disease.
- Adjuvant RAI.
- Consider EBRT dependent on disease extent.

112.19.4 Anaplastic Thyroid Cancer

It is the most aggressive sub-type of thyroid cancer; little progress has been made in the management of ATC. Diagnosis is critical as thyroid lymphoma can sometimes masquerade as ATC. Most patients will have locoregionally advanced disease with distant metastases and will therefore not be candidates for surgical resection. These patients should be supported and considered for clinical trials. Those patients who do present with localised disease may be candidates for resection with adjuvant therapy.

- Majority of patients not surgical candidates (extensive disease and poor performance status).
- Biopsy to exclude lymphoma is critical.
- Occasional patient with localised disease may benefit from surgery and adjuvant radiation.
- Majority of patients managed with best supportive care and consideration of available clinical trials.

112.20 Management of Persistent Disease

Persistent disease should be uncommon in thyroid cancer. Adequate pre-operative assessment should prevent clinically detectable disease from being overlooked. In the event that a surprise diagnosis is made on histology, or disease is more extensive than first expected, a thorough work-up is critical.

- Obtain accurate initial surgical reports.
- Patient assessment is critical (vocal cord check).
- Adequate cross-sectional imaging is essential.
- Balance risks of salvage surgery versus benefit.

112.21 Management of Locoregional Recurrence

Locoregional recurrence is not uncommon, particularly in the lymph nodes of the neck. Structural disease is best treated surgically, although this may represent a significant risk to the patient. Although some groups advocate percutaneous ablative therapy for small-volume recurrences, most authors agree that surgical resection should be considered the gold standard. An experienced surgeon should be involved, and the balance between risk and benefit considered prior to any re-operation for DTC.

- Surgical resection is gold standard.
- Determine any visceral involvement.
- Assess vocal cord and parathyroid function pre-operatively.
- Consider low-volume nodes (< 0.8 mm) in lateral neck for observation.
- Intervention for disease increasing in volume, involvement of critical structures and risk of local invasion causing imminent symptoms (proximity to RLN).

112.22 Management of Distant Metastases

Distant metastases present in 5 to 10% of patients with DTC. Most lesions will concentrate iodine and may be treated with RAI. As disease progresses, it may lose iodine avidity and therefore be RAI resistant. Such patients have poor outcomes. Recently, licenced targeted therapy agents (tyrosine kinase inhibitors [TKIs]) have shown promise in managing such patients. However, this class of drug is not without side effects and therapy continues lifelong or until the side effects can no longer be tolerated. As such, patient selection and clinical experience are critical when considering such treatment.

- Lung and bone most common.
- RAI should be used for treatment and assessment of RAI avidity.
- Isolated bony metastases can be considered for EBRT if unresponsive to RAI.
- Progressive RAI refractory disease may be suitable for targeted therapy (TKI).

Further Reading

Asimakopoulos P, Nixon IJ. Surgical management of primary thyroid tumours. Eur J Surg Oncol. 2018; 44(3):321–326

Haugen BR, Alexander EK, Bible KC, et al. 2015 American Thyroid Association Management Guidelines for Adult Patients with Thyroid Nodules and Differentiated Thyroid Cancer: The American Thyroid Association Guidelines Task Force on Thyroid Nodules and Differentiated Thyroid Cancer. Thyroid. 2016; 26(1):1–133

Mitchell AL, Gandhi A, Scott-Coombes D, Perros P. Management of thyroid cancer: United Kingdom National Multidisciplinary Guidelines. J Laryngol Otol. 2016; 130(S2):S150–S160

Newbold KL, Flux G, Wadsley J. Radioiodine for high risk and radioiodine refractory thyroid cancer: current concepts in management. Clin Oncol (R Coll Radiol). 2017; 29(5):307–309

Perros P, Boelaert K, Colley S, et al; British Thyroid Association. Guidelines for the management of thyroid cancer. Clin Endocrinol (Oxf). 2014; 81(Suppl 1):1–122

Related Topic of Interest

Thyroid disease—benign

T

113 Tinnitus

113.1 Definition

Tinnitus can be defined as the persistent perception of a sound that has no external physical source.

113.2 Epidemiology

Tinnitus is a common experience with up to one-third of the adult population experiencing it at some time in their life. Less than 1% of the adult population will have tinnitus of sufficient severity to seriously affect their quality of life (although up to 8% may seek medical advice about it). Rarely, tinnitus may be associated with suicide. This occurrence tends to be found in older men with recent-onset tinnitus and a previous history or tendency towards depression and anxiety. The prevalence of tinnitus increases in association with a high-frequency hearing loss although the association between severity of tinnitus and degree of hearing loss is very weak. Hyperacusis (as distinct from recruitment) is found as an associated symptom in about 40% of tinnitus sufferers. Hyperacusis can be defined as an undue sensitivity and distress to everyday sounds that would not normally trouble a 'normal-hearing' individual.

113.3 Pathophysiology

The cause of tinnitus is still not known with any certainty. In developing an understanding of tinnitus mechanisms, two points should be borne in mind: (a) there will be a generated potential somewhere in the auditory system, and (b) this signal will undergo extensive central auditory processing before it is perceived as tinnitus. It is felt that this signal is most commonly generated peripherally, but studies showing tinnitus in those with normal hearing, and after cochlear nerve section, suggest that this may not always be the case.

There are several hypotheses which attempt to explain aspects of this process:

1. *Altered auditory firing rate* There is some evidence that tinnitus is associated with an alteration in the spontaneous firing rate of auditory nerve fibres. Hence, the association is with a high-tone hearing loss.

2. *Crosstalk* It has been postulated that damage to the cochlea, by any mechanism, may cause damage to the myelin insulation between axons in the peripheral auditory system, leading to crosstalk between them and thus to phase locking of spontaneous neural activity, experienced subjectively as tinnitus.

3. *Central processing* Recent years have seen an increased appreciation of the role of central signal processing in tinnitus perception, specifically neural plasticity, overactivity in auditory pathway nuclei and altered levels of neurotransmitters. There is also evidence of increased central auditory gain in tinnitus sufferers and it may be this phenomenon that explains the frequently associated hyperacusis.

Like all sound perception, tinnitus has three components: auditory, attentional and emotional. Tinnitus begins with the auditory sensation, the actual sound perception. By itself, the tinnitus sound would seem to be without particular significance because its level is usually so low (< 15 dB SL). Indeed, many, if not most, people with tinnitus are not bothered by it. However, if the tinnitus captures a person's conscious awareness, this will lead to the attentional component where the subject listens to the tinnitus sound. To be a clinical problem, the tinnitus sound must attract a great deal of attention, so that the person focuses excessively on the presence of tinnitus. This 'over-focus' then leads to undesirable autonomic arousal and emotional reactions that are the clinical hallmarks of troublesome tinnitus: annoyance, frustration, depression, anxiety, insomnia and, in extreme cases, thoughts of suicide. It has become clear in recent years that the 'problem' of tinnitus relates far more to the individual's psychological response to the abnormal tinnitus signal than to the signal itself.

113.4 Associated Conditions

- *Local causes* Almost every ear disease and cause of deafness can be associated with tinnitus, and the great majority of tinnitus sufferers have some measurable hearing loss. Noise-induced hearing loss is frequently associated with tinnitus. Ménière's disease and age-associated hearing loss are also associated. Unilateral tinnitus may also be the only symptom of an acoustic neuroma.

- *General causes* include cardiovascular disease (hypertension, cardiac failure), a hyperdynamic circulation (as in anaemia) and fever and drugs (particularly salicylates). Neurological conditions (multiple sclerosis, neuropathy) may also lead to tinnitus. Objective tinnitus may be found in palatal myoclonus, vascular malformations, and exceptionally loud spontaneous otoacoustic emissions.

113.5 Clinical Assessment

From the patient's history confirm that the patient is truly suffering from tinnitus and determine the character of the sound (intermittent or constant, pulsatile or non-pulsatile). It is also important to establish how much trouble the patient is having because this will dictate appropriate management. Effects on sleep, mood and concentration are found most frequently. A number of instruments (such as the tinnitus handicap inventory [THI], the Tinnitus Reaction Questionnaire, the Tinnitus Functional Index or the Tinnitus Severity Index, for example) exist to try and provide a more objective assessment of tinnitus severity. Most tend to be used in a research or medicolegal setting and are uncommonly utilised in a more typical outpatient clinic setting. The THI is probably the most widely utilised.

A full ear, nose and throat (ENT) and cardiovascular examination should be performed to ensure the patient is not hearing transmitted sounds or does not have a potentially remedial cause of tinnitus.

113.6 Investigations

1. *Audiometric investigations*
   - A pure-tone audiogram is essential to document any hearing loss.
   - Tinnitus pitch and loudness matching may be performed. Usually, the pitch of the tinnitus is found to be at or around the frequency of the maximal hearing loss and the loudness is usually within 15 dB of the patient's pure-tone threshold at that frequency. These tests make the assumption that the characteristics of an external sound can be meaningfully related to those of an internally generated

sound. There is a consensus that psychoacoustic tests of this kind give no useful information regarding tinnitus severity nor is there any relationship between perceived loudness of tinnitus and complaint behaviour.
   - Loudness discomfort levels are useful if there is co-existent hyperacusis. When measured sequentially, they can indicate response to treatment.
   - Otoacoustic emissions are often abnormal but still occupy only a research role.
2. *Imaging*
   - Magnetic resonance imaging (MRI) scanning may be required as 10% of acoustic neuromas present with markedly asymmetrical or unilateral tinnitus. Many departments now have protocols on required duration, often 6 months or more.
   - Objective pulsatile tinnitus may require angiography if a specific vascular lesion is suspected.
3. *Blood tests*
   - In some cases, a full haematological screen to exclude anaemia, thyroid dysfunction, dyslipidemias and hypoglycemia can be helpful.

113.7 Management

Any underlying remedial cause should be treated first. Thereafter, if tinnitus persists, management is best undertaken by a dedicated team comprising of an otologist, hearing therapists, audiologists and ideally, a clinical psychologist. Access to a local self-help group is useful to provide emotional support, lay counselling and relaxation therapy.

Modern treatment is described as habituation-based therapy and consists of two main components: directive counselling and sound therapy. *Directive counselling* involves explaining the problem, countering negative beliefs and making efforts to ameliorate the tinnitus sufferer's reaction to the perception of his or her tinnitus signal. *Sound therapy* or sound enrichment involves the use of background sound, hearing aids and/or noise generators to raise the background 'sound floor' and thus reduce the prominence of the tinnitus signal.

- Hearing aids. These are useful for those patients who have a hearing loss. If an appropriate aid with maximal gain at around the frequency of the tinnitus is fitted, the increased awareness

T

of the background sound tends to make the tinnitus less apparent.

- Noise generators (NG). These produce a controllable and more palatable broadband sound. It is thought to act both by reducing the contrast between the tinnitus signal and background noise and improving the plasticity of the central auditory cortex and thereby facilitating adaptation and a reduction in perception. These are particularly useful for individuals with a minimal or no hearing loss.
- Combined hearing aid and NG unit. Useful for those with severe tinnitus and a hearing loss.
- A pillow radio or sound box, which produces repetitive neutral sounds such as wind, rain or waves, may help the patient with sleep.
- Pharmacotherapy may include sleeping tablets, anxiolytics and antidepressants, in more severe cases. Much recent research has looked at drugs to act on central neurotransmission, particularly drugs that act on N-methyl-d-aspartate (NMDA) receptors.
- Many other treatments have been tried (e.g. lignocaine, electrical, magnetic and ultrasonic stimulation, acupuncture, melatonin, Ginkgo biloba amongst others), but results have been inconsistent and success limited.

Further Reading

Ceranic B, Luxon LM. Tinnitus and other dysacuses. In: Gleeson M, ed. Scott-Brown's Otolaryngology, Head and Neck Surgery. 7th ed. London: Hodder Arnold; 2008;3:3594–3628

Martinez-Devesa P, Perera R, Theodoulou M, Waddell A. Cognitive behavioural therapy for tinnitus. Cochrane Database Syst Rev. 2010(9):CD005233

McCombe A, Baguley D, Coles R, McKenna L, McKinney C, Windle-Taylor P; British Association of Otolaryngologists, Head and Neck Surgeons. Guidelines for the grading of tinnitus severity: the results of a working group commissioned by the British Association of Otolaryngologists, Head and Neck Surgeons, 1999. Clin Otolaryngol Allied Sci. 2001; 26(5): 388–393

McFerran D. Tinnitus and hyperacusis. In: Graham J, Baguley D, eds. Ballantyne's Deafness. 7th ed. West Sussex, UK: Wiley Blackwell, 2009:175–188

Related Topics of Interest

Evoked response audiometry
Hearing aids
Pure-tone audiometry

114 Tonsil Disease

Most cases of acute tonsillitis are due to a viral aetiology, but some patients will develop a secondary bacterial infection and others will have a primary bacterial pharyngotonsillitis. GPs can determine which patients should be given antibiotics by using the Centor criteria. Patients with significantly enlarged tonsils should be considered for a 2- to 5-day course of intravenous (IV) steroids to reduce the risk of airway compromise.

114.1 Introduction

The tonsils are paired organs situated on the side of the oropharynx between the palatoglossal (anterior tonsillar pillar) and palatopharyngeal folds (posterior tonsillar pillar). They are part of Waldeyer's ring, a ring of lymphoid tissue consisting of the adenoids, the palatine tonsils and the lingual tonsils, which are embedded in the posterior third of the tongue. The ring is thought to act as a barrier against infection in the first few years of life. The tonsil is enclosed by a fibrous capsule, outside of which is a layer of areolar tissue. This separates the capsule from the pharyngobasilar fascia covering the superior constrictor muscle that forms the tonsil bed. The main blood supply of the tonsil is from the tonsillar branch of the facial artery.

114.2 Acute Tonsillitis

Acute tonsillitis is an infection which primarily affects the palatine tonsil. It may be the dominant feature of an upper respiratory tract infection when it is usually viral in aetiology, or it may present as a primary acute pharyngotonsillitis. The latter is also usually a viral infection involving the lymphoid tissue on the posterior pharyngeal wall and tonsil. Although acute tonsillitis is seen in adults, it is most frequent in childhood, presumably because immunity to common childhood organisms has not been fully established. Common cold and coryza viruses (e.g. influenza, parainfluenza, adenoviruses, enteroviruses and rhinoviruses) are the commonest cause of tonsillitis. An initial viral tonsillitis may predispose to a secondary bacterial tonsillitis (*Streptococcus pyogenes*, *Streptococcus pneumoniae*, *Haemophilus influenzae*, *Actinomyces*, found in so-called tonsillar debris) and anaerobic organisms.

114.3 Clinical Features

There may be a prodromal illness with pyrexia, malaise and headache for a day before the onset of the predominant symptom, a sore throat. Pain may radiate to the ears and suggest acute otitis media until the ears are examined (referred otalgia) and there may be tender cervical lymphadenopathy. Swallowing may be painful (odynophagia) and the patient's voice may sound muffled due to enlarged tonsils from acute tonsillar hyperplasia. Acutely enlarged tonsils may cause stertor (noisy breathing due to airway obstruction above the larynx) and acute obstructive sleep apnoea. There may be trismus and dribbling. Children may have abdominal pain and vomiting. Examination shows hyperaemic tonsils with pus and debris in the crypts. Patients with acute tonsillitis presenting to hospital usually have symptoms at the severe end of the spectrum, with significant systemic upset, inability to function normally and inability to maintain adequate hydration. Glandular fever, agranulocytosis, leukaemia and diphtheria are amongst the differential diagnoses in such cases. A full blood count, white cell differential, blood film and liver function tests should be performed in such cases and if diphtheria is suspected, a throat swab is taken.

Glandular fever tonsillitis is caused in more than 90% of cases by the Epstein–Barr virus (EBV) and in the remainder cytomegalovirus (CMV, another herpes virus). Tonsillar enlargement is particularly impressive. The tonsils are covered with a white/yellow exudate and the tender cervical lymphadenopathy is usually more marked than with other viral/bacterial causes. Hepatosplenomegaly and petechiae on the mucosa of the roof of the mouth may be seen in 50% of cases. There may be atypical lymphocytes on the blood film and raised liver enzymes.

The diagnosis of EBV (as opposed to CMV) glandular fever is confirmed with the heterophile antibody (monospot) test. This test is specific but not very sensitive with a false-negative rate of 25% during the first week of infection, 10% in the second week, and 5% in the third. Therefore, when a patient clinically has glandular fever but has a negative monospot, immunoglobulin G (IgG) and IgM tests for EBV are indicated.

T

114.4 Management

The first determinant is whether the tonsillitis is viral or bacterial. GPs can decide which patients should be given antibiotics by using the Centor criteria. These have been used to determine if an adult with a sore throat is likely to have a bacterial aetiology. They were produced in 1981 and modified in 2004 to highlight the possibility of a β-haemolytic group A streptococcal (*S. pyogenes*) tonsillitis/pharyngitis so that a course of antibiotics can be prescribed. A study published in the BMJ in 2013 concluded that the Centor criteria are ineffective in predicting the presence of group A streptococci on throat swab cultures in children.

There are four criteria each scoring one point:

1. A pyrexia.
2. Tonsillar exudate.
3. Tender anterior cervical lymphadenopathy.
4. Absence of a cough.

In the United Kingdom, there is no points modification for age, so the points score ranges from 0 to 4 and because the outcome of a throat swab depends on the expertise of the practitioner taking the swab, the time taken to reach the laboratory (may need to be stored overnight if a late afternoon or evening clinic), and the time taken to obtain a result thereafter (minimum 48 hours), there is no indication for routine swabs. Patients with a score of 3 or 4 should be treated with antibiotics.

In the United States, one point is added in a patient who is 14 years or younger and one point subtracted if a patient is 45 or older. The patient's score may therefore range from −1 to 5.

The management guidelines in the United States depend on the patient's score and are as follows:

-1 to 1 points	No antibiotics or throat swab needed (streptococcal risk < 10%).
2 or 3 points	Antibiotics prescribed only if a throat swab is positive (streptococcal risk 15% for a score of 2 and 32% for a score of 3).
4 or 5 points	The American Society of Internal Medicine no longer recommend empirical treatment but treatment based on a throat swab (streptococcal risk 56%).

Penicillin V is still the drug of choice, with erythromycin reserved for those patients allergic to penicillin. Amoxicillin should not be used to treat acute tonsillitis in case the patient has infectious mononucleosis, when a generalised maculopapular rash develops in 92% of patients (this can scar). If a quinsy is suspected, then metronidazole should be added because pus cultured from such patients often grows a mixed population of bacteria including anaerobes. Patients with significantly enlarged tonsils should be considered for a 2- to 5-day course of IV steroids to reduce the risk of airway compromise (dexamethasone) 6.6 mg bd or tds with a proton pump inhibitor [PPI] to reduce the gastritis risk. The patient should have paracetamol for analgesia. Aspirin is contraindicated in children because of the risk of Reye's syndrome. Fluid replacement and bed rest are important.

114.5 Complications of Acute Tonsillitis

1. Local
   a. Severe swelling causing respiratory obstruction.
   b. Abscess formation: Peritonsillar (quinsy).
      • Parapharyngeal.
      • Retropharyngeal.
   c. Acute otitis media.
   d. Recurrent acute tonsillitis (chronic tonsillitis).
2. General
   a. Septicaemia.
   b. Meningitis.
   c. Acute rheumatic fever.
   d. Acute glomerulonephritis.

114.6 Differential Diagnosis of Unilateral Tonsil Enlargement

a. Asymmetry in a patient with recurrent bouts of acute tonsillitis due to benign tonsillar hyperplasia.
b. Neoplasia (squamous cell carcinoma or lymphoma).
c. Apparent enlargement (peritonsillar abscess, parapharyngeal abscess, parapharyngeal mass such as a deep lobe pleomorphic adenoma).

114.7 Differential Diagnosis of Ulceration of the Tonsil

A working diagnosis can usually be determined from the history and clinical examination. Investigations include a full blood count, chest radiograph, serological tests, and biopsy. Possible causes include the following:

1. Infection
   a. Acute streptococcal tonsillitis.
   b. Diphtheria.
   c. Infectious mononucleosis.
   d. Vincent's angina.
2. Neoplasm
   a. Squamous cell carcinoma.
   b. Lymphoma.
   c. Salivary gland tumours (adenoid cystic carcinoma or mucoepidermoid tumour).
3. Blood diseases
   a. Agranulocytosis.
   b. Leukaemia.
4. Other causes
   a. Aphthous ulceration.
   b. Behçet's syndrome.
   c. Stevens–Johnson syndrome.
   d. Acquired immunodeficiency syndrome (AIDS).

Further Reading

Baugh RF, Archer SM, Mitchell RB, et al; American Academy of Otolaryngology-Head and Neck Surgery Foundation. Clinical practice guideline: tonsillectomy in children. Otolaryngol Head Neck Surg. 2011; 144(1, Suppl):S1–S30

Chiappini E, Regoli M, Bonsignori F, et al. Analysis of different recommendations from international guidelines for the management of acute pharyngitis in adults and children. Clin Ther. 2011; 33(1):48–58

Spektor Z, Saint-Victor S, Kay DJ, Mandell DL. Risk factors for pediatric post-tonsillectomy hemorrhage. Int J Pediatr Otorhinolaryngol. 2016; 84:151–155

Related Topics of Interest

Adenoids
Neck space infection
Tonsillectomy

T

115   Tonsillectomy

In 2010, the Scottish Intercollegiate Guidelines Network (SIGN) produced guidelines for consideration of tonsillectomy for recurrent significant episodes of sore throats, in both children and adults, which have been widely adopted. The Centor guidelines (see Chapter 114, Tonsil Disease) have been inappropriately used by some clinical commissioning groups to define a clinically significant episode of tonsillitis when applying SIGN guidelines. Tonsillectomy in the United Kingdom has reduced in frequency from 200,000 in 1995 to 31,000 in 2012. With this, the episodes of acute tonsillitis and complications of tonsillitis (such as quinsy or a parapharyngeal abscess) requiring acute hospital admission continue to rise.

115.1 Indications for Tonsillectomy

Indications for tonsillectomy fall into several categories.

1. Recurrent acute tonsillitis.
2. Upper airway obstruction or sleep disordered breathing due to enlarged tonsils.
3. To obtain histology in an abnormal-looking tonsil(s).
4. Part of another procedure (uvulopalatopharyngoplasty [UVPP], access to glossopharyngeal nerve or styloid process).
5. Previous episodes of peritonsillar abscess (quinsy).

115.2 The 2010 SIGN Guidelines

- Sore throats are due to tonsillitis.
- The sore throats are disabling and prevent normal functioning.
- There should be seven or more well-documented, clinically significant, adequately treated sore throats in the preceding year.
- Five or more such episodes in each of the preceding 2 years.
- Three or more such episodes in the preceding 3 years.

Note that the guidelines do not say the episodes of tonsillitis must be specifically due to a viral or a bacterial aetiology (i.e. can be due to either), and we know most cases of acute tonsillitis are due to a viral aetiology. Remember also, the Centor guidelines were produced to do the following:

a. Determine which patients with tonsillitis should be prescribed antibiotics.
b. To prevent unnecessary prescribing of antibiotics. Please see Chapter 118.

Unfortunately, while the SIGN guidelines are quite clear, many clinical commissioning groups in England have modified the guidelines to further ration surgery. The National Health Service (NHS) England has been the trigger for this. Perhaps through stealth or ignorance or perhaps through being confused by SIGN tonsillectomy guidelines and the Centor criteria, which are guidelines for two different issues, NHS England published an Interim Clinical Commissioning Policy: Tonsillectomy document (November 2013; ref: N-SC/033). This is the only tonsillectomy policy document available on their website. The policy refers to a significant episode of tonsillitis as an 'eligible episode'. It defines an 'eligible episode' as a score of at least 3 using the Centor criteria. Such a score is associated with a high likelihood that the episode of tonsillitis is due to a bacterial aetiology and using the Centor criteria antibiotics are recommended. In other words, this document, in effect, interprets 'clinically significant' in the SIGN guidelines to mean bacterial tonsillitis and 'adequately treated' in the SIGN guidelines to mean treated with antibiotics. This has allowed Clinical Commissioning groups in England to use the SIGN guidelines, but then add that each episode of tonsillitis should have been treated with antibiotics to count as an eligible episode. Clearly this is ridiculous because if one calculated that 50% of episodes of tonsillitis are bacterial (it is lower than this), then patients would need to have had twice the number of episodes recommended by the SIGN guidelines to be eligible for tonsillectomy. This means 14 episodes of tonsillitis in the preceding year or 10 episodes in each of the preceding 2 years to be eligible for tonsillectomy using NHS England's guidelines! ENTUK, in association with the Royal College of Surgeons and accredited by NICE, has published a commissioning guide (September 2016) which goes some way to address this. It

T

emphasises that 'adequately treated' does not mean 'treated with antibiotics' and from this it is reasonable to conclude 'clinically significant' does not mean only bacterial tonsillitis.

115.3 Contraindications

These contraindications are not absolute, but they need to be addressed before surgery. In some cases, the decision to proceed with surgery should be reconsidered in the context of the potential problems.

a. Recent episode of tonsillitis or upper respiratory tract infection (within 2 weeks).
b. Bleeding disorder.
c. Oral contraceptives. Each hospital should have its own policy for patients taking the oral contraceptive pill and who are undergoing surgery.
d. Cleft palate.
e. During certain epidemics (e.g. polio).

115.4 Complications of Tonsillectomy

1. Peri-operative
   a. Anaesthetic reaction.
   b. Damage to teeth.
   c. Trauma to the palate and posterior pharyngeal wall from the ear, nose and throat (ENT) surgeon (careless insertion of the tongue blade) or anaesthetist (insertion of pharyngeal airway or from suctioning).
   d. Straining or dislocation of the temporomandibular joint by over-opening the mouth gag.
2. Immediate
   a. Reactionary haemorrhage.
   b. Anaesthetic complications.
3. Early
   a. Secondary haemorrhage.
   b. Haematoma and oedema of the uvula. Nasal regurgitation and hyponasality (from traumatising or excising too much of the soft palate).
   c. Infection (may lead to secondary haemorrhage).
   d. Otalgia (referred otalgia or due to acute otitis media).
   e. Pulmonary complications (pneumonia and lung abscess are rare).
   f. Sub-acute bacterial endocarditis (if the patient has a cardiac defect).

4. Late
   a. Scarring of the soft palate (limiting mobility, possibly affecting the voice).
   b. Tonsillar remnants (which may be the site of recurrent acute infection).

115.5 Post-Tonsillectomy Haemorrhage

The most significant complication is haemorrhage, which occurs in approximately 2% of cases. Most of the deaths associated with tonsillectomy are directly or indirectly associated with this complication.

Reactionary (primary) haemorrhage is a haemorrhage occurring up to 24 hours post-operatively, but nearly all reactionary haemorrhages occur within the first 6 hours. It is one of the reasons why some surgeons are opposed to day case tonsillectomy.

It is essential to ensure adequate haemostasis at the end of the tonsillectomy procedure as blood in the airway at this time may cause laryngeal spasm or can occlude the airway. The post-nasal space should always be checked for a blood clot (the so-called 'coroner's clot'). Patients are nursed in the reverse Trendelenburg position (head down) so that blood trickles out of the mouth rather than being swallowed or aspirated. It would be very unusual for a patient to have had an uneventful post-operative recovery for the first 6 hours and then have a reactionary haemorrhage thereafter. It is therefore safe to discharge such patients home at 6 hours post-tonsillectomy.

The signs of reactionary haemorrhage are bleeding from the mouth, a gurgling sound in the throat on respiration, repeated swallowing, vomiting blood, a rising pulse rate and eventually a falling blood pressure, tachypnoea and circulatory failure (shock) from hypovolaemia. Blood must be cross-matched and a clotting screen performed. An intravenous infusion should be started. The tonsillar fossae should be inspected to identify a bleeding point. If clot is identified, some surgeons advise, if the patient is not shocked, clot removal and a gauze swab soaked in 1:1,000 adrenaline applied to the fossa. Others advise to leave the clot undisturbed and to give tranexamic acid at a maximum STAT dose (1.5 g IV in an adult) then 1 g tds for 3 to 5 days thereafter. If the patient is in circulatory failure, then tranexamic acid should be

T

given; the shock reversed by adequate and rapid fluid replacement, and the patient returned to theatre to ligate the bleeding point under general anaesthesia. The second anaesthetic is hazardous because the patient may have a compensated hypovolaemic which may then decompensate with provision of a general aanesthetic leading to acute hypovolaemic shock. A general anaesthetic for a secondary haemorrhage should therefore only be administered by an experienced anaesthetist.

Secondary haemorrhage occurs some 5 to 10 days post-tonsillectomy and is due to an infection within the tonsillar fossa or from separation of the false membrane that forms in the first 24 hours after surgery. A tonsillar vessel is exposed or necroses beyond its clotted segment and ruptures. The patient should be admitted to hospital for observation. A full blood count, clotting screen and at least a group and save (cross-match for shocked patients) should be performed. The infection and haemorrhage will usually settle after treatment with antibiotics (IV penicillin and metronidazole or erythromycin). It is unusual for such a patient to have to go back to theatre and when this is necessary, the tonsillar fossae are found to contain friable granulation tissue. It is usually straightforward to locate and ligate a specific bleeding point. Sometimes there is a widespread area of friable tissue and the bleeding point may not be obvious. It may then be necessary to suture the faucial pillars together, or over Kaltostat.

115.6 Follow-Up and Aftercare

No follow-up is required after a routine, uncomplicated tonsillectomy. Patients who have suffered a significant haemorrhage should be advised to have their haemoglobin checked at their GP. Patients who have a tonsillectomy for reasons other than recurrent acute tonsillitis should be followed up appropriately to their problem.

Further Reading

Commissioning guide: tonsillectomy. Royal College of Surgeons of England. 01 September 2016

De Luca Canto G, Pachêco-Pereira C, Aydinoz S, et al. Adenotonsillectomy complications: a meta-analysis. Pediatrics. 2015; 136(4):702–718

Marcus CL, Moore RH, Rosen CL, et al; Childhood Adenotonsillectomy Trial (CHAT). A randomized trial of adenotonsillectomy for childhood sleep apnea. N Engl J Med. 2013; 368(25):2366–2376

Related Topics of Interest

Adenoids
Neck space infection
Snoring and sleep-related breathing disorder
Tonsil disease

116   Tracheostomy

A tracheotomy is an operation to make an opening in the trachea, while a tracheostomy means converting this opening to a stoma on the skin surface. Tracheostomy should, whenever possible, be carried out as an elective procedure.

Obstructive airway problems were previously managed by surgical tracheostomy under local anaesthesia, but anaesthetists now tend to intubate the trachea directly or with fibre-optic guidance (with or without sedation). A temporary tracheostomy is commonly used during major head and neck surgery to mitigate against the risk of airway obstruction either immediately post-operatively (i.e. from haemorrhage and surgical reactive oedema) or when narrow airways are at risk of becoming more oedematous during radiation treatments. Overall, however, tracheostomy is now mainly used in intensive care patients to help provide temporary ventilator support for the lungs during periods of respiratory compromise and to minimise the risk of airway soiling. In most centres and situations, percutaneous dilational tracheostomy is the usual method for performing tracheostomy.

Although many disorders are now managed by endotracheal intubation, and this should always be carefully considered first, it is important that the decision for tracheostomy should not be left until it is too late. Children, especially, can deteriorate very suddenly. There is an old adage that states 'the time to do a tracheostomy is when you first think about it'. This should be tempered with thought of the alternatives but remains a poignant axiom.

116.1 Indications for Tracheostomy

The indications for open tracheostomy have tended to change over time, both because of modification in clinical practice and because of the relative ease or safety of techniques and performance. This has been most evident with the introduction of percutaneous tracheostomy.

1. Airway obstruction
Advances in anaesthetics, including improved alternatives for tracheal intubation and better tracheal tubes, have reduced the number of potential tracheostomies. Upper airway obstruction is now the least common indication for tracheostomy. Mitigation against risk of airway obstruction may be considered if there is a possibility of airway obstruction, usually in an iatrogenic sense. This includes patients who need temporary protection of their airway to cover surgical interventions. Some major head and neck procedures can result in post-operative airway obstruction, either from the nature of the surgery, post-operative haemorrhage or oedema. Likewise, there will be patients requiring radiotherapy or chemoradio-therapy of head and neck cancers where the airway is narrow to start with and risks being made worse because of an inflammatory oedematous reaction. Other indications can be remembered as follows:

- Congenital (subglottic stenosis, laryngeal web, laryngeal cysts).
- Trauma (foreign body, severe head and neck injury, swallowing corrosive, inhalation of irritants).
- Infection (acute epiglottitis, laryngotracheo-bronchitis, diphtheria, Ludwig's angina).
- Tumour (tongue, larynx, pharynx, trachea, thyroid).
- Neurological (vocal cord paralysis, e.g. thyroid-ectomy complication, bulbar palsy).

2. Protection of the tracheobronchial tree
Patients may benefit from a long-term tracheostomy if they suffer from any chronic condition (which are often neurological diseases) leading to inhalation of saliva, food, drink, gastric contents or blood or the stagnation of bronchial secretions. A cuffed tracheostomy tube will protect the airway from aspiration and allow easy access to the trachea for regular suction.

- Neurological diseases (motor neuron disease, polyneuritis, tetanus, myasthenia gravis, bulbar palsy, multiple sclerosis).
- Trauma (burns of the face and neck, multiple facial fractures).
- Coma (drug overdose, head injury, cerebrovascular accident).
- Head and neck surgery (oral or oropharyngeal resections, supraglottic laryngectomy).

3. Ventilatory support
Tracheostomy reduces upper respiratory dead space by about 70%, bypassing resistance to airflow in the nose, mouth and glottis, and allows the

T

use of various types of mechanically assisted respiration. Early tracheostomy may decrease the use of sedation needed compared with continuing with a tracheal tube and this tends to mean less cardiovascular compromise. The TracMan trial, however, found no difference in morbidity, mortality or length of critical care stay in patients randomised to early (within 4 days) or late (≥ 10 days) tracheostomy. Ventilatory support may be needed in the following:

- Pulmonary diseases (chronic bronchitis and emphysema, severe asthma, pneumonia).
- Neurological diseases (as above).
- Severe chest injury (e.g. traumatic lung injury).

116.2 Types of Tracheostomy

1. Cricothyroidotomy/mini-tracheostomy

Many different devices have been used for this procedure over the years. The procedure tends to be used as an emergency airway support (as an interim measure before a more secure method of airway control is established) or alternatively to deal with tracheal secretions in intensive care unit (ICU) or chest units. Many different kits have been used. These are based on either an initial needle or surgical blade penetration of the cricothyroid membrane. The patient should be positioned with the neck extended to facilitate access to the membrane. Identification of the cricothyroid membrane is more difficult in females and obese subjects. Increasing access to ultrasound has made bedside visualisation of the airway anatomy relatively straightforward. Once the trachea has been identified and opened, a hollow bougie or dilator then facilitates admittance for a larger cannula or tracheal tube. If this technique is being used to deal with upper airway obstruction and oxygen is applied to the tracheal tube, there must be a means of allowing the expired gas to escape to avoid 'gas trapping' and the risk of tension pneumothorax. In general, the main limitations are related to the size of cannula or tube used and its properties (e.g. cannulas kinking due to their thin walls). The technique has found some success as a temporary measure in the field with military applications.

2. Percutaneous tracheostomy

Percutaneous tracheostomy (PCT) is the current alternative to traditional surgical tracheostomy. Several techniques using a Seldinger needle and wire technique were described prior to the use of incremental dilators between adjacent tracheal rings by Ciaglia. The 'Blue Rhino' was introduced as a single tapered (horn-shaped) dilator to decrease the steps required and improve the overall efficacy. The operator should be particularly aware of the need to enter the trachea perpendicularly and to advance the curved dilator to avoid risk of damage to the posterior tracheal wall. Monitoring the process with synchronous bronchoscopic control from above the site of entry into the trachea should be considered mandatory. Once in place, it is important to confirm that all the tracheal tube cuff is in the trachea (i.e. not in the stomal tract) and the tube tip is above the carina. This has become the bedside norm for ICU tracheostomies, but it is still generally avoided in children and for emergency tracheal access. Extra care is obviously needed with enlarge thyroids, previous tracheostomy, cervical spine fractures, evidence of coagulopathy and previous laryngeal or neck surgery. Ultrasound may help identify the relevant structures and if the anatomy is normal. Benefits include reduced costs, increased speed and smaller and more aesthetic wounds which have lower rates of infection. While trauma can occur on insertion, the overall complication rates and risk of long-term tracheal stenosis is very low.

3. Surgical tracheostomy

The traditional surgical or open tracheostomy consists of an incision in the neck between the lower border of the cricoid and suprasternal notch is deepened to expose the trachea between the strap muscles. The thyroid gland is elevated superiorly by using a cricoid hook and the second to fourth tracheal rings exposed. Excision of cartilage is to be avoided as this promotes the risk of stenosis. There are, however, different accepted techniques for incision, which can be vertical or horizontal (with an inferiorly placed and shaped 'Bjork flap'). Most surgeons advocate using stay sutures to the incision which are secured to the chest. This is useful to control reposition of a dislodged tube. Catastrophic loss of the airway in the early post-operative period and mortality is a real risk and tubes should be secured to the skin as well as using straps around the neck.

116.3 Tracheostomy Tubes

The selection of tracheostomy tube depends on the reason for the procedure and the post-operative requirements. There are characteristics of tubes which will dictate their suitability.

- *A cuffed tube* is preferred if the patient needs protection of the lower airway from aspiration or haemorrhage. They will form a seal to prevent leakage of ventilating gases during prolonged mechanical ventilation.
- *Removable inner tubes* (double-lumen tubes) facilitate cleaning and removal of crusted secretions while the outer tube maintains the airway. This is a useful feature in patients with a recent tracheostomy while allowing the tract to mature. The inner tube decreases the internal diameter of the airway and increases airway resistance.
- *A fenestrated tube* permits the passage of air upwards through the glottis, thereby allowing the patient to speak. It allows potential aspiration and can't be used for positive pressure ventilation.

Most tubes are now made from PVC, silicone or other synthetic plastics that are non-toxic. Examples include the Portex, Shiley and Tracheo twist tubes. These tubes can be connected to an anaesthetic circuit or ventilator. Nowadays they have low-pressure cuffs which can remain inflated for weeks, preventing aspiration and pressure necrosis of the trachea. The cuff pressure should be checked daily using a manometer to check that safe pressure has been maintained. The recommended lower and upper limits for cuff pressures are 18 to 25 cm H_2O.

There are a range of longer tubes for the difficult airway that can assist in safe airway management. The tube used will be dependent on the patients' need. Portex flexiflange, Shiley XLT and Moores tubes can be used with the latter two tubes having the provision of an inner tube for safer long-term airway management. Occasionally, there is not a standard tube that can be provided for the patient and in that instance a customised tube can be made for the patient under the guidance of the medical team and the company to provide a custom-fit tube. The tube can be cuffed or fenestrated and have inner tubes for safer management.

116.4 Post-Operative Management

In response to a number of serious events and the 'National Tracheostomy Safety Project' involving the relevant stakeholders 'multi-disciplinary guidelines for the management of tracheostomy and laryngectomy airway emergencies' have been produced. The main recommendation concerned clarity as to whether a patient had a potentially patent upper airway or a laryngectomy. Bed-head signs are recommended for the attention of immediate responders in the event of an airway emergency. This information should also include when the procedure was formed, its nature (e.g. percutaneous or surgical tracheostomy) and how the tube was secured. Each sign continues with the relevant algorithm (for laryngectomy or tracheostomy, respectively) to help diagnose or manage airway compromise/obstruction.

116.5 Nursing Care

Constant nursing attention is essential for at least the first 24 hours following a tracheostomy. The patient should be in a well-supported upright position; care must be taken in infants that the chin does not occlude the tracheostomy. The patient's airway should be checked 4 hourly as a minimum, but this may change dependent on the patient's condition, secretions and suction needs. The tracheostomy site should be cleaned with Normasol and sterile gauze daily and a tracheostomy dressing applied to catch any exudate. The tapes should be checked daily and changed if soiled. The ward physiotherapist and speech therapist will assist in secretion management and communication.

1. Suction

The patient will be unable to cough and clear secretions so suction should be applied regularly, by aseptic technique, to prevent a buildup of secretions in the trachea and bronchi. A single-use sterile catheter is passed well down into each main bronchus in turn. The patient should be suctioned when clinically indicated and not as routine depending on the quantity and tenacity of the secretions. In the ICU, it is usual to use a dedicated 'closed system' suction to decrease the likelihood of contamination. The size of the suction catheter should not exceed more than half the internal diameter of the tracheostomy tube. The suction pressure applied should be between 14 and 16 kPa but may increase to 30 kPa if the secretions are tenacious.

2. Humidification

A tracheostomy bypasses the normal upper airway mechanisms for humidification, filtration and

T

warming of inspired air. Humidification of inspired air is essential to prevent drying of the airway, which encourages the formation of crusts and infection. Saline or sodium bicarbonate instillation into the trachea followed by immediate suction also helps to reduce the likelihood of such complications. Provision of a heat moisture exchanger (HME) will assist in filtration and warming of inspired air when the patient does not need any oxygen therapy. Various HME systems can be used and should be selected to suit the patient's needs.

3. Apnoea

Some patients with chronic obstructive airways disease may develop apnoea following restoration of their airway. This is due to lowering of their pCO_2, with loss of stimulation of their respiratory centre. These patients need monitoring and the administration of carbon dioxide via a flowmeter through the tracheostomy if necessary.

4. Speech

A notebook or erasable pad should be provided for the patient to communicate. Consideration to the patients' ability to read and write should be assessed and a picture communication aid could be used. If the larynx is still functioning, the patient can be shown how to speak by temporarily blocking the tube while exhaling or using a phonation valve.

Patients with a permanent tracheostomy should, if possible, have a fenestrated tube with a speaking valve incorporated with the inner tube.

5. Swallowing

Some patients with a tracheostomy experience swallowing difficulty, often because of the condition which necessitated the tracheostomy, but sometimes because the tracheostomy tube and cuff tethers the larynx, reducing its elevation when swallowing. Deflation of the cuff will sometimes improve laryngeal elevation, but some patients may not be able to swallow solids or liquids without aspirating and require a nasogastric tube for feeding. Assessment by a speech and language therapist can assist in the assessment of the patient's swallow and in the management of the nutritional status.

6. Care of the tube

If there is an inner tube, it should be taken out and cleaned whenever necessary, at least 4 hourly but may need to be done more frequently depending on the quantity and tenacity of the secretions. The outer tube must be held firmly while withdrawing the inner one. Replacement or cleaning of the outer tube is usually left for the first 5 days until a track has become established, then this should be done regularly, usually monthly or 2 monthly. If a cuffed tube has been used, it should be inflated with the minimum amount of air that prevents an air leak, and it must have a low-pressure cuff to minimise the risk of tracheal stenosis. A spare tube of identical size, plus the size below and a tracheostomy dilator must always be available at the bedside in case a quick change is necessary. A cuffed tube should be available in the event of an emergency when a cuffed tube may be needed for ventilation. The first tube change is usually done about 5 days after the tracheostomy and should always be performed by a doctor and preferably the surgeon who performed the procedure. Whenever the nursing staff perform subsequent tube changes, it should be done in the vicinity of a doctor trained in tracheostomy care in case of a problem.

7. Decannulation

The tracheostomy tube should be downsized, spigotted and removed as soon as feasible. A physiotherapist should assess the patient to ensure secretions can be expectorated safely prior to removal of the tube. Decannulation should only be carried out when it is obvious that it is no longer required. To test this is the case, the patient should be able to manage with the tube spigotted for a full 24-hour period, including a period of sleep. There may be difficulties in children who have had the tracheostomy for a long period of time, sometimes because of a psychological dependence on the tube. They also have a relatively smaller tracheal airway which may be partly blocked by granulation tissue. Surgical closure by excision of the scar tissue and the tracheocutaneous track may be required in some cases. After decannulation, the patient should remain in hospital under surveillance for at least 2 days, including overnight observation. An occlusive dressing should be used and the patient educated to splint his or her dressing when talking and coughing to assist in the fistula healing; an assessment should be made to ensure the wound is healing and a light dressing applied.

116.6 Complications of Tracheostomies

As with any operative procedure, the complications of tracheostomy can be immediate (during the first 24 hours), intermediate (1–14 days) or late (> 14 days). The following list can be a useful basis or plan for an examination answer.

1. Immediate

   - Anaesthetic complications (e.g. difficult ventilation due to poor alignment of the tube in the trachea).
   - Damage to local structures (cricoid cartilage, recurrent laryngeal nerve, oesophagus, brachiocephalic vein).
   - Cardiac arrest (e.g. secondary to hypoxia from loss of the airway due to initial paratracheal tube placement in a patient with a 'bull neck').
   - Primary haemorrhage.

2. Intermediate

   - Dislodgement/displacement of the tube.
   - Surgical emphysema.
   - Pneumothorax.
   - Obstruction of the tube or trachea (excessive crusting).
   - Infection (perichondritis, wound infection, secondary haemorrhage).
   - Tracheal necrosis (may lead to tracheal stenosis or tracheo-oesophageal fistula).
   - Tracheo-innominate artery fistula (sudden massive onset of bleeding 3 days to 6 weeks after tracheostomy).

3. Late

   - Subglottic and tracheal stenosis.
   - Decannulation difficulty.
   - Tracheo-cutaneous fistula.
   - Scar (hypertrophic or keloid).

Further Reading

Pracy P. Tracheostomy. In: Gleeson M, Browning GG, Burton MJ et al, eds. Scott-Brown's Otorhinolaryngology, Head and Neck Surgery. 7th ed, Vol 3. London: Hodder Arnold; 2008;3:2292–2304

Brass P, Hellmich M, Ladra A, Ladra J, Wrzosek A. Percutaneous techniques versus surgical techniques for tracheostomy. Cochrane Database Syst Rev. 2016; 7:CD008045

Feber T. Head and Neck Oncology Nursing. London: Whurr Publishers Ltd; 2000:245–252

McGrath BA, Bates L, Atkinson D, Moore JA; National Tracheostomy Safety Project. Multidisciplinary guidelines for the management of tracheostomy and laryngectomy airway emergencies. Anaesthesia. 2012; 67(9):1025–1041

Vyas D, Inweregbu K, Pittard A. Measurement of tracheal tube cuff pressure in critical care. Anaesthesia. 2002; 57(3):275–277

Young D, Harrison DA, Cuthbertson BH, Rowan K; TracMan Collaborators. Effect of early vs late tracheostomy placement on survival in patients receiving mechanical ventilation: the TracMan randomized trial. JAMA. 2013; 309(20):2121–2129

Related Topics of Interest

Paediatric airway problems
Paediatric endoscopy
Stertor and stridor

T

117 Tympanoplasty

117.1 Definition

- Tympanoplasty is an operation to treat disease in the middle ear and to reconstruct the hearing mechanism. It includes tympanic membrane grafting.
- Myringoplasty is defined as an operation to repair or reconstruct the tympanic membrane. It is the same as a type 1 tympanoplasty often used synonymously. The middle ear disease being treated is the hole in the eardrum.
- Ossiculoplasty is an operation to reconstruct the bones of hearing (the ossicles).
- Combined-approach tympanoplasty is the name given to a procedure where the 'disease' is approached via the ear canal and the mastoid. This is really a mastoidectomy and is described in Chapter 47, Mastoid Surgery.

117.2 Classification of Tympanoplasty

Horst Ludwig Wullstein (1906–1987) in 1956 described five tympanoplasty reconstruction techniques after eradication of middle ear disease. Garcia Ibanez added a sixth in 1961. These are generally academic but do get asked about in examinations and understanding them will give an idea of how to think about reconstruction when undertaking an operation. In Wullstein's paper most of the information he put forward has since been thought to be wrong, for instance, the movement of the eardrum hinged on the malleus and its ligaments has been proven to be far from the truth by laser Doppler interferometry measurements. However, the classification persists.

Type 1   Reconstruction of the tympanic membrane with a normal ossicular chain (myringoplasty), a common operation.

Type 2   The malleus handle is absent. The tympanic membrane is reconstructed over the malleus remnant and the long process of the incus (not very common).

Type 3   The incus and malleus have been removed (or eroded by disease). The tympanic membrane is repaired to lie directly on the stapes head (very commom).

Type 4   Only the mobile stapes footplate remains. The repaired tympanic membrane is placed onto the footplate and then the promontory but kept away from the round window creating a round window baffle or carva minorum (not common).

Type 5   The stapes footplate is fixed and a fenestration of the lateral semicircular canal is performed (now a historic operation as stapedotomy is now done).

Type 6   Otherwise known as sonoinversion. There is an ossicular discontinuity. The round window niche is left uncovered and the tympanic membrane reconstructed so that its inferior edge lies on the promontory above the round window, thereby creating an oval window baffle. (The author has never tried this or seen nature do this.)

117.3 Ossicular Chain Reconstruction

Autograft reconstruction using cortical bone or remodelled incus is the most reliable long-term ossicular reconstruction. Homograft tissue from bone banks is now contraindicated because of the risk of Creutzfeldt–Jakob disease (CJD) and other transmissible disease. Surgeons without the time or skill to remodel the incus or cortical bone use partial or total ossicular replacement prosthesis (PORPS/TORPS). The only artificial materials that have stood the test of time are hydroxyapatite and titanium although even they don't match bone. Hydroxyapatite has been shown to be replaced, at least in part, by osteogenic cells and host connective tissue and the oxides on the surface of titanium are disguised as bone and therefore not rejected chemically, but they are very ridged and are rejected biomechanically. All the plastic, ceramic, carbon and many other artificial materials fail in the medium term despite being placed in the immune-privileged middle ear and are now confined to history. The exception is the stapedotomy prosthesis, but these only work in ears that have got otosclerosis and no other disease.

T

Ossiculoplasty: loss and repair

1. *A stapes footplate remnant is present with or without the malleus.* A myringostapediopexy or malleostapediopexy is performed to create the tympanic membrane or malleus-to-footplate assembly. An incus body and short process can be remodelled for this.

2. *The stapes superstructure is intact, but there is an absent long process of incus.* The malleus handle may or may not be present. Autograft malleus-to-stapes assembly (incus transposition) is used. The incus body is used with a cup for the stapes head and a strut or hook to the malleus handle just below the tensor tympani insertion.

3. *There is an incudostapedial discontinuity secondary to an absent lenticular process and/or stapes head.* An incudostapediopexy using a cortical bone slither is the preferred method of reconstruction. Bone cement was used but has now been withdrawn because of safety issues and poor long-term results.

117.4 Cause of Perforation

Perforations may be traumatic (usually heal spontaneously), iatrogenic (after ventilation tube insertion), infective (often associated with eustasion tube disorders) or occasionally inflammatory. Multiple perforations indicate chronic inflammatory disease such as tuberculosis.

117.5 Cause of Ossicular Damage

This is usually infective but may be traumatic. The long process of the incus seems to have a tenuous blood supply and is easily eroded by the inflammatory effects of infectious disease. Cholesteatoma erodes the ossicles by inducing osteoclasts to absorb bone.

117.6 Consent for Surgery

Not doing surgery is the most important part of the consent. Most perforations or ossicular deficiencies are best left alone and no surgery done. Surgery should only be done if the results are definitively better than the natural history of the disease. If the hearing loss can be aided and the ear waterproofed, then no surgery is indicated.

If surgery is to be done, then a realistic prognosis has to be given and a detailed understanding of the course and outcome of the surgery in the normal course of events has to be understood by the patient.

The patient must consider the potential complications and their effects as well as their frequency. This includes the chances of failure of the procedure.

The patient must be warned of the following:

- Failure of operation: Graft failure and no hearing improvement, 20 to 50%, depending on the operation.
- Hearing loss including total loss of hearing in the operated ear (dead ear) (0.5%).
- Tinnitus: Disturbing or disabling noise in ear and brain (1%).
- Dizziness, which may be temporary (10%) and rarely permanent and disabling (0.1%).
- Taste change on side of tongue (5%) or loss of taste.
- The patient needs to be aware of the scar, risk of infection and the risks of the local or general anaesthetic.
- Most tympanic membrane perforations do not need any surgery.

117.7 Results of Conservative Management

No harm done unless the ear gets an infection that causes permanent sensorineural hearing loss!

117.8 Results of Surgery

Tympanoplasty: 38 to 80% success rate in the literature (probably about 75% in general).

Ossiculoplasty: 30 to 90% in the literature short term. Almost all artificial PORPS and TORPS have been shown to fail in the medium term. Homografts fair better and have results in the region of 70% if the stapes superstructure is present and 50% if it is absent. Complex reconstruction with plastic prostheses and Silastic bands may work better but in a few specialist hands only.

117.9 Surgical Approach

Tympanoplasty can be performed through the ear canal either endoscopically or microscopically, through an endaural incision in groove between the tragus inferiorly and helix superiorly (incisura terminalis) or through an incision behind the ear (post-auricular approach). The perforation has the edges freshened, the middle ear inspected and the graft inserted deep to the eardrum remnant. The most important thing in any tympanoplasty is having the graft tight up against the medial surface of the eardrum remnant. The most important thing in ossicular reconstruction is having the inserted bone (or artificial material) lightly touching the stapes and the eardrum and not touching the other middle ear structures. The factors beyond the surgeons control, that is, the middle ear aerations are also of great importance to the success of the procedures.

117.10 Graft Material

Fascia: Usually fibrous tissue from temporalis, pre-temporalis facia, incisura tissue, tragal perichondrium and occasionally vein.

Incisura tissue is the same collagen as temporalis fascia and is becoming a common graft material as it is easy to harvest.

Cartilage: This is harvested from the tragus or concha and can be used in patients with eustachian tube dysfunction who are more prone to develop recurrent retraction. It is also used to cover artificial ossicles to reduce extrusion through the tympanic membrane. It is also used in patients with a history of attic retraction cholesteatoma, as this disease commonly recurs if the lateral wall of the epitympanum is not reconstructed. Cartilage is used in the eardrum either as palisades or occasionally as a butterfly plug. Cartilage size and thickness dictate sound transfer and longevity. However thick the cartilage is, it does not prevent the effects of eustachian tube dysfunction in the long term.

Other grafts including xeroderm, made of pig gut, are coming back into fashion, particularly with endoscopic surgery and no incision is needed. This is ironic as the first recorded attempt at repairing the tympanic membrane was made by Marcus Banzer in 1640 using an ivory tube covered by pig's bladder. Early xeroderm results, however, suggest a high failure rate. Probably all successful tympanic membrane grafts work by being in effect, a scaffold which allows squamous epithelium from the freshened edge of the tympanic membrane perforation to grow across.

117.11 Follow-Up and Aftercare

The ear canal dressing is removed after 7 to 14 days. The ear may need repeated microsuction to compensate for the disrupted squamous migration and wax clearance that the surgery has temporally induced. Diving or repeated head injury (heading a football) may predispose to prosthesis displacement and should be avoided.

If artificial ossicle grafts are used, the patient should be followed up for the long term as displacement or rejection is likely and revision surgery or hearing aids are commonly required.

Further Reading

Grote JJ. Biomaterials in otology. Proceedings of the First International Symposium. Leiden, The Netherlands;1983

Kerr AG, Riley DN; Martinus Nijhoff Publishers. Disintegration of porous polyethylene prostheses. Clin Otolaryngol Allied Sci. 1999; 24(3):168–170

Wullstein H. Theory and practice of tympanoplasty. Laryngoscope. 1956; 66(8):1076–1093

Related Topics of Interest

Cholesteatoma
Mastoid surgery
Suppurative otitis media—chronic

118 Tympanosclerosis

Tympanosclerosis is an abnormal condition of the middle ear, characterised by calcareous deposits in the tympanic membrane, tympanic cavity and occasionally in the mastoid.

118.1 Aetiology

The exact cause is uncertain, but it appears likely that there is an abnormal healing process in response to single or multiple acute inflammatory episodes or due to chronic otitis media. Another important aetiological factor is tissue trauma, which is substantiated by the frequent occurrence of tympanosclerosis after myringotomy with or without insertion of ventilation tubes; this may be due to intra-epithelial haemorrhage.

118.2 Pathogenesis

Three stages are recognised. In the initial stage, inflammatory processes cause an exudate, the formation of granulation tissue and damage to collagen fibres. This phase is generally considered reversible. The second stage is the reparative phase, characterised by fibroblast invasion. This results in excessive collagen synthesis and hyalinisation, as a result of which fibres become indistinct, fusing into a homogeneous mass. Most authorities now consider this process to be irreversible, and in the third and final stage, calcification and occasionally ossification occurs. It has been established that the pathological changes of tympanosclerosis are situated in the lamina propria, which is the connective tissue component of the tympanic membrane and mucosa.

118.3 Clinical Features

The term myringosclerosis is used when the process is confined to the tympanic membrane and the term tympanosclerosis is used where the middle ear, ossicular chain and/or mastoid are affected. Morphologically, however, no differentiation can be made between tympanosclerosis in the drum or elsewhere in the middle ear. Furthermore, the occurrence of plaques in the tympanic membrane may indicate the presence of more extensive disease in the middle ear in patients with a history of chronic otitis.

1. *Tympanic membrane* Tympanosclerosis that is restricted to the tympanic membrane is most commonly seen, usually following myringotomy and ventilation tube insertion (occurring in around 60%). It occurs in all age groups. On otoscopy, deposits present as sharply demarcated areas of white opaque, chalk-like material. Plaques usually occur only in the pars tensa, mostly situated in the anterior or posterior segments, varying in size. The clinical importance of this calcification is dependent on its size. In most cases there is little, if any, effect on the patient's hearing, even with quite extensive plaques. However, with very large plaques and those that impinge across the annulus, a measurable conductive hearing loss may result (20–40 dB HL) because the rigid tympanic membrane is reducing transmission of sound to the ossicular chain. The condition occasionally occurs in children with otitis media with effusion who have had no previous surgery. There is, however, a natural tendency for resolution in this group.

2. *Middle ear* Middle ear involvement is much less common, but when it occurs, it usually accompanied by a perforation of the tympanic membrane. Interestingly, these ears are usually dry. The patients usually present when over 30 years of age and have had a long history of ear problems. The condition tends to be most prevalent around the round window niche, epitympanum and promontory. These patients often have a significant conductive hearing loss due to fixation of the ossicular chain.

118.4 Investigation

The clinical appearance of tympanosclerosis in either the middle ear cavity or tympanic membrane rarely presents any diagnostic difficulties although it may occasionally look like a cholesteatoma. Examination under a microscope will nearly always resolve the issue. In cases of tympanosclerosis, the involved ear is usually dry, whereas in an ear with cholesteatoma a perforation or retraction pocket is usually present and often there is keratin, granulation or malodorous otorrhoea. An audiogram to assess any degree of (conductive) hearing loss is always useful. High-resolution computed tomography (CT) scanning may help identify patients with ossicular fixation due to tympanosclerosis with good specificity but only around 50% sensitivity.

118.5 Management

Tympanic membrane tympanosclerosis (myringosclerosis) with an intact drum rarely requires treatment. Occasionally, removal of a plaque may be required to aid healing during myringoplasty for a co-existent perforation. Conductive hearing loss caused by tympanosclerosis can be treated with either a hearing aid or surgery. A hearing aid is safe and effective; surgery is controversial. The choice of procedure depends on the extent and location of middle ear involvement.

The incus and/or malleus may be fixed by tympanosclerosis in the attic. The resultant conductive hearing impairment can be corrected by removing the incus and head of malleus and performing a stapes to drum (or manubrium) reconstruction using a partial ossicular replacement prosthesis (PORP) and tragal/conchal cartilage.

Where tympanosclerosis affects the stapes, conductive losses can be corrected with stapes mobilisation or a stapedotomy. Results of stapes surgery in this situation are less successful than in otosclerosis. A post-operative air–bone gap within 20 dB is typically only achieved in 70% and with a higher incidence of a dead ear (around 4–5%).

118.6 Follow-Up and Aftercare

This should be appropriate to the patient's surgery and any active otological pathology.

Further Reading

Asiri S, Hasham A, al Anazy F, Zakzouk S, Banjar A. Tympanosclerosis: review of literature and incidence among patients with middle-ear infection. J Laryngol Otol. 1999; 113(12):1076–1080

Gurr A, Hildmann H, Stark T, Dazert S. [Treatment of tympanosclerosis] HNO. 2008; 56(6):651–657, quiz 658

Ho KY, Tsai SM, Chai CY, Wang HM. Clinical analysis of intratympanic tympanosclerosis: etiology, ossicular chain findings, and hearing results of surgery. Acta Otolaryngol. 2010; 130(3):370–374

Related Topics of Interest

Cholesteatoma
Otitis media with effusion
Tympanoplasty

T

119　Vertigo

Vertigo is the hallucination of movement. It is a cardinal symptom of a disorder of 'balance'. Dizziness is a vague term often used to describe either vertigo or the general unsteadiness. Patients may complain of this should they have an incompletely compensated vestibular hypofunction.

Normal function of the balance system is essential for most functions of daily living. It is required for the maintenance of posture, and for autonomic control of heart rate and blood pressure in response to these changes. It is particularly important for visual target fixation, as when hunting or fighting, from a teleological perspective and shopping or driving from a more modern perspective.

This chapter covers the background to balance and dizziness and the assessment of the patient presenting with vertigo. It is best read in conjunction with Chapter 120, Vestibular Function Tests.

119.1　Anatomy and Physiology

The sensory contributors to the balance system are the paired vestibular organs of the inner ear, the eyes and the visual information and proprioceptive information (position sense) provided by pressure sensors in the skin, tension sensors in muscle and position sensors in the various joints. Information from the neck and ankles seems particularly important in this regard. It is not possible in normal individuals with a normal input from all three systems, to apportion each system's contribution to balance. That the vestibular system is dominant can be seen from the fact that closing one's eyes when walking, if there is normal vestibular and proprioceptor input, it does not lead to collapse. An acute canal paresis in such circumstances, however, will cause profound symptoms of collapse and autonomic symptoms including nausea, vomiting and sweating.

This sensory information is collated and co-ordinated in various brainstem nuclei and with the involvement of the cerebellum, various reflex responses will then occur to maintain normal balance function. Particularly important reflex responses to be discussed further are the vestibulo-ocular reflex (VOR) and the vestibulospinal reflexes (VSRs). Further processing and input occur from higher centres of the central nervous system (CNS). For this system to work well, an adequate blood supply and normal neuropsychological function is required.

The vestibular organ consists of the three semi-circular canals and the otolithic organs, namely the saccule and the utricle. Its function is to translate information about head movements and position into electrical signals to be relayed to the appropriate brainstem nuclei.

The three semicircular canals are, as their name suggests, semicircular membranous tubes within the dense temporal bone, and are responsible for detecting angular acceleration (head movements). The membranes are fluid filled and at one end have an expansion or ampulla. On the 'floor' of the ampulla is the crista from which arise the stereocilia of the hair cells. These stereocilia are embedded in a gelatinous structure, the cupola, which largely fills the ampulla. As movement of the head occurs, there is a delay in the movement of the fluid of the canal due to inertia. This creates a relative movement of the cupola which causes a deflection of the stereocilia inserted in its base. This excites or inhibits the nerve cell, depending on the direction of deflection (excitatory if deflection is towards the kinocilium) and alters the tonic input to the relevant brainstem nucleus. The semicircular canals are at right angles to each other and their responses are complimentary. In other words, what creates excitation in one semicircular canal will create an equal but opposite response (inhibition) in the corresponding contralateral canal.

The utricle and saccule have otoconia (small crystals) attached to the ends of their stereocilia which are embedded in an overlying gel. They are positioned to detect linear acceleration: the utricle to detect tilt and lean (side/side and front/back) and the saccule to detect vertical movement (up/down). They are responsible for detecting changes of head position in relation to gravity.

119.2　Pathology and Clinical Syndromes

Non-vestibular disorders causing vertigo can arise from the following:

- Cardiovascular and metabolic disorders may cause patients to complain of dizziness. By this, they usually mean a sense of light-headedness, or unsteadiness, not vertigo. There may be features in the history to point in this direction such as palpitations, breathlessness, a history of diabetes, anaemia or renal failure.

- Disorders of the other systems that have input to maintain balance, that is, musculoskeletal disorders, particularly of the cervical spine, (causing reduced proprioceptor input) and visual and ocular disorders (causing reduced central ocular input) may cause vertigo. Cervicogenic vertigo is common and is due to disordered proprioceptive input from the neck. Most individuals over the age of 40 will have some degree of cervical spondylosis so that apportioning a contribution from cervical arthritis is not always simple. A standard optician's eye test can be a useful exercise in a dizzy patient.

- Central disease includes cerebrovascular disease, migraine, multiple sclerosis, brain tumours and, very rarely, vertebrobasilar insufficiency. The last hardly ever causes vertigo as a presenting symptom. Indeed, if the vertebral or basilar artery is constricted, dysarthria, visual phenomena, diplopia and weakness of one side of the body are usually the presenting signs. Of the central causes, vestibular migraine is far and away the commonest, and often has vague and atypical symptoms; nausea and photophobia are frequently associated.

- Iatrogenic vertigo may be caused by drugs (aminoglycosides, diuretics) due to either ototoxicity or a central effect. A past history of intensive care unit (ICU) admission may be significant.

- Non-organic dizziness and vertigo also exist. Anxiety and panic attacks can cause hyperventilation and subsequent vertigo. A situational precipitant may be volunteered.

- Because of its relatively slow rate of growth, which allows for adequate vestibular compensation, a vestibular schwannoma usually presents with a unilateral sensory hearing loss, but occasionally there can be vertigo from an acute reduction in vestibular function, or unsteadiness (a feeling of being on the deck of a ship) from poor compensation. Patients who are fully compensated may have episodes of decompensation if they are tired, stressed or unwell.

These causes aside, we are left with the peripheral causes of vertigo, of which there are four main symptom complexes.

1. Benign positional vertigo commonly occurs after a head injury or ear infection and is a short-lasting rotatory vertigo with specific head movements, such as rolling over to the trigger side in bed. It is diagnosed by the Dix–Hallpike manoeuvre.

2. Ménière's syndrome comprises paroxysmal fluctuating hearing loss, vertigo and tinnitus, each attack lasting many minutes or hours.

3. Acute vestibular failure consists of marked vertigo, associated with significant systemic upset including nausea and vomiting, and lasts for many hours or sometimes days before recovery and compensation occurs. It is most commonly preceded by an upper respiratory tract infection (viral labyrinthitis/vestibular neuronitis) but may be caused by perilymph leak, bacterial labyrinthitis complicating middle ear disease or vascular event, among other causes. Recovery is generally more rapid and complete in younger patients.

4. Chronic vestibular failure is the situation where following an acute disturbance of vestibular function, there is a failure to fully compensate for the deficit. This leads to a more generalised and persistent disequilibrium.

119.3 Clinical Features

The sense of balance is very basic and phylogenetically predates sight and hearing. When this basic system goes wrong, the patient is left disabled. Sir Terence Cawthorne once said 'labyrinthine disturbance may make one feel like the end of the world has arrived and I am told by sufferers from sea sickness, that in the acutest phase of their distress, they wish that it had!". Remembering this enables us to understand the distress of these patients. It also, in combination with the very basic nature of the sense of balance, explains the many frequently associated symptoms such as muzzy head, headache, loss of memory and confidence, autonomic disturbance (vomiting and bowel upset) and anxiety which may persist after the acute episode has settled but contribute to ongoing symptoms.

A full and thorough history is the most important part of the diagnostic process. Many patients focus in detail on certain aspects of their symptomatology which may or may not be relevant to the diagnosis. This is a function of their distress, anxiety and inability to function normally. Time and sympathy are therefore required.

It is therefore essential to clarify exactly what the patient means when he or she complains of vertigo or dizziness. It must be differentiated from fainting, light-headedness, anxiety, claustrophobia or peripheral (musculoskeletal) disequilibrium.

Once this is established, its frequency and duration and any associated symptoms or aggravating and relieving activities are important. A thorough description of the very first attack, if it can be recalled, is often very useful.

Useful diagnostic symptom associations:

- Other neurological symptoms such as diplopia, dysarthria, dysphagia and altered sensation may suggest a stroke or multiple sclerosis.
- Aural symptoms suggest an inner ear cause.
- Headache, nausea, photophobia and sound sensitivity suggest migraine.
- Syncope, or pre-syncopal symptoms associated with palpitations may suggest a cardiac rhythm disturbance.
- Dyspnoea, palpitations, sweating and anxiety may suggest a panic attack.

A full medical history, including medication and alcohol ingestion, is essential.

An otological and neurological examination is mandatory and a general medical examination may be required if the symptoms dictate.

In terms of clinical assessment, the following is a list of 'tests' that can be easily conducted in the general ear, nose and throat (ENT) clinic. Depending on the history and likely differential diagnosis, not all need to be conducted. More thorough and extensive testing may be undertaken in a specialist balance clinic facility. A thorough explanation of the various tests can be found in Chapter 120, Vestibular Function Tests.

- Tests of oculomotor control:
  Saccadic eye movements and smooth pursuit tracking. These tests are normally done while assessing eye movements as part of a cranial nerve assessment.
- Tests of the VOR:
  Halmagyi's head thrust.
  Head shake visual acuity.

- Tests of the VSR:
  Romberg's and Unterberger's testing.
  Gait assessment—straight line walking.
- The Dix–Hallpike manoeuvre for benign paroxysmal positional vertigo (BPPV).
- Additional general tests include erect and supine blood pressure measurement looking for postural hypotension, finger pointing and 'palm tapping' to look at cerebellar function. Hyperventilation is useful to identify anxiety-induced dizziness.

119.4 Investigations

Most cases of dizziness that present to the clinic will not require extensive investigation. Most should have a pure-tone audiogram. Subsequent specialised vestibular testing will be dictated by the details of the individual case and the suspected differential diagnoses.

A magnetic resonance imaging (MRI) scan is likely to be the radiological investigation of choice although high-resolution CT scanning may be indicated in certain conditions. A normal MRI scan can be therapeutic in patient management for the reassurance that it provides.

119.5 Management

Probably the most important aspect of the management of the vertiginous patient is an explanation of the nature of the problem and a reassurance of the absence of any life-threatening pathology. Vertigo is a symptom that severely affects self-confidence and ability to function normally. Concentrating on remaining stable, for patients in the recovery phase, can be exhausting and often affects their ability to work normally and their family life. A compassionate consultation and creation of a therapeutic plan can contribute to a significant improvement in the patient's feeling of well-being as they feel they are being listened to and their symptoms understood.

Other aspects of therapy include the following:

1. Vestibular rehabilitation. This is the mainstay of treatment in many vestibular disorders. The first step is to counsel the patients regarding their symptoms, to provide reassurance and to explain the importance of persisting with treatment. This is followed by a series of habituating exercises performed regularly to

V

enable tolerance mechanisms to occur in the brainstem. It is known that structural changes occur to allow vestibular compensation such as a modification of the distribution and sensitivity of cholinergic synapses. These allow a new equilibrium situation to occur. With adequate counselling, as many as 80% of patients with vestibular disorders will benefit from vestibular rehabilitation. Specific manoeuvres and exercises are used for BPPV. The Epley (liberatory) manoeuvre works as a single treatment on up to 80% of patients. Brandt–Daroff exercises encourage habituation (sometimes referred to as compensation) and succeed in 95% of cases in fully compliant patients.

In addition to vestibular rehabilitation, patients may also benefit from spectacles to improve their visual acuity or a walking stick to aid peripheral balance function and to give them more confidence.

2. Medical treatment. This may consist of lifestyle changes such as abstaining from alcohol and avoiding vestibular sedatives such as prochlorperazine, cinnarizine or antidepressants. The persistent use of labyrinthine sedatives can be counter-productive because they inhibit vestibular habituation (compensation) after recovery from the acute phase of vertigo. They are, however, useful in the acute phase of vertigo.

3. Surgery. This is rarely used in the dizzy patient. However, it does have a role in managing severe Ménière's disease that has proven unresponsive to all medical treatments and may involve endolymphatic sac shunting, vestibular neurectomy or labyrinthectomy. A middle ear infusion of an aminoglycoside via a cannula so it pools at the round window can be used to perform a 'chemical labyrinthectomy'. Occasionally, surgery is used for benign positional vertigo when posterior semicircular canal obliteration or singular neurectomy is done.

Further Reading

Hale T, Trahan H, Parent-Buck T. Evaluation of the patient with dizziness and balance disorders. In: Katz J, ed. Handbook of Clinical Audiology. 7th ed. Philadelphia, Baltimore, New York: Wolters Kluwer; 2015

Wuyts FL, Boudewyns A. Physiology of equilibrium, balance disorders. In: Gleeson M, Browning GG, Burton MJ, et al, eds. Scott-Brown's Otorhinolaryngology, Head and Neck Surgery. 7th ed, Vol 3. London: Hodder Arnold; 2008;3:3207–3244, 3673–3834

Related Topics of Interest

Caloric tests
Ménière's disease
Labyrinthitis
Vestibular function tests

V

120 Vestibular Function Tests

In most patients suffering with dizziness, a thorough history and neuro-otological examination will elucidate the diagnosis and enable a suitable management plan. Vestibular function tests are complimentary and serve to locate the site and may quantify the extent of a vestibular lesion, but do not always correlate with the functional deficit.

An individual maintains balance by co-ordinating sensory information provided by (1) the vestibular system, (2) the eyes and (3) various proprioceptors (primarily in the neck and ankles). These sensory organs connect directly with the brainstem and the cerebellum and then with the cerebrum. Having established the need for a general medical approach to the problem of unsteadiness, it is necessary to identify the presence or absence of a vestibular component.

There are many and various tests of vestibular function, some of which seem to be quite complicated. However, regardless of their apparent complexity, these tests are all just various ways of examining the following reflexes and their collective integration:

1. Oculomotor control.
2. Vestibulo-ocular reflex (VOR)—tests semicircular canal function.
3. Vestibulospinal reflex (VSR)—tests otoconial function (utricle and saccule) but may include some proprioceptive testing.

Many of the tests have developed as simple clinical tests but with the development of light-weight cameras and detector systems, and the benefit of computer analysis, they have progressed in terms of accuracy and application.

120.1 Oculomotor Control

There are several systems that control eye movements to maintain the target image on the fovea. The two main systems are as follows:

1. Smooth pursuit, where gaze is maintained on a moving target. The eye velocity is compared with that of the target velocity and produces a continuous match of eye and target position.
2. Saccades, which are extremely fast eye movements, where the vision is momentarily suppressed, that bring the target image back to the fovea when the eye has drifted. This is primarily a midbrain phenomenon.

Central nervous system disease may cause abnormalities of latency, accuracy or velocity of saccades. Bilaterally impaired smooth pursuit is usually a non-specific abnormality observed in a fatigued patient or one who is on certain medication (alcohol, antidepressants, anticonvulsants or benzodiazepines). Unilateral impairment is a more reliable marker of central nervous system pathology. Disorders of either of these two functions tend to localise the lesion to the midbrain.

120.1.1 Simple Tests

Following a moving finger as part of the standard cranial nerve assessment. It is best to trace a figure 'H' and observe what should be normal smooth pursuit. An alternative is to ask the patient to follow a pendulum. Asking the patient to alternately look at your right and left index fingers, held just wider than shoulder width apart, allows a simple assessment of saccadic eye movements.

120.1.2 Complex Tests—'Oculography'

These movements can also be assessed with Frenzel's glasses equipped with small infrared cameras (visual or video-oculography [VOG]) or electrodes, to detect extraocular muscle movement (electro-oculography [EOG], or sometimes called electronystagmography [ENG]), and computerised and appropriate targets projected onto a screen.

120.2 The Vestibulo-Ocular Reflex

Eye movements are generated in response to visual signals and vestibular activity. The central vestibulo-ocular and visuo-ocular pathways are intimately related, and both share the common final pathway of the oculomotor nerves. If visually controlled eye movements are normal (e.g. saccades and the smooth pursuit system), derangement of the VOR may correctly be ascribed to vestibular dysfunction. However, if visually controlled eye movements are abnormal, care must be taken in the interpretation of vestibulo-ocular responses.

Nystagmus is an involuntary, rhythmical oscillation of the eyes away from the direction of gaze, followed by a return of the eyes to their original position. It can be either physiological or pathological.

Physiological nystagmus refers to nystagmus observed in normal subjects. It will be present in most normal individuals if the irises of the eyes are deviated horizontally further than the punctum of the lacrimal sac, an important point to remember when testing for spontaneous nystagmus. Physiological nystagmus can also be induced by thermal (caloric) or rotational stimulation.

Pathological nystagmus may be congenital or acquired. Congenital nystagmus is nystagmus present from birth. It is nearly always dependent on optic fixation and so disappears when this is removed by asking the patient to wear Frenzel's glasses. Acquired nystagmus is described as ocular, vestibular or central in origin.

1. *Ocular nystagmus* This tends to be pendular, where the phases have equal speed (i.e. there is no slow and fast phase). It is common in congenital ocular disease such as bilateral cataract formation, optic nerve hypoplasia and aniridia but may occur without any defect of vision. Miner's nystagmus is a form of the ocular variety.

2. *Vestibular nystagmus* This consists of a slow movement of the eyes in one direction followed by a quick return in the opposite direction. The slow component is produced by impulses, or lack of them, from the vestibule. The fast component, or recovery movement, is a central correcting reflex. The direction of the nystagmus is named according to the direction of the fast component, for example, a nystagmus whose quick component is to the right is called a nystagmus to the right. Nystagmus is most marked when the patient looks in the direction of the fast component and is lessened or abolished when looking in the direction of the slow component. Vestibular nystagmus can be spontaneous or positional.

   a. Spontaneous nystagmus, when present, can be elicited by asking the patient to follow a finger held 60 cm away to the left and then to the right, and then up and down. Increasing degrees of severity of spontaneous nystagmus are recognised. First-degree nystagmus is present only when the eyes are deviated in the direction of the fast component. Second-degree nystagmus is present when the patient looks straight ahead and in the

direction of the fast component. Third-degree nystagmus is nystagmus that is still present when the patient looks in the direction of the slow component. Spontaneous nystagmus suggests pathology of the vestibular system, and the greater degree parallels the severity.

   b. Positional nystagmus may be rotatory and accompanied by rotatory vertigo. A nystagmus which is fatigable and short-lasting is associated with a peripheral pathology (e.g. benign paroxysmal positional vertigo [BPPV]). Nystagmus which is not associated with vertigo and does not fatigue is likely to be associated with a central lesion.

120.3 Tests Based on the Vestibulo-Ocular Reflex

120.3.1 Simple Tests

Head Impulse (Halmagyi and, the often neglected, Curthoys) Test

In this test, the patient's head is turned quickly through a small range (< 25 degrees) while maintaining focus on a distant target. A normal result is maintenance of target fixation. An abnormal result has the eyes move with the head and then a corrective saccade to bring the target back into focus. It suggests an abnormality of the side to which the head was turned that caused the saccade.

Head Shake Visual Acuity Test

In this test, the head is turned backwards and forwards, again through a small range and at a speed of approximately 1 Hz, while the subject is asked to read the lines of a Snellen chart. A difference of more than two lines between the test situation and with the head stationary suggests a disorder of the VOR.

Dix–Hallpike (Positional Testing)

Positional nystagmus is best elicited by this positional test. The patient is positioned sitting on a bed and the procedure is explained. This explanation should include a reassurance to the patient that he or she will not be allowed to fall whatever happens. The patient is told to keep his or her eyes open and look straight ahead. The head is held firmly between the examiner's hands and turned

V

45 degrees to the right or left. The patient is then rapidly laid backwards, with his or her head over the edge of the bed, 30 degrees below the horizontal. The patient is asked if this provokes symptoms similar to those he or she has been describing and the eyes are observed for nystagmus. If neither occurs after 30 seconds, then the patient is returned to the upright position and again asked if there is any vertigo and the eyes examined for nystagmus. If no symptoms or nystagmus are elicited, the process is repeated but with the head to the other side.

Benign paroxysmal positional nystagmus elicited by the Hallpike manoeuvre usually has a latent period of 5 seconds before the onset of rotatory nystagmus, a fast component of nystagmus directed towards the undermost ear, an associated vertigo which distresses the patient; and the nystagmus fatigues rapidly. This contrasts with nystagmus of central origin, which appears immediately, causes little or no vertigo, and persists indefinitely if the head position is maintained. If there are no symptoms or nystagmus after the Hallpike manoeuvre, it is still possible that head position has a role in the cause of the patient's vertigo. This is because canalolithiasis signs are a function of the volume of calcium debris within the semicircular canal at the moment of the Hallpike test. Volume of debris varies and therefore a history of a movement that will reliably and repeatedly cause fatigable vertigo (but which may fluctuate over weeks or months) is the most important factor in diagnosing BPPV.

120.3.2 Complex Tests

1. *Video head impulse test (vHIT)* It is argued that the clinical HIT only allows overt saccades to be seen. If pathology exists, it may also cause covert saccades. These are saccades that occur during the process of head movement. These can be detected using video-oculography. Analysis is of the visualised eye movements compared with the head movements as detected by inertial sensors in the goggles.

2. *Caloric tests* Despite improved imaging of the temporal bone and the advent of evoked response audiometry, this remains a popular investigation. It is still the only way of testing each vestibule independently and is also a popular topic in the Fellowship examination. Results can be measured by simply observing and timing the movement (nystagmus) of the eyes, but can also, and more accurately, be measured by VOG or EOG (also called ENG). This is a technique based on the positive potential which exists between the cornea and retina. Electrodes are attached to the skin at each outer canthus close to the eyes. Changes in the corneoretinal potential are recorded at the electrode sites as the eyes move from straight ahead gaze. The changes in electric potential are used to follow nystagmus, and after amplifications are recorded permanently on a moving paper strip.

3. *Rotational tests* The nystagmus induced by acceleration and deceleration in a rotating chair is recorded. Recording is normally done with ENG or videonystagmography (VNG). Rotational chairs are uncommon and expensive. There are standardised, computer-controlled, rotational strategies. Analysis of the results demands familiarity with the techniques. The test has the disadvantage of stimulating both labyrinths simultaneously (off axis rotation can be used to test otolith function—utricle and saccule).

120.4 Test of the Vestibulospinal Reflex

Tests based on the VOR are regarded as an essential part of investigation of the vestibular system. In contrast, tests of vestibulospinal function are commonly neglected in the evaluation of patients with balance dysfunction.

Clinically vestibulospinal function is tested by examining stance and gait.

120.4.1 Romberg's Test

The Romberg test is used to assess a patient's ability to stand, feet together, arms by the side, with eyes open and then closed. The patient may fall towards the side of a recent peripheral vestibular lesion. An additional aspect of this test is to elicit postural reflexes by gently and randomly pushing the patient to elicit corrective responses.

120.4.2 Unterberger's (Fukuda) Step Test

This is performed by asking the patient to walk up and down on the spot for 30 seconds, with eyes closed and arms outstretched in front, with hands clasped together. Body rotation of more than 30 degrees, or forward or backward displacement of more than 1 m is regarded as abnormal.

120.4.3 Gait Testing

Gait is assessed by watching the patient walk normally with eyes open and then closed. A hemiplegic gait, cerebellar ataxic gait, parkinsonian shuffle or high stepping gait with loss of proprioception may become apparent. With eye closure, some patients with uncompensated vestibular lesions will veer towards the affected side.

120.4.4 Subjective Visual Vertical

This test asks the subject to look at a vertical line and adjust it until he or she believes it represents true vertical. Simple methods include the use of a line drawn in the bottom of a bucket with a grid drawn on the base for the examiner. With acute vestibular failure, the line will tilt, by typically 10 degrees, towards the ipsilateral side. However, it is non-localising as central lesions can also affect the subjective visual vertical (SVV).

120.4.5 Posturography

Posturography is the recording of postural sway. Several techniques have been used to evaluate postural stability, but the most commonly used are computer-controlled force platforms (computerised dynamic posturography [CDP]). The data collected have enabled the effects of various sensory modalities upon balance to be identified, and some claim they allow various pathological conditions to be differentiated. A few of the more recent platforms have been used to rehabilitate patients with balance dysfunction by way of visual feedback. The high cost of many balance platforms has prohibited their use in both research and clinical practice. A cheaper clinical alternative is to perform the Romberg test with postural reflexes on both the floor and a cushioned mat.

120.4.6 Vestibular-Evoked Myogenic Potentials

It has been discovered that loud sounds can also stimulate the saccule and provoke a brief inhibition of ipsilateral cervical muscle contractions which can be measured by cervical electrodes adjacent to the sternocleidomastoid muscle, so-called cervical vestibular-evoked myogenic potential (cVEMP). In recent years, a similar response has been found with the extraocular muscles in response to acoustic or vibratory stimuli (contralateral excitation) and is thought to give an indication of utricular function, so-called ocular VEMP (oVEMP). The usefulness of these tests is still being developed although they do have the advantage of testing each ear separately.

Further Reading

Hale T, Trahan H, Parent-Buck T. Evaluation of the patient with dizziness and balance disorders. In: Katz J, ed. Handbook of Clinical Audiology. 7th ed. Philadelphia, Baltimore, New York: Wolters Kluwer; 2015

Wuyts FL, Boudewyns A. Physiology of equilibrium, Balance disorders. In: Gleeson M, Browning GG, Burton MJ, et al, eds. Scott-Brown's Otorhinolaryngology, Head and Neck Surgery. 7th ed, Vol 3. London: Hodder Arnold; 2008;3:3207–3244, 3673–3834

Related Topics of Interest

Caloric tests
Vertigo

V

121   Vestibular Schwannoma

Vestibular schwannoma represents 8% of all intracranial tumours and 80% of cerebellopontine angle tumours. They arise from Schwann's (neurilemmal) cells. The nerve of origin is usually the superior vestibular nerve. The term acoustic neuroma is still commonly used but is historic and factually incorrect and should be discarded.

121.1 Pathology

The medial portions of the cranial nerves are covered with glial stroma. Vestibular schwannomas originate at the junction of the glial and Schwann's cells (Redlich–Obersteiner zone), which for the vestibular nerve is usually within the internal auditory meatus (IAM). The sexes are equally affected and, whatever the time of onset and rate of progression, the presentation is most often between the ages of 40 and 60. The annual incidence is approximately 1 in 50,000. Sixty to seventy percent of vestibular schwannomas do not grow on serial imaging and this is particularly likely to be the case in tumours of less than 1.5 cm. The average rate of change in growing tumours is 2 mm per year although a proportion grows at significantly greater rates. The majority of these tumours are unilateral, and the small proportion that is bilateral (5%) is seen in neurofibromatosis type 2 (NF2). This is an autosomal dominant disease due primarily to mutations on the long arm of chromosome 22. In NF2, vestibular schwannomas often present at an earlier age than those without the gene.

Macroscopically, the tumour appears as a firm yellowish encapsulated mass with the vestibular nerve splayed out on its surface. Histologically, the tumour consists of packed sheaves of connective tissue cells (fasciculated) or may be composed of a disorderly loose network of cells with intercellular vacuoles and cysts (reticular pattern). Haemorrhage can occur (particularly in the reticular type), leading to a sudden increase in size and therefore marked symptoms such as acute vertigo or sudden deafness although in reality this is rare.

121.2 Clinical Features

Clinically, two phases can be recognised: an *otological phase in* which a small tumour compresses structures in the meatus, and a *neurological phase* as the tumour expands medially into the cerebellopontine angle.

1. *Otological symptoms* Gradual and progressive unilateral hearing loss is the usual presenting symptom (90%) and this is often associated with tinnitus (70%). Sudden-onset hearing loss can occur in 5 to 10%. A proportion of patients have normal hearing at presentation (5%). Associated significant vertigo is unusual as compensation for vestibular nerve damage usually keeps pace with the slow rate of loss of peripheral vestibular function. Many patients will, however, note previous episodes of short-lived vertigo or a longer period of imbalance (as if they were on a deck of a ship).
2. *Trigeminal nerve symptoms* Facial pain, numbness and paraesthesia may all occur.
3. *Headache* Discomfort and dull aching around the ear and mastoid area are probably caused by posterior fossa dura irritation.
4. *Late symptoms* Like most motor nerves, the facial nerve is resistant to slow pressure deformity and symptoms of facial weakness or hemifacial spasm are uncommon. Ataxia and unsteadiness develop with progressive brainstem displacement and cerebellar involvement. Diplopia due to pressure on the sixth cranial nerve, and hoarseness with dysphagia due to involvement of the ninth and tenth nerves is rare.
5. *Terminal symptoms* The raised cerebrospinal fluid (CSF) pressure causes failing vision due to papilloedema, headache, alteration in conscious level and eventually coma.

In the otological phase, general examination will usually reveal no abnormalities. The patient may have a unilateral sensorineural hearing loss. Hypo-aesthesia of the posterior external ear canal on the side of the hearing loss may be present (Hitselberger's sign). Loss of the corneal reflex is an early sign of trigeminal nerve impairment. Nystagmus when present may be vestibular or cerebellar in nature. Facial nerve impairment is usually of the sensory element and can be elicited as a lack of taste on electrogustometry or loss of lacrimation on Schirmer's test, although these tests are now rarely undertaken. Slight

V

facial weakness may show as a delay in the blink reflex. Neurological signs of the other cranial nerve palsies and ataxia may eventually become apparent.

121.3 Investigations

1. *Radiological investigations* The most accurate means of identifying small intracanalicular tumours is magnetic resonance imaging (MRI) of the brain and internal acoustic meatus. Standard practice in the United Kingdom is to perform a T2-weighted non-contrast MRI of the IAMs and brain. A T1-weighted MRI with gadolinium contrast is used for abnormal or equivocal scans. Gadolinium contrast is the gold standard in ongoing tumour surveillance. Computerised tomography (CT) scanning with high-definition and enhancement techniques will accurately diagnose and delineate most tumours above 1 cm in diameter and can be used when MRI is unavailable.

2. *Audiometry*
   a. A unilateral or asymmetrical sensorineural hearing loss can usually be demonstrated by a pure-tone audiogram. The hearing loss is classically a neural lesion with no loudness recruitment, abnormally rapid adaptation and disproportionately poor speech discrimination (rollover effect on speech audiogram). If the pure-tone threshold hearing loss is greater than 70 dB, the accuracy of audiometric testing is poor and these factors often restrict future rehabilitation with hearing aids.
   b. Stapedial reflex decay can be measured using impedance audiometry, and this gives a low false-negative rate of around 5%. Brainstem electric response audiometry has only a 3% false-negative rate. It demonstrates a retrocochlear lesion by an increased latency between N1 and N5 waves.

3. *Vestibular investigations* Caloric responses are usually reduced in or absent from the affected side, but there is no abnormality in some patients with small tumours. Special audiometric and vestibular testing are now rarely, if ever, used for the diagnosis of a vestibular schwannoma.

121.4 Differential Diagnosis of a Tumour at the Cerebellopontine Angle

1. Vestibular schwannomas (constitute 80% of cerebellopontine angle tumours).
2. Meningioma.
3. Neuroma of the seventh nerve.
4. Congenital cholesteatoma.
5. Aneurysm of the basilar or vertebral arteries.
6. Cholesterol granuloma of the petrous apex.
7. Cerebellar tumour.

121.5 Management

It is essential that these patients are assessed by a skull base multi-disciplinary team in determining optimum management. Careful consideration of the age and general condition of the patient and the size, hearing, site and rate of growth of the lesion are all factors to be considered. In view of tumour size contributing to the management of vestibular schwannomas, the British Skullbase Society has defined tumour size as meaning size in millimetres at the cerebellopontine angle and categorised the size as follows:

- Intracanalicular—0 mm.
- Small—1–15 mm.
- Medium—16–29 mm.
- Large—30–40 mm.
- Giant—> 40 mm.

1. *Conservative management* Small, slow-growing tumours in elderly patients can be watched by carrying out CT or MRI scanning at regular intervals to gauge the rate of growth. Following U.K. consensus, the largest extrameatal tumour diameter on axial MR imaging is recorded as the measurement of tumour size. Annual MRI shows that around 60% of vestibular schwannomas are not growing. Hearing rehabilitation in this patient group can be challenging, but it is important to offer support. Single-sided hearing loss may be helped with CROS aiding or bone conduction implants.

2. *Radiosurgery and radiotherapy* Stereotactic radiosurgery (Gamma Knife): Non-invasive treatment providing single fraction of high-dose ionising gamma radiation to the tumour

with the intention to arrest future tumour growth. The patient's head is fixed in a stereotactic frame, but it is performed as a 'single visit' relatively pain-free day-case procedure. The documented 'control' rate for tumours less than 2 cm is approximately 95%. Additionally, it may reduce the rate of hearing loss in some patients.

Traditional hyperfractionated radiotherapy (including more recently CyberKnife) is also used to treat vestibular schwannomas. This offers similar results in terms of tumour control yet requires multiple visits for treatment.

Radiosurgery may make future microsurgery more difficult and there is a theoretical risk of inducing future malignant change. It is used to control small tumours. It is associated with facial pain in approximately 3% of cases and facial nerve weakness in less than 1%. Initial swelling may be evident on post-treatment imaging prior to regression.

3. *Microsurgery* Removal of a vestibular schwannoma often results in hearing loss and carries a risk to cranial nerves IV to XI. This risk is determined by the size of the tumour and the expertise and experience of the team undertaking the surgery. Patients with tumours more than 25 to 30 mm or those with neurological signs will usually be advised to have microsurgery, even if they have excellent hearing in the affected ear. The morbidity and mortality from both tumour growth and its operative removal increase with large tumours. A small tumour can be extracted from the meatus with negligible risk and with preservation of the facial nerve, although such tumours are often managed conservatively.

There are three surgical approaches to the cerebellopontine angle and the choice depends on the position and size of the tumour and pre-operative assessment by the neuro-otologist and neurosurgeon.

1. *Translabyrinthine approach* This is one of the commonest approaches, but all residual hearing is lost. The approach has the highest rate of facial nerve preservation as the nerve is identified and controlled laterally, at the fundus of the IAM, early in the operation and tends to be used for patients with a severe sensorineural hearing loss (< 70% speech discrimination) and more lateral tumours.

2. *Retrosigmoid approach* This route provides wide exposure of the cerebellopontine angle and is often employed in larger tumours. The patient's hearing and facial nerve can be preserved, so this approach is also used for tumours when there is good hearing. The effect of cerebellar retraction is a potential concern, however.

3. *Middle fossa route* This gives limited access and was previously used for small intrameatal tumours as both hearing and the facial nerve can be preserved. It is now rarely used in the United Kingdom as such tumours are manged conservatively or with radiotherapy. There is a 15% risk of the patient developing epilepsy and in the United Kingdom, driving is banned for 1 year following this procedure.

121.6 Complications of Surgery

- Major/catastrophic: Death or stroke—1%
- Serious—CSF leak through the wound or nose via the often down the eustachian tube occurs in 2% in the senior author's experience although meningitis is rare. Deep vein thrombosis (DVT), pulmonary embolism (PE) and lower cranial nerve injury are rare too at about 1%.
- Facial nerve injury. This risk is proportionate to tumour size and the skill/experience of the surgical team. It is important that each surgeon knows his or her complication rate to provide accurate informed consent. As a guide, complication rates for skilled/experienced surgeons will be about in patients with up to a 20-mm tumour, 95% will have normal or near-normal facial nerve function post-operatively. Those with tumour size 20 to 30 mm have about an 80% chance of normal/near-normal facial nerve function, and those with a tumour more than 30 mm have a 70% chance of having normal/near-normal facial nerve function post-operatively.

▶ Fig. 121.1 shows the algorithm used by the senior author in the decision-making process of managing vestibular schwannoma.

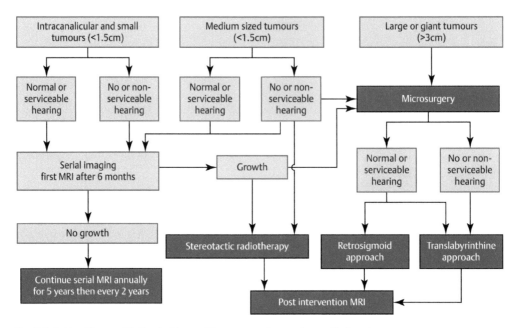

Fig. 121.1 Algorithm used in the decision-making process of managing vestibular schwannoma.

Further Reading

Battaglia A, Mastrodimos B, Cueva R. Comparison of growth patterns of acoustic neuromas with and without radiosurgery. Otol Neurotol. 2006; 27(5):705–712

Chandler CL, Ramsden RT. Acoustic schwannoma. Br J Hosp Med. 1993; 49(5):335–343, 335–343

Kanzaki J, Tos M, Sanna M, Moffat DA, Monsell EM, Berliner KI. New and modified reporting systems from the consensus meeting on systems for reporting results in vestibular schwannoma. Otol Neurotol. 2003; 24(4):642–648, discussion 648–649

Martin TPC, Senthil L, Chavda SV, Walsh R, Irving RM. A protocol for the conservative management of vestibular schwannomas. Otol Neurotol. 2009; 30(3):381–385

Related Topics of Interest

Evoked response audiometry

Imaging in ENT

Tinnitus

Vertigo

Vestibular function tests

V

122   Vocal Fold Paralysis

122.1 Anatomy

The roots of the vagus emerge from the pons and medulla to gain a trunk and exit the skull through the jugular foramen. The vagus gives two important branches for voice production: the superior and the recurrent laryngeal nerves. The superior laryngeal nerve branches into the external laryngeal nerve, supplying the cricothyroid muscle, the primary muscle increasing tension in the vocal folds (and hence increasing pitch), and the internal laryngeal nerve, which is sensory to the laryngeal mucosa above the vocal cords. The recurrent laryngeal nerve arises high in the chest on the right, looping around the subclavian artery to reach the tracheo-oesophageal groove, but on the left, arises at the level of and loops around the aortic arch to reach the same groove. On both sides, the nerve enters the larynx immediately behind the cricothyroid joint. It supplies the remaining intrinsic laryngeal muscles and is sensory to mucosa below the cords.

122.2 Pathology

A vocal fold paralysis (VFP) may be unilateral (UVFP) or bilateral (BVFP).

VFP may arise from pathology of the following:

1. The vagus and recurrent laryngeal nerve (RLN), for example, iatrogenic, pressure damage or a neuropathy.
2. The cricoarytenoid joint, for example, rheumatoid arthritis, iatrogenic trauma.
3. The intrinsic muscles which move the vocal cord, for example, a myopathy or infiltration by a malignancy.

In practice, the vast majority of cases are due to pathology of the RLN.

122.3 Aetiology

- Malignant disease, especially of the bronchus, oesophagus and thyroid.
- Iatrogenic, especially thyroid and parathyroid, oesophageal, carotid, cardiac and left lung surgery. Neurosurgical approaches to the cervical spine (e.g. anterior cervical discectomy and fusion) may also traumatise the RLN.
- External trauma, for example, from road traffic or sporting accidents and stab or gunshot injury.
- Idiopathic, in which no cause is identified but which may be related to infection with a neuropathic virus.
- Others, for example, neurological disorders, myopathies and inflammatory disease.

122.4 Unilateral Vocal Fold Paralysis

122.4.1 Clinical Features

UVFP may be relatively asymptomatic in some cases, but typical features of UVFP are a weak, breathy voice and an ineffective ('bovine') cough. Aspiration is common, causing the patient to cough on swallowing (especially liquids); this can sometimes lead to life-threatening pneumonia. Patients may complain subjectively of shortness of breath; in practice, this is usually because patients run out of breath frequently when speaking, giving them the sensation of dyspnoea.

122.4.2 Investigations

Having confirmed the diagnosis on laryngeal endoscopy, in non-iatrogenic cases, it is important to exclude malignancy as a cause. Hence, cross-sectional imaging from the skull base to the aortic arch is the first and most useful investigation. Further investigations are then chosen as appropriate to any identified underlying cause.

The use of electromyography (EMG) is controversial, but it may be helpful in determining the likely prognosis for recovery. This information may then help to direct management.

122.4.3 Management

Speech Therapy

This will be required in the majority of cases to help (a) improve the voice by encouraging compensation from the contralateral vocal fold; and (b) provide therapy techniques to avoid aspiration—these may include head-turning, chin tuck or double swallow. In some cases, fluid thickeners

V

will be recommended to reduce the risk of aspiration on thin liquids.

Monitoring

In some cases, it may be acceptable simply to monitor the patient's progress while awaiting resolution of the UVFP or compensation from the contralateral vocal fold.

Medialisation Procedures

The purpose of medialising a paralysed vocal fold is to move it closer to the midline to allow for better glottic closure on phonation. It was previously suggested that a patient should be made to wait for a period of up to 12 to 18 months before offering medialisation; this was to allow for recuperation or compensation. However, with newer injection techniques and materials, it is no longer reasonable to leave a patient to languish for so long with vocal difficulties.

Medialisation may be achieved in a number of ways:

1. Injection in the clinic under local anaesthetic. This technique has the advantage of being relatively quick and simple to perform. It is particularly suited to patients with co-morbidities which would preclude a general anaesthetic. Patients requiring a rapid improvement (such as those who are terminally ill) are also good candidates. Injection materials may be temporary (e.g. Restylane or Radiesse Voice Gel) or semi-permanent (e.g. Radiesse Voice). Injections may be performed transcutaneously (via the cricothyroid or thyrohyoid membrane), transorally or via a channeled flexible nasendoscope.

2. Injection under general anaesthetic in the operating theatre. Using suspension laryngoscopy, the vocal cords are exposed and a medialisation material is injected. Materials can include fat, Vox, Radiesse Voice or others.

3. Thyroplasty (Isshiki type 1 thyroplasty; medialisation laryngoplasty). Under local anaesthetic (often with sedation), a skin incision over the thyroid cartilage is made. The strap muscles are retracted laterally and a window is fashioned in the cartilage at the level of the vocal fold. The position of the window is confirmed with a flexible endoscope and a medialisation material (e.g. Silastic, Gore-Tex, Montgomery implant) is inserted through the window in the thyroid lamina and into the paraglottic space. This technique has the advantage of using a permanent implant rather than a resorbable injection substance. It can also be reversed if necessary.

4. Arytenoid re-positioning procedures. In cases of UVFP where the arytenoid is sitting in a very lateral position, it may be necessary to re-position it. These arytenoid procedures are relatively complex and are less frequently performed than thyroplasty.

Re-Innervation

Trials of re-innervation techniques are showing promising results. Branches of the ansa cervicalis may be used to anastomose to the RLN. This generally restores tone in the vocal fold (and hence improves bulk), but rarely restores normal vocal fold movement.

122.5 Bilateral Vocal Fold Paralysis

122.5.1 Clinical Features

In cases where both vocal folds are immobile, the position of the vocal folds will determine the clinical picture. If the vocal cords are abducted, the patient will have a weak and breathy voice; it is also very likely that they will be aspirating. However, given that the vocal folds are lateralised, the airway may be adequate.

Conversely, if the vocal folds are paralysed in the paramedian position, the voice may be relatively good; however, in this situation, the airway is likely to be compromised.

122.5.2 Management

If the airway is compromised, intervention will be required. Inevitably in this clinical situation, there will be a compromise between airway calibre and voice quality.

1. Tracheostomy. This has the advantage of not interfering with the vocal folds; the voice will therefore be unchanged. However, there is clearly significant morbidity associated with a tracheostomy.

2. Airway widening procedures
   a. Cordotomy. A laser may be used to produce a cut across the membranous vocal fold. These destructive procedures are usually significantly deleterious to the voice.
   b. Laser arytenoidectomy. This procedure aims to preserve the membranous part of the vocal fold to maintain voice, while opening the posterior glottis by removing some of the arytenoid cartilage.
   c. Lateralisation techniques. A suture may be passed through the skin and into the arytenoid cartilage to pull it laterally. This is reversible.

3. Re-innervation. Roots of the phrenic nerve are taken and implanted (via an interposition nerve graft) into the posterior cricoarytenoid (PCA) muscle. Thus, on inspiration, the phrenic nerve activates the PCA muscle, causing the vocal folds to abduct.

Further Reading

Rosen CA, Simpson CB. Operative Techniques in Laryngolofy. Springer-Verlag Berlin Heidelberg; 2008

Costell D, Sandhu G. Practical Laryngology. Boca Raton, FL: CRC Press; 2016

Misono S, Merati AL. Evidence-based practice: evaluation and management of unilateral vocal fold paralysis. Otolaryngol Clin North Am. 2012; 45(5):1083–1108

Snyder SK, Angelos P, Carty SE, et al. Injection of bulking agents for laryngoplasty. Surgery. 2018; 163(1):6–8

Vila PM, Bhatt NK, Paniello RC. Early-injection laryngoplasty may lower risk of thyroplasty: A systematic review and meta-analysis. Laryngoscope. 2018; 128(4):935–940

Related Topics of Interest

Laryngeal carcinoma
Neck swellings
Thyroid disease—benign
Thyroid disease—malignant
Anaesthesia—local
Anaesthesia—sedation

V

123 Voice Disorders

This chapter focuses on disorders of the larynx causing dysphonia, rather than pathologies, usually of the oral cavity, leading to dysarthria. One of the key components of human interaction is vocal communication. Normal speech is important for this and can be essential in a number of occupations.

123.1 Functions of the Larynx

The primary function of the larynx is to protect the lower airways by fulfilling a sphincteric action during swallowing. During deglutition, the true vocal folds adduct firmly to close the glottis; the false cords then also close. Further functions of the larynx are voice production, coughing and the Valsalva manoeuvre.

From a practical point of view, a 'normal' voice is one that is audible in a wide range of settings, is appropriate for the gender and age of the individual, is absent of any hoarseness or breathiness, is not easily fatigued and is not associated with any discomfort.

123.2 Voice Assessment

A patient's voice may be assessed in a number of different ways:

- Firstly, the patient can self-rate his or her voice using a questionnaire such as the voice handicap index (VHI). This is a 30-question assessment (VHI-30), but a shorter 10-question version has been developed and is equally applicable (VHI-10).
- Secondly, the voice is assessed by the clinicians using perceptual grading scales. The most commonly used of these is the GRBAS (grade, roughness, breathiness, asthenia and strain) tool developed by Hirano.
- Thirdly, the larynx is examined (see later).
- Finally, the voice may be assessed on a variety of parameters (jitter, shimmer, noise-to-harmonic ratio, etc.) using computer software.

Examination of the larynx is usually undertaken with a flexible transnasal endoscope (either fibre-optic or distal chip). Examination of the larynx with a mirror is now considered a historical modality. Rigid (70- or 90-degree Hopkins' rod)

endoscopy gives an outstanding view in patients who will tolerate it. Detailed laryngeal examination in the voice clinic should also include stroboscopy; this technique gives the illusion of slow motion movement of the vocal folds; by using a stroboscopic light source, the cyclical periodic vibration of the vocal folds is captured at a different point in the cycle from one cycle to the next. Thus, there is an illusion of slow motion.

123.3 Voice Production—Normal and Pathological

Production of a normal voice relies on three components: vocal folds with straight medial edges; adequate glottic closure; and normal vocal fold pliability. Also required are an ability to produce controlled airflow through the larynx, and good neuromuscular control of the 'articulators' (mouth, teeth, tongue, palate and lips).

In most instances, any treatment by an ear, nose and throat (ENT) surgeon should be supplemented with voice therapy. This is not only to address the underlying cause, but also to deal with issues of vocal hygiene, and to reinforce instructions with regards to voice usage around the time of any surgery. Voice clinics should therefore be staffed by an ENT surgeon and a speech therapist.

123.3.1 Voice Disorders

Voice disorders can be divided into four broad categories:

1. Neoplastic/structural.
2. Inflammatory.
3. Neuromuscular conditions.
4. Muscle tension imbalance disorders.

Neoplastic/Structural

Vocal Fold Nodules

These chronic lesions occur as a consequence of long-term vocal abuse. At the point of maximal collision of the vocal folds (the junction of the anterior third and the posterior two-thirds), sub-epithelial thickening gives rise to swellings. Nodules are always bilateral—any unilateral lesion must be due to another pathology. They cause the voice to sound rough and breathy in quality. Singers will also complain of a loss of upper singing registers. Treatment is with voice therapy, focusing on reducing vocal loading and avoiding hard glottal attack in the voice. In children, this will involve education of the wider family of the importance of limiting extraneous noise at home. With appropriate voice production changes, the vast majority of patients will improve significantly. Very rarely, surgical excision is indicated.

Reinke's Oedema (Polypoid Corditis, Polypoid Degeneration)

Chronic exposure to cigarette smoke can result in an accumulation of thick fluid in Reinke's space—hence 'Reinke's oedema'. In this condition, the voice is typically rough in quality and low in pitch. For female patients, this latter symptom can be problematic as they are frequently mistaken for men on the telephone. Cessation of smoking is mandatory, and may result in significant improvement in early cases; however, these changes can take many months. Surgery is reserved for those patients who have given up smoking, as the oedema will recur (often within weeks) if smoking is resumed after laryngeal surgery.

Polyp

A vocal fold polyp will typically arise as a consequence of a single episode of phonotrauma such as yelling. The patient will notice a sudden onset of a change in voice quality. There is no pain, but in the longer term, compensatory muscle tension patterns can give rise to muscular ache and discomfort. Polyps rarely resolve spontaneously, so surgery is usually required.

Cyst

The aetiology of cysts is not clear, but they occasionally occur as a consequence of a single episode of phonotrauma. Blockage of a mucus-secreting gland results in a mucous retention cyst. Alternatively, an epidermoid cyst may be found. Both these types sit in Reinke's space (superficial lamina propria). Cysts present with hoarseness and (as with a polyp) long-term muscle tension issues that can then give rise to throat and neck discomfort. On stroboscopic examination, a swelling will be seen, and the mucosal wave (pliability

of the vocal fold) will be reduced as a consequence of the interference with Reinke's space. Surgery is often required to resolve vocal fold cysts.

Laryngeal Papillomatosis

Laryngeal papillomatosis (recurrent respiratory papillomatosis) is caused by human papilloma virus (HPV) types 6 and 11. Accumulations of HPV cause irregularity of the vocal fold surfaces, resulting in hoarseness. In some cases, the papilloma can enlarge to the point of airway compromise.

Treatment is with repeated excision, but the papillomata invariably recur. Various modalities have been used, including steel instruments, laser, microdebrider, and coblation. In recent years, adjuvant therapies have been suggested (indole-3-carbinol, interferon, cidofovir), but their long-term effectiveness is not known. Immunization against HPV6 and 11 (e.g., with the Gardasil vaccine) may be beneficial in some patients.

Intracordal Hemorrhage

An isolated episode of phonotrauma may result in a bleed into Reinke's space along the whole length of a vocal fold. This may be due to a prominent vessel, but at the time of presentation, this will not be evident because of the discoloration of the vocal fold. The major consideration is to ensure that the vocal fold heals with minimal scarring to ensure that the mucosal wave returns. For this reason, most laryngologists advocate complete voice rest. Serial examinations will chart the resolution of the hemorrhage, and if a prominent vessel is found to be the cause, this can be ablated (usually with a potassium titanyl phosphate [KTP] laser).

Anterior Glottic Web

Any surgery on the vocal folds should aim to avoid trauma at the anterior commissure; if surgery causes exposure of the subepithelial layer on both anterior vocal folds, a web may form. This can result in profound voice changes, and is very difficult to treat.

Vocal Process Granuloma

If cartilage is denuded of its perichondrium and mucosa, the exposed cartilage can produce a florid reaction known as a granuloma. In the larynx, these typically occur on the vocal process of one or other arytenoid. In most patients, the symptoms are of throat irritation, unilateral pain (and sometimes otalgia), and voice change. The aetiology is usually traumatic (sometimes due to intubation with an endotracheal tube), and treatment rests on removing any ongoing irritation. Hence, treating any laryngopharyngeal reflux is paramount. Patients should also see a voice therapist to reinforce good vocal hygiene and to eliminate vocally abusive behaviors such as throat clearing and yelling.

Surgical excision is not recommended unless malignancy is suspected; any attempts to excise granulomas usually result in recurrence—and they frequently recur more aggressively than their original presentation.

Inflammatory

Infective Laryngitis

The commonest cause of infection of the larynx is a viral pathogen. This will usually present with a mild degree of hoarseness and pain that lasts for a few days. Bacterial laryngitis will give rise to a similar illness, but with more pronounced and longer-lasting symptoms. Viral and bacterial laryngitis rarely present to ENT surgeons as they are self-limiting and are usually treated in primary care.

Fungal laryngitis (e.g., with *Candida albicans*) results in painless voice change; laryngeal examination will usually show plaques (or scattered small deposits) of *Candida* around the larynx. Treatment is usually with a short course of antifungals. Fungal laryngitis is frequently seen in patients taking steroid inhalers; they should be advised to gargle after using their inhalers to prevent the steroid from accumulating on the vocal folds and leaving them prone to such infection. Patients on systemic steroids or with immunodeficiency are also at risk of developing fungal infections of the upper aerodigestive tract.

Reflux

Laryngopharyngeal reflux (LPR, extraesophageal reflux) is a controversial topic. Its presentation, clinical findings, investigation, manifestations, and treatment are all the subjects of much debate.

Manifestations of LPR are said to range from the "typical" reflux symptoms of dyspepsia, heartburn,

acid brash, and belching through to throat clearing, globus pharyngeus, dysphagia, voice change, and cough.

Laryngeal examination is not diagnostic of LPR, and many clinicians will use dual-probe pH monitoring, manometry, and/or impedance to establish the diagnosis. Empirical treatment with proton pump inhibitors (PPIs) is widely used, although alginates have been demonstrated to be more efficacious in reducing nonacid reflux (e.g., pepsin).

Trauma

Physical trauma (e.g., phonotrauma or coughing) can cause inflammatory changes to the larynx, as can chemical and smoke inhalation.

Certain autoimmune conditions (e.g., rheumatoid, Sjögren's) may produce a variety of changes, from dehydration to isolated mucosal lesions.

Neuromuscular Conditions

Vocal Fold Paralysis

This condition is discussed in Chapter 122.

Parkinson's Disease

The hypofunctional voice of Parkinson's disease is characterized by a quiet and breathy quality combined with indistinct articulation and a monotone production (lack of pitch inflection). In addition to systemic treatment (with levodopa), voice therapy is the mainstay of treatment—particularly the (very intensive) Lee Silverman Voice Therapy (LSVT).

Other Neurological Conditions

Many generalized neurological conditions can give rise to voice changes; these include mysasthenia gravis, motor neuron disease, and multiple sclerosis.

Spasmodic Dysphonia

Spasmodic dysphonia (SD) is a rare focal dystonia of the larynx. It is a task-specific dystonia, only occurring in speech (never on vegetative tasks such as coughing or laughing) and is significantly more common in women than men.

Two types of SD are recognized: adductor and abductor. Adductor SD is the more common of the two, and results in a staccato quality of the voice, characterized by abrupt cessations in the flow of speech. Adductor SD occurs as a result of spasmodic activation of the adductor muscles of the larynx, hence repeatedly cutting off the flow of air from the lungs during phonation. Conversely, abductor SD occurs when there is spasm of the posterior cricoarytenoid muscle (the only abductor of the vocal folds). The flow of the voice is broken up by breathy pauses. In both types of SD, injections of botulinum toxin can give relief from symptoms for a few months, but repeated treatments are required, indefinitely.

Tremor

Laryngeal/vocal tremor is more common in older age, and may coexist with spasmodic dysphonia. A more widespread tremor may be seen (in, e.g., head, hands, or face), and treatment in the first instance should be with systemic medications such as β-blockers.

Muscle Tension Imbalance Disorders

Muscle Tension Dysphonia

This is a broad category of conditions, and probably represents the commonest group of voice disorders presenting to the general ENT clinic. In such cases there is no definable organic issue, but laryngeal tension is either heard in the voice, or seen in the larynx, or both. Depending on the patterns of muscle recruitment, the voice may sound strained, breathy, or altered in pitch. Speech therapy is the primary treatment modality and is used to reeducate and "train"the patient. If present, and required, any other pathological processes (e.g., a polyp) are treated. Stress, fatigue, anxiety, depression, and conversion disorders are all known to overlap with muscle tension dysphonia, and these other factors should also be addressed.

Puberphonia

In the adolescent boy, the rapid enlargement of the larynx results in a drop in pitch of the voice. However, some boys fail to utilize this lower register, and continue to speak in a high-pitched falsetto quality of voice. This can become a deeply entrenched pattern of behavior and may present to the voice clinic. In all cases, the secondary sexual characteristics are normal, and voice therapy (possibly supplemented with psychological therapy) is successful in those patients who are keen to effect a change in their voice.

Conversion Aphonia

This is a particular variant of muscle tension dysphonia, in which the patient has normal laryngeal anatomy and physiology, but fails to adduct the vocal folds on phonation, and hence produces no audible voice. There is frequently an underlying psychological trigger, and voice therapy combined with psychological therapy is required.

123.4 Conclusion

There are many different pathologies that may produce a disorder of voice. A thorough history and examination, with appropriate investigation, will identify the etiology of most. Regardless of any specific treatment for the condition in question, the vast majority of patients will also require input from speech therapy services. However, with appropriate treatment and support, most patients can achieve significant benefits.

Further Reading

Merati AL. Bielamowicz SA. Textbook of Laryngology. Plural Publishing Inc; 2006

Rosen CA, Simpson CB. Operative Techniques in Laryngolofy. Springer-Verlag Berlin Heidelberg; 2008

Costello D,Sandhu G. Practical Laryngology. Boca Raton, FL: CRC Press; 2016

Related Topics of Interest

Globus pharyngeus
Speech and swallow rehabilitation following head and neck surgery
Vocal fold paralysis

V

Index

Note: Page numbers set in **bold** or *italic* indicate headings or figures/tables, respectively.